FROM THE EXPERTS IN ENDO

ENDO 2020
MEET THE PROFESSOR

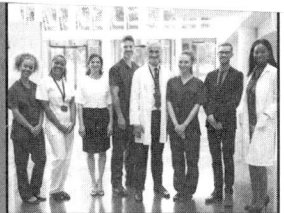

ENDOCRINE
CASE MANAGEMENT

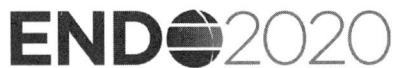

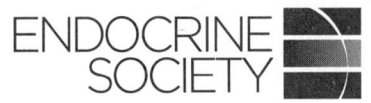

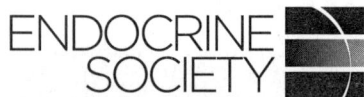

2055 L Street, NW, Suite 600
Washington, DC 20036
www.endocrine.org

Other Publications:
endocrine.org/publications

The Endocrine Society is the world's largest, oldest, and most active organization working to advance the clinical practice of endocrinology and hormone research. Founded in 1916, the Society now has more than 18,000 global members across a range of disciplines.

The Society has earned an international reputation for excellence in the quality of its peer-reviewed journals, educational resources, meetings, and programs that improve public health through the practice and science of endocrinology.

Clinical Practice Chair, ENDO 2020:
Maralyn Druce, MA, FRCP, PhD

The statements and opinions expressed in this publication are those of the individual authors and do not necessarily reflect the views of the Endocrine Society. The Endocrine Society is not responsible or liable in any way for the currency of the information, for any errors, omissions or inaccuracies, or for any consequences arising therefrom. With respect to any drugs mentioned, the reader is advised to refer to the appropriate medical literature and the product information currently provided by the manufacturer to verify appropriate dosage, method and duration of administration, and other relevant information. In all instances, it is the responsibility of the treating physician or other health care professional, relying on independent experience and expertise, as well as knowledge of the patient, to determine the best treatment for the patient.

ISBN: 978-1-879225-66-4
eISBN: 978-1-879225-67-1
Library of Congress Control Number: 9781879225664

ENDO 2020 CONTENTS

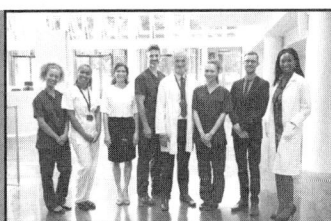

ADIPOSE TISSUE, APPETITE, AND OBESITY

ADRENAL

BONE AND MINERAL METABOLISM

DIABETES MELLITUS AND GLUCOSE METABOLISM

NEUROENDOCRINOLOGY AND PITUITARY

PEDIATRIC ENDOCRINOLOGY

REPRODUCTIVE ENDOCRINOLOGY

THYROID

MISCELLANEOUS

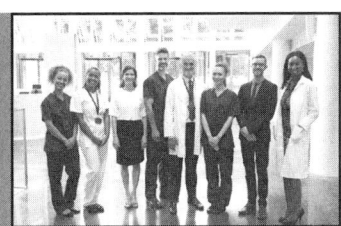

2020 Endocrine Case Management: Meet the Professor Faculty

Craig A. Alter, MD
Children's Hospital of Philadelphia
Pearlman School of Medicine at
the University of Pennsylvania

Bradley D. Anawalt, MD
University of Washington
School of Medicine

Richard J. Auchus, MD, PhD
University of Michigan

Laura K. Bachrach, MD
Stanford University
School of Medicine

**Stephen G. Ball, MBBS,
BSc, PhD, FRCP**
Manchester University Foundation Trust
University of Manchester
United Kingdom

Irina Bancos, MD
Mayo Clinic – Rochester

Diana Barb, MD
University of Florida

Andrew J. Bauer, MD
The Children's Hospital of Philadelphia

Petter Bjornstad, MD
University of Colorado
School of Medicine

Kristien Boelaert, MD, PhD, FRCP
University of Birmingham
United Kingdom

Elizabeth O. Buschur, MD
Ohio State University
Wexner Medical Center

Marcelle I. Cedars, MD
University of California – San Francisco

Philippe Chanson, MD, MS
Paris-Saclay University Hospital
France

Marc-Andre Cornier, MD
University of Colorado
School of Medicine

**Mehul T. Dattani, MBBS,
DCH, FRCPCH, FRCP, MD**
UCL GOS Institute of Child Health
United Kingdom

Chrysoula Dosiou, MD, MS
Stanford University School of Medicine

Richard Eastell, MD
University of Sheffield
United Kingdom

Rossella Elisei, MD
University of Pisa
Italy

Ghada El-Hajj Fuleihan, MD, MPH
American University of Beirut
Lebanon

Mary C. Frates, MD
Brigham and Women's Hospital,
Boston Children's Hospital

Neil J. Gittoes, BSc, PhD, FRCP
University of Birmingham,
University Hospitals Birmingham
United Kingdom

Whitney S. Goldner, MD
University of Nebraska
Medical Center

Jennifer B. Green, MD
Duke University Medical Center

**Ashley Grossman, BA BSc,
MD, FRCP, FMedSci**
Churchill Hospital, University of Oxford
Barts and the London School of
Medicine, University of London
United Kingdom

Mathis Grossmann, MD, PhD, FRACP
University of Melbourne,
Austin Health
Australia

Mark Gurnell, MD, PhD
University of Cambridge and
Addenbrooke's Hospital
Wellcome Trust-MRC Institute
of Metabolic Science
United Kingdom

Claire Higham, DPhil, FRCP
Christie Hospital
United Kingdom

Sacha Howell, PhD, FRCP
Manchester University
United Kingdom

Erick Hung, MD
University of California – San Francisco

Channa Jayasena, MD, PhD
Imperial College London
United Kingdom

Electron Kebebew, MD
Stanford University

Marta Korbonits, MD, PhD
Barts and the London
School of Medicine
United Kingdom

Andrea L. Kossler, MD, FACS
Stanford University
School of Medicine

E. Michael Lewiecki, MD
University of New Mexico
Health Sciences Center

Matthew Lewis, MD, MPH
Stanford University
School of Medicine

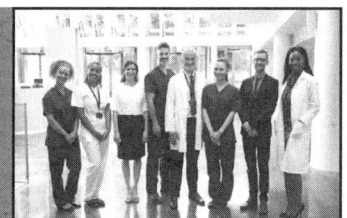

OVERVIEW

Endocrine Case Management: Meet the Professor is designed to provide physicians with a concise and high-quality review of more than 50 common and rare endocrine disorders to help you keep your practice current. It consists of case-based clinical vignettes and rationales written by experts in all areas of endocrinology, diabetes, and metabolism.

ACCREDITATION STATEMENT

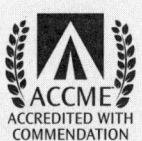

The Endocrine Society is accredited by the Accreditation Council for Continuing Medical Education to provide continuing medical education for physicians. The Endocrine Society has received Accreditation with Commendation.

The Endocrine Society designates this enduring material for a maximum of 30.0 *AMA PRA Category 1 Credits™*. Physicians should claim only the credit commensurate with the extent of their participation in the activity.

LEARNING OBJECTIVES

Endocrine Case Management: Meet the Professor will allow learners to assess their knowledge of all aspects of endocrinology, diabetes, and metabolism.

Upon completion of this educational activity, learners will be able to:

- Recognize clinical manifestations of endocrine and metabolic disorders and select among current options for diagnosis, management, and therapy.

- Identify risk factors for endocrine and metabolic disorders and develop strategies for prevention.

- Evaluate endocrine and metabolic manifestations of systemic disorders.

- Use existing resources pertaining to clinical guidelines and treatment recommendations for endocrine and related metabolic disorders to guide diagnosis and treatment.

TARGET AUDIENCE

Endocrine Case Management: Meet the Professor provides case-based education to clinicians interested in improving patient care.

STATEMENT OF INDEPENDENCE

As a provider of CME accredited by the Accreditation Council for Continuing Medical Education, the Endocrine Society has a policy of ensuring that the content and quality of this educational activity are balanced, independent, objective, and scientifically rigorous. The scientific content of this activity was developed under the supervision of the Endocrine Society's Annual Meeting Steering Committee.

DISCLOSURE POLICY

The faculty, committee members, and staff who are in position to control the content of this activity are required to disclose to the Endocrine Society and to learners any relevant financial relationship(s) of the individual or spouse/partner that have occurred within the last 12 months with any commercial interest(s) whose products or services are related to the CME content. Financial relationships are defined by remuneration in any amount from the commercial interest(s) in the form of grants; research support; consulting fees; salary; ownership interest (eg, stocks, stock options, or ownership interest excluding diversified mutual funds); honoraria or other payments for participation in speakers' bureaus, advisory boards, or boards of directors; or other financial benefits. The intent of this disclosure is not to prevent CME planners with relevant financial relationships from planning or delivering content, but rather to provide learners with information that allows them to make their own judgments of whether these financial relationships may have influenced the educational activity with regard to exposition or conclusion. The Endocrine Society has reviewed all disclosures and resolved or managed all identified conflicts of interest, as applicable.

The following faculty reported relevant financial relationships, as identified below, as of January 1, 2020:
Craig A. Alter, MD, Advisory Board Member: Novo

Nordisk; Consulting Fee: Pfizer, Inc. **Bradley D. Anawalt, MD**, UptoDate Author; **Richard J. Auchus, MD, PhD**, Consulting Fee: Novartis Pharmaceuticals, Corcept Therapeutics, Jansen Pharmaceuticals, Adrenas Therapeutics, Selenity Therapeutics, Quest Diagnostics; Research Investigator: Novartis Pharmaceuticals, Corcept Therapeutics, Strongbridge Biopharma, Neurocrine Biosciences, Spruce Biosciences. **Irina Bancos, MD**, Advisory Board Member: Corcept. **Andrew J. Bauer, MD**, Other, Sandoz. **Petter M. Bjornstad, MD**, Speaker: Horizon Pharm; Other: Boehringer Ingelheim. **Philippe Chanson, MD, MS**, Advisory Board Member: Tiburio; Research Investigator: Tiburio. **Mehul T. Dattani, MD, DCH, FRCPCH, FRCP, MBBS**, Advisory Board Member: Novo Nordisk; Consulting Fee: Ipsen; Speaker: Novo Nordisk. **Chrysoula Dosiou, MD, MS**, Advisory Board Member: Horizon Therapeutics. **Richard Eastell, MD, MBChB**, Consulting Fee: Roche Diagnostics, Immunodiagnostic Systems, Nittobo; Grant Recipient: Roche Diagnostics, Immunodiagnostic Systems, Nittobo. **Rossella Elisei, MD**, Advisory Board Member: Bayer, Inc, Loxo, Ipsen; Consulting Fee: Genzyme Corporation, Eli Lilly & Company, Exelixis, Inc. **Neil J. Gittoes, PhD, FRCP, MBCB, BSc**, Advisory Board Member: Shire, Amgen, Inc; Consulting Fee: Shire, Takeda; Speaker: Shire. **Whitney S. Goldner, MD**, Research Investigator: Roche Diagnostics. **Jennifer B. Green, MD**, Advisory Board Member: AstraZeneca, Boehringer Ingelheim; Consulting Fee: Novo Nordisk; Research Investigator: Boehringer Ingelheim, Sanofi. **Mathis Grossmann, MD, PhD, FRACP**, Speaker: Besins Health Care. **Mark Gurnell, PhD, FRCP, MBBS, MA**, Speaker: Ipsen. **Channa N. Jayasena, MD, PhD**, Speaker: BES 2016: Speaking against motion for androgen therapy in older men, during debate sponsored by Besins healthcare. **Marta Korbonits, MD, PhD**, Advisory Board Member: ONO-Pharma, Novo Nordisk; Research Investigator: ONO-Pharma; Speaker: Ipsen, Pfizer, Inc. **Andrea L. Kossler, MD**, Advisory Board Member: Horizon Therapeutics. **E. Michael Lewiecki, MD**, Advisory Board Member: Amgen, Inc; Grant Recipient: Amgen, Inc, Radius Health, Inc; Speaker: Alexion Pharmaceuticals, Inc, Radius Health, Inc; Advisory Board Member (Spouse): Radius Health, Inc, Alexion Pharmaceuticals, Inc, Sandoz. **Mark E. Molitch, MD**, Advisory Board Member: Jansen Pharmaceuticals, Sanofi; Consulting Fee: Merck, Novartis Pharmaceuticals, Pfizer, Inc; Grant Recipient: Novartis Pharmaceuticals, Bayer, Inc, Strongbridge, Novo Nordisk. **Robert D. Murray, MD, FRCP, BSc**, Grant Recipient: Sandoz, Takeda, Pfizer,

Inc. **Simon H.S. Pearce, MD, FRCP, MBBS**, Research Investigator: Apitope; Speaker: Sanofi-Aventis, Quidel. **Ian Reid, FRACP**, Advisory Board Member: Amgen, Inc; Research Investigator: Amgen, Inc; Speaker: Eli Lilly & Company, Amgen, Inc. **Molly O. Regelmann, MD**, Consulting Fee: Bluebird Bio; Speaker: Bluebird Bio. **Phyllis W. Speiser, MD**, Advisory Board Member: Spruce Biosciences; Consulting Fee: Gerson Lehman Group; Research Investigator: Boehringer Ingelheim; **Peter J. Tebben, MD**, Research Investigator: Ultragenyx. **Christopher J. Thompson, MD, PhD**, Speaker: Otsuka. **Steven D. Wittlin, MD**, Advisory Board Member: Senseonics; Consulting Fee: Novo; Speaker: Medtronic-Diabetes. **Philip S. Zeitler, MD, PhD**, Consulting Fee: Merck, Eli Lilly & Company, Boehringer Ingelheim, Novo Nordisk; Research Investigator: Jansen Pharmaceuticals.

The following faculty reported no relevant financial relationships as of January 1, 2020: **Stephen G. Ball, PhD, FRCP; Diana Barb, MD; Laura K. Bachrach, MD; Elizabeth O. Buschur, MD; Kristien Boelaert, MD, PhD; Marcelle I. Cedars, MD; Mary C. Frates, MD; Marc-Andre Cornier, MD; Ghada El-Hajj Fuleihan, MD, MPH; Ashley Grossman, MD, FRCP; Claire E. Higham, DPhil, MBBS; Sacha J. Howell, PhD, FRCP; Erick Hung, MD; Electron Kebebew, MD; Pedro Marques, MD; Rochelle N. Naylor, MD; Genevieve S. Neal-Perry, MD, PhD; Elizabeth J. Murphy, MD, DPhil; Lillian R. Meacham, MD; Matthew Lewis, MD, MPH; Joy Y. Wu, MD, PhD; Carole A. Spencer, PhD, FACB, MT; Jenny Tong, MD, MPH; William F. Young, Jr., MD, MSc; Vin Tangpricha, MD, PhD; Peter J. Trainer, MD, FRCP, MBChB, BSc; David J. Torpy, PhD, FRACP, MBBS; Greet Van den Berghe, MD, PhD; David Saxon, MD, MSc; Micol S. Rothman, MD; Thomas Weber, MD; Marzieh Salehi, MD, MS**

The following AMSC peer reviewers reported relevant financial relationships as of January 1, 2020: **Anders Juul, MD, PhD, DMSC**, Novo Nordisk, Pfizer, Ferring, Merck, Bayer, speakers bureau, honorarium; Novo Nordisk, pharmaceutical industry, sponsor and principal investigator of a clinical multicenter trial (NESGAS), unrestricted research grant; Ferring, pharmaceutical industry; clinical co-investigator in a Ferring-sponsored clinical trial (PORIYA); Diurnal, pharmaceutical industry; principal investigator in Denmark, financial support for participation in a multicenter study (RCT) on long-actinghydrocortisone (Chronocort) in CAH. **Antonio Bianco, MD, PhD**, paid consultant for Allergan, BLA Technology, IBSA Foudnation,

Synthonics. **Daniel Dumesic, MD**, NIH, Study Section member, per diem fee; NIH, P50 grantee, 10% FTE. **David D'Alessio, MD**, American Diabetes Association, Associate Editor for *Diabetes and Diabetes Care*; Lilly, consultant and research grant; Merck, research grant; Intarcia, consultant. **Eliot Brinton, MD**, Akcea, advisor and speaker; Amarin, advisor and speaker; Amgen, advisor and speaker; Boehringer-Ingelheim, speaker; Esperion, advisor; Kowa, advisor and speaker; Medicure, advisor; Merck, advisor and speaker; Novo-Nordisk, speaker; Regeneron, advisor and speaker; Sanofi-Aventis, advisor and speaker. **Francesco Celi, MD, MHSc**, IBSA, Acella. **Jennifer Sherr, MD, PhD**, Medtronic Diabetes, consultant; Bigfoot Biomedical, advisory board; Lilly, advisory board; Insulet, advisory board; JDRF, grantee; Cecelia Health, advisory board; Sanofi, consultant. **Marie Demay, MD**, Syros Pharmaceuticals CMO (spouse); NIH reviewer and grantee (self). **Nicola Napoli, MD, PhD**, UCB; LILLY, advisory board; consulting fees, Abiogen, Lilly; speaker fee, Lilly. **Richard Feelders, MD, PhD**, Novartis, research grants; Ipsen, research grants. **Robin Peeters, MD, PhD**, Berlin-Chemie, lecture fee; Goodlife Fertility BV, lecture fee; Institut Biochimique SA (IBSA), lecture fee; Sanofi Genzyme, lecture fee, advisory board; Bayer, lecture fee, advisory board; EISAI, advisory board. **Veronica Mericq, MD**, Grant of growth innovation (GGI grant) scientific committee member; Yearly Prize, funded by Merck; Scientific committee of EDGe; educational pediatric endocrinology activity funded by Novartis/Sandoz since 2014; Pfizer global advisory board for SGA specific subject; advisory board for Latin America–based Sandoz, Merck, and Novo Nordisk.

The following AMSC peer reviewers reported no relevant financial relationships as of January 1, 2020: **Bassil Kublaoui, MD, PhD; Dawn Davis, MD, PhD; Jennifer Sipos, MD; Larry Fox, MD; Lauren Fishbein, MD, PhD; Margareta Pisarska, MD; Mark Cooper, MD, PhD; Matthew Freeby, MD; Niki Karavitaki, FRCP, PhD; Robert Wermers, MD; Selma Witchel, MD**

The Endocrine Society staff associated with the development of content for this activity reported no relevant financial relationships.

DISCLAIMERS
The information presented in this activity represents the opinion of the faculty and is not necessarily the official position of the Endocrine Society.

USE OF PROFESSIONAL JUDGMENT:
The educational content in this enduring activity relates to basic principles of diagnosis and therapy and does not substitute for individual patient assessment based on the health care provider's examination of the patient and consideration of laboratory data and other factors unique to the patient. Standards in medicine change as new data become available.

DRUGS AND DOSAGES:
When prescribing medications, the physician is advised to check the product information sheet accompanying each drug to verify conditions of use and to identify any changes in drug dosage schedule or contraindications.

POLICY ON UNLABELED/OFF-LABEL USE
The Endocrine Society has determined that disclosure of unlabeled/off-label or investigational use of commercial product(s) is informative for audiences and therefore requires this information to be disclosed to the learners at the beginning of the presentation. Uses of specific therapeutic agents, devices, and other products discussed in this educational activity may not be the same as those indicated in product labeling approved by the Food and Drug Administration (FDA). The Endocrine Society requires that any discussions of such "off-label" use be based on scientific research that conforms to generally accepted standards of experimental design, data collection, and data analysis. Before recommending or prescribing any therapeutic agent or device, learners should review the complete prescribing information, including indications, contraindications, warnings, precautions, and adverse events.

PRIVACY AND CONFIDENTIALITY STATEMENT
The Endocrine Society will record learner's personal information as provided on CME evaluations to allow for issuance and tracking of CME certificates. The Endocrine Society may also track aggregate responses to questions in activities and evaluations and use these data to inform the ongoing evaluation and improvement of its CME program. No individual performance data or any other personal information collected from evaluations will be shared with third parties.

ACKNOWLEDGMENT OF COMMERCIAL SUPPORT
This activity is not supported by educational grant(s) or other funds from any commercial supporter.

AMA PRA CATEGORY 1 CREDIT (CME) INFORMATION

To receive a maximum of 30.0 *AMA PRA Category 1 Credits*™, participants must complete the online interactive module and activity evaluation located at **https://education.endocrine.org/MTP2020**. Participants must achieve a minimum score of 70% to claim CME credit. After initially completing the module, if participants do not achieve a minimum score of 70%, they have the option to change their answers and make additional attempts to achieve a passing score. Learners also have the option to clear all answers and start over.

METHOD OF PARTICIPATION

This enduring material is presented online and in print format. The estimated time to complete this activity, including review of material, is 30 hours. Participants must achieve a minimum score of 70% to claim CME credit. After initially completing the module, if participants do not achieve a minimum score of 70%, they have the option to change their answers and make additional attempts to achieve a passing score. Participants also have the option to clear all answers and start over.

SYSTEM REQUIREMENTS

To complete this activity, participants must have access to a computer or mobile device with an Internet connection and use an up to date version of any major Web browser, such as Internet Explorer 10+, Firefox 32+, Safari, or Google Chrome 37+. In addition, cookies and Javascript must be enabled in the browser's options.

LAST REVIEW DATE: January 2020

ACTIVITY RELEASE DATE: March 28, 2020

ACTIVITY EXPIRATION DATE:
March 30, 2022 (date after which this enduring material is no longer certified for *AMA PRA Category 1 Credits*™)

For questions about content or obtaining CME credit, please contact the Endocrine Society at http://education.endocrine.org/contact.

COMMON ABBREVIATIONS

ACTH = corticotropin

ACE inhibitor = angiotensin-converting enzyme inhibitor

ALT = alanine aminotransferase

AST = aspartate aminotransferase

BMI = body mass index

CNS = central nervous system

CT = computed tomography

DHEA = dehydroepiandrosterone

DHEA-S = dehydroepiandrosterone sulfate

DNA = deoxyribonucleic acid

DPP-4 inhibitor = dipeptidyl-peptidase 4 inhibitor

DXA = dual-energy x-ray absorptiometry

FDA = Food and Drug Administration

FGF-23 = fibroblast growth factor 23

FNA = fine-needle aspiration

FSH = follicle-stimulating hormone

GH = growth hormone

GHRH = growth hormone–releasing hormone

GLP-1 receptor agonist = glucagonlike peptide 1 receptor agonist

GnRH = gonadotropin-releasing hormone

hCG = human chorionic gonadotropin

HDL = high-density lipoprotein

HIV = human immunodeficiency virus

HMG-CoA reductase inhibitor = 3-hydroxy-3-methylglutaryl coenzyme A reductase inhibitor

IGF-1 = insulinlike growth factor 1

LDL = low-density lipoprotein

LH = luteinizing hormone

MCV = mean corpuscular volume

MIBG = *meta*-iodobenzylguanidine

MRI = magnetic resonance imaging

NPH insulin = neutral protamine Hagedorn insulin

PCSK9 inhibitor = proprotein convertase subtilisin/kexin 9 inhibitor

PET = positron emission tomography

PSA = prostate-specific antigen
PTH = parathyroid hormone

PTHrP = parathyroid hormone–related protein

SGLT-2 inhibitor = sodium-glucose cotransporter 2 inhibitor

SHBG = sex hormone–binding globulin

T$_3$ = triiodothyronine

T$_4$ = thyroxine

TPO antibodies = thyroperoxidase antibodies

TRH = thyrotropin-releasing hormone

TRAb = thyrotropin-receptor antibodies

TSH = thyrotropin

VLDL = very low-density lipoprotein

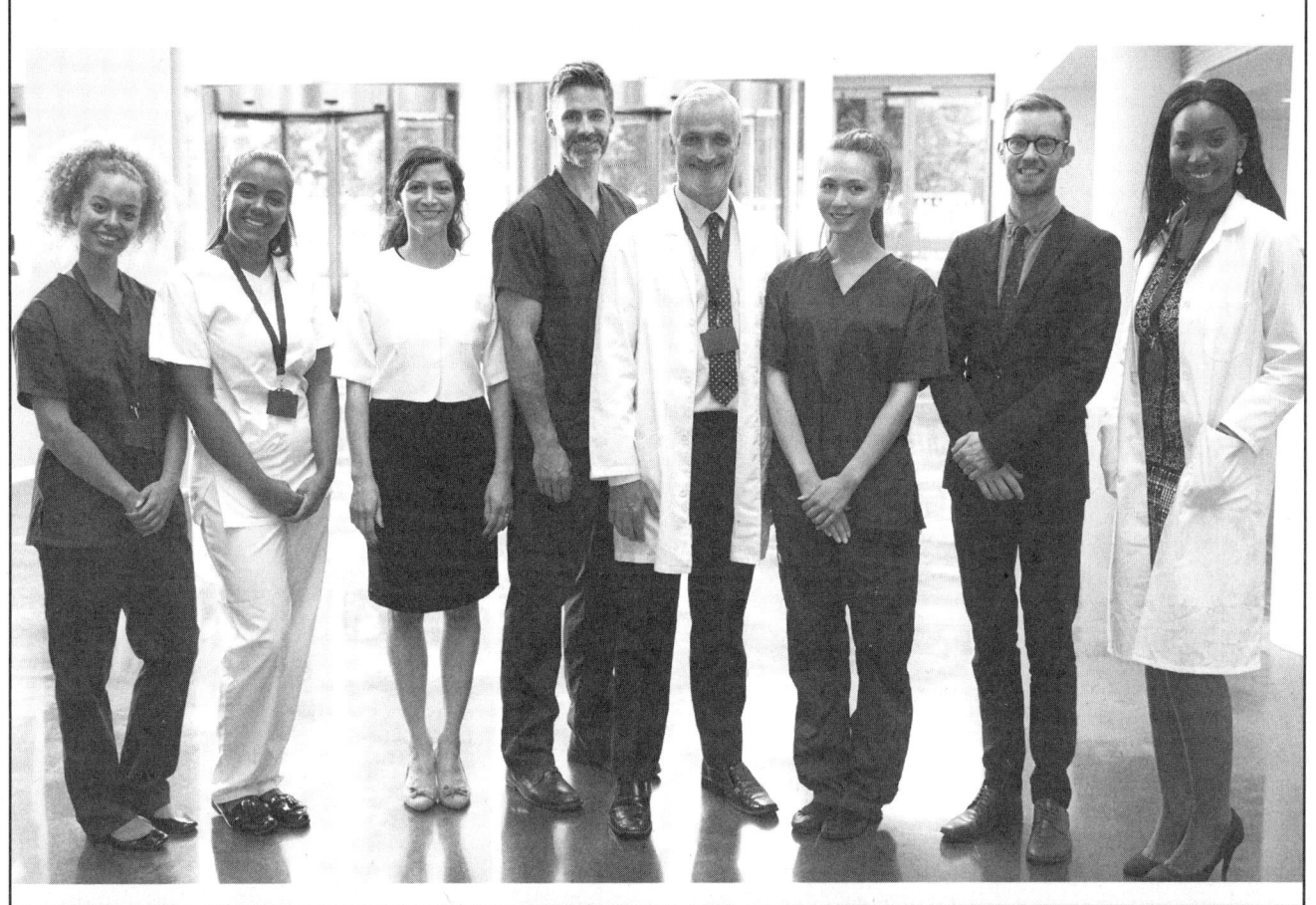

ADIPOSE TISSUE, APPETITE, AND OBESITY

Controversies in Bariatric Surgery

Jenny Tong, MD, MPH. Division of Metabolism, Endocrinology, and Nutrition, Department of Medicine, University of Washington, VA Puget Sound Health Care Systems, Seattle, WA; E-mail: tongj@uw.edu

Marzieh Salehi, MD, MS. Department of Medicine, Diabetes Division, University of Texas Health at San Antonio, Audie Murphy Hospital, San Antonio, TX; E-mail: salehi@uthscsa.edu

Learning Objectives

As a result of participating in this session, learners should be able to:

- Explain differential effects of Roux-en-Y gastric bypass (RYGB) vs sleeve gastrectomy on weight loss, diabetes mellitus remission, and long-term metabolic outcomes.

- Describe the controversy in performing bariatric surgery in elderly patients and the impact of bariatric surgery on psychiatric conditions, renal function, and bone health.

- Diagnose and treat the late complication of hypoglycemia after weight-loss surgery.

Main Conclusions

While bariatric surgery has emerged to be the most effective treatment for obesity and type 2 diabetes mellitus (T2DM), many controversies remain regarding its durability, applications, and outcomes in specific patient populations and the best approach to managing its complications.

Significance of the Clinical Problem

The number of bariatric surgeries has markedly increased in the last 2 decades. Endocrinologists are at the front line in deciding whether a patient should be referred for bariatric surgery, discussing with patients the expectations and managing their complications. Many areas of controversy exist regarding the use of bariatric surgery in the treatment of obesity and related complications. This chapter highlights a few controversies related to factors (ie, age, psychiatric conditions, renal function) that affect referral decisions and reviews how surgery type affects outcome of weight loss and diabetes resolution. The chapter also summarizes the current concepts in diagnosis and treatment of the life-threatening condition of hypoglycemia after RYGB.

Barriers to Optimal Practice

- Lack of public and medical community awareness of available evidence.

- Lack of longitudinal trials beyond 10 years to address the long-term effects of weight-loss/metabolic surgeries.

- Lack of high-level evidence to guide decision making in individualized treatment for obesity and diabetes.

Clinical Case Vignettes

Case 1

A 40-year-old woman presents with a BMI of 40 kg/m^2. She has been heavy all her life. T2DM was diagnosed 2 years after pregnancy. Oral medication was initially prescribed, but she had to start insulin a year ago. Her hemoglobin A_{1c} level is 8.0% (64 mmol/mol). She is in tears and is concerned about her risk of having similar problems to those experienced by her father, who had renal dysfunction and a myocardial infarction in his 50s. She is fed up with her lack of success in weight loss and diabetes treatment.

Which of the following would be the most effective treatment for weight loss and diabetes?

A. Intensive medical therapy and lifestyle interventions

B. RYGB

C. Sleeve gastrectomy

D. B or C

Answer: D) B or C

Treatment of obesity and related complications, such as T2DM, remains a challenge. To date, weight-loss surgery is the most effective treatment for obesity and T2DM. Among these procedures, RYGB, rerouting the gastrointestinal tract by connecting the surgically reduced stomach pouch to the jejunal limb of a Roux-en-Y enterotomy, and sleeve gastrectomy, creating a tube-like stomach by surgically removing a large portion of stomach's greater curvature, are the most commonly performed procedures in the United States. Longitudinal data on the effectiveness of these procedures to treat T2DM beyond 10 years are lacking. However, remission of T2DM following bariatric surgeries has been well documented. Several randomized clinical trials have demonstrated that a larger proportion of patients with uncontrolled diabetes achieve target glycemic control (estimated based on hemoglobin A_{1c} level) 2 to 5 years after RYGB[1,2]

and sleeve gastrectomy[3,4] than those who receive medical intervention with or without lifestyle interventions. While weight loss induced by these surgeries has a significant role in diabetes resolution, it is now being recognized that glycemic improvement after RYGB, and to a lesser degree after sleeve gastrectomy, is partly independent of the amount of weight loss.[5-8] Between the 2 procedures, RYGB has been shown to be more effective than sleeve gastrectomy[9] in inducing complete diabetes remission after surgery.[10]

Whether glycemic improvement after these procedures translates into improved survival or reduction in the incidence of diabetes-related complications has been studied using various methodologies in recent years. The STAMPEDE trial randomly assigned 150 obese patients with diabetes to gastric bypass, sleeve gastrectomy, or intensive medical intervention and reported a lower urinary albumin-to-creatinine ratio in the sleeve gastrectomy group at 5 years.[9] More recently, larger, retrospective, population database studies matching patients with T2DM treated with and without bariatric surgery have collectively demonstrated that bariatric surgery can reduce mortality by 40% to 60%, the incidence of microvascular complications by 50% to 60%,[11,12] and macrovascular complications by 30% to 40%[12,13] at median follow-up of 4 to 5 years.

Main Takeaway Points

- Both RYGB and sleeve gastrectomy induce significant and durable weight loss.

- RYGB is superior to sleeve gastrectomy in inducing diabetes remission.

- Long-term beneficial effects of these procedures on diabetes-related complications and survival, particularly in those with T2DM,[14] have been documented.

Case 1 (Continued)

The patient also has a history of major depression and binge eating. She takes an antidepressant and is under the care of a behavioral psychologist. She has not had any suicidal thoughts or attempts.

Which of the following statements is true?

A. She cannot have bariatric surgery because she has major depression

B. Her depressive symptoms will get worse within the first few years after bariatric surgery

C. Self-harm behavior and suicide rates might increase a few years after bariatric surgery

D. The prevalence of mental health disorders is lower in the bariatric surgery population

Answer: C) Self-harm behavior and suicide rates might increase a few years after bariatric surgery

The prevalence of depression is higher among patients seeking surgical treatment for obesity than in the general US population (19% vs 8%) according to one systemic review.[15] There is conflicting evidence regarding the association between preoperative mental health conditions and postoperative weight loss. Neither depression nor binge eating disorder has been consistently associated with differences in weight outcomes. Moderate-quality evidence suggests that bariatric surgery is associated with postoperative reduction in the prevalence, frequency, and severity of depressive symptoms, at least during the first 3 years after surgery. There is some evidence for increased rates of suicide, self-harm behavior, and alcohol abuse after bariatric surgery, but the level of evidence is low to moderate.

Main Takeaway Points

- Mental health conditions are common among bariatric surgery patients.

- Depressive symptoms are likely to improve after bariatric surgery.

- Increased self-harm behaviors and substance abuse have been reported in cohort studies.

Case 1 (Continued)

The patient undergoes RYGB with normal recovery. She loses 120 lb (54.5 kg) in 1 year, her diabetes goes into remission, and her triglycerides normalize. Two years after surgery, she starts having episodic palpitations and sweating. While she is at work one day, she passes out. Her glucose is checked, and it is 39 mg/dL (2.2 mmol/L). She regains consciousness immediately after intravenous glucose infusion.

Which of the following is the most likely diagnosis and what is the best next step?

A. Insulinoma; perform 72-hour fasting test

B. Hypoglycemia after RYGB; obtain a complete medical history to confirm and exclude any fasting hypoglycemia, initiate dietary modification and acarbose therapy

C. Adrenal insufficiency; perform cosyntropin-stimulation test

D. B and C

Answer: B) Hypoglycemia after RYGB, obtain a complete medical history to confirm and exclude any fasting hypoglycemia, initiate dietary modification and acarbose therapy

Postprandial hyperinsulinemic hypoglycemia is a late complication of bariatric surgery. Hypoglycemic symptoms that occur mainly during 1 to 3 hours after eating generally manifest after 1 year from surgery. Causes other than RYGB should be considered for clinical hypoglycemia manifesting less than 6 months from surgery and beyond 4 to 5 hours from meal ingestion. Given the lack of consensus in diagnostic criteria, the true incidence remains unknown. Diagnosis relies on detecting a low glucose concentration (plasma glucose <54 mg/dL [<3.0 mmol/L]) associated with symptoms or signs that are relieved by raising glucose values (Whipple triad). Hypoglycemic symptoms are traditionally divided into autonomic and neuroglycopenic symptoms. Since symptoms of dumping cannot be distinguished with autonomic symptoms of hypoglycemia, it is recommended that the diagnosis be based on neuroglycopenic symptoms. When clinical hypoglycemia cannot be documented in free-living conditions, a provocative test can be used to induce hypoglycemia in individuals with a history suggesting this condition. The provocative test for diagnosis of prandial hypoglycemia is a mixed-meal test rather than an oral glucose challenge.[16]

Bypassing the foregut alters the balance between the total glucose delivery (ingested glucose and hepatic glucose production) and total glucose use from circulation, improving glycemia in most patients with T2DM. However, when the glucose delivery falls behind glucose use in those with susceptibility to glucose abnormality, hypoglycemia occurs. Experimental studies have shown that the exaggerated appearance of ingested glucose into circulation, enhanced β-cell secretory response to food intake (likely due to exaggerated GLP-1 action), as well as diminished prandial insulin clearance contribute to the hypoglycemia in this condition.[17]

Therefore, the most effective treatment strategies for this condition are those that selectively delay intestinal glucose delivery/absorption or suppress prandial insulin secretion. Currently, treatment is limited to dietary and medical interventions based on their effectiveness in other conditions such as insulinoma. Dietary modification consisting of lowering the amount of carbohydrate for every meal, avoiding simple carbohydrates, adding fat and protein to every meal, and modifying carbohydrate composition from glucose to fructose has been tried with some success. Among the available pharmacotherapeutic options, acarbose, an α-glucosidase blocker, has been used as the first-line agent along with dietary modification. When dietary modification and acarbose fail to improve severity or frequency of hypoglycemia, other therapeutic options targeting insulin secretion are considered. Among these agents, diazoxide and somatostatin analogues have been tried with limited success. Investigational drugs that are in different phases of development are GLP-1 receptor antagonists (exendin-9-39), glucagon, and insulin receptor antibody.[16]

Main Takeaway Points

- Postprandial hypoglycemia is a devastating late complication of bariatric surgery.

- Diagnosis is complex and requires documentation of the Whipple triad either during free-living conditions or with use of a provocative test.

- Dietary and pharmacologic interventions that reduce prandial glucose spikes and insulin levels are the most effective strategies to treat this condition.

Case 2

A 70-year-old man presents with a BMI of 45 kg/m². He has a history of hypertension, obstructive sleep apnea, arthritis of the knees, and stage 4 chronic kidney disease from uncontrolled hypertension. He has no history of diabetes. He is quite independent, plays golf once a week, and lives with his wife. His weight has been bothering him for a long time. He has joined weight-loss programs and tried liraglutide in the past, but he was unable to lose more than 10% of his body weight. He asks, "Can I have surgery to help me lose more weight, doc? Is it safe for my kidneys? Will it break my bones?"

Which of the following statements is true?

A. Bariatric surgery–related morbidity and mortality rates are the same for persons older than 70 years and those younger than 70 years

B. Within a few years after bariatric surgery, proteinuria increases and the glomerular filtration rate decreases in obese patients with impaired renal function

C. DXA can provide accurate measurement of bone mineral density during the acute weight-loss phase after surgery

D. Increased bone turnover, decreased bone mineral density, and increased fracture risk have been observed after gastric bypass surgery

Answer: D) Increased bone turnover, decreased bone mineral density, and increased fracture risk have been observed after gastric bypass surgery

Current evidence is insufficient to assess the balance of benefits and harms of offering bariatric surgery as an adjunct to comprehensive lifestyle intervention for weight loss or to improve some obesity-associated conditions to patients older than 65 years. While bariatric surgery has a low risk of complications and mortality, higher rates of morbidity and mortality have been reported for patients older than 70 years who had bariatric surgery compared with those younger than 70.[18] This could be due to the higher morbidity and mortality risk in the over-70 group preoperatively. Sleeve gastrectomy may be a safer option for elderly patients. More research is needed.

In general, proteinuria, albuminuria, and glomerular hyperfiltration decline after bariatric surgery in obese patients with impaired renal function.[19] One study in the Medicare population reported that patients with stage 3 or 4 chronic kidney disease who underwent either RYGB or sleeve gastrectomy had a higher estimated glomerular filtration rate than did nonsurgically treated control participants at up to 3 years after surgery. Between the 2 procedures, RYGB achieved a higher estimated glomerular filtration rate than did sleeve gastrectomy.[20] Adverse renal sequelae such as increased frequency of oxalate stones after bariatric surgery have also been reported. Lack of randomized controlled trials and long-term follow-up are the limits of existing literature.

Available data suggest that fracture risk after bariatric surgery varies depending on the bariatric procedure. Mixed restrictive and malabsorptive procedures are associated with an increased risk of fracture at osteoporotic sites and the risk starts to increase between 2 and 5 years after surgery.[21-23] However, the low number of fracture events does not allow assessment of fracture risk by site in most studies. Increase in bone turnover markers; decline in areal and volumetric bone mineral density at the lumbar spine, total hip, and appendicular skeleton sites; and endocortical absorption and decrease in bone strength have all been reported in literature. The effects of bariatric surgery on bone mass may particularly impact postmenopausal women. It is worth noting that assessment of bone mineral density changes by DXA may be inaccurate in the context of acute weight loss.[24]

Main Takeaway Points

- High-level evidence is needed to guide appropriate recommendations for bariatric surgery in older adults.

- Bariatric surgery has a positive impact on renal function but also potential harm in selected patients.

- Increased bone turnover and decreased bone mineral density have been reported in the literature, but their relationship to fracture risk has not been firmly established.

References

1. Ikramuddin S, Korner J, Lee WJ, et al. Roux-en-Y gastric bypass vs intensive medical management for the control of type 2 diabetes, hypertension, and hyperlipidemia: the Diabetes Surgery Study randomized clinical trial. *JAMA.* 2013;309(21):2240-2249. PMID: 23736733

2. Mingrone G, Panunzi S, De Gaetano A, et al. Bariatric surgery versus conventional medical therapy for type 2 diabetes. *N Engl J Med.* 2012;366(17):1577-1585. PMID: 22449317

3. Peterli R, Wolnerhanssen BK, Vetter D, et al. Laparoscopic sleeve gastrectomy versus Roux-Y-gastric bypass for morbid obesity-3-year outcomes of the prospective randomized Swiss Multicenter Bypass or Sleeve Study (SM-BOSS). *Ann Surg.* 2017;265(3):466-473. PMID: 28170356

4. Yang J, Wang C, Cao G, et al. Long-term effects of laparoscopic sleeve gastrectomy versus roux-en-Y gastric bypass for the treatment of Chinese type 2 diabetes mellitus patients with body mass index 28-35 kg/m(2). *BMC Surg.* 2015;15:88. PMID: 26198306

5. Schauer PR, Ikramuddin S, Gourash W, Ramanathan R, Luketich J. Outcomes after laparoscopic Roux-en-Y gastric bypass for morbid obesity. *Ann Surg.* 2000;232(4):515-529. PMID: 10998650

6. Ferrannini E, Camastra S, Gastaldelli A, et al. Beta-cell function in obesity: effects of weight loss. Diabetes. 2004;53(Suppl 3):S26-S33. PMID: 15561918

7. Jorgensen NB, Jacobsen SH, Dirksen C, et al. Acute and long-term effects of Roux-en-Y gastric bypass on glucose metabolism in subjects with type

2 diabetes and normal glucose tolerance. *Am J Physiol Endocrinol Metab.* 2012;303(1):E122-E131. PMID: 22535748

8. Peterli R, Wolnerhanssen B, Peters T, et al. Improvement in glucose metabolism after bariatric surgery: comparison of laparoscopic Roux-en-Y gastric bypass and laparoscopic sleeve gastrectomy: a prospective randomized trial. *Ann Surg.* 2009;250(2):234-241. PMID: 19638921

9. Schauer PR, Bhatt DL, Kashyap SR. Bariatric surgery or intensive medical therapy for diabetes after 5 years. *N Engl J Med.* 2017;376(20):1997. PMID: 28514616

10. Salminen P, Helmio M, Ovaska J, et al. Effect of laparoscopic sleeve gastrectomy vs laparoscopic Roux-en-Y gastric bypass on weight loss at 5 years among patients with morbid obesity: the SLEEVEPASS randomized clinical trial. *JAMA.* 2018;319(3):241-254. PMID: 29340676

11. O'Brien R, Johnson E, Haneuse S, et al. Microvascular outcomes in patients with diabetes after bariatric surgery versus usual care: a matched cohort study. *Ann Intern Med.* 2018;169(5):300-310. PMID: 30083761

12. Aminian A, Zajichek A, Arterburn DE, et al. Association of metabolic surgery with major adverse cardiovascular outcomes in patients with type 2 diabetes and obesity. *JAMA* [Epub ahead of print]

13. Fisher DP, Johnson E, Haneuse S, et al. Association between bariatric surgery and macrovascular disease outcomes in patients with type 2 diabetes and severe obesity. *JAMA.* 2018;320(15):1570-1582. PMID: 30326126

14. Lent MR, Benotti PN, Mirshahi T, et al. All-cause and specific-cause mortality risk after Roux-en-Y gastric bypass in patients with and without diabetes. *Diabetes Care.* 2017;40(10):1379-1385. PMID: 28760742

15. Dawes AJ, Maggard-Gibbons M, Maher AR, et al. Mental health conditions among patients seeking and undergoing bariatric surgery: a meta-analysis. *JAMA.* 2016;315(2):150-163. PMID: 26757464

16. Salehi M, Vella A, McLaughlin T, Patti ME. Hypoglycemia after gastric bypass surgery: current concepts and controversies. *J Clin Endocrinol Metab.* 2018;103(8):2815-2826. PMID: 30101281

17. Honka H, Salehi M. Postprandial hypoglycemia after gastric bypass surgery: from pathogenesis to diagnosis and treatment. *Curr Opin Clin Nutr Metab Care.* 2019;22(4):295-302. PMID: 31082828

18. Pechman DM, Munoz Flores F, Kinkhabwala CM, et al. Bariatric surgery in the elderly: outcomes analysis of patients over 70 using the ACS-NSQIP database. *Surg Obes Relat Dis.* 2019;15(11):1923-1932. PMID: 31611184

19. Li K, Zou J, Ye Z, et al. Effects of bariatric surgery on renal function in obese patients: a systematic review and meta analysis. *PLoS One.* 2016;11(10):e0163907. PMID: 27701452

20. Imam TH, Fischer H, Jing B, et al. Estimated GFR before and after bariatric surgery in CKD. *Am J Kidney Dis.* 2017;69(3):380-388. PMID: 27927587

21. Rousseau C, Jean S, Gamache P, et al. Change in fracture risk and fracture pattern after bariatric surgery: nested case-control study. *BMJ.* 2016;354:i3794. PMID: 27814663

22. Yu EW, Lee MP, Landon JE, Lindeman KG, Kim SC. Fracture risk after bariatric surgery: Roux-en-Y gastric bypass versus adjustable gastric banding. *J Bone Miner Res.* 2017;32(6):1229-1236. PMID: 28251687

23. Gagnon C, Schafer AL. Bone health after bariatric surgery. *JBMR Plus.* 2018;2(3):121-133. PMID: 30283897

24. Yu EW, Bouxsein ML, Roy AE, et al. Bone loss after bariatric surgery: discordant results between DXA and QCT bone density. *J Bone Miner Res.* 2014;29(3):542-550. PMID: 23929784

Pharmacotherapy in Obesity

Marc-Andre Cornier, MD. University of Colorado School of Medicine, Denver, CO; E-mail: marc.cornier@cuanschutz.edu

David R. Saxon, MD. University of Colorado School of Medicine, Denver, CO; E-mail: david.saxon@cuanschutz.edu

Learning Objectives

As a result of participating in this session, learners should be able to:

- Recognize the potential benefits and roles of antiobesity medications in clinical practice.

- Feel comfortable discussing available prescription antiobesity medications with patients.

- Decide which antiobesity medication best fits a given patient.

Main Conclusions

Pharmacotherapy is indicated as an adjunct to caloric restriction and increased physical activity in adults with a BMI greater than 30 kg/m^2 or between 27 and 29.9 kg/m^2 with at least 1 weight-related comorbidity. The rationale for pharmacologic treatment of obesity is that weight loss and maintenance of weight loss are difficult for most patients because caloric restriction is counteracted by adaptive biologic responses of increased appetite and decreased basal metabolic rate, which promote weight regain.

Antiobesity medications have a checkered past that make many clinicians uncomfortable with their use. Specifically, the experience with fenfluramine, a serotonin-releasing agent that acted on 5-HT2B receptors and was found to cause valvular heart disease and pulmonary hypertension resulting in its removal from the US market in 1997, gives many clinicians and patients pause about the use of antiobesity medications. Fortunately, over the past several years, a number of pharmacologic options for the treatment of obesity have become available and approvals have been granted supporting their long-term use and safety.

Barriers exist to prescribing these medications and they are underutilized in relation to patients' desires to try antiobesity medications to lose weight with the support of their health care providers. Endocrinologists can improve their patients' weight-loss success by incorporating FDA-approved weight-loss medications into their clinical practices.

Significance of the Clinical Problem

In the United States, the prevalence of obesity has trended upwards over recent decades, and as of 2015-2016, rates were 39.8% in adults and 18.5% in children.[1] Worldwide in 2008 an estimated 1.46 billion adults had a BMI greater than 25 kg/m^2 and 205 million men and 297 million women were obese.[2] It is projected that by the year 2030, obesity prevalence in the United States will have grown by another 65 million adults.[3] The obesity epidemic has resulted in the drastic rise in other chronic metabolic conditions such as type 2 diabetes and an overall loss in quality-adjusted life years across all US demographic categories from 1993 to 2008.[4] Similarly, reductions in the rate of rise in overall life expectancy in the United States may be attributable to rising obesity.[5]

Despite the availability of 5 antiobesity medications that are FDA approved for long-term use, rates of pharmacologic treatment of obesity are low. In a cohort of more than 2.2 million adults eligible for antiobesity medications by current guidelines across 8 health care organizations, only 1.3% filled even 1 antiobesity medication prescription between 2009 and 2015.[6] Interestingly, among the small group of health care providers who wrote at least 1 antiobesity medication prescription during that same period, 24% were "frequent prescribers" who wrote 90% of all filled prescriptions. One barrier for patients to obtaining antiobesity medications seems to be that primary care providers tend to overvalue exercise relative to medications as an effective method for weight loss.[7] Other barriers include lack of formal training in weight management and limited time during routine clinic visits. Finally, one of the most important factors is the high cost of antiobesity medications in conjunction with very limited insurance coverage.

Barriers to Optimal Practice

- Lack of insurance coverage and high out-of-pocket costs for available antiobesity medications.

- Modest degree of efficacy of antiobesity medications relative to degree of excess weight in most patients.

- Bias among health care providers towards patients with obesity.

- Inadequate formal training in obesity management for endocrinologists and other clinicians.

- Complexity of obesity management.

- Competing, often more apparently urgent, interests during brief clinical visits.

Strategies for Diagnosis, Therapy, and/or Management

FDA-Approved Pharmacotherapy for Obesity

Pharmacotherapy for weight management should be considered and is FDA approved for use as an adjunct to comprehensive lifestyle modification in patients with a BMI greater than or equal to 27 kg/m^2 who have a weight-related comorbidity or in patients with a BMI greater than 30 kg/m^2. Antiobesity medications can improve adherence to dietary strategies that lead to weight loss and are also beneficial to prevent the weight regain commonly seen with diet alone. Antiobesity medications are considered by the FDA to be effective if shown to cause greater than or equal to 5% of body weight loss after 3 months use (*Table 1*).

A number of professional societies and organizations have promoted the use of antiobesity medications, including but not limited to the Endocrine Society, American Association of Clinical Endocrinologists, The Obesity Society, American Heart Association, American College of Cardiology, and Veterans Health Administration.

The Endocrine Society Clinical Practice Guideline on the Pharmacological Management of Obesity was published in 2015.[8] This guideline emphasizes that a central point of caring for patients with overweight or obesity, or at patients risk for these conditions, is to review their concurrent use of medications that may promote weight gain. Many medications used to treat psychiatric conditions, seizure disorders, diabetes, and inflammatory conditions are commonly associated with weight gain. When possible, clinicians should consider switching patients to alternative medications that are weight neutral or that promote weight loss.

In a systematic review and meta-analysis of 257 randomized controlled trials, weight gain was associated with the use of a number of commonly used medications (*Table 2*).[9]

Table 1. Summary of FDA-Approved Antiobesity Medications

Agent	Mechanism of Action	Typical Maintenance Dose	Average Price for 30-Day Supply*	Weight Loss**	Patients Losing ≥5% of Initial Weight	Patients Losing ≥10% of Initial Weight	Key Points
Phentermine	Norepinephrine release	8-37.5 mg daily	$34.78 ($4.12)	~5%	X	X	Approved for short-term use
Orlistat	Lipase inhibitor	60 mg TID (OTC); 120 mg TID (Rx)	OTC (Alli): ~$60; RX (Xenical): $800 ($599.58)	3%-4%	~21%	~12%	Available over-the-counter, gastrointestinal adverse side effects
Lorcaserin	Serotonin receptor agonist	10 mg BID (also 20 mg XR daily version)	$366.52 ($305)	3%-4%	27%	15%	Least adverse effects, cardiovascular disease safety
Naltrexone ER/ bupropion ER	Opioid antagonist/ antidepressant (dopamine) reuptake inhibitor	16 mg/180 mg BID	$308 ($272.10)	5%-6%	35%	20%	Intermediate in effectiveness and adverse effects (nausea/vomiting)
Liraglutide, 3.0 mg	GLP-1 receptor agonist	3.0 mg daily	$1492.06 ($1243.17)	6%-7%	36%	23%	Intermediate effectiveness and side effects, ?cardiovascular disease benefit, very high cost
Phentermine/ topiramate ER	Sympathomimetic/ GABA	7.5-15 mg/ 46-92 mg daily	$231.07 ($191.47)	8%-11%	41%-49%	30%-41%	Most effective, intermediate adverse effects

US FDA. Drugs@FDA. http://www.accessdata.fda.gov/Scripts/cder/DrugsatFDA/

US FDA. Safety alerts for human medical products. http://www.fda.gov/safety/medwatch/safetyinformation/safetyalertsforhumanmedicalproducts/ucm391013.htm.

*Average retail price (discounted price) as listed on GoodRx the week of November 11, 2019.

** 1-year efficacy, difference vs placebo (P<.05 for all). Note: Such results are not available for phentermine alone.

Phentermine

Phentermine is the most widely prescribed antiobesity medication in the United States. Available in the United States since 1959, phentermine is a sympathomimetic that is FDA approved only for short-term use (≤3 months); however, many patients are prescribed the medication on a long-term basis.[6] While there are no long-term cardiovascular outcome studies assessing the safety of phentermine, a recent retrospective analysis of real-world data did not identify an increase in cardiovascular risk with longer exposure to phentermine.[10] Phentermine regimens include 8 mg 3 times daily and 15 mg, 30 mg, or 37.5 mg taken once daily. Potential adverse effects include increased heart rate and blood pressure, insomnia, agitation, dry mouth, headache, tremor, constipation. Typical weight loss with phentermine is about 5% of total body weight. Advantages of phentermine include a long historical experience with the medication and low cost.

Orlistat

Orlistat is a gastric and pancreatic lipase inhibitor that has been FDA approved for long-term use for weight management since 1999. Both over-the-counter and prescription formulations are available. Typical weight loss is about 3% to 4%. The gastrointestinal adverse effects of orlistat often

In February 2020, the medication lorcaserin was voluntarily removed from the US market.

limit its use, as steatorrhea, flatulence, increased defecation, and fecal incontinence are common, and malabsorption of fat-soluble vitamins may also occur. Despite these limitations, orlistat has been shown to decrease the incidence of diabetes in a prediabetes population over a 4-year period.[11]

Lorcaserin

Lorcaserin is a selective serotonin 2C receptor agonist that was FDA approved in 2012 for chronic weight management. Given that agonism of the 5-HT2B receptor by fenfluramine and dexfenfluramine resulted in cardiac valvulopathy (leading to their removal from the market in 1997), lorcaserin was developed with 5-HT2C as a target because the serotonin 2C receptor is only located in the brain. In the preapproval trial of lorcaserin, patients were monitored with echocardiography at the screening visit and at weeks 24, 52, 76, and 104. Among 2472 patients evaluated at 1 year and 1127 patients evaluated at 2 years, the rate of cardiac valvulopathy was not increased with the use of lorcaserin.[12] Subsequently, in CAMELLIA TIMI-61, a postmarketing cardiovascular safety trial that enrolled 12,000 patients, the primary endpoint of noninferiority compared with placebo for major cardiovascular was met.[13] In that trial at 1 year, weight loss of at least 5% occurred in 1986 of 5135 patients (38.7%) in the lorcaserin group and in 883 of 5083 patients (17.4%) in the placebo group (odds ratio, 3.01; 95% confidence interval, 2.74-3.30; $P<.001$). Average weight loss is typically around 4%. Lorcaserin decreases the risk of incident diabetes by 19% in patients with prediabetes and by 23% in patients without diabetes.[14] The medication is available as 10 mg taken twice daily or 20 mg extended-release taken once daily. Adverse effects may include headache, nausea, dry mouth, fatigue, constipation, and dizziness.

Phentermine/Topiramate ER

Topiramate has had FDA approval for seizures since 1996 and for migraine prevention since 2004. When used in combination with phentermine, weight loss is greater than with either medication alone.

In February 2020, the medication lorcaserin was voluntarily removed from the US market.

Table 2. Medications Associated With Weight Gain and Weight Loss

Weight Gain	Weight Loss
tolbutamide (+2.8 kg)	zonisamide (−7.7 kg)
pioglitazone (+2.6 kg)	topiramate (−3.8 kg)
glyburide (+2.6 kg),	pramlintide (−2.3 kg)
olanzapine (+2.4 kg)	liraglutide (−1.7 kg)
glipizide (+2.2 kg)	bupropion (−1.3 kg)
gabapentin (+2.2 kg)	fluoxetine (−1.3 kg)
glimepiride (+2.1 kg)	exenatide (−1.2 kg)
amitriptyline (+1.8 kg)	metformin (−1.1 kg)
gliclazide (+1.8 kg)	miglitol (−0.7 kg)
mirtazapine (+1.5 kg)	acarbose (−0.4 kg)
quetiapine (+1.1 kg)	
risperidone (+0.8 kg)	
sitagliptin (+0.55 kg)	
nateglinide (+0.3 kg)	

Adapted from: Domecq JP, et al. Clinical review: drugs commonly associated with weight change: a systematic review and meta-analysis. *J Clin Endocrinol Metab*. 2015;100(2):363-370.[9]

In the CONQUER trial, a 56-week phase 3 trial, 2487 adults who were overweight or obese (age 18-70 years, BMI 27-45 kg/m^2) and had 2 or more comorbidities (hypertension, dyslipidemia, diabetes or prediabetes, or abdominal obesity) were randomly assigned to placebo, once-daily phentermine 7.5 mg/topiramate 46 mg, or once-daily phentermine 15 mg/topiramate 92 mg in a 2:1:2 ratio.[15] At 56 weeks, body weight change was −1.4 kg, −8.1 kg, and −10.2 kg in those respective groups. Five percent weight loss was achieved in 21% of patients on placebo, 62% of patients on phentermine 7.5 mg/topiramate 46 mg daily, and 70% of patients on phentermine 15 mg/92 mg daily. The corresponding percentages of patients achieving 10% weight loss were 7%, 37%, and 48%.

Potential adverse effects from this medication combination are increased blood pressure and heart rate, paresthesias, insomnia, agitation, acute angle glaucoma (rare), metabolic acidosis, and cognitive impairment ("brain fog"). Because topiramate may cause orofacial clefts in infants exposed in utero, a Risk Evaluation Mitigation Strategy (REMS) exists for phentermine/topiramate with the purpose of informing prescribers and female patients of the potential for this teratogenic effect, the importance of pregnancy prevention in women of reproductive age receiving this medication, and the need to discontinue the medication immediately if pregnancy occurs.

Naltrexone/Bupropion SR

Naltrexone is an opioid antagonist approved for the treatment of opioid and alcohol dependence. Bupropion is a reuptake inhibitor of dopamine and norepinephrine that is FDA approved for depression and smoking cessation. Of the available antidepressants, it is least likely to produce weight gain. In combination, these medications suppress appetite and food-related reward to produce weight loss; however, the exact mechanism is not understood.

The LIGHT trial was a randomized, multicentered, placebo-controlled noninferiority trial meant to assess the cardiovascular safety of naltrexone/bupropion; however, the trial was terminated prematurely after Orexigen disclosed favorable interim analysis findings for the drug after only 25% of expected vascular events had accrued.[16] Typical weight loss seen with this combination is in the range of 5% to 6%.

Medication adverse effects may include increased blood pressure and heart rate, nausea, vomiting, constipation, and headache. Precautions should be taken in patients with a history of suicidal thoughts and behaviors, seizures, and glaucoma.

Liraglutide, 3.0 mg

GLP-1 receptor agonists are FDA approved primarily for the treatment of type 2 diabetes; however, liraglutide, 3.0 mg, is approved for the treatment of patients with obesity in the United States and many other countries. GLP-1 receptor agonists produce weight loss by slowing gastric emptying and by increasing satiety.

The SCALE trial enrolled 3731 patients without type 2 diabetes (61.2% had prediabetes) who had either a BMI of 27 kg/m^2 with treated or untreated dyslipidemia or hypertension, or a BMI greater than 30 kg/m^2, and randomly assigned them to once-daily injections of liraglutide, 3.0 mg, or placebo.[17] At 56 weeks, the mean weight loss was 8.4 ± 7.3 kg with liraglutide vs 2.8 ± 6.5 kg with placebo (−5.6 kg difference; confidence interval −6.0 to −5.1; $P<.001$). In total, 63.2% lost 5% of body weight and 33.1% lost 10% of body weight with liraglutide (vs 27.1% and 10.6%, respectively, in the placebo group).

Gastrointestinal adverse effects are common with all GLP-1 receptor agonists and risk of medication discontinuation because of this issue is higher at the 3.0 mg dosage of liraglutide than with lower dosages. Liraglutide results in dose-dependent, reversible increases in amylase and lipase. Specifically with liraglutide, 3.0 mg, 9.4% of patients had increases in amylase and 43.5% had increases in lipase that were greater than or equal to the upper normal limit. However, the rates of enzyme elevations greater than 3 times the upper normal limit were low, and routine monitoring of these enzymes is not recommended.[18] Acute pancreatitis did occur more often in the SCALE trial in patients on liraglutide, 3.0 mg, and it is possible that gallstones contributed to 50% of cases.

Comparison of the 5 Antiobesity Medications Approved for Long-Term Use

Comparative effectiveness data for the 5 medications that are FDA approved for the long-term management of obesity are limited. In a systematic review and meta-analysis of 28 randomized clinical trials of antiobesity medications that included more than 29,000 patients, 5% weight loss was achieved with a median of 23% of placebo participants vs 75% of participants taking phentermine/topiramate, 63% taking liraglutide,

---

In February 2020, the medication lorcaserin was voluntarily removed from the US market.

55% taking naltrexone/bupropion, 49% taking lorcaserin, and 44% taking orlistat.[19]

Other Medications That Produce Weight Loss

Zonisamide is another anticonvulsant medication that can produce significant weight loss, but it is not FDA approved for this indication. In a small randomized controlled trial of 60 patients given either zonisamide vs placebo over 16 weeks, zonisamide resulted in 6% weight loss when combined with a hypocaloric diet compared with 1% weight loss in the placebo group.[20]

Setmelanotide is an investigational selective agonist of the MC4R receptor that has shown promising results in small, highly selected populations of patients with rare genetic obesity disorders. In 2 patients with proopiomelanocortin (POMC) (a disease characterized by extreme early-onset obesity, hyperphagia, hypopigmentation, and hypocortisolism), setmelanotide resulted in 51.0-kg weight loss after 42 weeks in one patient and 20.5-kg weight loss after 12 weeks in a second patient.[21] This peptide is currently being studied in patients with Bardet-Biedl syndrome, Alström syndrome, and leptin receptor deficiency, and it has received orphan drug approval for the treatment of Prader-Willi syndrome.

Few studies have evaluated the combination of antiobesity medications with diabetes medications. In one small randomized, double-blinded phase 2a trial, canagliflozin plus phentermine resulted in statistically superior weight loss compared with placebo (mean difference –6.9%) and was generally well tolerated.[22]

Clinical Case Vignettes

Case 1

A 54-year-old woman with hyperlipidemia, hypertension, prediabetes, and obesity seeks help for weight loss. She is taking atorvastatin and amlodipine. She went through menopause at age 51 years. Her BMI is 33 kg/m². Her blood pressure is 128/76 mm Hg. She has tried calorie-counting programs, meal replacement shakes, and several other diets, but has always had weight regain after some temporary weight-loss success. She has recently re-enrolled in an online diet program. She goes to the gym 3 times weekly and generally does strenuous cardiovascular exercise for 30 to 45 minutes at a time. She is frustrated that despite her efforts, she has been unable to lose weight. She identifies snacking as a behavior she has not been able to break, as she often feels hungry. She is interested in trying an antiobesity medication and you discuss multiple options.

Which antiobesity medication, on average, would be expected to provide the best weight-loss results if trialed in combination with continued lifestyle modification in this patient?

A. Naltrexone/bupropion SR

B. Lorcaserin

C. Phentermine/topiramate ER

D. Liraglutide, 3.0 mg

E. Orlistat

Answer: C) Phentermine/topiramate ER

Phentermine/topiramate ER (Answer C) on average produces the most weight loss compared with the other antiobesity medication options listed. It is a reasonable option in this patient, and her postmenopausal status means that monthly monitoring for pregnancy, which is required through a REMS program for women of reproductive age, would not be needed. Although less expensive than most of the other options, phentermine/topiramate ER is still expensive; therefore, generic phentermine could also be offered.

Case 2

A 47-year-old man with a history of obesity (BMI = 39 kg/m²), uncontrolled hypertension (blood pressure = 165/94 mm Hg today), kidney stones,

---

In February 2020, the medication lorcaserin was voluntarily removed from the US market.

and bipolar disorder presents to discuss weight management. He experienced a 50-lb (22.7-kg) weight gain 5 years ago during an episode of major depression that resulted in an inpatient psychiatry admission after a suicide attempt and treatment with olanzapine. Since then he has been on a selective serotonin reuptake inhibitor with good control of his depression. However, he has struggled to lose weight despite his best efforts. He has never been on an antiobesity medication, but he is very interested in trialing one.

Which of the following antiobesity medications would be best to recommend for this patient?

A. Naltrexone/bupropion SR

B. Lorcaserin

C. Phentermine/topiramate ER

D. Liraglutide, 3.0 mg

E. Orlistat

Answer: E) Orlistat

Orlistat (Answer E) is the best option for this patient. Phentermine/topiramate ER (Answer C) should be avoided in this patient because of his uncontrolled hypertension and kidney stone history. In studies involving various anticonvulsants, an increased risk of suicidal thoughts and behavior has been observed; therefore, it is recommended that use of phentermine/topiramate be avoided in such patients. In a pooled analysis of the SCALE trial of liraglutide, 3.0 mg (Answer D), no neuropsychiatric safety concerns arose; however, this was an idealized trial population and caution should still be taken to monitor for worsening depression and suicidal ideation, especially in patients with a history of psychiatric disease.[23] Furthermore, the cost could be prohibitive. Lorcaserin (Answer B) when used in combination

with a selective serotonin reuptake inhibitor has the potential to produce serotonin syndrome, and patients on lorcaserin in general should be monitored for mood changes. Naltrexone/bupropion SR (Answer A) should be avoided given concurrent use of a selective serotonin reuptake inhibitor and can raise blood pressure. Phentermine should also not be considered at this time in light of the uncontrolled hypertension.

Case 3

A 56-year-old woman with obesity (BMI = 32 kg/m^2) presents to discuss antiobesity medication treatment options. She has a medical history of type 2 diabetes, glaucoma, irritable bowel syndrome, a distant episode of pancreatitis due to hypertriglyceridemia, and seizures. Her blood pressure has always been controlled. She has tried several behavioral lifestyle modification programs and exercises 5 days per week for 40 minutes each session, but she has struggled to lose weight and maintain any weight loss she achieves.

Which of the following is the best long-term antiobesity medication choice for her?

A. Naltrexone/bupropion SR

B. Lorcaserin

C. Phentermine/topiramate ER

D. Liraglutide, 3.0 mg

E. Orlistat

Answer: B) Lorcaserin

Lorcaserin (Answer B) is the safest and best long-term medication for this patient with a history of type 2 diabetes, glaucoma, pancreatitis, and seizures because her comorbidities are contraindications for the other listed options. Naltrexone/bupropion (Answer A) should not be used in patients with a history of seizures. Phentermine/topiramate ER (Answer C) is

---

In February 2020, the medication lorcaserin was voluntarily removed from the US market.

contraindicated in patients with glaucoma. Liraglutide, 3.0 mg (Answer B), is for use in patients with a history of obesity without diabetes and her pancreatitis history should give pause to clinicians about use of a GLP-1 receptor agonist.

Orlistat (Answer E) should not be used in patients with irritable bowel syndrome. While not approved for long-term use, generic phentermine could also be considered and offered.

References

1. Hales CM, Carroll MD, Fryar CD, Ogden CL. Prevalence of obesity among adults and youth: United States, 2015-2016. *NCHS Data Brief*. 2017;(288):1-8. PMID: 29155689

2. Finucane MM, Stevens GA, Cowan MJ, et al; Global Burden of Metabolic Risk Factors of Chronic Diseases Collaborating Group (Body Mass Index). National, regional, and global trends in body-mass index since 1980: systematic analysis of health examination surveys and epidemiological studies with 960 country-years and 9·1 million participants. *Lancet*. 2011;377(9765):557-567. PMID: 21295846

3. Wang YC, McPherson K, Marsh T, Gortmaker SL, Brown M. Health and economic burden of the projected obesity trends in the USA and the UK [*Lancet*. 2011;378(9805):1778]. *Lancet*. 2011;378(9793):815-825. PMID: 21872750

4. Jia H, Lubetkin EI. Obesity-related quality-adjusted life years lost in the U.S. from 1993 to 2008. *Am J Prev Med*. 2010;39(3):220-227. PMID: 20709253

5. Preston SH, Vierboom YC, Stokes A. The role of obesity in exceptionally slow US mortality improvement. *Proc Natl Acad Sci U S A*. 2018;115(5):957-961. PMID: 29339511

6. Saxon DR, Iwamoto SJ, Mettenbrink CJ, et al. Antiobesity medication use in 2.2 million adults across eight large health care organizations: 2009-2015. *Obesity (Silver Spring)*. 2019;27(12):1975-1981. PMID: 31603630

7. Iwamoto S, Saxon D, Tsai A, et al. Effects of education and experience on primary care providers' perspectives of obesity treatments during a pragmatic trial. *Obesity (Silver Spring)*. 2018;26(10):1532-1538. PMID: 30257072

8. Apovian CM, Aronne LJ, Bessesen DH, et al; Endocrine Society. Pharmacological management of obesity: an Endocrine Society clinical practice guideline. *J Clin Endocrinol Metab*. 2015;100(2):342-362. PMID: 25590212

9. Domecq JP, Prutsky G, Leppin A, et al. Clinical review: drugs commonly associated with weight change: a systematic review and meta-analysis. *J Clin Endocrinol Metab*. 2015;100(2):363-370. PMID: 25590213

10. Lewis KH, Fischer H, Ard J, et al. Safety and effectiveness of longer-term phentermine use: clinical outcomes from an electronic health record cohort. *Obesity (Silver Spring)*. 2019;27(4):591-602. PMID: 30900410

11. Torgerson JS, Hauptman J, Boldrin MN, Sjöström L. XENical in the prevention of diabetes in obese subjects (XENDOS) study: a randomized study of orlistat as an adjunct to lifestyle changes for the prevention of type 2 diabetes in obese patients [published correction appears in Diabetes Care. 2004;27(3):856]. *Diabetes Care*. 2004;27(1):155-161. PMID: 14693982

12. Smith SR, Weissman NJ, Anderson CM, et al. Multicenter, placebo-controlled trial of lorcaserin for weight management. *N Engl J Med*. 2010;363(3):245-256. PMID: 20647200

13. Bohula EA, Wiviott SD, McGuire DK, et al; CAMELLIA-TIMI 61 Steering Committee and Investigators. Cardiovascular safety of lorcaserin in overweight or obese patients. *N Engl J Med*. 2018;379(12):1107-1117. PMID: 30145941

14. Bohula EA, Scirica BM, Inzucchi SE, et al; CAMELLIA-TIMI 61 Steering Committee Investigators. Effect of lorcaserin on prevention and remission of type 2 diabetes in overweight and obese patients (CAMELLIA-TIMI 61): a randomised, placebo-controlled trial. *Lancet*. 2018;392(10161):2269-2279. PMID: 30293771

15. Gadde KM, Allison DB, Ryan DH, et al. Effects of low-dose, controlled-release, phentermine plus topiramate combination on weight and associated comorbidities in overweight and obese adults (CONQUER): a randomised, placebo-controlled, phase 3 trial [published correction appears in *Lancet*. 2011;377(9776):1494]. *Lancet*. 2011;377(9774):1341-1352. PMID: 21481449

16. Nissen SE, Wolski KE, Prcela L, et al. Effect of naltrexone-bupropion on major adverse cardiovascular events in overweight and obese patients with cardiovascular risk factors: a randomized clinical trial. *JAMA*. 2016;315(10):990-1004. PMID: 26954408

17. Pi-Sunyer X, Astrup A, Fujioka K, et al; SCALE Obesity and Prediabetes NN8022-1839 Study Group. A randomized, controlled trial of 3.0 mg of liraglutide in weight management. *N Engl J Med*. 2015;373(1):11-22. PMID: 26132939

18. Steinberg WM, Rosenstock J, Wadden TA, Donsmark M, Jensen CB, DeVries JH. Impact of liraglutide on amylase, lipase, and acute pancreatitis in participants with overweight/obesity and normoglycemia, prediabetes, or type 2 diabetes: secondary analyses of pooled data from the SCALE Clinical Development Program. *Diabetes Care*. 2017;40(7):839-848. PMID: 28473337

19. Khera R, Murad MH, Chandar AK, et al. Association of pharmacological treatments for obesity with weight loss and adverse events: a systematic review and meta-analysis. *JAMA*. 2016;315(22):2424-2434. PMID: 27299618

20. Gadde KM, Franciscy DM, Wagner HR 2nd, Krishnan KR. Zonisamide for weight loss in obese adults: a randomized controlled trial. *JAMA*. 2003;289(14):1820-1825. PMID: 12684361

21. Kühnen P, Clément K, Wiegand S, et al. Proopiomelanocortin deficiency treated with a melanocortin-4 receptor agonist. *N Engl J Med*. 2016;375(3):240-246. PMID: 27468060

22. Hollander P, Bays HE, Rosenstock J, et al. Coadministration of canagliflozin and phentermine for weight management in overweight and obese individuals without diabetes: a randomized clinical trial. *Diabetes Care*. 2017;40(5):632-639. PMID: 28289041

23. O'Neil PM, Aroda VR, Astrup A, et al; Satiety and Clinical Adiposity - Liraglutide Evidence in individuals with and without diabetes (SCALE) study groups. Neuropsychiatric safety with liraglutide 3.0 mg for weight management: results from randomized controlled phase 2 and 3a trials. *Diabetes Obes Metab*. 2017;19(11):1529-1536. PMID: 28386912

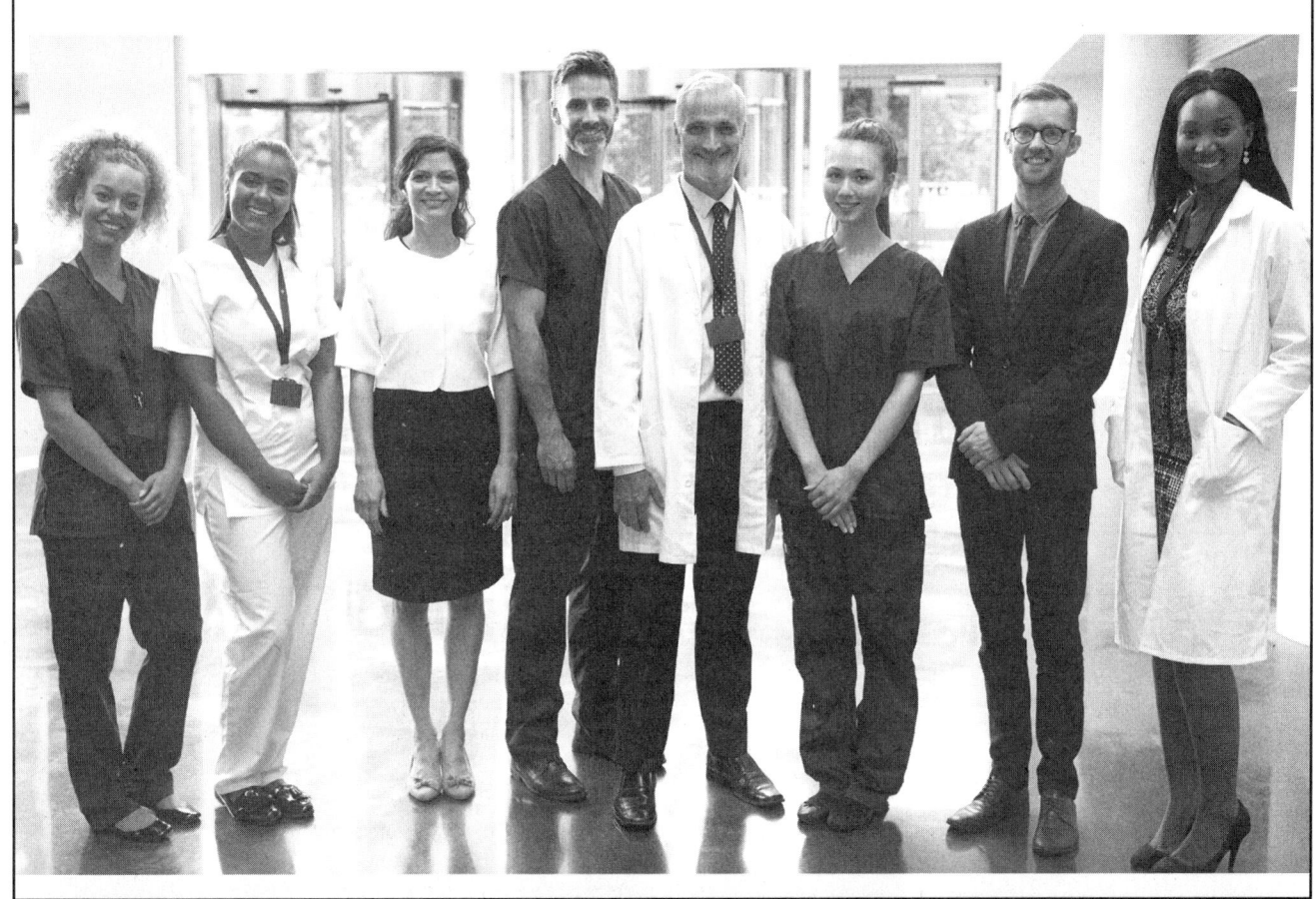

ADRENAL

Selection, Dosing, and Monitoring of Steroid Replacement in the Patient With Adrenal Failure

Irina Bancos, MD. Division of Endocrinology, Metabolism, and Nutrition, Mayo Clinic, Rochester, MN; E-mail: bancos.irina@mayo.edu

Richard Auchus, MD, PhD. Division of Metabolism, Endocrinology, and Diabetes, University of Michigan, Ann Arbor, MI; E-mail: rauchus@med.umich.edu

Learning Objectives

As a result of participating in this session, learners should be able to:

- Illustrate the optimal approach to glucocorticoid, mineralocorticoid, and androgen replacement therapy and monitoring through a case-based approach.

- Review types of glucocorticoid replacement therapies based on potency, pharmacokinetics, delivery, and impact on clinical and biochemical outcomes.

Main Conclusions

Management of adrenal insufficiency includes glucocorticoid replacement therapy (for all types of adrenal insufficiency) and mineralocorticoid replacement (for primary adrenal insufficiency only). Androgen replacement therapy could be considered in women with adrenal insufficiency. Replacement therapy may need to be adjusted in special situations such as shift work, pregnancy, insulin-dependent diabetes mellitus, prolonged intense exercise, and end-stage renal disease. Glucocorticoid potency and circadian delivery need to be considered when deciding on the glucocorticoid type, dose, and frequency of administration. Both clinical and biochemical parameters are helpful in monitoring of optimal replacement therapy.

Significance of the Clinical Problem

Adrenal insufficiency is an endocrine disorder characterized by lack of cortisol.[1] Primary adrenal insufficiency occurs when the adrenal cortex is destroyed by an autoimmune attack (Addison disease) or infiltrative disease (tuberculosis, bilateral fungal infection, or bilateral metastases).[2] Secondary adrenal insufficiency occurs in pituitary dysfunction leading to insufficient production of corticotropin, such as in pituitary macroadenomas, hypophysitis, Sheehan syndrome, or use of certain medications (glucocorticoids and opioids).[3] Prompt recognition, diagnosis, and management of adrenal insufficiency are key to avoid poor quality of life, adrenal crisis, and even death.[4,5]

Optimal management of adrenal insufficiency includes education on glucocorticoid and mineralocorticoid therapy, sick day rules, and instruction in injection and situations requiring an injectable steroid. Selecting a regimen that works with a patient's lifestyle is important to ensure adherence and optimal quality of life.[1]

Barriers to Optimal Practice

- Poor specificity of symptoms and signs of adrenal insufficiency.
- Lack of biomarkers to monitor glucocorticoid replacement therapy.
- Poor access to certain therapies for adrenal insufficiency.

Strategies for Diagnosis, Therapy, and/or Management

Glucocorticoid Replacement Therapy

The goal of glucocorticoid replacement therapy is providing physiological replacement therapy that mimics circadian rhythm as closely as possible. Choice of glucocorticoid therapy, including type and frequency of administration, must be balanced against individual preferences and circumstances.

Currently available glucocorticoid preparations demonstrate different glucocorticoid potencies and half-lives that affect both dosing and frequency of administration (*Table 1*).

Hydrocortisone is the most commonly used glucocorticoid, with a starting dosage of 15 to 25 mg daily in divided (2 to 3) doses. Prednisone and prednisolone are used less frequently at 4 to 6 mg daily, each morning. Dexamethasone should not be used in the treatment of adrenal insufficiency for several reasons. It has a long half-life, which does not allow for diurnal replacement. Given dexamethasone's high potency, even the smallest dose tablet currently available is excessive for most patients, providing little opportunity for dose adjustment and high likelihood of overtreatment with development of iatrogenic Cushing syndrome.

Monitoring of glucocorticoid replacement therapy includes history and physical examination (*Table 2*). Manifestations of cortisol excess include weight gain, fatigue, and development of features consistent with iatrogenic Cushing syndrome. Patients on insufficient glucocorticoid replacement therapy may complain of fatigue, anorexia or nausea, and weight loss (*Table 2*).

Androgen replacement therapy has been described in women with either primary or secondary adrenal insufficiency with a starting dehydroepiandrosterone (DHEA) dosage of 25 mg daily. The goal of therapy is improved libido, mood, and energy, as well as DHEA-S concentrations in mid-normal range (*Table 2*).[6] Several approaches to initiation of DHEA may be considered. One approach is to consider initiation of DHEA only in women experiencing low libido and sexual dissatisfaction (symptoms most likely to improve with DHEA). Another approach is to discuss DHEA with every woman who has adrenal insufficiency after stabilization of glucocorticoid and mineralocorticoid therapy. Emphasis must be placed on review of current evidence, which describes small but statistically significant improvement in quality of life, fatigue, mood, and libido in women treated with DHEA, as well as highlights that younger women may experience a more substantial benefit than postmenopausal women.[6]

Mineralocorticoid replacement therapy consists of fludrocortisone, 100 mcg daily (usually

Table 1. Glucocorticoid Type and Potency[1]

Drug	Hydrocortisone Equivalent	Number of Doses per Day	Total Daily Dose
Hydrocortisone = cortisol	1	2 to 3	15 to 25 mg
Cortisone acetate = cortisone	1.6	2	30 to 40 mg
Prednisolone, methylprednisolone	0.2	1	5 mg
Prednisone	0.25	1	5 mg

Table 2. Monitoring Steroid Replacement Therapy

Replacement Therapy	Usual Starting Dosage	Clinical Monitoring	Laboratory Monitoring	Manifestations of Excessive Therapy	Manifestations of Suboptimal Therapy
Glucocorticoid replacement therapy	Hydrocortisone, 15 to 25 mg daily, in divided doses (2 to 3)	Clinical exam: weight, energy level, sleep quality History: use of stress dose steroids, hospital admissions, circumstances around adrenal crises	No bloodwork is needed for monitoring of therapy, but can measure post-dose cortisol to confirm exposure	Weakness Weight gain Metabolic abnormalities Decrease in bone density	Fatigue Weight loss Nausea Hyperpigmentation Adrenal crisis
Mineralocorticoid replacement therapy	Fludrocortisone, 100 mcg daily	Clinical exam: blood pressure, orthostatic vitals, lower extremities (for edema)	Potassium, sodium, renin, or renin plasma activity	Hypertension Lower-extremity edema Hypokalemia Low renin/renin plasma activity	Hypotension Dizziness Salt craving Hyperkalemia Elevated renin/renin plasma activity
Androgen replacement therapy (women)	DHEA, 25 mg daily	Clinical exam: hirsutism, acne, other signs of androgen excess	DHEA-S and testosterone concentrations in the morning, before taking DHEA supplement	Signs of androgen excess Elevated DHEA-S	Low DHEA-S Nonspecific: no symptoms vs fatigue, low sex drive

50-300 mcg daily), and is required in 95% of patients with primary adrenal insufficiency. The goal of therapy is to achieve absence of orthostatic hypotension and normal electrolytes and renin plasma activity. Monitoring includes assessment of orthostatic vitals during each visit, electrolytes, and renin plasma activity at least yearly or 3 months after each dosage adjustment (*Table 2*). In a patient with hypertension and optimal mineralocorticoid replacement therapy, effective antihypertensive agents include calcium-channel blockers and α-adrenergic blockers (*Table 3*).

Glucocorticoid and mineralocorticoid therapy should be adjusted in certain circumstances. For example, in shift workers, the larger dose of glucocorticoid should be taken on waking, and the second dose 6 to 8 hours later. In pregnancy, given that physiologically cortisol production increases, consider increasing the hydrocortisone dosage by about 20% in each trimester (*Table 3*). The decision to increase the dosage should be made depending on the starting baseline dosage and the clinical evaluation. Other special situations are listed in Table 3.

Adrenal crisis usually occurs during a viral illness, such as gastroenteritis or an upper respiratory infection.[4] However, nonadherence, improper glucocorticoid management in the perioperative period, and severe psychological crisis have also been reported to lead to adrenal crisis.[4] As such, comprehensive education, instruction on injection, and provision of proper supplies are important interventions for adrenal crisis prevention (*Table 4*).

Clinical Case Vignettes
Case 1

A 31-year-old woman with a history of primary autoimmune adrenal insufficiency diagnosed at age 22 years presents for follow-up. She shares that she is 8 weeks pregnant. Her medical history includes vitiligo and autoimmune primary hypothyroidism. She has no concerns and no new symptoms. Her medical therapy consists of hydrocortisone, 15 mg on waking, and 5 mg at noon; fludrocortisone, 100 mcg daily; levothyroxine, 112 mcg daily; and a multivitamin. Over the last 12 months, she had to increase the hydrocortisone dosage for several days during an upper respiratory illness. She is comfortable self-administering her injectable glucocorticoid and has sufficient supplies. Laboratory workup reveals normal electrolytes, normal thyroid function, and renin plasma activity at goal.

Table 3. Special Circumstances in Steroid Replacement Therapy[1]

Shift worker	Change glucocorticoid and mineralocorticoid replacement according to schedule (take the larger dose of hydrocortisone on waking, the second dose 6 to 8 hours after the first one)
Pregnancy	Glucocorticoids • 2nd → 3rd trimester: increase in cortisol-binding globulin, total cortisol, and free cortisol • Consider an increase in hydrocortisone dosage (20%-40% of total daily dose) Mineralocorticoids • Consider change in mineralocorticoid dosage in the last trimester, as progesterone is anti-mineralocorticoid • Monitor with sodium and potassium (plasma renin is physiologically increased in pregnancy and thus not useful)
Prolonged intense exercise	Small carbohydrate meal before exercising Additional salt requirement to replace sweat losses, consider small dose increases in glucocorticoid and mineralocorticoids when undertaking extraordinarily strenuous exercise (eg, consider 2.5 to 5 mg hydrocortisone every 3 hours during a marathon run or triathlon)
Hot environment	Additional salt requirement to replace sweat losses Consider increasing fludrocortisone by 50 to 100 mcg daily to compensate for salt and water loss
Travel	No routine increase, but be prepared for stress dosing and emergency
Insulin-dependent diabetes mellitus	Consider longer-acting glucocorticoids (eg, prednisolone) to avoid cortisol-driven peaks and troughs in blood glucose
Dialysis	Stop fludrocortisone (no longer needed) Plan glucocorticoid replacement (substantial amounts of the morning glucocorticoid dose might be lost through hemodialysis)
Hypertension	Consider decreasing fludrocortisone Add calcium-channel blockers Note: ACE inhibitors and angiotensin-receptor blockers are less effective

The patient is counseled on adrenal crisis prevention and her comfort level and knowledge are confirmed regarding self-injection.

Which of the following adjustments would also be recommended?

A. No adjustments in either hydrocortisone or fludrocortisone are needed throughout the pregnancy

B. Double the hydrocortisone dosage during third trimester, continue the same fludrocortisone dosage

C. Increase the hydrocortisone dosage to 25 mg daily in the second trimester and to 30 mg daily in the third trimester; monitor the need for fludrocortisone adjustment

D. Increase the hydrocortisone and fludrocortisone dosages by 20% now

Answer: C) Increase the hydrocortisone to 25 mg daily in the second trimester and to 30 mg daily in the third trimester. monitor the need for fludrocortisone adjustment

Cortisol production increases during pregnancy, possibly due to increased placental production of corticotropin-releasing hormone, which results in hypertrophy of the adrenal cortex and increased cortisol. To mimic this physiological increase in cortisol, the typical practice is to increase the

Table 4. Adrenal Crisis Prevention

Identification	Steroid emergency card AND/OR medical alert bracelet or necklace
Education	Sick day rule 1: double daily glucocorticoid dose in times of illness until well for 1 day Sick day rule 2: inject glucocorticoid in times of inability to take oral glucocorticoid or severe illness AND proceed to emergency care Special attention: explain reasons for dosage adjustment, discuss the situations needing adjustment, teach self-administration of injectable glucocorticoid
Supplies	Sufficient supply of glucocorticoid/mineralocorticoid Emergency injection kits/vials/syringes/needles
Follow-up	Reinforce the education during each visit

hydrocortisone dosage by 20% in second and third trimesters (Answer C).[7] The increased progesterone concentration during pregnancy has an antimineralocorticoid effect, and thus, adjustment of fludrocortisone is occasionally needed in the third trimester.[7] There is no clinical indication to increase her hydrocortisone dosage at this time in early pregnancy (Answer D). Making no adjustments (Answer A) is unlikely to be correct and is premature to conclude. Doubling the hydrocortisone dosage in the third trimester (Answer B) is an excessive increase.

Case 2

A 23-year-old woman with a history of primary autoimmune adrenal insufficiency diagnosed 2 years ago presents for evaluation of insomnia, afternoon fatigue, and decreased libido. She has no other symptoms or signs of glucocorticoid or mineralocorticoid underreplacement or overreplacement. Her menstrual cycle is normal. Her weight is stable, and she has no orthostasis. She is currently taking hydrocortisone, 15 mg on waking and 5 mg at bedtime. She takes fludrocortisone, 50 mcg each morning. On physical examination, she has normal sitting and standing blood pressure. Her laboratory workup demonstrates normal electrolytes, renin plasma activity, and TSH. There is no evidence of pernicious anemia or celiac disease.

Which of the following changes in therapy should be considered?

A. No adjustments in current therapy are needed; refer the patient to the sleep medicine team for further evaluation

B. Add another 5 mg of hydrocortisone at noon and reevaluate in 3 months

C. Trial of DHEA supplementation

D. Move the bedtime hydrocortisone dose to the early afternoon

E. Both C and D

Answer: E) Trial of DHEA supplementation AND move the bedtime hydrocortisone dose to the early afternoon

This patient could benefit from a change in glucocorticoid replacement therapy to mimic circadian rhythm. Adding another 5 mg of hydrocortisone at noon (Answer B) may improve her afternoon fatigue, but it would not help her insomnia and would increase her total glucocorticoid replacement leading to potential signs and symptoms of cortisol excess. Moving the bedtime hydrocortisone dose to the early afternoon (Answer D) is most likely to both improve insomnia and help with afternoon fatigue.

DHEA replacement therapy (Answer C) in women with adrenal insufficiency (especially younger women)[1,6] has been reported to potentially help with libido and could be tried for at least 6 months (usual dosage of 25 mg daily, with a goal of mid-normal DHEA-S concentrations).

Referring the patient to sleep medicine (Answer A) would be premature until the timing of the bedtime hydrocortisone dose, which is the likely cause, is moved earlier.

Case 3

A 40-year-old man is status post bilateral adrenalectomy for incurable pituitary Cushing disease of 5 years' duration following 2 unsuccessful transsphenoidal surgeries. He also received pituitary radiation and is now panhypopituitary. He takes levothyroxine, testosterone, and growth hormone in addition to hydrocortisone, 15 mg on rising plus 5 mg after lunch, and fludrocortisone, 200 mcg at bedtime. His physical examination findings and laboratory data confirm adequate adrenal replacement, but he has concerns of chronic fatigue and mental clouding. He heard on an Internet chat group that he should try subcutaneous hydrocortisone delivered by insulin infusion pump, and he would like a prescription for this treatment.

Which of the following should be conveyed to this patient regarding this treatment?

A. Subcutaneous hydrocortisone is superior to oral hydrocortisone for quality of life

B. Hydrocortisone sodium succinate is not FDA approved for subcutaneous infusion

C. Cortisol exposure from subcutaneous hydrocortisone infusion is milligram-for-milligram identical to oral hydrocortisone

D. The data regarding patient satisfaction with subcutaneous hydrocortisone are mixed

E. Both B and D

Answer: E) Hydrocortisone sodium succinate is not FDA approved for subcutaneous infusion AND the data regarding patient satisfaction with subcutaneous hydrocortisone are mixed

Limited data on continuous subcutaneous hydrocortisone in patients with adrenal insufficiency showed some improvement in the vitality domain on quality-of-life scores, but not sleep in one study.[8] No differences were observed in another small study (thus, Answer A is incorrect).[9] Problems related to pump gear can occur.[8] Overall patient satisfaction with subcutaneous hydrocortisone was mixed (Answer D) in a study of 10 patients when 5 preferred subcutaneous hydrocortisone, 4 preferred oral hydrocortisone, and 1 was uncertain.[9] Hydrocortisone is not FDA approved for subcutaneous infusion (Answer B), and evidence on long-term improvement in quality of life in patients with adrenal insufficiency is scarce. The bioavailability of hydrocortisone is usually high but incomplete and more prone to first-pass metabolism via CYP3A4 and drug-drug interactions than parenteral administration (thus, Answer C is incorrect).

References

1. Bancos I, Hahner S, Tomlinson J, Arlt W. Diagnosis and management of adrenal insufficiency. *Lancet Diabetes Endocrinol.* 2015;3(3):216-226. PMID: 25098712

2. Herndon J, Nadeau AM, Davidge-Pitts CJ, Young WF, Bancos I. Primary adrenal insufficiency due to bilateral infiltrative disease. *Endocrine.* 2018;62(3):721-728. PMID: 30178435

3. Donegan D, Bancos I. Opioid-induced adrenal insufficiency. *Mayo Clin Proc.* 2018;93(7):937-944. PMID: 29976376

4. Hahner S, Loeffler M, Bleicken B, et al. Epidemiology of adrenal crisis in chronic adrenal insufficiency: the need for new prevention strategies. *Eur J Endocrinol.* 2010;162(3):597-602. PMID: 19955259

5. Hahner S, Spinnler C, Fassnacht M, et al. High incidence of adrenal crisis in educated patients with chronic adrenal insufficiency: a prospective study. *J Clin Endocrinol Metab.* 2015;100(2):407-416. PMID: 25419882

6. Alkatib AA, Cosma M, Elamin MB, et al. A systematic review and meta-analysis of randomized placebo-controlled trials of DHEA treatment effects on quality of life in women with adrenal insufficiency. *J Clin Endocrinol Metab.* 2009;94(10):3676-3681. PMID: 19773400

7. Lebbe M, Arlt W. What is the best diagnostic and therapeutic management strategy for an Addison patient during pregnancy? *Clin Endocrinol (Oxf).* 2013;78(4):497-502. PMID: 23153216

8. Oksnes M, Bjornsdottir S, Isaksson M, et al. Continuous subcutaneous hydrocortisone infusion versus oral hydrocortisone replacement for treatment of addison's disease: a randomized clinical trial. *J Clin Endocrinol Metab.* 2014;99(5):1665-1674. PMID: 24517155

9. Gagliardi L, Nenke MA, Thynne TR, et al. Continuous subcutaneous hydrocortisone infusion therapy in Addison's disease: a randomized, placebo-controlled clinical trial. *J Clin Endocrinol Metab.* 2014;99(11):4149-4157. PMID: 25127090

Complexities in the Diagnosis and Treatment of Cushing Syndrome

Ashley B. Grossman, BA BSc, MD, FRCP, FMedSci. Oxford Centre for Diabetes, Endocrinology and Metabolism, Churchill Hospital, University of Oxford; Centre for Endocrinology, Barts and the London School of Medicine, University of London, United Kingdom; E-mail: Ashley.grossman@ocdem.ox.ac.uk

Learning Objectives

As a result of participating in this session, learners should be able to:

- Describe the problems and complexities in diagnosing Cushing syndrome and in localizing its source.

- Explain the various therapeutic approaches to the treatment of Cushing syndrome, including surgery, radiotherapy, and medical therapy, and describe their advantages, disadvantages, and sequential use when required.

Main Conclusions

Cushing syndrome is a rare but important condition that can be problematic in both diagnosis and successful management. The original diagnostic tests were devised for the most obvious cases, but the endocrinologist is increasingly faced with patients who have mild disease, which is difficult to distinguish from a variety of common clinical conditions. The optimal approach is to (1) use a series of biochemical tests, ranging from those with high sensitivity to those with increasing specificity, (2) determine whether the disorder is ACTH-dependent, and (3) when appropriate, locate the source of ACTH. Imaging is part of this paradigm, but biochemical assessment is paramount. Finally, in severe cases, the metabolic abnormalities should be dealt with as a matter of urgency. If necessary, serum cortisol levels should be lowered to normal safe concentrations. The most appropriate long-term management is surgery. It cannot be overemphasized that the management of these patients requires experience and expertise of a dedicated clinical team, and the investigation and management often benefit from the input of a center of excellence.

Significance of the Clinical Problem

Cushing syndrome is a rare condition, once exogenous sources of Cushing syndrome have been excluded. However, it is almost always eminently treatable, as long as certain basic rules and considerations are accepted in both making the diagnosis and identifying the source of the problem. It is vital to assess any test procedures in the light of a clinical suspicion of Cushing syndrome, and then to proceed in that direction. The diagnosis is based on the demonstration of an autonomous source of excess cortisol production, most apparent and demonstrable by loss of the normal circadian rhythmicity and failure to show adequate feedback regulation. Thus, the usual investigative techniques are based on the recognition of an increase in the 24-hour production of cortisol (urinary free cortisol), a failure to show a fall in cortisol after the corticosteroid dexamethasone is administered (dexamethasone-suppression test), and an absence of the usual decease in hypothalamic-pituitary-adrenal axis activity at night (midnight cortisol measurement, late-night salivary cortisol). Unfortunately, all of the investigatory techniques have pitfalls and require careful interpretation.

Once the diagnosis of Cushing syndrome is established, effective treatment depends on demonstration of the source. Around 80% of cases are ACTH-dependent, which effectively means either a pituitary corticotroph tumor (Cushing disease) or an ectopic source. Contrary to earlier publications, such ectopic sources may not be grossly obvious. The classic ectopic ACTH syndrome due to small cell lung carcinoma, presenting in an older patient with severe metabolic defects and an obvious malignancy, is now being increasingly replaced in practice by small bronchial, thymic, pancreatic, or other carcinoids, best referred to as neuroendocrine tumors, occurring at almost any age. In the presence of low or undetectable ACTH levels, an adrenal source should be sought, usually an adrenal adenoma or carcinoma, although there are the very rare patients with bilateral adrenal hyperplasia (sometimes part of Carney complex) or bilateral macronodular hyperplasia.

Barriers to Optimal Practice

- Many urinary free cortisol assays are based on plasma assays and lack sufficient sensitivity for mild cases of Cushing syndrome.

- Dexamethasone-suppression tests are varied in application, and dose regimens depend on the effective absorption and metabolism of dexamethasone.

- Loss of circadian rhythmicity of serum cortisol requires an in-patient admission.

- MRI may fail to detect a corticotroph tumor even with optimal imaging protocols; especially in older patients, incidental pituitary lesions may be mistaken for a corticotroph tumor.

- Late-night salivary cortisol necessitates a well-validated salivary cortisol assay with extensive normal ranges.

- Low levels of plasma ACTH with adrenal autonomy may overlap with mild cases of Cushing disease.

Strategies for Diagnosis, Therapy, and/or Management

While the classic clinical presentation of Cushing syndrome is usually beyond doubt, the endocrinologist is increasingly faced with mild cases where patients may present with obesity, depression, hypertension, or diabetes, problems widespread in the general population. Various attempts have been made to screen at-risk populations, but it has generally been concluded that the rarity of Cushing syndrome precludes any special screening program, at least in most situations. However, it should be emphasized that in Cushing syndrome the catabolic changes are most useful in the differential diagnosis; these include thinning of the skin with associated easy bruising, myopathy, osteoporosis, and, in children, short stature and/or a fall in growth velocity. Thus, the clinician will see many patients with a Cushing-like presentation, and some may have mildly abnormal biochemistry, so-called pseudo-Cushing states, including patients with anorexia, depression, and obstructive sleep apnea (although this term of pseudo-Cushing is not generally recommended). Every type of investigation will have a significant false-positive and false-negative rate. The approach and one's interpretation of test results depend on the *a priori* likelihood of the diagnosis.

It is therefore essential to investigate the diagnosis in stages, beginning with a test that is simple to use and has very high sensitivity.[1] Then, if this test indicates possible Cushing syndrome, more specific tests can be used. Many clinicians start with the overnight dexamethasone-suppression test, administering 1 mg of dexamethasone orally at midnight followed by a 9-AM serum cortisol measurement. A cortisol concentration less than 1.8 µg/dL (<50 nmol/L) has a greater than 95% sensitivity and approximately 80% specificity. With all dexamethasone-suppression tests, it is important to be aware that false-positive results may occur with any form of poor absorption or the presence of drugs that increase dexamethasone catabolism, such as rifampicin or phenytoin.

With a clinical suspicion and some biochemical evidence in favor of hypercortisolism, many clinicians move on to an extended low-dose 48-hour dexamethasone-suppression test, using dexamethasone, 0.5 mg given strictly at 6-hour intervals for 48 hours. A 48-hour serum cortisol concentration less than 1.8 µg/dL (<50 nmol/L) excludes Cushing syndrome, with approximately 95% probability and very high specificity. Alternative tests include measurement of 24-hour urinary free cortisol and late-night salivary cortisol.

Urinary free cortisol has classically been the screening test most used, but it has many drawbacks.[2] The collection is complex and sometimes difficult for patients, and incomplete collections are not uncommon. Furthermore, it relies on the fact that only 5% of serum cortisol is excreted in the urine and, at least in the past, most assays were simply based on assays for serum samples, which were then applied to urine. In general, 3 to 4 completely normal urine collections can (almost) always be interpreted to exclude Cushing syndrome, while a cortisol level greater than 4 times the upper normal limit is very confirmatory of Cushing syndrome. However, it is possible, but not yet definitively shown, that when using the newer mass spectrometric assay, an elevated urinary free cortisol measurement would be more suggestive of the diagnosis, and a value more than 2 times the upper normal limit would be diagnostic. The problem remains of the very large number of patients whose values lie slightly above normal or fluctuate in and out of the normal range. The introduction of more accurate assays, especially those based on mass spectrometry, may allow for more specific and sensitive assays (with

a much lower limit of "normal"), but it is probably best to reserve urinary free cortisol measurement for those patients whose other test results are indeterminate, although it may be more useful in children.[3]

The loss of circadian rhythmicity is a critical feature of Cushing syndrome, but it can also be difficult to ascertain. For many years, a sleeping midnight cortisol measurement was used, but it required hospitalization for at least 2 days and required the patient to be asleep, at least when the sample was beginning to be drawn. Again, a concentration less than 1.8 µg/dL (<50 nmol/L) excludes Cushing syndrome, while a concentration greater than 7.5 µg/dL (>208 nmol/L) renders the diagnosis highly probable. Unfortunately, the "grey" area (1.8-7.5 µg/dL [50-208 nmol/L]) is indeterminate. There is now increasing evidence that a midnight salivary cortisol measurement can also readily differentiate Cushing syndrome from noncushingoid states, and the sample can be collected at home and then brought or mailed to the laboratory. With an appropriate assay and reliable normative values, this test approaches greater than 95% sensitivity and specificity. However, the normal ranges tend to be assay specific, and there is some evidence for lesser reliability in older patients, so experience in its use is important.

Assuming that a firm clinical and biochemical diagnosis of Cushing syndrome has been made, the next step is to identify a source: approximately 20% of patients have an adrenal source, and this can be confirmed with a 9-AM plasma ACTH measurement. It is important to collect the sample correctly, and in such a situation, a concentration less than 10 pg/mL (<2.2 pmol/L) indicates an adrenal source, a concentration greater than 30 pg/mL (>6.6 pmol/L) indicates ACTH dependence. Two to three samples should be collected to ensure the reliability of the results. If the ACTH concentration is persistently in the range of 10 to 30 pg/mL (2.2-6.6 pmol/L), then many clinicians perform a corticotropin-releasing hormone test (100 mcg of human or ovine-sequence corticotropin-releasing hormone intravenously, with sampling every 15 minutes for 2 hours). A clear rise above 30 pg/mL (>6.6 pmol/L) confirms ACTH-dependence. When the test suggests ACTH-independence, imaging of the adrenals with CT or occasionally MRI is used to identify an adrenal tumor (benign or malignant), bilateral macronodular hyperplasia (bilaterally enlarged adrenal glands), or primary pigmented nodular adrenal dysplasia (a disorder with often entirely normal or slightly nodular adrenal glands, usually seen in young adults and frequently in the context of Carney complex). If corticotropin-releasing hormone is unavailable, then one could proceed directly to adrenal imaging, with the caveat that longstanding Cushing disease may lead to asymmetric adrenal enlargement and a false diagnosis of an adrenal tumor.

With ACTH-dependent Cushing syndrome, the differential diagnosis consists of a corticotroph tumor, Cushing disease, or an ectopic source. Generally, the higher the levels of ACTH and cortisol, the more severe the metabolic upset and the presence of hypokalemia, and the more likely there is an ectopic source, but no biochemical or clinical feature is pathognomonic.[4] A young woman with a long history of symptoms and mild Cushing syndrome is much more likely to have Cushing disease, while an older man with severe biochemistry is more likely to have an ectopic source, but there is considerable overlap, and such features merely alter the *a priori* probability of the cause. For this reason, many dynamic tests have been introduced to differentiate among these possibilities, but none has a major clinically useful discriminatory power. Many clinicians use the responses to a low-dose 48-hour dexamethasone-suppression test (a fall in cortisol >20%) and the corticotropin-releasing hormone test (a rise in cortisol >20%) to be very highly suggestive of Cushing disease. In the presence of a clear pituitary lesion on MRI, this may be enough to mandate pituitary surgery. Equally, extreme biochemistry in an older man with a mass lesion in the chest would suggest thoracic surgery. However, in almost all cases, it is best to consider

bilateral inferior petrosal sinus sampling, where an experienced interventional neuroradiologist inserts catheters into the petrosal veins directly draining the pituitary; corticotropin-releasing hormone (or desmopressin if corticotropin-releasing hormone is unavailable) is injected intravenously, and the gradient in ACTH between the central and simultaneous peripheral venous samples is compared. A central-to-peripheral ACTH gradient greater than 3 after corticotropin-releasing hormone is 95% sensitive and almost 100% specific for the diagnosis of Cushing disease. If the bilateral inferior petrosal sinus sampling shows no central gradient, then the probability of Cushing disease moves from a 90% to a 50% likelihood, and more detailed imaging should be pursued. Most ectopic sources are in the neck or chest, and CT of the neck, chest, and abdomen often reveals a bronchial carcinoid (the most common source), a thymic carcinoid, medullary thyroid carcinoma, a pancreatic islet-cell tumor, or a pheochromocytoma (other sites have also been identified in large case series). Radionuclide scanning with ^{68}Ga-DOTATATE PET can be very useful,[5] although tumors can still be missed: *overt* sources are those revealed on initial cross-sectional scanning, and *covert* sources are those that eventually are diagnosed with more detailed imaging. *Occult* sources are those that defy identification, even with the most sophisticated imaging techniques.

Not infrequently, the biochemical changes in Cushing syndrome are highly fluctuant, and variability by more than 100% in 15% of patients with all causes of Cushing syndrome has been noted.[6] This is—probably incorrectly—known as periodic or cyclic Cushing syndrome. Rarely, there may indeed be a regular intermittency of cortisol secretion. However, for Cushing syndrome to truly "switch off" for prolonged periods, while recognized, is very rare. In such situations, in the face of uncertainty, it may be appropriate to wait and then reassess when the disease is in an active phase.

Finally, while in most patients a careful and analytic approach will lead to the correct diagnosis and appropriate management, it must be emphasized that the diagnosis of Cushing syndrome and the identification of its source remains essentially probabilistic and not algorithmic. In cases of ongoing uncertainty, a pragmatic wait-and-see approach may be reasonable, while the lack of identification of a source may require medical or surgical (bilateral adrenalectomy) therapy to at least diminish the harm from ongoing cortisol excess. In addition, great attention should be given to the metabolic complications, such as hypertension and diabetes and the ever-present risk of sepsis. Many clinicians advise anticoagulation with subcutaneous heparin as soon as the diagnosis is confirmed.

For confirmed Cushing disease, transsphenoidal surgery by an experienced surgeon should have a high cure rate, approaching 90%, while a repeat surgery when initially unsuccessful can still lead to cure in around 50% of patients.[7,8] Failed surgery can be followed by external beam radiotherapy if there is no obvious tumor, or radiosurgery or proton-beam therapy when there is a discrete lesion, but normalization of serum cortisol levels may take several years (faster in children, often <1 year). Medical therapy with metyrapone, ketoconazole, or mifepristone may be used while awaiting normalization. A minority of patients with Cushing disease respond to cabergoline, while those with mild disease may respond to the somatostatin analogue pasireotide, although with a substantial risk of diabetes mellitus and long-term suppression of growth hormone. Ectopic sources should be removed where possible, or the patient should undergo bilateral laparoscopic adrenalectomy when cure is not possible, and this option should also be considered for occasional patients with residual or recurrent Cushing disease.

Adrenal tumors should generally be removed laparoscopically, and patients with bilateral disease should be treated with bilateral adrenalectomy, although unilateral adrenalectomy has been proposed in milder cases.

Patients with overwhelming metabolic complications of Cushing syndrome of any cause should be treated with intravenous etomidate, which rapidly and effectively lowers cortisol when administered with due care.[9]

In any but the most straightforward case, patients should be treated in a center of excellence. The diagnosis and treatment of Cushing syndrome remains one of the most satisfying, as well as frustrating, problems in endocrinology.

Clinical Case Vignettes
Case 1

A 26-year-old man with a 5-year history of significant symptoms and signs highly suggestive of Cushing syndrome is referred for evaluation. Several serum cortisol measurements have all been greater than 63 μg/dL (>1750 nmol/L), with plasma ACTH levels of 300 to 350 pg/mL (66-77 pmol/L). CT chest shows left lower collapse/consolidation.

Which of the following should be the next investigation?

A. Low-dose dexamethasone-suppression test
B. Corticotropin-releasing hormone test
C. Bilateral inferior petrosal sinus sampling
D. Bronchoscopy
E. ^{68}Ga-DOTATATE PET scanning

Answer: D) Bronchoscopy

The diagnosis of Cushing syndrome in this patient is clear and does not require further confirmation. There are very high levels of both cortisol and ACTH, so there is no need to confirm Cushing syndrome with a dexamethasone-suppression test (Answer A). The differential diagnosis is an ectopic source or Cushing disease. The corticotropin-releasing hormone test (Answer B) can sometime add useful information, but with such high levels of cortisol and ACTH, ectopic ACTH is more likely and responses to corticotropin-releasing hormone will not shift this to any extent. The ^{68}Ga-DOTATATE PET scan (Answer E) can be positive with any sort of inflammation, so in this instance, finding positive uptake in the lung would be unhelpful. Bilateral inferior petrosal sinus sampling (Answer C) is often extremely useful, but as there is already evidence for a lung abnormality with an abnormal CT scan, bronchoscopy (Answer D) to look for a bronchial tumor is the most useful and expeditious investigation at this stage.

Case 1 (Continued)

Bronchoscopy demonstrates a combined bacterial, fungal, and cytomegalovirus infection. This considerably improves with appropriate antibiotics, antiviral treatment, and antifungal treatment. There is no abnormal cytology, and the patient experiences complete resolution. Pituitary MRI shows slight enlargement of the right side of the pituitary, while a ^{68}Ga-DOTATATE PET scan shows no abnormal uptake.

Which of the following should be the next investigation?

A. Bilateral inferior petrosal sinus sampling

B. Thoracic surgery

C. A combined dexamethasone–corticotropin-releasing hormone test

D. A high-dose dexamethasone-suppression test

E. Pituitary exploration

Answer: A) Bilateral inferior petrosal sinus sampling

There is no obvious ectopic source, and further dynamic tests are unlikely to be helpful at this stage. The dexamethasone–corticotropin-releasing hormone test (Answer C) is a cumbersome test to diagnose Cushing syndrome and would not add useful information, while the high-dose dexamethasone-suppression test (Answer D) has significant false-positive and false-negative results, plus the added danger of adding a further steroid load to an already compromised patient. The source remains uncertain, and there is no clear evidence for a thoracic origin, so chest surgery (Answer B) is not indicated. Patients with Cushing syndrome are at considerable risk of infections with a variety of organisms, as in this case, due to profound immunosuppression. Much of the biochemical data are indicative of an ectopic source, and many healthy patients have minor pituitary abnormalities on MRI, such that pituitary exploration (Answer E) would be premature. Bilateral inferior petrosal sinus sampling (Answer A) should clarify whether the high levels of ACTH are likely to be ectopic or pituitary in origin.

Indeed, bilateral inferior petrosal sinus sampling in this patient confirmed a central source, mainly lateralized to the left side. During transsphenoidal surgery, a left-sided corticotroph tumor was identified and removed, and the patient was cured by surgery. Postoperative 9-AM serum cortisol concentrations were less than 1.8 μg/dL (<50 nmol/L).

References

1. Nieman LK, Biller BM, Findling JW, et al. The diagnosis of Cushing's syndrome: an Endocrine Society clinical practice guideline. *J Clin Endocrinol Metab.* 2008;93(5):1526-1540. PMID: 18334580

2. Alexandraki KI, Grossman AB. Is urinary free cortisol of value in the screening of patients with Cushing's syndrome? *Curr Opin Endocrinol Diabet.* 2011;18(4):259-263. PMID: 21681089

3. Shapiro L, Elahi S, Riddoch F, et al. Investigation for paediatric Cushing's syndrome using twenty-four-hour urinary free cortisol determination. *Horm Res Paediatr.* 2016;86(1):21-26. PMID: 27287747

4. Hayes RA, Grossman AB. The ectopic adrenocorticotropic hormone syndrome: rarely easy, always challenging. *Endocrinol Metab Clin North Am.* 2018;47(2):409-425. PMID: 29754641

5. Isidori AM, Sbardella E, Zatelli MC, et al; ABC Study Group. Conventional and nuclear medicine imaging in ectopic Cushing's syndrome: a systematic review. *J Clin Endocrinol Metab.* 2015;100(9):3231-3244. PMID: 26158607

6. Alexandraki KI, Kaltsas GA, Isidori AM, et al. The prevalence and characteristic features of cyclicity and variability in Cushing's disease. *Eur J Endocrinol.* 2009;160(6):1011-1018. PMID: 19289537

7. Nieman LK, Biller BM, Findling JW, et al; Endocrine Society. Treatment of Cushing's syndrome: an Endocrine Society clinical practice guideline. *J Clin Endocrinol Metab.* 2015;100(8):2807-2831. PMID: 26222757

8. Pivonello R, De Leo M, Cozzolino A, Colao A. The treatment of Cushing's disease. *Endocr Rev.* 2015;36(4):385-486. PMID: 26067718

9. Preda V, Sen J, Karavitaki N, Grossman AB. Etomidate in the management of hypercortisolaemia in Cushing's syndrome [published correction appears in *Eur J Endocrinol.* 2013;168(2):X1]. *Eur J Endocrinol.* 2012;167(2):137-143. PMID: 22577107

Diagnosis and Management of Endocrine Hypertension: Deciding Who to Screen for Genetic Causes

William F. Young, Jr., MD, MSc. Division of Endocrinology, Diabetes, Metabolism, and Nutrition, Department of Internal Medicine, Mayo Clinic, Rochester, MN; E-mail: young.william@mayo.edu

Learning Objectives

As a result of participating in this session, learners should be able to:

- Recognize the key signs, symptoms, biochemical testing, and adrenal imaging findings that should raise suspicion for pheochromocytoma.

- Consider the role for genetic testing in patients with pheochromocytoma.

- Recognize the key signs, symptoms, and clinical circumstances that should trigger case-detection testing for primary aldosteronism.

- Consider the role for genetic testing in patients with primary aldosteronism.

Main Conclusions

Hypertension affects approximately 25% of all adults. In most, hypertension is primary (essential or idiopathic), but a subgroup of approximately 15% of patients has secondary hypertension. More than 50% of children and 30% of young adults (<40 years) have secondary hypertension. The secondary causes of hypertension include renal causes (eg, renal parenchymal disease) and endocrine causes. Hypertension may be the initial clinical presentation for at least 15 endocrine disorders (*Table*).[1] An accurate diagnosis of endocrine hypertension provides clinicians with the opportunity to recommend a surgical cure or treat with effective targeted pharmacologic therapy. During this Meet the Professor session, we will focus on the 2 main causes of adrenal-dependent hypertension: pheochromocytoma and primary aldosteronism. We will also include commentary on genetic testing in patients who have these disorders.

Significance of the Clinical Problem

Major problems related to the diagnosis of adrenal-dependent hypertension:

- Clinicians think about and test for pheochromocytoma a lot! However, because of the false-positive rate of plasma normetanephrine and the rarity of pheochromocytoma, 97% of patients with elevated plasma normetanephrine do not have a pheochromocytoma. This leads to additional downstream testing and, occasionally, surgical misadventures.

- Even though primary aldosteronism affects 5% to 10% of all persons with hypertension, clinicians do not think about it very much and do not test for it. The delayed or missed diagnosis of primary aldosteronism leads to suboptimal quality of life and cardiac- and renal-related morbidities.

Barriers to Optimal Practice

Clinical practice barriers related to pheochromocytoma:

- Lack of awareness of the medications associated with false-positive biochemical testing.

Table. Endocrine Causes of Hypertension

Etiology

Adrenal-dependent causes

   1. Pheochromocytoma and sympathetic paraganglioma

   2. Primary aldosteronism

   3. Hyperdeoxycorticosteronism

      a. Congenital adrenal hyperplasia

         i. 11β-Hydroxylase deficiency

         ii. 17α-Hydroxylase deficiency

      b. Deoxycorticosterone-producing tumor

      c. Primary cortisol resistance

   4. Cushing syndrome

Apparent mineralocorticoid excess/11β-hydroxysteroid dehydrogenase deficiency

   1. Genetic

   2. Acquired

      a. Licorice or carbenoxolone ingestion

      b. Cushing syndrome

Parathyroid-dependent causes

   1. Hyperparathyroidism

Pituitary-dependent causes

   1. Acromegaly

   2. Cushing syndrome

Secondary hyperaldosteronism

   1. Renovascular hypertension

Thyroid-dependent causes

   1. Hypothyroidism

   2. Hyperthyroidism

Complex effects

   1. Obstructive sleep apnea

- Not recognizing that 3% to 5% of all adrenal incidentalomas prove to be pheochromocytomas and that 60% of pheochromocytomas are discovered as incidental adrenal masses on computed cross-sectional imaging.

- Unawareness of the key role of imaging phenotype when determining whether an adrenal mass may be a pheochromocytoma and the concept of "prebiochemical pheochromocytoma."

- Determining which patients with pheochromocytoma or paraganglioma should have genetic testing for germline pathogenic variants.

Clinical practice barriers related to primary aldosteronism:

- Lack of case-detection testing worldwide—primary aldosteronism is one of the most underdiagnosed endocrine disorders.

- Clinicians thinking that primary aldosteronism is rare or difficult to diagnose.

- Confusion regarding which medications a patient can or cannot be taking when case-detection testing is performed for primary aldosteronism.

- Determining which patients with primary aldosteronism should have genetic testing for germline pathogenic variants.

Strategies for Diagnosis, Therapy, and/or Management
Pheochromocytoma

Pheochromocytoma is a frequently sought, but rarely found, catecholamine-secreting tumor usually localized to the adrenal gland.[2] When pheochromocytoma is correctly diagnosed and properly treated, it is curable; when undiagnosed or improperly treated, it can be fatal. The prevalence of pheochromocytoma in the hypertensive population is 0.01% to 0.1% and it occurs equally in men and women—primarily in the third through fifth decades of life. In 2020, a symptomatic presentation occurs in less than 40% of patients because the mode of diagnosis has changed dramatically over the past 90 years.[3] In the most recent series of patients with pheochromocytoma reported from Mayo Clinic (271 patients from 2005 to 2016), 61% were detected as adrenal incidentalomas and 12% were detected because of genetic or family testing.[3] Whereas in the initial Mayo Clinic series (138 patients from 1926 to 1970), pheochromocytoma was diagnosed based on paroxysmal symptoms or refractory hypertension in 90% of patients.[3] Clinicians should suspect pheochromocytoma in the following clinical scenarios:

- Hyperadrenergic spells (eg, episodes of forceful palpitations, diaphoresis, headache, tremor, pallor)—but recognizing that most patients with spells do not have pheochromocytoma

- Treatment-resistant hypertension

- A familial syndrome that predisposes to pheochromocytoma or paraganglioma (eg, multiple endocrine neoplasia type 2, neurofibromatosis type 1, von Hippel–Lindau syndrome, pathogenic variants in the *SDHx* genes)

- A family history of pheochromocytoma

- An incidentally discovered adrenal mass (3% to 5% of all adrenal incidentalomas prove to be pheochromocytoma)

- A pressor response to anesthesia, surgery, angiography, high-dose corticosteroid, or β-adrenergic blocker

- Onset of hypertension at a young age (<30 years)

Case-detection testing can be accomplished by measurement of fractionated catecholamines (dopamine, norepinephrine, and epinephrine) and fractionated metanephrines (metanephrine and normetanephrine) by high-performance liquid chromatography or tandem mass spectrometry. At Mayo Clinic, the most reliable case-detection strategy is measuring fractionated metanephrines

and catecholamines in a 24-hour urine collection. If clinical suspicion is high, then plasma fractionated metanephrines are also measured. Although it is preferred that patients not be on any medications at the time of laboratory testing, treatment with most medications may be continued (all blood pressure–related medications are OK!). Tricyclic antidepressants (TCAs) interfere most frequently with the interpretation of 24-hour urinary fractionated catecholamines and metanephrines. Cyclobenzaprine is a TCA. Treatment with TCAs and antipsychotic agents should be tapered and discontinued at least 4 weeks before testing. Frequently this is not possible, and in that setting, testing should proceed and if the results are normal, no further testing is needed. It is also important to recognize that catecholamine secretion may be appropriately increased in situations of physical stress or illness (eg, stroke, myocardial infarction, acute congestive heart failure). Medications that may increase measured levels of catecholamines and metanephrines include TCAs (including cyclobenzaprine); levodopa; drugs containing adrenergic receptor agonists (eg, decongestants); amphetamines; buspirone and most psychoactive agents (but not selective serotonin reuptake inhibitors); selective norepinephrine reuptake inhibitors (may cause 2-fold increases above upper limit of reference range); prochlorperazine; reserpine withdrawal from clonidine and other drugs (eg, illicit drugs); and ethanol. However, with current assay methodology (tandem mass spectrometry, high-performance liquid chromatography), antihypertensive medications and acetaminophen do not interfere with testing.

Genetic testing should be considered in all patients with pheochromocytoma, especially if a patient has 1 or more of the following: paraganglioma; bilateral adrenal pheochromocytoma; unilateral adrenal pheochromocytoma and a positive family history for pheochromocytoma; unilateral adrenal pheochromocytoma and young age (<60 years); or other clinical findings suggestive of a related syndromic disorder. Genetic testing can be complex, and testing of one family member has implications for related individuals. Genetic counseling is recommended to help families understand the implications of genetic test results, to coordinate testing of at-risk individuals, and to help families work through the psychosocial issues that may arise before, during, or after the testing process. An asymptomatic person at risk for disease on the basis of family history of pheochromocytoma or paraganglioma should have genetic testing only if an affected family member has a known pathogenic variant.

Primary Aldosteronism

Primary aldosteronism is usually diagnosed in patients between 20 and 60 years of age. Current prevalence estimates for primary aldosteronism are 5% to 10% of all patients with hypertension. There is no reliable clinical phenotype to guide the clinician on which patients should be tested for primary aldosteronism. The degree of hypertension is typically moderate to severe and may be resistant to usual pharmacologic treatments. In general, patients with aldosterone-producing adenomas tend to have higher aldosterone levels and higher blood pressures than do patients with bilateral idiopathic hyperplasia. Because hypokalemia is present in only 28% of patients with primary aldosteronism, all patients with hypertension are potential candidates for this disorder. There is a unique subset of young patients (typically <35 years) who present with marked hypokalemia but are not technically hypertensive with systolic/diastolic blood pressures of 130s/80s mm Hg. These patients usually have prior baseline blood pressures that average 100/60 mm Hg. Thus, although they do not meet the criteria for hypertension, there is a clinically significant change from baseline, and presumably their young age and blood pressure counter-regulatory mechanisms prevent hypertension, at least in the first year or two of the disease.

The prevalence of target-organ damage to the heart and kidney is increased in patients with primary aldosteronism compared with the prevalence in those with essential hypertension. Longstanding, undiagnosed primary aldosteronism frequently leads to chronic kidney disease. In a recent meta-analysis of 31 studies, including 3838 patients with primary aldosteronism and 9284 patients with essential hypertension, patients with aldosterone-producing adenomas and bilateral hyperplasia had an increased risk of stroke (odds ratio [OR], 2.58), coronary artery disease (OR, 1.77), atrial fibrillation (OR, 3.52), and heart failure (OR, 2.05).[4] In addition, the diagnosis of primary aldosteronism increased the risk of diabetes (OR, 1.33), metabolic syndrome (OR, 1.53), and left ventricular hypertrophy (OR, 2.29).[4] Thus, the cardiovascular toxicity in primary aldosteronism extends beyond hypertension; there is an aldosterone-specific toxicity. In addition, several studies have demonstrated the negative impact of primary aldosteronism on quality of life.

Before 1981, primary aldosteronism was thought to be a rare cause of hypertension. Over time, it has been shown that most patients with primary aldosteronism are not hypokalemic and that case-detection testing can be completed without stopping antihypertensive medications. Case-detection testing is performed with a morning venipuncture for the measurement of plasma aldosterone concentration and plasma renin activity or plasma renin concentration.

Familial primary aldosteronism should be considered when primary aldosteronism is diagnosed before age 20 years or when primary aldosteronism is diagnosed in more than one family member. In nearly all cases, patients with familial primary aldosteronism have bilateral adrenal disease and would not be cured with unilateral adrenalectomy.

Clinical Case Vignettes
Case 1

You see two 50-year-old women with adrenal incidentalomas. Axial CT images of their adrenal masses are shown (*see images*).

Patient 1

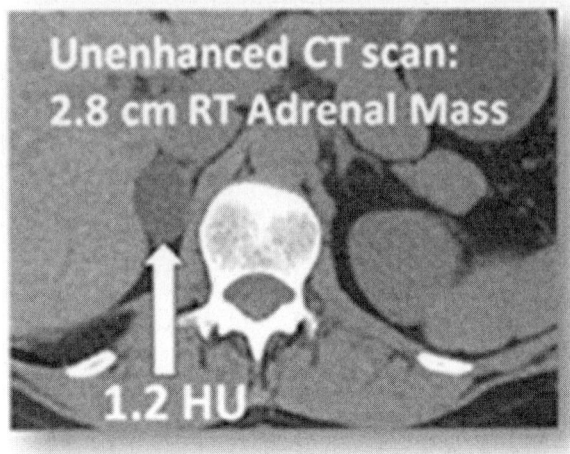

Patient 2

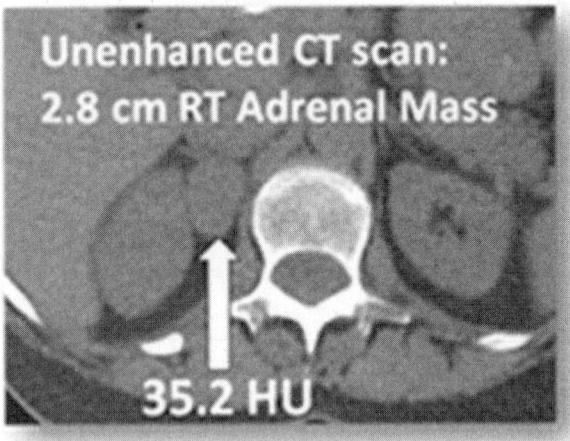

Which patient(s) should be screened for pheochromocytoma?

A. Patient 1

B. Patient 2

C. Both patients

D. Neither patient

Answer: B) Patient 2

In this clinical vignette, you are provided with the unenhanced CT images from 2 patients with nearly identical 2.8-cm right adrenal masses. The one difference is the unenhanced CT attenuation measured in Hounsfield units (HU). In a multicenter retrospective study of 533 patients with 548 histologically confirmed pheochromocytomas, among the 376 pheochromocytomas for which unenhanced CT attenuation data were available, 374 had an attenuation value greater than 10 HU (99.5%).[5] In the 2 exceptions (0.5%), the unenhanced CT attenuation was exactly 10 HU. An adrenal incidentaloma with an unenhanced CT attenuation of 1.2 HU simply cannot be a pheochromocytoma. The smart clinician can avoid the conundrum of false-positive biochemical testing in Patient 1 by not testing for pheochromocytoma, as biochemical testing is not needed if the unenhanced CT attenuation is less than 10 HU. The CT image for Patient 2 is highly suspicious for pheochromocytoma, and this patient should be screened (Answer B).

Case 2

You are asked to see a 49-year-old man for an incidentally discovered, lipid-poor, vascular, 1.6-cm left adrenal mass. The patient has been troubled by intermittent right upper-quadrant pain, which was thought to be related to gallbladder dysfunction. In the process of imaging, the 1.6-cm mass was incidentally discovered (*see images, arrows*). The unenhanced CT attenuation is 40.5 HU.

Biochemical testing documents normal plasma concentrations of fractionated metanephrines:

Metanephrine = 39 pg/mL (<99 pg/mL)
(SI: <0.2 nmol/L [<0.5 nmol/L])
Normetanephrine = 101 pg/mL (<165 pg/mL)
(SI: 0.55 nmol/L [<0.9 nmol/L])

In addition, 24-hour urine shows normal excretion of the following:

Metanephrine = 151 μg/24 h (<400 μg/24 h)
(SI: 766 nmol/d [<2028 nmol/d])
Normetanephrine = 447 μg/24 h (<900 μg/24 h)
(SI: 2441 nmol/d [<4914 nmol/d])
Epinephrine = 7.6 μg/24 h (<21 μg/24 h)
(SI: 41 nmol/d [<115 nmol/d])
Norepinephrine = 61 μg/24 h (<80 μg/24 h)
(SI: 361 nmol/d [<473 nmol/d])
Dopamine = 201 μg/24 h (<400 μg/24 h)
(SI: 1311 nmol/d [<2610 nmol/d])

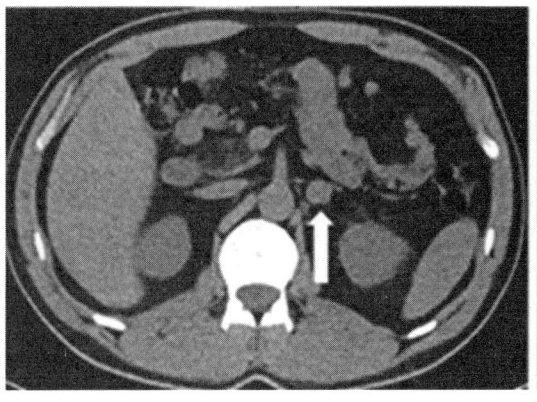 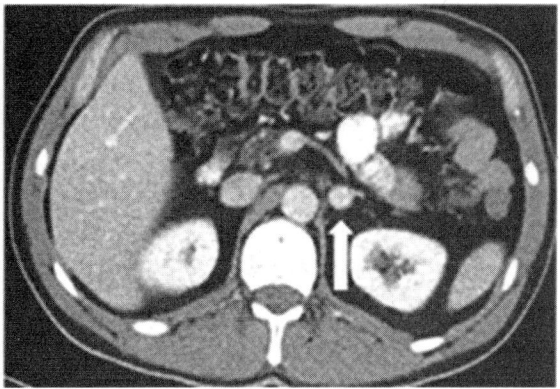

Do the normal plasma fractionated metanephrines and normal 24-hour urine results for fractionated metanephrines and catecholamines exclude the diagnosis of pheochromocytoma in this patient?

A. Yes

B. No

C. Umm, maybe

Answer: B) No

At laparoscopic left adrenalectomy, this patient proved to have a 2.1 × 1.7 × 1.3-cm pheochromocytoma. The key learning point here is that all pheochromocytomas are "prebiochemical" when small. Pheochromocytomas need a "big factory" (typically >1.5 cm in diameter) to be biochemically detectable. Lipid-poor and vascular adrenal masses should be considered as suspicious for pheochromocytoma or small adrenocortical carcinoma. They should either be resected (assuming you have an expert adrenal surgeon) or followed closely.

Case 3

With regard to genetic testing in the 49-year-old man in Case 2, which of the following is the best next step?

A. *SDHx* panel

B. *RET* gene testing

C. *NF1* gene testing

D. Next-generation sequencing panel for 12 genes

E. Genetic testing is not indicated in this patient

Answer: D) Next-generation sequencing panel for 12 genes

The pathogenesis of pheochromocytoma can be separated into 2 general pathways:

- Hypoxic signaling pathway—"Cluster 1" (noradrenergic tumors): *SDHx* (*SDHA, SDHAF2, SDHB, SDHC, SDHD*); *VHL*; *FH*; *EPAS1* (*HIF2A*); *EGLN1* (*PHD2*), *EGLN2* (*PDH1*); *KIF1B*; *IDH1*; *MDH2*; *SLC25A11*; *DNMT3A*

- Kinase signaling pathway—"Cluster 2" (adrenergic tumors): *RET*; *NF1*; *MAX*; *TMEM127*

The prevalence of a detectable germline pathogenic variant decreases with each decade of life. For example, when pheochromocytoma is diagnosed in the first decade of life, 90% of children have a detectable pathogenic variant (most commonly in the *VHL* gene).[2] When pheochromocytoma is diagnosed in the seventh to ninth decades of life, only 20% of patients have a detectable pathogenic variant.[2] The patient in this vignette is 49 years old, and he has a 32% probability of carrying a germline pathogenic variant. Due to that risk, genetic testing is indicated. Multigene testing with next-generation sequencing (Answer D) is indicated in this case because of the small size of this patient's pheochromocytoma and thus normal biochemistry, one does not know if it is adrenergic or noradrenergic and selective or targeted testing would be costly and time consuming.

Genetic testing should be considered in all patients with pheochromocytoma, especially if a patient has one or more of the following: paraganglioma; bilateral adrenal pheochromocytoma; unilateral adrenal pheochromocytoma and a positive family history for pheochromocytoma; unilateral adrenal pheochromocytoma and young age (<60 years); or other clinical findings suggestive of one of the syndromic disorders. Genetic testing can be complex, and testing of one family member has implications for related individuals. Genetic counseling is recommended to help families understand the implications of genetic test results, to coordinate testing of at-risk individuals, and to help families work through the psychosocial issues that may arise before, during, or after the testing process. An asymptomatic person at risk for disease on the basis of family history of pheochromocytoma or paraganglioma should have genetic testing only if an affected family member has a known pathogenic variant.

Case 4

Which of the following patients should be screened for primary aldosteronism?

A. 56-year-old man with hypertension controlled with 3 drugs and a serum potassium concentration of 3.3 mEq/L (3.3 mmol/L)

B. 23-year-old woman with new-onset hypertension controlled with 2 medications and a serum potassium concentration of 4.0 mEq/L (4.0 mmol/L)

C. Both patients

D. Neither patient

Answer: C) Both patients

Answer A is technically correct because it follows the 2016 Endocrine Society clinical practice guideline on primary aldosteronism.[6] However, several studies have documented that clinicians are not testing for primary aldosteronism.[7,8] It is likely that less than 2% of the 1.5 billion people in the world with hypertension are being tested

for primary aldosteronism; most of the 75 million people with primary aldosteronism go undetected. Primary care providers think that primary aldosteronism is an uncommon and complicated disorder and do not test for it or treat it. Primary care providers (and probably most physicians— including endocrinologists!) are not following the Endocrine Society guidelines on primary aldosteronism—where high-probability subsets of patients are recommended to have case-detection testing. It is frustrating to see patients who were not tested for primary aldosteronism when they were first diagnosed with hypertension, but rather only after they have developed irreversible stage 4 to 5 chronic kidney disease. Clinical practice guidelines have not been effective in driving more clinicians to consider case-detection testing for primary aldosteronism.[7,8] Could the guidelines be too complicated with regard to rules on medications and by focusing on recommending subsets of patients for testing? The diagnostic algorithm should be simplified, and case-detection testing for primary aldosteronism should be recommended at least once for all patients with hypertension.[8] In this clinical vignette, it would be a shame to miss the diagnosis of primary aldosteronism in a 23-year-old woman with new-onset hypertension. The lack of hypokalemia is meaningless—70% of patients with primary aldosteronism have a normal serum potassium concentration. Thus, both patients should be tested (Answer C).

Case 5

You see a 56-year-old man with 20-year history of hypertension, poorly controlled for the past year on 5 drugs: lisinopril, 20 mg daily; spironolactone, 50 mg daily; hydrochlorothiazide, 25 mg daily; metoprolol, 100 mg daily; and amlodipine, 10 mg daily. Despite those 5 medications, his current blood pressure is 165/110 mm Hg.

Which medication(s) should be stopped before screening for primary aldosteronism in this patient?

A. Lisinopril (ACE inhibitor)

B. Spironolactone (mineralocorticoid receptor antagonist)

C. Hydrochlorothiazide (thiazide diuretic)

D. Metoprolol (β-adrenergic blocker)

E. All of the above

F. None of the above

Answer: F) None of the above

In this patient with severe hypertension, no reasonable clinician should stop these medications and switch to doxazosin and verapamil. Most clinicians simply would not test this patient for primary aldosteronism because they think they cannot due to the "interfering" medications. The facts are these: (1) no medication causes false-positive testing if you use a cutoff for the plasma aldosterone concentration (eg, >10 ng/dL [>277 pmol/L]); (2) in most patients with primary aldosteronism, you cannot budge plasma renin activity (or plasma renin concentration) with these medications; (3) most patients treated with mineralocorticoid receptor antagonists are on subtherapeutic dosages and if the patient has primary aldosteronism, plasma renin activity will be suppressed; and (4) endocrinologists have created a barrier to diagnosing primary aldosteronism, leading to increased morbidity.[9] Patients can be on any sodium diet and any blood pressure medication, including spironolactone and eplerenone, when performing case-detection testing for primary aldosteronism.[8] If renin is not suppressed in that setting and the clinician is still suspicious of primary aldosteronism, then simply stop what are viewed as the offending medications, keep blood pressure controlled, and repeat case-detection testing.

Case 6

The 56-year-old patient from Case 5 proved to have primary aldosteronism due to a unilateral aldosterone-producing adenoma and was cured with unilateral adrenalectomy.

Should this patient have genetic testing for familial hyperaldosteronism?

A. Yes

B. No

C. Umm, maybe

Answer: B) No

There are 6 familial forms of primary aldosteronism:[8]

- Glucocorticoid-remediable aldosteronism (GRA) or familial hyperaldosteronism type I—*CYP11B1/CYP11B2* germline chimeric gene

- Familial hyperaldosteronism type II—germline *CLCN2* pathogenic variants

- Familial hyperaldosteronism type III—germline *KCNJ5* pathogenic variants

- Familial hyperaldosteronism type IV—germline *CACNA1H* pathogenic variants

- Primary aldosteronism with seizures and neurologic abnormalities (PASNA)—germline *CACNA1D* pathogenic variants

- Familial hyperaldosteronism and *ARMC5* pathogenic variants, causing bilateral macronodular adrenal hyperplasia

However, all forms of familial hyperaldosteronism are rare; type II is the most common. Familial hyperaldosteronism should be considered when primary aldosteronism is diagnosed before age 20 years or when primary aldosteronism is diagnosed in more than one family member. In nearly all cases, patients with familial hyperaldosteronism have bilateral adrenal disease and would not be cured with unilateral adrenalectomy. Thus, there is no role for genetic testing in the patient described in this clinical vignette. What would be recommended to patients such as this one is to encourage any blood relatives who have hypertension to be screened for primary aldosteronism by measuring plasma aldosterone and plasma renin activity.

References

1. Young WF Jr, Calhoun DA, Lenders JWM, et al. Screening for endocrine hypertension: an Endocrine Society scientific statement. *Endocr Rev.* 2017;38(2):103-122.

2. Neumann HPH, Young WF Jr, Eng C. Pheochromocytoma and paraganglioma. *N Engl J Med.* 2019;381(6):552-565. PMID: 31390501

3. Gruber LM, Hartman RP, Thompson GB, et al. Pheochromocytoma characteristics and behavior differ depending on method of discovery. *J Clin Endocrinol Metab.* 2019;104(5):1386-1393. PMID: 30462226

4. Monticone S, D'Ascenzo F, Moretti C, et al. Cardiovascular events and target organ damage in primary aldosteronism compared with essential hypertension: a systematic review and meta-analysis. *Lancet Diabetes Endocrinol.* 2018;6(1):41-50. PMID: 29129575

5. Canu L, Van Hemert JAW, Kerstens MN, et al. CT characteristics of pheochromocytoma: relevance for the evaluation of adrenal incidentaloma. *J Clin Endocrinol Metab.* 2019;104(2):312-318. PMID: 30383267

6. Funder JW, Carey RM, Mantero F, et al. The management of primary aldosteronism: case detection, diagnosis, and treatment: an Endocrine Society clinical ppractice guideline. *J Clin Endocrinol Metab.* 2016;101(5):1889-1916. PMID: 26934393

7. Rossi E, Perazzoli F, Negro A, Magnani A. Diagnostic rate of primary aldosteronism in Emilia-Romagna, Northern Italy, during 16 years (2000-2015). *J Hypertens.* 2017;35(8):1691-1697. PubMed PMID: 28410304

8. Mulatero P, Monticone S, Burrello J, Veglio F, Williams TA, Funder J. Guidelines for primary aldosteronism: uptake by primary care physicians in Europe. *J Hypertens.* 2016;34(11):2253-2257. PMID: 27607462

9. Young WF Jr. Diagnosis and treatment of primary aldosteronism: practical clinical perspectives. *J Intern Med.* 2019;285(2):126-148. PMID: 30255616

Difficulties in Diagnosis and Management of Adrenal Insufficiency in the Critically Ill Patient

David J. Torpy, MBBS, PhD, FRACP. Endocrine and Metabolic Unit, Royal Adelaide Hospital and University of Adelaide, Adelaide, SA, Australia; E-mail: david.torpy@sa.gov.au

Learning Objectives

As a result of participating in this session, learners should be able to:

- Describe the current status of adjunctive hydrocortisone therapy in critical illness.

- Explain the clinical options for management of adrenal insufficiency in the light of evidence from physiological studies and clinical trials in critical illness.

Main Conclusions

Patients with critical illness are subject to profound physiological stress with multiple stimuli such as fever, elevation of inflammatory cytokines, pain, and hypovolemia leading to activation of the hypothalamic-pituitary-adrenal (HPA) axis. Cortisol has a pivotal role in maintaining homeostasis and in immunomodulation in critical illness. Routine measurements of serum cortisol may not reflect end-organ glucocorticoid sufficiency due to tissue resistance to cortisol and reduced concentrations of the principal carrier proteins for cortisol, corticosteroid-binding globulin (CBG) and albumin.

Septic shock, a common state and important cause of mortality, with a 30% to 40% mortality rate despite standard antibiotics, fluids, and catecholaminergic vasopressors, has been studied extensively over the past 2 decades from the point of view of glucocorticoid therapy. Earlier studies of high-dose, short-term synthetic glucocorticoids for septic shock showed increased mortality. Continuing clinical observations of benefit from hydrocortisone in septic shock led to a succession of small trials revealing salutary effects such as a pressor response and reduced inflammatory cytokines, ultimately leading to progressively larger multicenter randomized controlled trials of "low-dose" hydrocortisone. The general conclusion is that randomized hydrocortisone, generally 200 mg daily, leads to reduced time-to-withdrawal of vasopressor support (1-2 days) and a possible small benefit in mortality. Sicker patients and curiously those treated with fludrocortisone may benefit more in terms of mortality. It may be that a subset of patients benefits more from hydrocortisone. A state of reduced cortisol response to cosyntropin, 250 mcg (<9 μg/dL [<248 nmol/L] at 60 minutes) may identify a state of relative adrenal insufficiency, later referred to as critical illness–related corticosteroid insufficiency (CIRCI). Initial studies suggested CIRCI predicted mortality benefit from parenteral hydrocortisone, but this was not confirmed in larger trials. At present, hydrocortisone, 200 mg daily, 50 mg every 6 hours or by intravenous infusion for 7 days without taper, perhaps with fludrocortisone, 0.05 mg enterally via nasogastric tube daily, is indicated in patients with hypotension despite fluid resuscitation and vasopressor treatment. Other conditions for which hydrocortisone therapy may be clinically indicated include community-acquired pneumonia requiring hospitalization, acute respiratory distress syndrome, and bacterial meningitis. A place for hydrocortisone in severe trauma is not established. The decisions regarding hydrocortisone in these conditions are generally not made by endocrinologists, but awareness of the trials and limitations of the evidence is of value, particularly among endocrinologists in hospital practice.

Significance of the Clinical Problem

The use of glucocorticoids in critical illness has been controversial for decades. Endocrinologists will find the area challenging, as the notion of corticosteroid insufficiency (ie, a lack of glucocorticoid sufficiency at the tissue level without obvious deficits in random or cosyntropin-stimulated cortisol) requires reference to clinical trial data and consideration of patient status where many variables may affect the primary feature of CIRCI (ie, hypotension unresponsive to fluids and vasopressors). Previous operational definitions of CIRCI, including the 60-minute rise in serum cortisol of less than 9 μg/dL (<248 nmol/L), remain controversial. A measure of tissue glucocorticoid sufficiency relevant to CIRCI is not available. Even the initial pressor response to glucocorticoids is not known to be predictive of benefits such as mortality and time to vasopressor withdrawal. Endocrinologists may be asked to comment on serum cortisol values and the use of hydrocortisone in the intensive care unit, and a working knowledge of the current data is useful.

Barriers to Optimal Practice

- Conventional measurements of serum cortisol, performed on a random or postcosyntropin basis, are not strong predictors of response to exogenous glucocorticoids, although they may still identify patients with conventional adrenal insufficiency.

- Immediate response to exogenous glucocorticoids may not reflect mortality or ultimate pressor benefit in critical illness.

Strategies for Diagnosis, Therapy, and/or Management

Definitions

Adrenal insufficiency is defined as the inability to produce sufficient glucocorticoids and mineralocorticoids for tissue requirements.[1] Biochemically, it is defined by a suboptimal cortisol response to cosyntropin, 250 mcg (eg, peak cortisol at 30 minutes <18 μg/dL [<500 nmol/L] [assay dependent]) and subclassified by ACTH level into primary and secondary forms. Primary forms may have aldosterone deficiency as determined by plasma aldosterone and renin measurements. CIRCI is a concept, developed in critical care medicine, of impaired HPA response to the stress of critical illness.[2] CIRCI is operationally defined as a serum cortisol increment of less than 9 μg/dL (<248 nmol/L) 60 minutes after administration of 250 mcg cosyntropin.

Critical Illness Stress Response

Critical illness such as sepsis is associated with central stimulation of the HPA axis as a response to multiple stimuli, including the following: inflammatory cytokines IL-1, TNF-α, and IL-6 acting at all HPA levels; pain; psychic stress of many stimuli; reduced cortisol metabolism through inhibition of 5α/5β reductases[3] and 11β-hydroxysteroid dehydrogenase type 2 (11BHSD2),[4] explaining the prolonged serum half-life of cortisol in sepsis, only moderately elevated cortisol production rate, and lack of elevation of ACTH in many cases; reductions in the concentrations of cortisol-binding proteins in plasma (CBG and albumin); redirection of adrenal steroidogenesis from androgens towards cortisol; tissue resistance to cortisol based on the activation of NFκB pathways, which antagonize intracellular pathways used by the glucocorticoid receptor and reduced levels and transcription of GRα and increased levels of the dominant negative GRβ;[5,6] corticostatins reducing ACTH receptor activity;[7] and drug effects on the HPA axis such as the inhibitory effects of opioids, benzodiazepines, and in some cases etomidate. In addition, concomitant activation of the sympathetic nervous system at the central level is augmented by cortisol's action, increasing conversion of norepinephrine to epinephrine at the adrenal medulla and cortisol's augmentation of norepinephrine's effects on the vasculature to sustain and redirect blood flow. Given the complexity of these influences on the HPA axis, especially the variable degree of tissue resistance that accompanies systemic inflammation and the fall in serum binding proteins that alter the relationship between total and free cortisol, serum cortisol concentrations may not reflect tissue glucocorticoid status.

Sepsis is a life-threatening organ dysfunction caused by a dysregulated host response to infection. The American College of Chest Physicians and Society of Critical Care Medicine Consensus Conference criteria in 1992 defined septic shock as the presence of systemic inflammatory response syndrome, documented infection or positive blood culture and the presence of organ dysfunction, hypoperfusion abnormality, or sepsis-induced hypotension refractory to adequate fluid resuscitation or vasopressor agents.[8] The systemic inflammatory response was manifested by 2 or more of the following: fever (temperature >100.4°F [>38°C]) or hypothermia (temperature <95.9°F [<35.5°C]), tachycardia (>90 beats/min), tachypnea (>20 breaths/min), leukocytosis or leukopenia (white blood cell count >12,000 or <4000 cells/μL),

or immature neutrophils (bands >10%). The criteria for organ dysfunction or hypoperfusion abnormality are 1 of the following: altered mental status, hypoxemia (PaO_2 <75 mm Hg), oliguria (urine output <30 mL/h), and elevated plasma lactate (>2 mmol/L). The definition for hypotension is systolic blood pressure less than 90 mm Hg or a reduction of systolic blood pressure by 40 mm Hg or more from baseline. More recent criteria have used definitions that incorporate sepsis-related organ failure assessment (SOFA) scores.[9]

The chief vasopressor used in septic shock is noradrenaline, which acts through vasoconstriction to elevate blood pressure. Reducing the time-to-withdrawal of vasopressor support reduces costs and complications from prolonged intensive care unit stays. Anecdotally, patients with septic shock may experience a beneficial rise in blood pressure when given exogenous glucocorticoid, resulting in shock reversal, confirmed by systematic analyses.[10,11] However, early studies of high-dosage, short-course synthetic glucocorticoids (equivalent to hydrocortisone, 40,000 mg daily, often in a single dose) in septic shock showed increased mortality.[12]

Effects of Stress-Dose Hydrocortisone in Septic Shock

Hydrocortisone, 10 mg hourly, increases plasma cortisol levels around 4-fold, to a mean of 109 μg/dL (3000 nmol/L) after the first day, which is above the upper end of the normal range for patients with septic shock at diagnosis.[13,14] The effects of cortisol concentrations at this level include attenuation of the inflammatory cytokines IL-6 and IL-8; soluble E-selectin, a factor important in endothelial-granulocyte interactions; and expression of the neutrophil activation markers CD11b and CD64, while the antiinflammatory cytokines IL-10 and soluble TNF receptor I and II are also attenuated. Markers of monocyte function such as HLA-DR antigen expression and in vitro phagocytosis are not affected, nor are the Th1 function markers,

IL-12 and IFN-γ.[13] Overall, these hydrocortisone responses are considered antiinflammatory rather than immunosuppressive.

Longer treatment (7 days) with lower-dosage hydrocortisone approximating the normal adrenocortical cortisol output in severe stress (200-300 mg daily) shortens the need for vasopressor support. Basal cortisol values in sepsis/septic shock are not useful predictors of mortality except at extremely high cortisol levels (>45 μg/dL [>1242 nmol/L]).[15] The term relative adrenal insufficiency was developed to describe a deleteriously attenuated cortisol response to exogenous ACTH without a deficient basal cortisol level.[16] In the Rothwell study of 32 patients with septic shock, 13 had a cortisol response to ACTH of less than 9 μg/dL (<250 nmol/L), of whom none (0/13) survived, compared with 13 of 19 survivors among those with cortisol responses greater than 9 μg/dL (>250 nmol/L). Hence, a total plasma cortisol response to cosyntropin, 250 mcg, of less than 9 μg/dL (<248 nmol/L) empirically defines relative adrenal insufficiency. A single center, double-blind, randomized study of 40 patients with septic shock patients found that hydrocortisone, 0.18 mg/kg per h after a 100-mg loading dose reduced the time-to-withdrawal of vasopressor support from 7 to 2 days (P = .005).[17] Forty-one patients with early septic shock given a 50-mg loading dose of intravenous hydrocortisone followed by 0.18 mg/kg per h had a reduced time-to-withdrawal of vasopressor from a median 120 to 53 hours (P = .02) with lowered serum cytokines.[18] A relationship between relative adrenal insufficiency and survival was noted in 189 patients with septic shock with the lowest survival rate seen in those with a basal cortisol concentration greater than 34 μg/dL (>935 nmol/L) and a cortisol response to cosyntropin at 60 minutes less than 9 μg/dL (<248 nmol/L).[19] Relative adrenal insufficiency is associated with a blunted response to vasopressors that can be reversed by hydrocortisone.[20,21]

These precepts were tested over 2 decades in clinical trials of critical illness, mostly in septic shock but also in sepsis and major trauma.[22] A 2002 randomized controlled trial of hydrocortisone, 50 mg every 6 hours, and fludrocortisone, 0.05 mg daily, vs placebo revealed a 28-day mortality benefit for treatment in the 229 nonresponders to cosyntropin, 250 mcg (cortisol response at 30 and 60 minutes less than 9 μg/dL [<248 nmol/L], indicative of relative adrenal insufficiency; confidence interval, 0.47-0.95; P = .02), but no mortality benefit in 70 responders.[23] Similarly a reduced time-to-vasopressor-withdrawal in the treatment group was apparent in nonresponders (expressed as withdrawal rates of 57% vs 40% at 28 days), but not in responders. This study was criticized, as 72 of 99 patients received etomidate, an adrenal 11-hydroxylase inhibitor that reduces cortisol synthesis, and 68 of these had relative adrenal insufficiency.[24] The use of etomidate may explain the high rate of relative adrenal insufficiency in the Annane et al study (77%) compared with only 33%. There was also a relatively high mortality rate of 55% to 61%; most studies have lower mortality rates (30%-40%) despite similar selection criteria. The results of this study increased interest and use of hydrocortisone in patients with septic shock, especially those in whom shock is refractory to fluids and catecholaminergic vasopressors.

The CORTICUS trial, however, did not reveal any 28-day mortality benefit from hydrocortisone, 50 mg every 6 hours in 499 patients with septic shock (233 nonresponders and 266 responders to cosyntropin, 250 mcg at 60 minutes; 251 treated patients, 248 patients placebo) relative to randomized placebo.[25] Hydrocortisone, however, was associated with more rapid resolution of shock. Risks of hydrocortisone included hyperglycemia, hypernatremia, and new infection. The CORTICUS trial was under-enrolled (500 vs planned 800 patients) and was criticized for being underpowered and had a relatively low mortality, suggesting less sick patients were enrolled.[26] The relevance of nonadministration of fludrocortisone in the CORTICUS trial is still debated, although hydrocortisone in dosages of 200 mg daily has full mineralocorticoid traditional effects on fluid and electrolyte status, effects of fludrocortisone on central or immune function, perhaps particularly relevant in sepsis, are mooted based on animal studies.[27] After these and other trials (totaling 33 randomized controlled trials of 4268 patients), a Cochrane systematic review concluded that corticosteroids significantly reduced mortality at 28 days compared with placebo.[28] Most recently, 2 large trials have further defined the utility of hydrocortisone in patients with septic shock.[29,30] Venkatesh et al administered 200 mg intravenous hydrocortisone via continuous infusion for 7 days, no taper) to 3658 ventilated patients with septic shock (1832 hydrocortisone, 1826 placebo). No difference in 28-day mortality was observed, but a 1-day reduction in time to shock resolution (3 vs 4 days) and a 1-day reduction in initial time of mechanical ventilation (5 vs 7 days) was noted, with no increase in rates of bacteremia or fungemia.[29] In contrast, Annane et al administered hydrocortisone, 50 mg intravenously every 6 hours, and fludrocortisone, 50 mcg daily via nasogastric tube, or placebo to 1241 patients with septic shock and achieved a lower 90-day (but not 28-day) mortality in the treatment group (43% vs 49.1%), as well as fewer days requiring vasopressor support. There were similar adverse events, apart from increased hyperglycemia, in the treatment group.[30]

Potential for Plasma Free Cortisol and CBG Measurements to Improve Diagnosis of CIRCI

Serum cortisol is approximately 80% bound to high-affinity CBG, 15% bound to low-affinity albumin, and 5% free. Cortisol levels above 20 to 25 µg/dL (>552 to 690 nmol/L) saturate CBG, leading to an exponential rise in free cortisol concentration.[31] In sepsis, TNFα and IL-6 reduce hepatic CBG synthesis. When comparing control patients with patients who have sepsis and septic shock, free cortisol increments correspond to illness severity more closely than total cortisol.[14] CBG may be cleaved at inflammatory sites by neutrophil elastase, reducing the CBG to cortisol binding affinity by 90%.[32] This liberates cortisol to tissues where the immunomodulatory effects of

cortisol may protect tissues from immune damage, thereby reducing the risk of multiorgan failure, the sine qua non of septic shock. Depletion of high-affinity CBG is a feature of sepsis, with the extent of depletion relating to categorical sepsis illness severity and mortality.[33,34] Routine measurements of serum cortisol do not allow assessment of free cortisol or that bound to specific carrier proteins, especially that fraction bound to high-affinity CBG. Hence, routine cortisol measurements may not reflect that portion of circulating cortisol most relevant to tissue action in the setting of sepsis.

Current Intensive Care Practice

The major critical care medicine societies guidelines regarding CIRCI[22,35] appeared before the recent published large trials; however, these trials still suggest that there are positive pressor effects of hydrocortisone, perhaps augmented by fludrocortisone, in septic shock.[29,30] The effects of hydrocortisone administration on mortality (relative risk 0.91-0.96; upper limit 95% confidence interval, 0.98-1.03) are modest if deployed randomly to patients with septic shock after fluid resuscitation and vasopressor therapy.[36] Current total cortisol measurements at baseline or after corticotropin are not considered reliably predictive of a response to adrenal corticosteroids.

The Society of Critical Care Medicine and European Society of Intensive Care Medicine[22,35] include the following points regarding CIRCI:

- No recommendation for routine use of the 250-mcg cosyntropin test

- Suggest against use of free cortisol (very low-quality evidence) or salivary cortisol (very low-quality evidence) for diagnosis

- Use of 250 mcg over 1 mcg cosyntropin (low-quality evidence) for diagnosis

- Suggested use of cosyntropin 250 mcg over a hemodynamic response test to bolus hydrocortisone 50-300 mg (very low-quality evidence)

- Suggest against use of ACTH levels for CIRCI diagnosis (low-quality evidence)

These guidelines make the following treatment recommendations:

- Suggest against use of corticosteroids for adults with sepsis without shock

- Suggest use of corticosteroids in adults septic shock unresponsive to fluid and moderate- to high-dosage vasopressor therapy (low-quality evidence)

- Use of long course, low-dosage intravenous hydrocortisone (<400 mg daily, >3 days) (low-quality evidence)

- Use of corticosteroids in patients with early acute respiratory distress syndrome (moderate-quality evidence)

- Suggest against use of corticosteroids in major trauma (low-quality of evidence)

- Recommendations were made for the use of corticosteroids in hospitalized patients with early moderate to severe acute respiratory distress syndrome (conditional recommendation [ie, benefits of adherence probably outweighs risks]) (moderate-quality evidence); community-acquired pneumonia (<400 mg hydrocortisone or equivalent daily, 5-7 days) (conditional, moderate-quality evidence)

- Recommend corticosteroid use in bacterial meningitis (strong recommendation, low-quality evidence)

- Suggest use in coronary bypass surgery (conditional recommendation, moderate-quality evidence)

- Suggest use in cardiac arrest (conditional recommendation, very low-quality evidence)

Clinical Case Vignettes
Case 1

A 58-year-old man with metastatic melanoma being treatment with the immune checkpoint inhibitor ipilimumab presents with low-grade fever, hypotension (blood pressure 80/50 mm Hg), severe postural hypotension, anorexia, and profound fatigue. Routine blood tests reveal mild hyponatremia, normal serum potassium, and a serum cortisol concentration of 4 μg/dL (110 nmol/L).

Which of the following statements is true?

A. Cosyntropin-stimulation testing is needed to determine whether he has adrenal insufficiency or CIRCI

B. Current use of synthetic glucocorticoid therapy may be the cause of this clinical situation

C. Past use of synthetic glucocorticoid therapy is a likely cause of this situation

D. Checkpoint inhibitor–related adrenal insufficiency is the likely cause of the presentation, and parenteral glucocorticoids should be administered without delay

E. Most patients with checkpoint inhibitor–related adrenal insufficiency recover with time and this process is aided by high-dosage corticosteroid administration

Answer: D) Checkpoint inhibitor–related adrenal insufficiency is the likely cause of the presentation, and parenteral glucocorticoids should be administered without delay

Baseline cortisol and clinical features are sufficiently diagnostic of adrenal insufficiency. Synthetic glucocorticoid therapy would not be consistent with clinical features. Past glucocorticoid therapy rarely produces clinical features of this severity. Ipilimumab (CTLA-4 inhibitor) produces hypophysitis in up to 20% of patients. HPA axis recovery is rare, and there is no recovery benefit from high-dosage glucocorticoids.

Case 2

A 75-year-old man is admitted to the hospital with septic shock 2 weeks after a 3-vessel coronary bypass graft procedure. Fluid resuscitation is administered, as well as a norepinephrine infusion at a rate of 2.0 mcg/kg per min. However, there is persistent hypotension. A random serum cortisol measurement is 18 μg/dL (497 nmol/L) and a 250-mcg cosyntropin test reveals a baseline cortisol value of 14 μg/dL (386 nmol/L) with a rise to 17 μg/dL (469 nmol/L) at 60 minutes.

Which of the following statements is true?

A. Administration of intravenous hydrocortisone is not indicated, as the evidence in trials does not show a consistent mortality benefit and the risks of treatment are excessive

B. This patient meets the criteria for treatment with hydrocortisone for presumed CIRCI and cosyntropin testing was mandatory before consideration of intravenous hydrocortisone therapy

C. The results of testing may reflect low cortisol-binding proteins (corticosteroid-binding globulin and albumin) and these should be measured to clarify the pathophysiology and guide treatment

D. Salivary free cortisol measurement may assist with diagnosis

E. The clinical circumstances warrant the use of low-dosage hydrocortisone such as intravenous 200 mg daily for 7 days without taper

Answer: E) The clinical circumstances warrant the use of low-dosage hydrocortisone such as intravenous 200 mg daily for 7 days without taper

Hydrocortisone use is recommended in septic shock unresponsive to fluid resuscitation and inotropes. Pressor effects are well demonstrated to reduce vasopressor requirement and time to withdrawal of vasopressor. The CIRCI operational definition is not required for hydrocortisone treatment. Risks of 7-day hydrocortisone treatment do not outweigh benefit. Cortisol-binding protein measurements have not been shown to be useful to guide treatment to date.

Case 3

A 33-year-old woman with Addison disease has a cystoscopy for the investigation of microscopic hematuria (sterile urine). Twenty-four hours later, she presents with fever 102°F (39°C), rigors, neutrophilia, and weakness. Her blood pressure is 110/70 mm Hg. Antimicrobial therapy directed at urosepsis is initiated.

Which of the following statements is true?

A. Glucocorticoid stress dosing (hydrocortisone, 100 mg intravenously every 6 hours, and 200 mg daily for 2 days) was necessary perioperatively to prevent adrenal crisis

B. No glucocorticoid stress doses were required with the procedure

C. Given the circumstances, full glucocorticoid stress dosing (50 mg every 6 hours) should be implemented to prevent adrenal crisis, as well as appropriate antibiotic therapy

D. The patient has sepsis and even without a history of Addison disease, hydrocortisone, 200 mg daily, is indicated given that sepsis connotes a clear risk of progression to septic shock

E. The administration of supraphysiologic dose glucocorticoids in this circumstance risks hyperglycemia and hypernatremia and may promote infection and is therefore contraindicated

Answer: C) Given the circumstances, full glucocorticoid stress dosing (50 mg every 6 hours) should be implemented to prevent adrenal crisis, as well as appropriate antibiotic therapy

This patient has sepsis with severe manifestations. She is at risk of adrenal crisis and stress-dose hydrocortisone is required. Sepsis without shock in a patient without Addison disease would not mandate use of hydrocortisone. Hydrocortisone, 100 mg intravenously/intramuscularly with the procedure and double-dose oral glucocorticoids for 48 hours was required.

Case 4

A 24-year-old man had a motorcycle crash with a head injury resulting in unconsciousness for 4 days, requiring several months of inpatient rehabilitation. He was treated with dexamethasone, 4 mg every 6 hours, for 2 weeks after the head injury. Six months after his injuries, he presents with severe dyspnea and hypoxemia that have been present for several hours. He is hypotensive (blood pressure 90/60 mm Hg), and chest x-ray shows lobar pneumonia. Tests of pituitary function document the following:

> Serum cortisol = 16 μg/dL (SI: 440 nmol/L)
> Serum total testosterone = 173 ng/dL
> (230-865 ng/dL) (SI: 6 nmol/L [8-30 nmol/L])
> LH = 2.0 mIU/mL (1.0-10.0 mIU/mL) (SI: 2.0 IU/L [1.0-10.0 IU/L])
> Free T_4 = 0.9 ng/dL (0.8-1.6 ng/dL) (SI: 11 pmol/L [10-20 pmol/L])
> Free T_3 = 1.8 pg/mL (2.0-3.5 pg/mL) (SI: 2.8 pmol/L [3.1-5.4 pmol/L]
> TSH = 0.2 mIU/L (0.4-4.0 mIU/L)

Which of the following statements is true?

A. The serum cortisol is adequate; administration of hydrocortisone is not indicated

B. Thyroid hormone replacement is required, and this may reduce cortisol concentrations through increased cortisol metabolism

C. The previous dexamethasone administration may explain the relatively low cortisol in the setting of acute respiratory distress syndrome

D. The low testosterone level makes structural hypothalamic-pituitary injury from trauma a likely diagnosis, hence reinforcing the likelihood that the cortisol response to illness is likely to be inadequate

E. Hydrocortisone administration may be indicated for the community-acquired pneumonia on clinical grounds alone and reassessment of the hypothalamic-pituitary axis can be performed outside of the setting of acute illness where testing and clinical assessment is likely to be more relevant to long-term therapy considerations

Answer: E) Hydrocortisone administration may be indicated for the community-acquired pneumonia on clinical grounds alone and reassessment of the hypothalamic-pituitary axis can be performed outside of the setting of acute illness where testing and clinical assessment is likely to be more relevant to long-term therapy considerations

This patient needs standard fluid resuscitation, antibiotics, and supportive measures. His serum cortisol measurement does not indicate severe adrenal insufficiency; however, he has community-acquired pneumonia requiring hospitalization. Low TSH and free T_3 may reflect illness, and levothyroxine is not indicated. Increased cortisol metabolism may result from higher doses if used. Dexamethasone use was too remote to influence serum cortisol. Low testosterone may reflect illness and does not necessarily indicate a defect of hypothalamic-pituitary-gonadal function. Hydrocortisone at a dosage less than 400 mg daily or the equivalent for 5 to 7 days is suggested for community-acquired pneumonia based on results from 13 trials, 12 of which showed reduced mortality. Most of the trials also showed reduced ventilator use and reduced incidence of acute respiratory distress syndrome. The principal adverse effect was more frequent hyperglycemia.

References

1. Bornstein SR, Allolio B, Arlt W, et al. Diagnosis and treatment of primary adrenal insufficiency: an Endocrine Society clinical practice guideline. *J Clin Endocrinol Metab.* 2016;101(2):364-389. PMID: 26760044

2. Marik PE, Pastores SM, Annane D et al. Recommendations for the diagnosis and management of corticosteroid insufficiency in critically ill adult patients: consensus statements from an international task force by the American College of Critical Medicine. *Crit Care Med.* 2008;36(8):1937-1949. PMID: 1896365

3. Boonen E, Vervenne H, Meersseman P, et al. Reduced cortisol metabolism during critical illness. *N Engl J Med.* 2013;368(16):1477-1488. PMID: 23506003

4. Tomlinson JW, Moore J, Cooper MS, et al. Regulation of the expression of 11beta-hydroxysteroid dehydrogenase type 1 in adipose tissue: tissue-

specific induction by cytokines. *Endocrinology.* 2001;142(5):1982-1989. PMID: 11316764

5. Ledderose C, Mohnle P, Limbeck E, et al. Corticosteroid resistance in sepsis is influenced by microRNA-124-induced downregulation of glucocorticoid receptor-α. *Crit Care Med.* 2012;40(10):2745-2753. PMID: 22846781

6. Annane D, Pastores SM, Arlt W, et al. Critical illness-related corticosteroid insufficiency (CIRCI): a narrative review from a multispeciality task force of the Society of Critical Care Medicine (SCCM) and the European Society of Intensive Care Medicine (ESICM). *Crit Care Med.* 2017;45(12):2089-2098. PMID: 28938251

7. Tominaga T, Fukata J, Naito Y, et al. Effects of corticostatin-I on rat adrenal cells in vitro. *J Endocrinol.* 1990;125(2):287-292. PMID: 2165121

8. American College of Chest Physicians/Society of Critical Care Medicine Consensus Conference Committee. American College of Chest Physicians/Society of Critical Care Medicine Consensus Conference Committee: definitions for sepsis and organ failure and guidelines for the use of innovation therapies in sepsis. *Crit Care Med.* 1992;20(6):864-874. PMID:1597042

9. Singer M, Deutschman CS, Seymour CW, et al. The third international consensus defiintions for sepsis and septic shock (Sepsis-3). *JAMA.* 2016;315(8):801-810. PMID: 26903338

10. Annane D, Bellissant E, Bollaert PE, et al. Corticosteroids in the treatment of severe sepsis and septic shock in adults: a systematic review. *JAMA.* 2009;301(22):2362-2375. PMID: 19509383

11. Sligl WI, Milner DA Jr, Sundar S, Mphatswe W, Majumdar SR. Safety and efficacy of corticosteroids for the treatment of septic shock: a systematic review and meta-analysis. *Clin Infect Dis.* 2009;49(1):93-101. PMID: 19489712

12. Minneci PC, Deans KJ, Banks SM, Eichacker PQ, Natanson C. Meta-analysis: the effect of steroids on survival and shock during sepsis depends on the dose. *Ann Intern Med.* 2004;141(1):47-56. PMID: 15238370

13. Keh D, Boehnke T, Weber-Cartens S, et al. Immunologic and hemodynamic effects of "low-dose" hydrocortisone in septic shock: a double-blind, randomized, placebo-controlled, crossover study. *Am J Respir Crit Care Med.* 2003;167(4):512-520. PMID: 12426230

14. Ho JT, Al-Musalhi H, Chapman MJ, et al. Septic shock and sepsis: a comparison of total and free plasma cortisol levels. *J Clin Endocrinol Metab.* 2006;91(1):105-114. PMID: 16263835

15. Sam S, Corbridge TC, Mokhlesi B, Comellas AP, Molitch ME. Cortisol levels and mortality in severe sepsis. *Clin Endocrinol (Oxf).* 2004;60(1):29-35. PMID: 14678284

16. Rothwell PM, Udwadia ZF, Lawler PG. Cortisol response to corticotropin and survival in septic shock. *Lancet.* 1991;337(8741):582-583. PMID: 1671944

17. Briegel J, Forst H, Haller M, et al. Stress doses of hydrocortisone reverse hyperdynamic septic shock: a prospective, randomized, double-blind, single-center study. *Crit Care Med.* 1999;27(4):723-732. PMID: 10321661

18. Oppert M, Schindler R, Husung C, et al. Low-dose hydrocortisone improves shock reversal and reduces cytokine levels in early hyperdynamic septic shock. *Crit Care Med.* 2005;33(11):2457-2464. PMID: 16276166

19. Annane D, Sebille V, Troche G, Raphael JC, Gajdos P, Bellissant E. A 3-level prognostic classification in septic shock based on cortisol levels and cortisol response to corticotropin. JAMA. 2000;283(8):1038-1045. PMID: 10697064

20. Annane D, Bellissant E, Sebille V, et al. Impaired pressor sensitivity to noradrenaline in septic shock patients with and without impaired adrenal function reserve. *Br J Clin Pharmacol.* 1998;46(6):589-597. PMID: 9862249

21. Bellissant E, Annane D. Effect of hydrocortisone on phenylephrine--mean arterial pressure dose-response relationship in septic shock. *Clin Pharmacol Ther.* 2000;68(3):293-303. PMID: 11014411

22. Annane D, Pastores SM, Rochwerg B, et al. Guidelines for the diagnosis and management of critical illness related corticosteroid insufficiency (CIRCI) in critically ill patients (Part 1): Society of Critical Care Medicine (SCCM) and European Society of Intensive Care Medicine (ESICM) 2017. 2017;45(12):2078-2088. PMID: 28938253

23. Annane D, Sebille V, Charpentier C, et al. Effect of treatment with low doses of hydrocortisone and fludrocortisone on mortality in patients with septic shock. *JAMA.* 2002;283(7):862-871. PMID: 12186604

24. Anonymous. Corticosteroids for patients with septic shock. *JAMA.* 2003;289(1):41-44.

25. Sprung CL, Annane D, Keh D, et al; CORTICUS Study Group. Hydrocortisone therapy for patients with septic shock. *N Engl J Med.* 2008;358(2):111-124. PMID: 18184957

26. Mason PE, Al-Khafaji A, Milbrandt EB, Suffoletto BP, Huang DT. CORTICUS: the end of unconditional love for steroid use. *Crit Care.* 2009;13(4):309. PMID: 19691813

27. Heming N, Sivavandamoorthy S, Meng P, Bounab R, Annane D. Immune effects of corticosteroids in sepsis. *Front Immunol.* 2018;9:1736. PMID: 30105022

28. Annane D, Bellissant E, Bollaert PE, Briegel J, Keh D, Kupfer Y. Corticosteroids for treating sepsis. *Cochrane Database Syst Rev.* 2015;12:CD002243. PMID: 26633262

29. Venkatesh B, Finfer S, Cohen J, et al; ADRENAL trial investigators and the Australian--New Zealand Intensive Care Society Trials Group. Adjunctive glucocorticoid therapy in patients with septic shock. *N Engl J Med.* 2018;378(9):797-808. PMID: 29347874

30. Annane D, Renault C, Brun-Buisson B, et al. Hydrocortisone plus fludrocortisone for adults with septic shock. *N Engl J Med.* 2018;378(9):809-818. PMID: 29490185

31. Ballard PL. Delivery and transport of glucocorticoids to target cells. *Monogr Endocrinol.* 1979;12:25-48. PMID: 386085

32. Pemberton PA, Stein PE, Pepys MB, Potter JM, Carrell RW. Hormone binding globulins undergo serpin conformational change in inflammation. *Nature.* 1988;336(6196):257-258. PMID: 314075

33. Nenke MA, Rankin W, Chapman MJ, et al. Depletion of high-affinity corticosteroid-binding globulin corresponds to illness severity in sepsis and septic shock: clinical implications. *Clin Endocrinol (Oxf).* 2015;82(6):801-807. PMID: 25409953

34. Meyer EJ, Nenke MA, Rankin W, et al. Total and high affinity corticosteroid-binding globulin depletion in septic shock is associated with mortality. *Clin Endocrinol (Oxf).* 2019;90(1):232-240. PMID: 30160799

35. Pastores SM, Annane D, Rochwerg B; Corticosteroid Guideline Task Force of SCCM and ESICM. Guuidelines for the diagnosis and management of critical illness related corticosteroid insufficiency (CIRCI) in critically ill patients (Part II): Society of Critical Care Medicine (SCCM) and European Society of Intensive Care Medicine (ESICM) 2017. 2018;46(1):146-148. PMID: 29095205

36. Annane D. Why my steroid trials in septic shock were "positive." *Crit Care Med.* 2019;47(12):1789-1793. PMID: 31259754

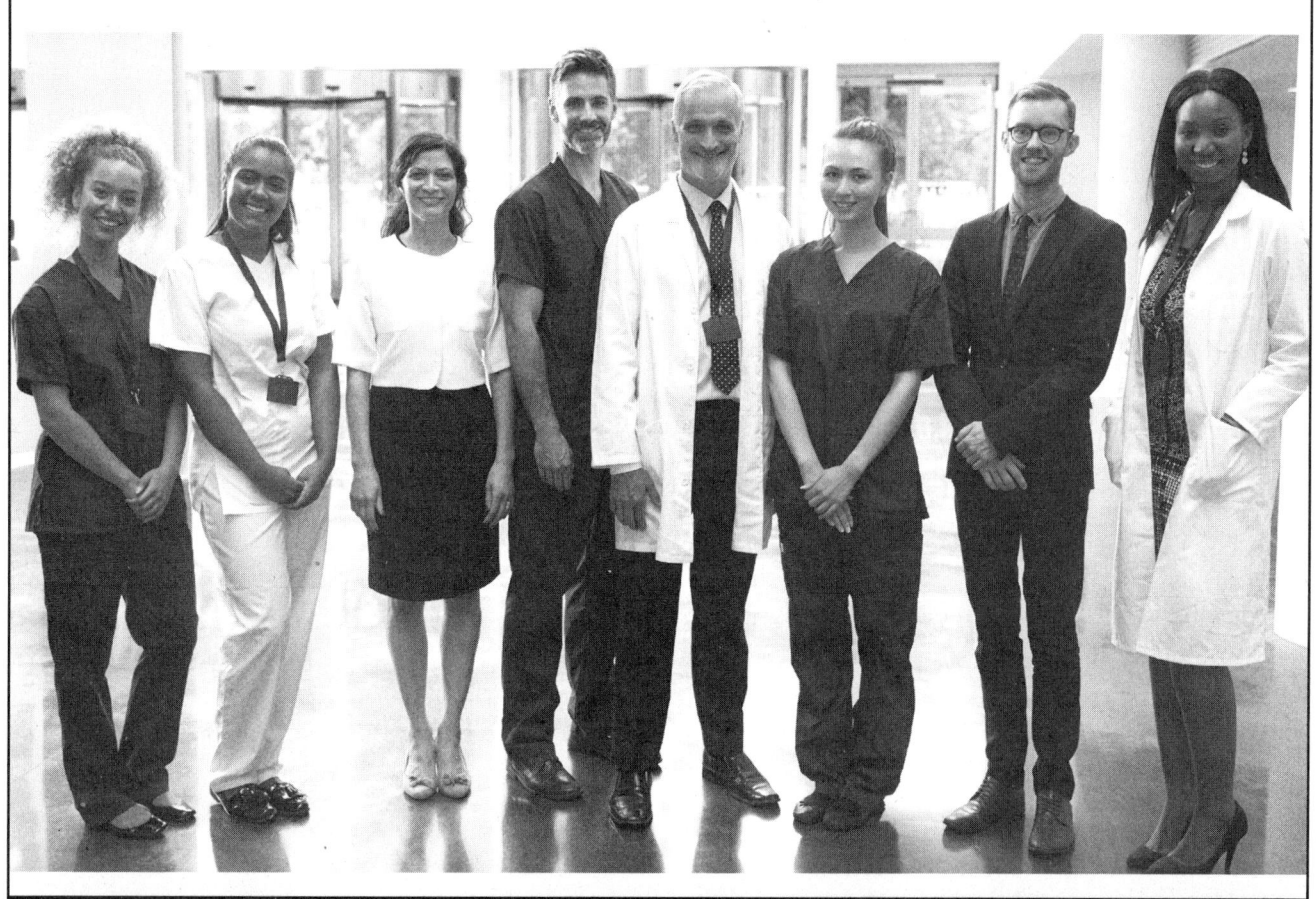

BONE AND MINERAL METABOLISM

Evaluation of the Patient With Hypophosphatemia

Peter J. Tebben, MD. Division of Endocrinology, Diabetes, Metabolism, and Nutrition, Department of Internal Medicine and Department of Pediatrics and Adolescent Medicine, Mayo Clinic, Rochester, MN; E-mail: tebben.peter@mayo.edu

Learning Objectives

As a result of participating in this session, learners should be able to:

- Identify clinical manifestations of acute and chronic hypophosphatemia.

- Explain phosphate homeostasis and identify an approach for evaluation of patients with hypophosphatemia.

- Describe therapeutic options for the management of various causes of hypophosphatemia.

Main Conclusions

- Measure serum phosphate and apply the age-appropriate reference range when evaluating patients with unexplained musculoskeletal complaints.

- History and limited laboratory evaluation can establish the underlying etiology of hypophosphatemia.

- Treatment for hypophosphatemia due to poor intake or malabsorption includes phosphate supplementation, dietary changes, and/or treatment of underlying malabsorption disorders.

- Treatment options for hypophosphatemia due to renal phosphate wasting includes active vitamin D and phosphorus replacement or anti-fibroblast growth factor 23 antibody therapy for those with X-linked hypophosphatemic rickets.

- Patients treated with active vitamin D and phosphorus require close monitoring to avoid complications of therapy including secondary/tertiary hyperparathyroidism and nephrocalcinosis/nephrolithiasis.

Significance of the Clinical Problem

Hypophosphatemia is a common clinical abnormality identified in hospitalized patients and has been associated with poor outcomes.[1] Chronic hypophosphatemia is less common and requires a systematic approach to determine the underlying etiology and formulate an effective treatment plan. The biological role of phosphorus is diverse, and it is essential for the proper function of a multitude of systems, including having a critical role in skeletal mineralization.[2] Disorders that lead to chronic hypophosphatemia are associated with abnormal mineralization and manifest as rickets in children or osteomalacia in adults.[3,4]

Symptoms of acute hypophosphatemia can be nonspecific and generally reflect the severity and acuity of the decline of the serum phosphate concentration.[5] Muscle weakness and fatigue are common symptoms, particularly in those with acquired hypophosphatemia. Cardiac and respiratory dysfunction, as well as rhabdomyolysis and hemolysis, may occur with severe, acute hypophosphatemia.[5] However, patients with chronic hypophosphatemia due to heritable causes such as X-linked hypophosphatemic rickets (XLH) generally do not experience these severe symptoms and typically present with skeletal manifestations of rickets and osteomalacia. Serum phosphorus is an important mineral that is frequently overlooked in the evaluation of patients with musculoskeletal complaints, which can lead to significant delays in diagnosis and treatment.[6,7]

Barriers to Optimal Practice

- Symptoms of hypophosphatemia can be nonspecific and serum phosphate concentrations are not part of routine chemistry panels. Therefore, the diagnosis of hypophosphatemic conditions may go unrecognized or delayed.

- Serum phosphate concentrations are significantly higher in infants and younger children than in adults. As a result, hypophosphatemia may be overlooked if the adult reference range is applied to the pediatric population.

- Understanding the goals and potential adverse effects of therapy for chronic hypophosphatemia are not always appreciated and can lead to adverse outcomes.

Strategies for Diagnosis, Therapy, and/or Management

The majority of total body phosphate is found in the skeleton, with the remainder distributed in other tissues and the extracellular space. Many factors affect intestinal absorption and renal reabsorption of phosphorus that influence concentrations measured in the in the blood (*Figure 1*). The major hormones involved in phosphate homeostasis include $1\alpha\text{-}25(OH)_2D_3$ and PTH. However, phosphaturic peptides such as fibroblast growth factor 23 (FGF-23) also have an important role in disorders of phosphate metabolism and this has provided a target for

Figure 1. Major Factors in Phosphate Homeostasis

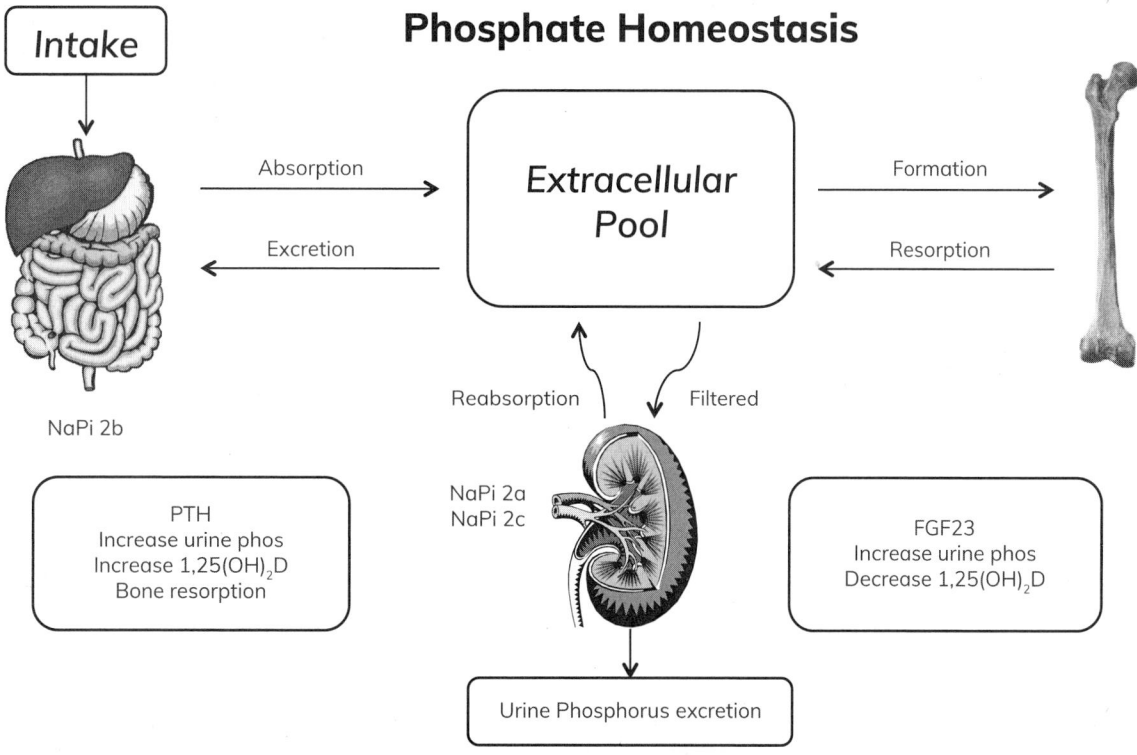

therapeutic intervention in patients with excess FGF-23 due to XLH.[8-12]

Hypophosphatemia is defined as a serum phosphate concentration below the lower end of normal and is dependent on age. The normal range of serum phosphate in adults is approximately 2.5 to 4.5 mg/dL (0.8-1.5 mmol/L). Infants and children have significantly higher serum phosphate concentrations than adults. It is imperative to use the appropriate reference range in this younger population or the diagnosis of hypophosphatemia may be overlooked.

Hypophosphatemia can be divided into 3 main categories (*Table*):

1. Decreased intake and/or malabsorption
2. Redistribution within the body
3. Renal phosphate wasting

   - FGF-23 mediated
   - Non–FGF-23 mediated

      □ Hyperparathyroidism
      □ Other

These 3 categories provide a useful framework for evaluation and management of patients with hypophosphatemia (*Figure 2*).

Decreased Intake and/or Malabsorption

Intestinal absorption of phosphorus is largely dependent on the amount of phosphorus consumed. Absorption takes place primarily in the proximal small bowel with both active and passive mechanisms.[13] Decreased intake or malabsorption should be considered in patients with primary malabsorption disorders such as inflammatory bowel disease or short gut syndrome. In addition, patients receiving phosphate binders such as calcium, sevelamer, or lanthanum carbonate can develop hypophosphatemia due to reduced intestinal phosphate availability. Metabolic bone disease (fractures and/or rickets) has been identified in some children receiving an elemental-based infant and child formula thought to be related to low phosphate bioavailability.[14,15]

Table. Conditions Associated with Hypophosphatemia

Low Intake or Impaired Absorption	Redistribution	Renal Phosphate Wasting

Low phosphate intake
Vitamin D deficiency
• Nutritional
• 1α-hydroxylase deficiency
• Vitamin D receptor pathogenic variant
Malabsorption
• Inflammatory bowel disease
• Short bowel syndrome
• Chronic diarrhea
Phosphate binders
• Calcium
• Sevelamer
• Lanthanum carbonate
	• Insulin therapy for diabetic ketoacidosis
	• Refeeding syndrome
	• Acute respiratory alkalosis
	• Hungry bone syndrome
		PTH mediated
		• Hyperparathyroidism
		• Vitamin D deficiency
		  □ Nutritional
		  □ 1α-hydroxylase deficiency
		  □ Vitamin D receptor pathogenic variant
		FGF-23 mediated
		• X-linked hypophosphatemic rickets
		• Autosomal dominant hypophosphatemic rickets
		• Fibrous dysplasia
		• Tumor-induced osteomalacia
		• Iron infusions
		• DMP1 pathogenic variant
		• ENPP1 pathogenic variant
		Non–FGF-23 mediated
		• Renal Fanconi syndrome
		• Renal sodium-phosphate cotransporter pathogenic variant

Laboratory Assessment

Figure 2 outlines an approach to the clinical investigation of patients with hypophosphatemia. Most patients can be categorized based on widely available tests, including measurement of serum calcium, phosphate, PTH, creatinine, and vitamin D metabolites. Urinary calcium, phosphate, and creatinine should also be measured. Low urine phosphate with a low fractional excretion of phosphate (less than 5%) is a hallmark of hypophosphatemia caused by inadequate intake or malabsorption. Elevated $1\alpha,25(OH)_2D_3$ concentration is also expected in this category of patients.

Treatment

Treatment for this group of patients is primarily directed at identification and correction of the underlying pathology. If dietary restriction or phosphate binders are the culprit, adjusting the diet or reducing/discontinuing phosphate binders will resolve the hypophosphatemia. Patients with malabsorption due to severe inflammatory bowel disease or short bowel syndrome may require phosphate supplementation if the underlying gastrointestinal pathology cannot be fully corrected. Caution must be exercised in this group, and a low initial dose of phosphorus should be used to avoid worsening gastrointestinal symptoms. Stomach upset and diarrhea are the most common adverse effects of phosphate supplementation.

Redistribution

Hypophosphatemia due to redistribution is typically apparent based on history alone and generally does not require extensive evaluation to establish the etiology. Diabetic ketoacidosis (DKA) and severe malnutrition are states of whole-body

Figure 2. Algorithm for Evaluation of Patients With Hypophosphatemia

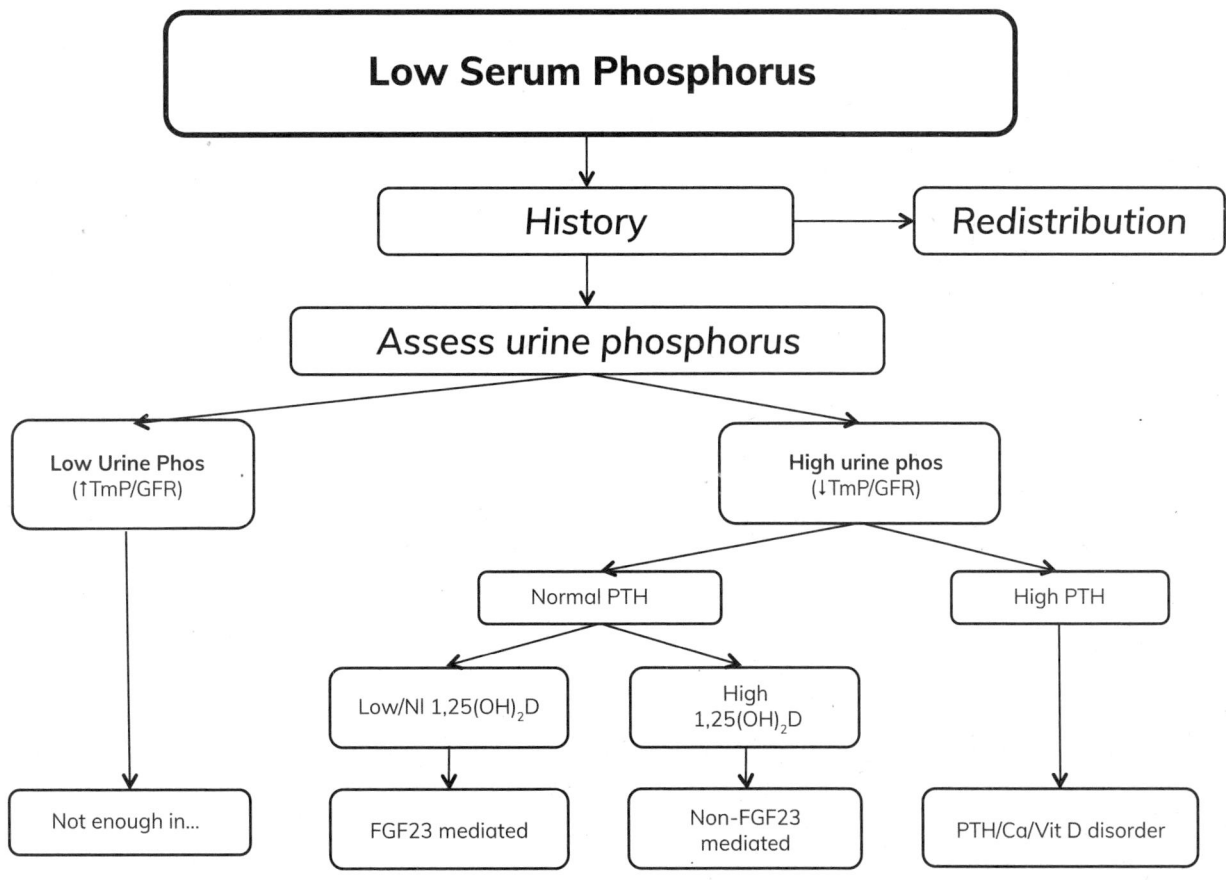

phosphate depletion. Serum phosphate is often normal before initiation of treatment for these conditions. However, when insulin is administered to patients with DKA or when feeding is introduced in malnourished patients, cellular uptake of phosphorus ensues, causing hypophosphatemia that is sometimes severe.

Hungry bone syndrome is a consequence of calcium and phosphate uptake into bone following surgery for primary hyperparathyroidism. Although most patients do not experience hungry bone syndrome following parathyroidectomy, larger parathyroid adenoma volume, higher alkaline phosphatase, and older age are risk factors for this condition.[16]

Acute respiratory alkalosis can cause transient hypophosphatemia due to transcellular shifts, is self-limited, and does not require phosphate replacement therapy.

Laboratory Assessment

Limited laboratory testing is needed to establish the cause of hypophosphatemia due to redistribution. However, management of these patients may require more extensive laboratory monitoring. In addition to hypophosphatemia, refeeding syndrome and treatment of DKA are associated with other electrolyte abnormalities that require monitoring and replacement. Vitamin D status should be evaluated in all malnourished patients. Patients with hungry bone syndrome require close monitoring of serum calcium, phosphate, and magnesium, as well as assessment for vitamin D deficiency.

Treatment

Patients with severe malnutrition require a team experienced with refeeding syndrome to identify those at risk and to implement strategies to minimize the ensuing electrolyte disturbances. Correction of baseline electrolyte abnormalities before initiating the refeeding process is recommended.[17] Oral phosphate replacement is preferred when tolerated. Intravenous phosphate replacement is reserved for patients with severe symptomatic hypophosphatemia. If intravenous phosphate is required, serum calcium must be closely monitored due to the risk of hypocalcemia.

Although hypophosphatemia occurring with treatment of DKA can be severe, it is not clear that replacement improves outcomes.[18] Despite this, many DKA protocols include potassium phosphate in the intravenous fluid therapy.

Treatment of hungry bone syndrome is focused primarily on correction of hypocalcemia. Active vitamin D metabolites can be helpful not only to address hypocalcemia, but they also have a salutary effect on serum phosphate concentration via increased intestinal absorption. Phosphorus administration will exacerbate hypocalcemia and should only be considered in patients with severe hypophosphatemia.

Renal Phosphate Wasting

Renal phosphate wasting is caused by a wide variety of conditions (*Table*). These disorders can be further divided into FGF-23–mediated and non–FGF-23–mediated disease. Renal reabsorption of phosphorus is sodium-dependent and is mediated by sodium-phosphate cotransporters (NaPi IIa and NaPi IIc).[19,20] PTH and FGF-23 both inhibit renal phosphate reabsorption via reduced sodium-phosphate transporter abundance in the proximal tubule.[20]

Vitamin D deficiency can lead to hypophosphatemia via 2 mechanisms: decreased intestinal absorption and increased urinary output due to the phosphaturic effect of secondary hyperparathyroidism that often ensues in a state of vitamin D deficiency.

Laboratory Assessment

Measurement of serum calcium, phosphate, PTH, creatinine, and vitamin D metabolites, as well as urinary calcium, phosphate, and creatinine narrows the differential diagnosis substantially. Although FGF-23 concentrations can be measured, the assay is clinically available in a limited number of reference laboratories. However, patients with hypophosphatemia due to renal phosphate wasting have characteristic biochemical patterns that distinguish

FGF-23–mediated from non–FGF-23–mediated disease:

- FGF-23 mediated:

  □ Normal serum calcium

  □ Normal or low urinary calcium

  □ Low or inappropriately normal $1\alpha,25(OH)_2D_3$

- Non–FGF-23 mediated

  □ Normal or elevated serum calcium

  □ Elevated $1\alpha,25(OH)_2D_3$

  □ Hypercalciuria

Treatment

FGF-23–Mediated Disease

Optimal treatment for patients with tumor-induced osteomalacia includes identification of the offending tumor and surgical removal. Tumors are notoriously difficult to locate and often require extensive advanced whole-body imaging techniques.[6] After surgical intervention, patients with tumor-induced osteomalacia require ongoing monitoring for recurrence. When tumor location is elusive or not resectable, calcitriol and phosphate supplementation is required. Although not part of usual treatment, improved phosphate balance with use of the calcimimetic agent cinacalcet has been described in small numbers of patients with FGF-23–mediated disease (tumor-induced osteomalacia and XLH).[21-23] The presumed mechanism is reduced PTH-mediated phosphaturia.

Until recently, the most effective treatment for XLH was calcitriol and phosphate supplementation. Phosphate must be given in 3 to 5 divided doses. Calcitriol can be given daily or twice daily. More recently, anti-FGF-23 antibody therapy (burosumab) has become available and has reduced the treatment burden. Treatment goals in children with XLH include improvement in rickets (radiographic and biochemical), improved linear growth, straightening of legs, and avoidance of complications due to therapy. In adults, treatment goals include healing of osteomalacia, reduced bone pain, and healing/prevention of fractures. It should be noted that not all adults with XLH require pharmacologic intervention.

Treatment with calcitriol and phosphate supplementation requires vigilant monitoring to avoid complications such as secondary/tertiary hyperparathyroidism, hypercalciuria, nephrocalcinosis, and nephrolithiasis. A comprehensive review of conventional therapy for patients with XLH has previously been published.[24]

Burosumab treatment results in reduced renal phosphate wasting and increased $1\alpha,25(OH)_2D_3$ concentrations. Burosumab is given as a subcutaneous injection every 2 weeks in children and every 4 weeks in adults and improves radiographic changes of rickets in children and improves healing of fractures in adults.[11,25] Monitoring of serum phosphate is recommended with the dosage adjusted to maintain serum phosphate within the age-appropriate reference range. Burosumab has not been approved for treatment of other FGF-23–mediated conditions.

PTH-Mediated Disease

Treatment of primary hyperparathyroidism is surgical. Secondary hyperparathyroidism is most commonly caused by vitamin D and or calcium deficiency. Treatment is focused on replacement of vitamin D and optimizing calcium intake, which will lead to correction of the secondary hyperparathyroidism and restoration of phosphate balance. Secondary hyperparathyroidism related to genetic abnormalities in vitamin D production (1α-hydroxylase deficiency) or action (vitamin D receptor pathogenic variant) is rare. 1α-Hydroxylase deficiency is treated with active vitamin D metabolites and calcium. Therapy in patients with a vitamin D receptor pathogenic variant is more challenging and requires high-dosage calcium supplementation.

Other

Patients with renal Fanconi syndrome or the rare patient with a sodium-phosphate cotransporter defect are treated with phosphate supplementation. Because these are not FGF-23–mediated conditions, calcitriol is not indicated as it would worsen the hypercalciuria and lead to nephrocalcinosis and nephrolithiasis.

Clinical Case Vignettes

Case 1

A 21-year-old woman with XLH presents for evaluation of recent-onset hypercalcemia. She was diagnosed with XLH at age 2 years based on typical radiographic findings and laboratory abnormalities. She had been treated with calcitriol, 0.5 mcg twice daily, and phosphorus, 5 g daily in divided doses. She presented to her local emergency department with a chief concern of abdominal pain. Laboratory studies at that time identified hypercalcemia (13.2 mg/dL [3.3 mmol/L]) with an elevated PTH concentration. Calcitriol and phosphorus supplements were discontinued and furosemide was initiated. Her medical history is notable for nephrolithiasis with nephrocalcinosis and abscessed teeth. Her laboratory studies 1 month after discontinuation of phosphorus and calcitriol are shown:

> Calcium = 11.2 mg/dL (8.2-10.2 mg/dL)
>   (SI: 2.8 mmol/L [2.1-2.6 mmol/L])
> Phosphate = 2.2 mg/dL (2.5-4.5 mg/dL)
>   (SI: 0.7 mmol/L [0.8-1.5 mmol/L])
> Creatinine = 0.8 mg/dL (0.6-1.1 mg/dL)
>   (SI: 70.2 μmol/L [53.0-97.2 μmol/L])
> 25-Hydroxyvitamin D = 35 ng/mL (30-80 ng/mL
>   [optimal]) (SI: 87.4 nmol/L [74.9-199.7 nmol/L])
> 1,25-Dihydroxyvitamin D = 46 pg/mL (16-65 pg/mL)
>   (SI: 119.6 pmol/L [41.6-169.0 pmol/L])
> Bone-specific alkaline phosphatase = 13 μg/L
>   (<22 μg/L)
> PTH = 244 pg/mL (10-65 pg/mL) (SI: 244 ng/L
>   [10-65 ng/L])
> Urinary calcium = 380 mg/24 h (100-300 mg/24 h)
>   (SI: 9.5 mmol/d [2.5-7.5 mmol/d])

Which of the following is the best initial management?

A. Restart phosphorus supplementation to correct the hypophosphatemia and reduce serum calcium

B. Continue furosemide to prevent worsening hypercalcemia

C. Order genetic testing for multiple endocrine neoplasia given her hyperparathyroidism at a young age

D. Consult a parathyroid surgeon

Answer: D) Consult a parathyroid surgeon

This patient has developed tertiary hyperparathyroidism as a result of overzealous phosphate supplementation. Hyperparathyroidism from any cause will worsen the renal phosphate wasting and contribute to hypophosphatemia. Surgery is therefore indicated (Answer D). Restarting phosphorus supplementation before addressing her hyperparathyroidism (Answer A) would only exacerbate the hyperparathyroidism. Furosemide (Answer B) should only be used transiently in treating severe hypercalcemia and would be inappropriate for long-term treatment. In addition, a loop diuretic would worsen her hypercalciuria and nephrocalcinosis.

Case 1 (Continued)

The patient's calcium and PTH concentrations normalize after 3 and 1/2 gland parathyroidectomy. She has completed linear growth, has no recent fractures, and has no bone pain.

Which of the following would be the best treatment of her XLH?

A. Resume phosphate and calcitriol therapy

B. Start burosumab, 1 mg/kg every 4 weeks

C. Observe without specific bone targeted therapy

Answer: A, B, or C) Resume phosphate and calcitriol therapy, or start burosumab, 1 mg/kg every 4 weeks, or observe without specific bone targeted therapy

All 3 options could be considered. Not all adults with XLH are symptomatic and therefore not all require pharmacologic intervention. After linear growth is completed, it is difficult to predict which patients will benefit from ongoing therapy. Significant clinical variability exists even within the same family.

Case 1 (Continued)

The patient elects to remain off therapy due to previous adverse effects and lack of symptoms of hypophosphatemia or osteomalacia. She returns to clinic 2 years later with multiple fractures after a fall on ice. She develops 2 abscessed teeth and mild pain related to enthesopathy and osteoarthritis in her hips. Radiographs identify pseudofractures in both femurs. She elects to reinitiate treatment with burosumab.

Which of the following is expected to occur as a result of therapy with anti-FGF-23 antibody treatment (burosumab)?

A. Reduced bone pain and healing of her pseudofractures

B. Improvement in pain related to osteoarthritis

C. Improvement in pain related to enthesopathy

D. Reduction in frequency of abscessed teeth

Answer: A) Reduced bone pain and healing of her pseudofractures

A reasonable expectation from treatment with anti-FGF-23 antibody therapy (or conventional therapy) includes healing of pseudofractures and reduced bone pain related to osteomalacia (Answer A). Currently, there is no evidence that anti-FGF-23 antibody therapy improves pain associated with osteoarthritis (Answer B) or enthesopathy (Answer C) or reduces the frequency of dental abscess (Answer D). In one randomized controlled trial, burosumab-treated children with XLH developed dental abscess more frequently than those treated with conventional therapy.[26]

Case 2

A 40-year-old man presents for evaluation of progressive pelvic, lower-extremity, back, and rib pain. Imaging identifies several rib fractures and stress fractures of his pelvis and bilateral femur. Bone density assessment reveals T-scores in the osteoporosis range. He is of average height and weight with no lower-extremity deformity. Examination findings are notable for an antalgic gait, muscle weakness, and a 2.5×3-cm firm lesion at the base of his neck on his left shoulder. He has no family history of bone disorders. His medications include calcium, 500 mg once daily; vitamin D, 5000 IU once daily; and over-the-counter pain medication.

Initial laboratory test results:

> Calcium = 9.7 mg/dL (8.2-10.2 mg/dL)
> (SI: 2.4 mmol/L [2.1-2.6 mmol/L])
> Creatinine = 0.9 mg/dL (0.7-1.3 mg/dL)
> (SI: 79.6 μmol/L [53.0-97.2 μmol/L])
> 25-Hydroxyvitamin D = 69 ng/mL
> (30-80 ng/mL [optimal]) (SI: 172.2 nmol/L
> [74.9-199.7 nmol/L])
> Phosphate = 1.8 mg/dL (2.5-4.5 mg/dL)
> (SI: 0.6 mmol/L [0.8-1.5 mmol/L])
> Bone-specific alkaline phosphatase = 2-fold upper
> normal limit
> PTH = 69 pg/mL (10-65 pg/mL) (SI: 69 ng/L
> [10-65 ng/L])

Which of the following is the best next step in this patient's evaluation and management?

A. Initiate alendronate, 70 mg once weekly, to treat his low bone density and fractures

B. Refer to medical genetics to assess for heritable hypophosphatemic disorders

C. Obtain urine studies to assess tubular reabsorption of phosphorus

D. Perform parathyroid scan due to possible eucalcemic primary hyperparathyroidism

E. Schedule a tetracycline-labeled bone biopsy

Answer: C) Obtain urine studies to assess tubular reabsorption of phosphorus

This patient has clinical and biochemical evidence of osteomalacia with low serum phosphate, fractures, and elevated alkaline phosphatase. His low bone density is related to osteomalacia and not osteoporosis. Assessing urine phosphate status (Answer C) is the most important next step in identifying the underlying cause of his hypophosphatemia. The mild elevation in PTH with normal serum calcium would not be expected to result in this degree of hypophosphatemia and alkaline phosphatase elevation.

Case 2 (Continued)

His fractional excretion of phosphorus is inappropriately elevated. Urinalysis does not reveal excess protein or glucose. You suspect an FGF-23–mediated process such as tumor-induced osteomalacia.

Which of the following laboratory parameters is most consistent with hypophosphatemia due to elevated FGF-23?

A. Elevated 1,25-dihydroxyvitamin D

B. High urinary calcium

C. Low 1,25-dihydroxyvitamin D

D. Elevated serum creatinine

Answer: C) Low 1,25-dihydroxyvitamin D

FGF-23 not only reduces renal phosphate reabsorption but also inhibits 1α-hydroxylase activity. This results in low or inappropriately normal 1,25-dihydroxyvitamin D concentrations (Answer C). Elevated 1,25-dihydroxyvitamin D (Answer A) and hypercalciuria (Answer B) is seen in non-FGF23–mediated renal phosphate wasting disorders. Elevated creatinine (Answer D) due to chronic kidney disease is associated with elevated FGF-23; however, chronic kidney disease leads to hyperphosphatemia, not hypophosphatemia.

Case 2 (Continued)

This patient's history and laboratory studies are consistent with the diagnosis of tumor-induced osteomalacia.

Which of the following is the best next step in this patient's management?

A. Initiate treatment with calcitriol and phosphorus supplementation

B. Start anti-FGF-23 antibody therapy (burosumab) and monitor serum phosphate concentration

C. Perform whole-body imaging such as FDG-PET or ^{68}Ga DOTATATE PET scan

D. Perform biopsy of skin lesion at the base of his neck

Answer: D) Perform biopsy of skin lesion at the base of his neck

Lesions causing tumor-induced osteomalacia are notoriously difficult to locate and can occur in nearly any part of the body. Cutaneous lesions causing tumor-induced osteomalacia have been described, and this patient has such a lesion at the base of his neck. Biopsy of the lesion (Answer D) is the best next step. Excision of this lesion was not only diagnostic but also therapeutic. Calcitriol and phosphate (Answer A) can be used in patients for whom the tumor is not identified or not resectable. Anti-FGF-23 antibody therapy (Answer B) is not approved for treatment of tumor-induced osteomalacia. If the cutaneous lesion was not the offending tumor or if metastatic disease was suspected, whole-body imaging (Answer C) would be appropriate.

Case 2 (Continued)

The offending tumor was identified and removed, which led to correction of his serum phosphate, alkaline phosphatase, and osteomalacia.

Regarding follow-up, which of the following is the best recommendation?

A. Return to clinic if symptoms recur

B. Periodic serum phosphate measurement

C. Annual whole-body imaging with FDG-PET or ^{68}Ga DOTATATE PET scan

D. No follow-up is required after surgical cure

Answer: B) Periodic serum phosphate measurement

Patients with tumor-induced osteomalacia should be monitored proactively after apparent surgical cure. The best recommendation is periodic serum phosphate measurement (Answer B). When disease recurs, it is frequently local, but it may also be found at distant sites if malignant transformation with metastases occurs. Several years after his initial surgery, this patient developed recurrence of hypophosphatemia with sarcomatous transformation and metastases. Hypophosphatemia is often present before symptoms occur or osteomalacia develops. It would therefore be inappropriate to only reassess if symptoms recur.

References

1. Brunelli SM, Goldfarb S. Hypophosphatemia: clinical consequences and management. *J Am Soc Nephrol.* 2007;18(7):1999-2003. PMID: 17568018

2. Neuman WF. Bone material and calcification mechanisms. In: Urist MR, ed. *Fundamental and Clinical Bone Physiology.* Philadelphia, PA: Lippincott; 1980:83-107.

3. Berry JL, Davies M, Mee AP. Vitamin D metabolism, rickets, and osteomalacia. Semin Musculoskelet Radiol. 2002;6(3):173-182. PMID: 12541194

4. Econs MJ, McEnery PT. Autosomal dominant hypophosphatemic rickets/osteomalacia: clinical characterization of a novel renal phosphate-wasting disorder. *J Clin Endocrinol Metab.* 1997;82(2):674-681. PMID: 9024275

5. Imel EA, Econs MJ. Approach to the hypophosphatemic patient. *J Clin Endocrinol Metab.* 2012;97(3):696-706. PMID: 22392950

6. Boland JM, Tebben PJ, Folpe AL. Phosphaturic mesenchymal tumors: what an endocrinologist should know. *J Endocrinol Invest.* 2018;41(10):1173-1184. PMID: 29446010

7. Hodgson SF, Clarke BL, Tebben PJ, Mullan BP, Cooney WP 3rd, Shives TC. Oncogenic osteomalacia: localization of underlying peripheral mesenchymal tumors with use of Tc 99m sestamibi scintigraphy. *Endocr Pract.* 2006;12(1):35-42. PMID: 16524861

8. Imel EA, Econs MJ. Fibroblast growth factor 23: roles in health and disease. *J Am Soc Nephrol.* 2005;16(9):2565-2575. PMID: 16033853

9. Schiavi SC, Kumar R. The phosphatonin pathway: new insights in phosphate homeostasis. Kidney Int. 2004;65(1):1-14. PMID: 14675031

10. Berndt TJ, Schiavi S, Kumar R. "Phosphatonins" and the regulation of phosphorus homeostasis. *Am J Physiol Renal Physiol.* 2005;289(6):F1170-F1182. PMID: 16275744

11. Carpenter TO, Whyte MP, Imel EA, et al. Burosumab therapy in children with X-linked hypophosphatemia. *N Engl J Med.* 2018;378(21):1987-1998. PMID: 29791829

12. Insogna KL, Briot K, Imel EA, et al; AXLES 1 Investigators. A randomized, double-blind, placebo-controlled, phase 3 trial evaluating the efficacy of burosumab, an anti-FGF23 antibody, in adults with X-linked hypophosphatemia: week 24 primary analysis. *J Bone Miner Res.* 2018;33(8):1383-1393. PMID: 29947083

13. Hernando N, Wagner CA. Mechanisms and regulation of intestinal phosphate absorption. Compr Physiol. 2018;8(3):1065-1090. PMID: 29978897

14. Creo AL, Epp LM, Buchholtz JA, Tebben PJ. Prevalence of metabolic bone disease in tube-fed children receiving elemental formula. *Horm Res Paediatr.* 2018;90(5):291-298. PMID: 30497080

15. Gonzalez Ballesteros LF, Ma NS, Gordon RJ, et al. Unexpected widespread hypophosphatemia and bone disease associated with elemental formula use in infants and children. *Bone.* 2017;97:287-292. PMID: 28167344

16. Brasier AR, Nussbaum SR. Hungry bone syndrome: clinical and biochemical predictors of its occurrence after parathyroid surgery. *Am J Med.* 1988;84(4):654-660. PMID: 2400660

17. Boateng AA, Sriram K, Meguid MM, Crook M. Refeeding syndrome: treatment considerations based on collective analysis of literature case reports. *Nutrition.* 2010;26(2):156-167. PMID: 20122539

18. Fisher JN, Kitabchi AE. A randomized study of phosphate therapy in the treatment of diabetic ketoacidosis. *J Clin Endocrinol Metab.* 1983;57(1):177-180. PMID: 6406531

19. Murer H, Hernando N, Forster I, Biber J. Molecular aspects in the regulation of renal inorganic phosphate reabsorption: the type IIa sodium/inorganic phosphate co-transporter as the key player. *Curr Opin Nephrol Hypertens.* 2001;10(5):555-561. PMID: 11496046

20. Gattineni J, Bates C, Twombley K, et al. FGF23 decreases renal NaPi-2a and NaPi-2c expression and induces hypophosphatemia in vivo predominantly via FGF receptor 1. *Am J Physiol Renal Physiol.* 2009;297(2):F282-F291. PMID: 19515808

21. Geller JL, Khosravi A, Kelly MH, Riminucci M, Adams JS, Collins MT. Cinacalcet in the management of tumor-induced osteomalacia. *J Bone Miner Res.* 2007;22(6):931-937. PMID: 17352646

22. Alon US, Levy-Olomucki R, Moore WV, Stubbs J, Liu S, Quarles LD. Calcimimetics as an adjuvant treatment for familial hypophosphatemic rickets. *Clin J Am Soc Nephrol.* 2008;3(3):658-664. PMID: 18256372

23. Yavropoulou MP, Kotsa K, Gotzamani Psarrakou A, et al. Cinacalcet in hyperparathyroidism secondary to X-linked hypophosphatemic rickets: case report and brief literature review. *Hormones (Athens).* 2010;9(3):274-278. PMID: 20688626

24. Carpenter TO, Imel EA, Holm IA, Jan de Beur SM, Insogna KL. A clinician's guide to X-linked hypophosphatemia [*J Bone Miner Res.* 2015;30(2):394]. *J Bone Miner Res.* 2011;26(7):1381-1388. PMID: 21538511

25. Portale AA, Carpenter TO, Brandi ML, et al. Continued beneficial effects of burosumab in adults with X-linked hypophosphatemia: results from a 24-week treatment continuation period after a 24-week double-blind placebo-controlled period. *Calcif Tissue Int.* 2019;105(3):271-284. PMID: 31165191

26. Imel EA, Glorieux FH, Whyte MP, et al. Burosumab versus conventional therapy in children with X-linked hypophosphataemia: a randomised, active-controlled, open-label, phase 3 trial. *Lancet.* 2019;393(10189):2416-2427. PMID: 31104833

Challenging Cases in Bone and Mineral Disease

Neil J. L. Gittoes, BSc, PhD, FRCP. Centre for Endocrinology, Diabetes and Metabolism, University of Birmingham and University Hospitals Birmingham, Birmingham, West Midlands, United Kingdom; E-mail: n.j.gittoes@bham.ac.uk

Learning Objectives

As a result of participating in this session, learners should be able to:

- Recognize key clinical and biochemical parameters signifying that a case is challenging and requires specific attention.

- Select appropriate investigations to differentially diagnose challenging cases in bone and mineral metabolism.

Main Conclusions

- Pathologies in bone and mineral metabolism are common and may require a formulaic approach, such as protocolized assessment of facture risk in osteoporosis.

- Assessment and management of rarer bone and mineral diseases, or rare events in common conditions, require a considered and individualized approach.

- Evaluation of bone and mineral metabolism disorders relies on a limited set of investigations; with clear understanding and appropriate interpretation of these, most conditions can be reliably diagnosed and managed.

Significance of the Clinical Problem

Disorders of bone and mineral include prevalent public health conditions such as osteoporosis and vitamin D deficiency, as well as ultra-rare diseases of the skeleton and mineral handling. Although most clinical presentations of these conditions are subacute and managed through outpatient pathways, acute, severe, and life-threatening presentations of mineral homeostasis also occur. Given the spectrum of prevalence and acuity of bone and mineral diseases, there is great scope for challenge to clinicians managing such patients, within endocrinology and beyond. Challenging cases may arise through difficulties in diagnosis and acute or long-term management.

Recognizing that a case is challenging is the first step to addressing that challenge. Some rare conditions in this arena have a poor evidence base, and management can be largely experiential. It is important to concentrate experience for such cases and to use clinical networks to share best practice for the benefit of patients. Rapidly expanding developments in genomics, new treatments, and technologies in bone and mineral diseases offer new challenges, as well as opportunities.[1,2]

Barriers to Optimal Practice

- Cases are often challenging because of rarity and lack of objective data and high-quality evidence. Experience is required to extrapolate information from analogous clinical situations but always using the principle of first do no harm. Individualized care can be highly variable and opinion based.

- Lack of robust discriminatory investigations may hinder diagnosis or management such as in the case of familial hypocalciuric hypercalcemia and tumor-induced osteomalacia (localization), respectively. Use of genomic techniques may be engaged later than ideal in the diagnostic odyssey.[3]

- Awareness of thresholds of intervention for treatment and rare adverse effects of commonly used drugs may be overlooked, potentially causing patient harm, such as bisphosphonate-associated atypical femoral fractures and rebound vertebral fractures with denosumab.[4]

- Lack of awareness of complexities in cases with multiple comorbidities may promote less appropriate prescribing such as inappropriate use of bisphosphonates in the setting of chronic kidney disease–mineral and bone disorder due to low bone turnover.[5]

Strategies for Diagnosis, Therapy, and/or Management

Initial assessment of patients with potential bone and mineral disorders should include a detailed history that incorporates early-life developmental milestones and clinical events. Skeletal, dental, soft-tissue, and systemic features should be explored and particular attention should be paid to family history of illnesses. Findings on physical examination may be unremarkable but in some instances they may offer subtle or even obvious clues to an underlying diagnosis. The expression of bone and mineral pathologies is not confined to musculoskeletal features but can be diverse, cutting across all major systems (eg, renal calcification as a manifestation of hypercalciuria, neuropsychiatric presentations in chronic hypoparathyroidism, and blue sclerae in some forms of osteogenesis imperfecta).

Mineral Disease

Evaluation of mineral metabolism disorders relies on a limited set of investigations and most conditions can be reliably diagnosed and managed using these. Serum calcium adjusted for albumin, phosphate, alkaline phosphatase, PTH, and 25-hydroxyvitamin D usually provide pointers to underlying disorders of mineral homeostasis. Plasma magnesium measurement and assessment of urinary calcium excretion also provide useful additional information.

Traditionally, estimating the ratio of renal clearance of calcium to that of creatinine in the fasting state has been central to distinguishing familial hypocalciuric hypercalcemia (FHH) from primary hyperparathyroidism. However, with genetic panel testing for FHH being more readily accessible, this approach can also be used to help distinguish the condition from primary hyperparathyroidism.[6]

Measurement of the active form of vitamin D, 1,25-dihydroxyvitamin D, is very rarely indicated, but it occasionally can be useful in rare conditions of extrarenal synthesis of 1,25-dihydroxyvitamin D, such as sarcoidosis. Similarly, measurement of PTHrP in serum is very rarely indicated. The utility of calcitonin measurement is confined to the diagnosis and monitoring of medullary carcinoma of the thyroid. There is no role for calcitonin measurement in the routine investigation of calcium and bone metabolism.

Bone Disease

Biochemical markers of bone turnover (resorption markers such as CTX and NTX and formation markers such as P1NP and osteocalcin) may be useful in assessing overall risk of osteoporotic fracture and accelerated bone loss and in judging response to treatments for osteoporosis and hence poor adherence to therapy. However, the clinical utility of *routine* measurements of bone turnover markers is yet to be established.

Bone imaging using basic skeletal radiology is still useful to detect fractures, diagnose specific diseases such as Paget disease of bone, and identify bone dysplasias. Basic x-rays are not useful for assessing bone density, but the appearance of "osteopenia" on a plain film is an indication for a DXA scan.

Isotope bone scans are useful to characterize the entire skeleton for evidence of localized areas of bone disease, such as fractures, Paget disease, and metastases. Uptake on such imaging is not selective, however, and is not diagnostic of specific bone diseases. Therefore, further triangulation with additional clinical, biochemical, and imaging information is required to reach a diagnosis.

Measurement of bone mass using DXA scanning is a reliable measure of bone strength that allows prediction of fracture risk. It is important not to consider T-score values in isolation and use them as isolated thresholds for treatment; DXA-determined data should always be contextualized to the full fracture risk profile of the patient.

Bone biopsy is not a routine test, but it can be helpful in patients with complex metabolic bone diseases, particularly when there is unexplained osteomalacia or a need for detailed assessment of renal osteodystrophy. Bone biopsies must only be undertaken in highly specialized centers with appropriate expertise.

Clinical Case Vignettes

Case 1

A 42-year-old man presents with acute disturbance of vision bilaterally. His mood has become very low, and there has been substantial change in his personality. In the emergency department, he has hyperventilation, paraesthesia, and carpopedal spasm and is diagnosed with panic attacks. There is no relevant medical or family history, and his only medication is low-dosage aspirin and sertraline.

On physical examination, he is an anxious but well-appearing man with no features of systemic disease. Visual acuity is 6/12 on the right side and 6/6 on the left side. Visual fields show gross constriction of both fields. Fundoscopy reveals a pale optic disc on the right and a grossly swollen disc on the left. Cranial MRI shows no pathology, and cerebrospinal fluid examination documents a normal opening pressure and normal composition.

Which of the following is the most likely cause for this patient's presentation?

A. Anterior ischemic optic neuropathies

B. Hypocalcemia

C. Primary affective disorder

D. Pheochromocytoma

E. Normal pressure hydrocephalus

Answer: B) Hypocalcemia

This patient's laboratory test results were as follows:

> Serum adjusted calcium (repeated measurements) = 5.3 mg/dL (8.4-10.4 mg/dL) (SI: 1.33 mmol/L [2.10-2.60 mmol/L])
> Phosphate = 4.67 mg/dL (2.48-4.33 mg/dL) (SI: 1.51 mmol/L [0.80-1.40 mmol/L])
> Alkaline phosphatase = 159 U/L (73-330 U/L) (SI: 2.66 µkat/L [1.22-5.51 µkat/L])
> Magnesium = 1.70 mg/dL (1.82-2.55 mg/dL) (SI: 0.70 mmol/L [0.75-1.05 mmol/L])
> PTH = 2.0 pg/mL (12.0-72.0 pg/mL) (SI: 2.0 ng/L [12.0-72.0 ng/L])
> Urinary calcium = 56 mg/24 h (100-300 mg/24 h) (SI: 1.4 mmol/d [2.5-7.5 mmol/d])

Results of other investigations were normal and an autoantibody screen was negative. Chvostek and Trousseau signs were both absent and electrocardiography documented a normal QT interval. Idiopathic hypoparathyroidism was diagnosed, and the patient was treated with calcium carbonate and alfacalcidol. With correction of his serum calcium, there was a marked improvement in vision, paraesthesia, and personality traits. Fundoscopy showed full resolution of optic disc swelling. His visual fields enlarged dramatically. Sertraline was discontinued and his premorbid personality returned.

Neuropsychiatric presentations, including mood disturbance, are recognized features of hypocalcemia. There is also a rare but recognized association between hypocalcemia and papilledema. The mechanism is unclear, but it may be linked to reversible reduction in cerebrospinal fluid absorption due to hypocalcemia.

Classic signs of hypocalcemia (eg, Chvostek sign) may be absent despite significant hypocalcemia. Optimal care in hypoparathyroidism is still to be defined.[7]

Anterior ischemic optic neuropathies (Answer A) do not explain the breadth of symptoms at presentation. A primary affective disorder (Answer C) does not account for chronic changes in visual acuity and fields. Pheochromocytoma (Answer D) may have complex presentations, but persistent changes in vision make this an unlikely unifying explanation of all the presenting features. The absence of headaches in the history make normal pressure hydrocephalus (Answer E) unlikely.

Case 2

A 64-year-old woman with osteogenesis imperfecta type 4 was commenced on bisphosphonates after a low-trauma fracture of her ankle. After having received pamidronate for 3 years and zoledronic acid for 2 years, she describes a 10-month history of right lateral thigh and groin pain. She is able to bear weight with only minimal discomfort, and there is no limitation of movement. Plain radiographs demonstrate an incomplete subtrochanteric fracture of the lateral cortex of the right femur and a similar finding at the mid-diaphysis on the left femur. Nuclear medicine bone scanning with single-photon emission CT combined with CT reveals intense uptake in the regions corresponding to those identified on plain x-rays. Orthopedic opinion is that the risk of completed fractures is low, and because of the shape of the femora, nailing would be technically challenging.

DXA scan lumbar spine T-score is –2.7, and total hip T-score is –1.7.

Which of the following is the most appropriate next step in pharmacologic management?

A. Continue zoledronic acid
B. Continue calcium and vitamin D only
C. Switch to denosumab
D. Switch to romosozumab
E. Switch to teriparatide

Answer: E) Switch to teriparatide

Further bisphosphonate treatment was withheld. Teriparatide (Answer E), a bone anabolic agent, was commenced to promote fracture healing (non-licensed indication).

Osteogenesis imperfecta is typically associated with frequent fractures in childhood and adolescence. However, with age-associated decline in bone density, affected patients may enter a second period of heightened fracture risk. This patient had a genetic predisposition to fractures and was treated with bisphosphonates with an intention to ameliorate fracture risk. Paradoxically, in this case, such treatment is linked to the evolution of bilateral incomplete subtrochanteric fractures. Even in patients with unequivocally increased fracture risk (such as in osteogenesis imperfecta), close clinical scrutiny and follow-up are required when using bisphosphonates to provide individualized treatment. Careful and sequential reassessments of risks and benefits must be made when managing all patients taking bisphosphonates.

Persisting with an antiresorptive agent such as zoledronic acid (Answer A) or denosumab (Answer C) is incorrect, as such treatments exacerbate suppression of bone turnover, thought to be causally linked to atypical femoral fractures. Continuing calcium and vitamin D (Answer B) is reasonable, but given the patient's predicament of impending complete fractures, this would be regarded as rather noninterventional drug therapy. Romosozumab (Answer D) may have a role in situations such as that presented, but there are no data to support its use in this scenario. Limited data exist for teriparatide (Answer E) in this setting, but it is the most appropriate pharmacologic therapy listed.

Case 3

A 42-year-old man presents with a 3-year history of progressive pain in his feet and ankles. He describes progressive difficulty walking due to pain and muscle weakness. He has been evaluated by multiple specialists. The progressive neurogenic or myogenic weakness has affected all 4 limbs to the extent that he stopped working. Plain x-rays, MRI, and electromyelography have revealed no pathology, and routine laboratory tests have documented mildly elevated alkaline phosphatase. At today's appointment, he is severely myopathic.

Current laboratory test results:

> Alkaline phosphatase = 495 U/L (73-330) U/L
> (SI: 8.27 µkat/L [1.22-5.51 µkat/L])
> Phosphate = 1.64 mg/dL (2.48-4.33 mg/dL)
> (SI: 0.53 mmol/L [0.80-1.40 mmol/L])
> Serum adjusted calcium = 9.08 mg/dL (8.4-
> 10.4 mg/dL) (SI: 2.27 mmol/L [2.10-
> 2.60 mmol/L])
> Serum urea nitrogen = 10.9 mg/dL (9.5-21.3 mg/dL)
> (SI: 3.9 mmol/L [3.4-7.6 mmol/L])
> Creatinine = 1.00 mg/dL (0.68-1.43 mg/dL)
> (SI: 88.4 µmol/L [60-126 µmol/L])
> 25-Hydroxyvitamin D = 15 ng/mL (20-
> 68 ng/mL) (SI: 37.4 nmol/L [50-170 nmol/L])
> [15 (20-68) ng/ml]
> PTH = 68.5 pg/mL (12-65 pg/mL) (SI: 68.5 ng/L
> [12-65 ng/L])
> Urine phosphate excretion = 0.94 g/24 h
> (SI: 30.4 mmol/d)
> 1,25-Dihydroxyvitamin D = 14.6 pg/mL
> (7.7-46.2 pg/mL) (SI: 38 pmol/L [20-
> 120 pmol/L])
> FGF-23 = 251 U/L (<100 U/L)

Which of the following is the most likely diagnosis causing this patient's symptoms?

A. Secondary hyperparathyroidism

B. Tumor-induced osteomalacia

C. Vitamin D deficiency

D. Vitamin D resistance

E. X-linked hypophosphatemic rickets

Answer: B) Tumor-induced osteomalacia

This patient had little symptomatic benefit from treatment with phosphate and activated vitamin D. MRI showed a right ethmoid sinus mass that, following successful excision, histologically revealed a hemangiopericytoma. Immediately following surgery, the patient experienced a dramatic improvement in symptoms, and all biochemical parameters rapidly normalized.

Hypophosphatemic conditions are rare.[8] Tumor-induced osteomalacia (Answer B) is a potentially reversible form of such pathology that has a typical biochemical pattern. Some laboratories do not include phosphate as part of a standard blood panel, so the diagnosis can be missed and symptoms can be profound and progressive. While surgical excision of the causal tumor (usually benign and of mesenchymal origin) provides relief and full reversal of the manifestations of tumor-induced osteomalacia, localizing the tumor can be particularly challenging, although multiple imaging modalities have been explored. Medical therapy with phosphate and activated vitamin D can be effective in ameliorating symptoms, but phosphate supplements are often poorly tolerated. Surgical removal should be pursued if feasible.

The biochemical picture does not substantiate a diagnosis of secondary hyperparathyroidism (Answer A) that may be causally linked to the clinical presentation. While the 25-hydroxyvitamin D level is low, PTH is not correspondingly elevated and phosphate is disproportionately low. For the duration and degree of symptomatology, one may also expect to see x-ray bone changes consistent with osteomalacia if vitamin D deficiency (Answer C) or resistance (Answer D) were the primary cause. The biochemical picture is compatible with X-linked hypophosphatemic rickets (Answer E), but this condition typically presents clinically much earlier in life.

Case 4

A 31-year-old woman from South East Asia has been diagnosed with celiac disease. She has iron deficiency anemia with an adjusted calcium value of 8.68 mg/dL (8.4-10.4 mg/dL) (SI: 2.17 mmol/L [2.25-2.60 mmol/L]) and an alkaline phosphatase value of 1607 U/L (35-104 U/L) (SI: 26.84 μkat/L [0.58-1.74 μkat/L]) with otherwise normal liver function. She commences a gluten-free diet with ferrous sulfate and calcium/vitamin D supplementation. She next presents to an orthopedic clinic when she is 21 weeks pregnant, with a large swelling over her left proximal tibia following minor trauma 3 months previously. X-ray of the leg shows a 5 × 2-cm destructive lesion in the anterior tibia with an associated soft-tissue mass (*see left image*). MRI shows localized destruction with extension into the soft tissues. Referral is made to a specialized orthopedic oncology unit. Needle biopsy show loose fibrous tissue containing several osteoclast-type giant cells. A month later, she develops a pathologic fracture through the lesion (*see right image*).

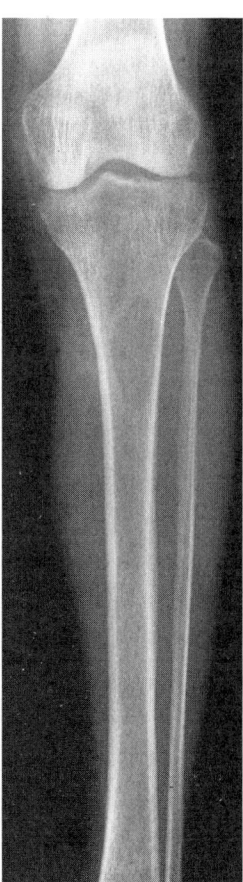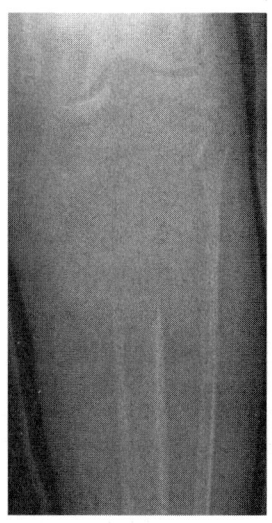

Which of the following is the most likely cause of the x-ray appearance?

A. Brown tumor

B. Aneurysmal bone cyst

C. Fibrous dysplasia

D. Giant-cell tumor

E. Simple bone cyst

Answer: A) Brown tumor

In this case, repeated investigations showed the following:

> Adjusted calcium = 7.8 mg/dL (8.4-10.4 mg/dL) (SI: 1.95 mmol/L [2.25-2.60 mmol/L])
> Alkaline phosphatase = 2011 U/L (35-104 U/L) (SI: 33.58 μkat/L [0.58-1.74 μkat/L])
> PTH = 482 pg/mL (12-65 pg/mL) (SI: 482 ng/L [12-65 ng/L])
> 25-Hydroxyvitamin D = <6 ng/mL (20-68 ng/mL) (SI: <15 nmol/L [50-170 nmol/L])

Osteomalacia with secondary hyperparathyroidism caused brown tumors (Answer A) (a contralateral lesion also developed). Vitamin D with calcium was initiated and recalcified the "bone tumors," but she had 2 cm loss of leg length. Biochemical markers returned to normal, suggesting poor prior adherence to treatment. Celiac disease and pregnancy had contributed to the severe expression of osteomalacia.

Frank osteomalacia is uncommon but is seen more frequently in developing countries throughout the world. Brown tumors are very rare pseudotumoral manifestations of hyperparathyroidism. High PTH levels (can also be seen in primary hyperparathyroidism) increase osteoclast activity and produce irregular bone resorption resulting in microfractures and hemorrhage. Microscopically, these lesions are indistinguishable from giant-cell tumors or aneurysmal bone cysts and a diagnosis of brown tumor of hyperparathyroidism is based on abnormal biochemistry. Most brown tumors due to secondary hyperparathyroidism are seen in renal osteodystrophy, and other causes are rare.

The biochemical picture provides context to the radiograph. Aneurysmal bone cyst (Answer B) or giant-cell tumor (Answer D) are within the x-ray differential diagnosis, but the biochemical tests point clearly to a metabolic origin as a brown tumor. One would not expect this degree of biochemical abnormalities in a patient with fibrous dysplasia (Answer C) or a simple bone cyst (Answer E). The rapidly progressive nature would also not support the latter 2 diagnoses. The cystic area is too large and dynamic for a simple bone cyst.

References

1. Kishnani PS, Rockman-Greenberg C, Rauch F, et al. Five-year efficacy and safety of asfotase alfa therapy for adults and adolescents with hypophosphatasia. *Bone.* 2019;121:149-162. PMID: 30576866

2. Carpenter TO, Whyte MP, Imel EA, et al. Burosumab therapy in children with X-linked hypophosphatemia. *N Engl J Med.* 2018;378(21):1987-1998. PMID: 29791829

3. Hannan FM, Newey PJ, Whyte MP, Thakker RV. Genetic approaches to metabolic bone diseases. *Br J Clin Pharmacol.* 2019;85(6):1147-1160. PMID: 30357886

4. Black DM, Abrahamsen B, Bouxsein ML, Einhorn T, Napoli N. Atypical femur fractures: review of epidemiology, relationship to bisphosphonates, prevention, and clinical management. *Endocr Rev.* 2019;40(2):333-368. PMID: 30169557

5. Damasiewicz MJ, Nickolas TL. Rethinking bone disease in kidney disease. *JBMR Plus.* 2018;2(6):309-322. PMID: 30460334

6. Hannan FM, Kallay E, Chang W, Brandi ML, Thakker RV. The calcium-sensing receptor in physiology and in calcitropic and noncalcitropic diseases. *Nat Rev Endocrinol.* 2018;15(1):33-51. PMID: 30443043

7. Mannstadt M, Bilezikian JP, Thakker RV, et al. Hypoparathyroidism. *Nat Rev Dis Primers.* 2017;3:17080. PMID: 28980621

8. Christov M, Jüppner H. Phosphate homeostasis disorders. *Best Pract Res Clin Endocrinol Metab.* 2018;32(5):685-706. PMID: 30449549

Bone Turnover Markers in the Management of Osteoporosis

Richard Eastell, MD. Department of Oncology and Metabolism, University of Sheffield, Sheffield, South Yorkshire, England; E-mail: r.eastell@sheffield.ac.uk

Learning Objectives

As a result of participating in this session, learners should be able to:

- Identify poor response to treatment using bone turnover markers.

- After stopping treatment, identify offset of effect using bone turnover markers.

Main Conclusions

Bone turnover markers (BTMs) can be measured reliably in the serum or urine and are widely available. BTMs respond rapidly and by a lot after starting the usual treatments for osteoporosis, such as bisphosphonates. The greater the response, the greater the reduction in fracture risk. The goal in the individual patient is for the change in BTMs to exceed the least significant change into the lower half (or below) of the reference interval for healthy young women.

BTMs increase after stopping bisphosphonates, but not to the levels found before starting them. An increase beyond the least significant change or to a level in the upper half (or above) of the reference range for healthy young women indicates the need to restart therapy.

Significance of the Clinical Problem

The decision to treat a patient with osteoporosis is based on their future risk of fracture and this is usually assessed based on bone mineral density (BMD), the prior occurrence of a fracture (such as spine or hip), or a high 10-year fracture risk.[1] The most commonly used drugs are oral bisphosphonates, particularly alendronate. Up to 10% of older women in the United Kingdom take alendronate. However, the adherence to the medication is poor and after 1 year of treatment, only about 50% of patients continue the drug. There is a big need to assess adherence. A working group of the International Osteoporosis Foundation and the European Calcified Tissue Society proposed that the measurement of BTMs before and then 3 months after starting treatment could be a successful strategy to identify poor drug response, most likely caused by poor adherence.[2]

After 5 years of an oral bisphosphonate such as alendronate, there is an increased risk of atypical femur fractures. A "drug holiday" at this time could be considered if the patient is at low risk of further fracture (hip BMD T-score above −2.5 and no prior spine fracture).[3] There is not a clear approach to restarting treatment, but one method to determine no further antiresorptive effect of the bisphosphonate is to measure BTMs.

Barriers to Optimal Practice

- How should clinicians provide personalized care for the individual patient to monitor treatment response? One could count the number of fractures a patient suffers, but these are uncommon events and can occur even with effective treatment. One could measure BMD, but the changes are small and slow to occur.

- How should clinicians provide personalized care for the individual patient to monitor when it is time to restart treatment? One could measure BMD, but the changes are small and slow to occur.

Strategies for Diagnosis, Therapy, and/or Management

Bone Turnover Markers

BTMs can be measured in the serum and the urine, and they can reflect bone resorption or bone formation. The bone resorption markers include degradation products of type I collagen such as serum CTX (C-telopeptide) or urinary NTX (N-telopeptide) or the enzyme tartrate resistant acid phosphatase type 5b. The bone formation markers include matrix proteins such as PINP (procollagen I N-propeptide) or osteocalcin, or the enzyme bone-specific alkaline phosphatase.

The International Osteoporosis Foundation and the International Federation of Clinical Chemistry have proposed using CTX and PINP as the reference markers.[4] When conducting research, these 2 BTMs should always be included. This does not mean that NTX, TRACP5b, osteocalcin, and bone alkaline phosphatase are not useful in clinical practice.

These BTMs are easy to measure using manual (ELISA) or automated immunoassays, and the latter method has low precision error (less than 5%) and gives consistent results. Automated immunoassays are available for most of the BTMs worldwide and are to be recommended. The only exception is that in the United States the automated assays for PINP have not been approved by the FDA.

Sources of Variability in BTMs

The most common reason for confusion in the use of BTMs is their variability.[5] BTM levels change throughout the day. For example, CTX is twice as high in the morning as in the afternoon, so it is recommended to draw the patient's blood in the fasting state, first thing in the morning.

Different reference ranges should be used based on age. Children often have BTM levels about 10-times higher than those of adults. After menopause, women's levels are about twice as high as those of premenopausal women. A recent fracture results in a large increase in BTMs with a peak after 3 months and levels not returning to normal for a year. This is particularly striking for the bone formation markers.

Drugs can affect BTMs. The most commonly encountered problem is the use of glucocorticoids. These suppress BTM, especially bone formation markers, so if the dose has been increased in the last few days BTMs would be reduced. Thus, BTMs are only helpful in patients with glucocorticoid-induced osteoporosis if the glucocorticoid dosage remains unchanged.

Clinical Uses of BTMs—Identification of Treatment Response

There is some evidence to support the idea that higher BTM levels are associated with higher rates of bone loss, greater fracture risk, the presence of secondary osteoporosis, and better response to any forms of osteoporosis treatment. However, the evidence is not strong enough for use in the individual patient.[6]

The best use of BTMs is in the identification of treatment response and in monitoring the offset of treatment.

The TRIO study was set up to evaluate the clinical utility of BTM in postmenopausal osteoporosis.[7] The study included a formal assessment of the 2 treatment targets:

1. The least significant change. This is the least change that can be considered to be significant (at $P<.05$) based on 2 measurements in an individual patient. This was estimated to be around 10 µg/L for PINP and 120 ng/L for CTX.

2. The median value for BTM in a healthy young woman. This second target is useful if there is only 1 BTM measurement documented while on treatment. If the BTM is below the premenopausal median value (or below the reference interval), then the patient is considered to have responded. These mean values are 35 µg/L for PINP and 280 ng/L for CTX.

The TRIO study included 3 commonly used oral bisphosphonates (alendronate, ibandronate, and risedronate), and the percentage of responders using least significant change in this research study at 12 weeks of treatment was around 90% for CTX and 85% for PINP. The percentage of responders using a value below the premenopausal mean in this research study at 12 weeks of treatment was around 95% for CTX and 90% for PINP. Of course, in clinical practice fewer patients respond.

Clinical Uses of BTMs— Identification of Treatment Offset of Effect

Patients taking oral bisphosphonates are recommended to stop treatment after 5 years if they are at relatively low fracture risk (BMD T-score above –2.5 at the hip and no recent fracture) to reduce the risk of atypical femur fractures. The rate of bone loss after stopping these drugs is very low, as the drugs continue to prevent bone loss for several years after stopping them, particularly in the spine. BTMs are more useful, as they reflect the way in which these drugs work.[8] An increase in BTM above the least significant change or a BTM level (off treatment) above the premenopausal median signify offset of response and therefore treatment would be recommended to restart.

Clinical Uses of BTMs—Monitoring Drugs Other Than Bisphosphonates

The principles shown here for bisphosphonates can apply to other antiresorptive drugs such as denosumab and raloxifene. The response rate will be even higher for denosumab, but lower for raloxifene, as denosumab is much more potent. Indeed, it could be argued that everyone responds to denosumab, so there is no need to monitor efficacy.[9] However, after stopping denosumab, there is a rebound increase in BTMs and the timing of the rebound might help dictate the optimal time to give a bisphosphonate to prevent accelerated bone loss.

The principles also apply to anabolic agents such as teriparatide, abaloparatide, and romosozumab. These drugs all cause an early and large increase in BTMs, particularly PINP. This marker can be measured as early as a month after treatment initiation to identify response and it should increase. An increase above the least significant change (>10 µg/L) to above the upper limit of the reference range (>65 µg/L) indicates good response.[6] There is no role for monitoring offset of effect, as all these agents should be followed by treatment with antiresorptive drugs.

Clinical Case Vignettes
Case 1

A 70-year-old woman has osteopenia noted in spinal radiographs. She is treated with alendronate, 70 mg once weekly, calcium, and vitamin D. The BMD T-score at the total hip and lumbar spine is –3. BTMs are measured at baseline and after 6 months of treatment. The patient takes alendronate for 5 years (60 months) and BTMs are measured again and then 1 year later.

Time Point	CTX	PINP
0 months	500 ng/L	60 µg/L
6 months	120 ng/L	20 µg/L
60 months	120 ng/L	20 µg/L
72 months	400 ng/L	40 µg/L

Did the patient respond to treatment? Has the treatment effect worn off?

A. She responded to treatment and the effect has worn off

B. She did not respond to treatment and the effect has not worn off

C. She responded to treatment and the effect has not worn off

D. The results cannot be interpreted as there is too much variability

Answer: A) She responded to treatment and the effect has worn off

For CTX, she responded, as she exceeded the least significant change (decrease by more than 120) and the value fell below the median for premenopausal women (280 ng/L). For PINP, she responded, as she exceeded the least significant change (decrease by more than 10) and the value fell below the median for premenopausal women (35 µg/L).

She had evidence for offset of effect for CTX, as she exceeded the least significant change (increase by more than 120) and the value increased above the median for premenopausal women (280 ng/L). She had evidence for offset of effect for PINP, as she exceeded the least significant change (increase by more than 10) and the value increased above the median for premenopausal women (35 µg/L).

She exceeds the least significant change and this takes into account any month-by-month variability, so the results can indeed be interpreted.

Case 2

An 87-year-old woman had previous fractures of the left femur, left shoulder, right wrist, and the spine (vertebrae L3, L4). She was treated with alendronate, 70 mg once weekly for 10 years, which was stopped 2 years ago. She is now receiving calcium and vitamin D alone. A vertebral fracture assessment reveals a fracture at L2, confirmed by radiographs. Workup for secondary causes of osteoporosis is negative. Her PINP concentration is 140 µg/L.

Which of the following would be the best treatment now?

A. None, just watch and wait

B. Anabolic therapy (eg, teriparatide, abaloparatide, romosozumab)

C. Restart alendronate at half the usual dosage

D. Zoledronate or denosumab

Answer: D) Zoledronate or denosumab

This patient is no longer having suppression of bone turnover from the prior alendronate therapy. She has high bone turnover and is likely to have a good BMD response to zoledronate or denosumab (Answer D).

She is at risk for further fractures, so watching and waiting (Answer A) would be a high-risk strategy. Anabolic therapy (Answer B) is not an unreasonable approach, as the BMD response to anabolic drugs is greater if BTMs are high. It is more expensive than zoledronate or denosumab, though. The use of the licensed dosage of alendronate (for osteoporosis) is not an unreasonable approach. However, low-dosage treatment (Answer C) for such high bone turnover is unlikely help this patient reach the BTM target.

References

1. Eastell R, Rosen CJ, Black DM, Cheung AM, Murad MH, Shoback D. Pharmacological management of osteoporosis in postmenopausal women: an Endocrine Society clinical practice guideline. *J Clin Endocrinol Metab.* 2019;104(5):1595-1622. PMID: 30907953

2. Diez-Perez A, Naylor KE, Abrahamsen B, et al; Adherence Working Group of the International Osteoporosis Foundation and the European Calcified Tissue Society. International Osteoporosis Foundation and European Calcified Tissue Society Working Group. Recommendations for the screening of adherence to oral bisphosphonates. *Osteoporos Int.* 2017;28(3):767-774. PMID: 28093634

3. Adler RA, El-Hajj Fuleihan G, Bauer DC, et al. Managing osteoporosis in patients on long-term bisphosphonate treatment: report of a task force

of the American Society for Bone and Mineral Research. *J Bone Miner Res.* 2016;31(1):16-35. PMID: 26350171

4. Vasikaran S, Eastell R, Bruyere O, et al; IOF-IFCC Bone Marker Standards Working Group. Markers of bone turnover for the prediction of fracture risk and monitoring of osteoporosis treatment: a need for international reference standards. *Osteoporos Int.* 2011;22(2):391-420. PMID: 21184054

5. Szulc P, Naylor K, Hoyle NR, Eastell R, Leary ET; National Bone Health Alliance Bone Turnover Marker Project. Use of CTX-I and PINP as bone turnover markers: National Bone Health Alliance recommendations to standardize sample handling and patient preparation to reduce pre-analytical variability. *Osteoporos Int.* 2017;28(9):2541-2556. PMID: 28631236

6. Eastell R, Pigott T, Gossiel F, Naylor KE, Walsh JS, Peel NFA. Diagnosis of endocrine disease: bone turnover markers: are they clinically useful? *Eur J Endocrinol.* 2018;178(1):R19-R31. PMID: 29046326

7. Naylor KE, Jacques RM, Paggiosi M, et al. Response of bone turnover markers to three oral bisphosphonate therapies in postmenopausal osteoporosis: the TRIO study. *Osteoporos Int.* 2016;27(1):21-31. PMID: 25990354

8. Kim TY, Bauer DC, McNabb BL, et al. Comparison of BMD changes and bone formation marker levels 3 years after bisphosphonate discontinuation: FLEX and HORIZON-PFT Extension I Trials. *J Bone Miner Res.* 2018;34(5):810-816. PMID: 30536713

9. Eastell R, Christiansen C, Grauer A, et al. Effects of denosumab on bone turnover markers in postmenopausal osteoporosis. *J Bone Miner Res.* 2011;26(3):530-537. PMID: 20839290

Using the Best Available Evidence to Personalize Osteoporosis Treatment

E. Michael Lewiecki, MD. University of New Mexico Health Sciences Center, Albuquerque, NM; E-mail: mlewiecki@gmail.com

Micol S. Rothman, MD. University of Colorado School of Medicine, Aurora, CO; E-mail: micol.rothman@cuanschutz.edu

Learning Objectives

As a result of participating in this session, learners should be able to:

- Recognize the variability and limitations of clinical practice guidelines for osteoporosis.

- Apply the best available medical evidence to the care of individual patients for whom guidelines may not be appropriate.

Main Conclusions

Many clinical practice guidelines address the management of patients with osteoporosis.[1-4] These are often developed by societies or organizations that address specific patient populations using divergent approaches to analyze and interpret the medical evidence, with or without consideration of cost-effectiveness, and differing views on inclusion of expert opinion. Guidelines that rely exclusively on data derived from large, randomized, placebo-controlled clinical trials are scientifically rigorous but tend to be restrictive, complex, and lacking the flexibility required to address the needs of some patients. Many or most patients seen in clinical practice would not qualify for participation in the clinical trials supporting the approval of the medications used to treat them,[5] casting into doubt the applicability of the studies for some patients. Guidelines developed by experts interpreting the best available medical evidence may be simpler, more intuitive, and easier to apply in clinical practice, but are open to criticism that they are overly subjective and based on a lower level of evidence. The application of any guideline when making decisions for individual patients must consider all available clinical information, including comorbidities, previous experiences, and patient preferences.

Significance of the Clinical Problem

Osteoporosis is a common disorder characterized by low bone density and poor bone quality resulting in increased risk of fractures. Despite the availability of excellent tools to assess fracture risk and approved medications that reduce fracture risk, most patients at risk for fractures are not being treated.[6] The large treatment gap is now recognized as a global crisis in the care of patients with osteoporosis.[7]

Barriers to Optimal Practice

Many factors contribute to the treatment gap, including fear of medication adverse effects, poor understanding of the balance of benefits and risks with treatment, inadequate communication skills to quantify risk, lack of appreciation of the potentially serious consequences of fractures, failure to recognize that a prior fracture is due to osteoporosis, reductions in reimbursement for bone density testing (United States) resulting in the closure of many office-based DXA facilities, conflicting clinical practice guidelines, limited available time for physician-patient encounters, and competing health care priorities.

Strategies for Diagnosis, Therapy, and/or Management

Accordingly, many strategies to reduce the treatment gap have been proposed,[8] including technology-enabled collaborative learning, the prototype of which is Bone Health TeleECHO.[9] Tools and algorithms have been developed to help patients and providers alike better quantify the risks and benefits of osteoporosis therapy. However, providers must recognize that there is not a "one size fits all" answer for many patients. At times, more than one visit and a variety of materials may be needed for patients to understand their diagnosis of osteoporosis and feel comfortable with initiation of medication. Clinical judgment, patient preference, and other factors are key aspects of managing complex cases of osteoporosis.

Clinical Case Vignettes

Case 1

A 62-year-old woman presents after a painful vertebral compression fracture. She has a history of chronic obstructive pulmonary disease with frequent courses of oral glucocorticoids and long-term inhaled steroids. She undergoes bone mineral density testing that shows osteopenia based on lowest T-score. Secondary workup is otherwise negative with adequate vitamin D levels and normal renal function.

Which of the following is the best option to reduce the risk of another vertebral fracture in this patient?

A. Calcium and vitamin D with no other pharmacologic agent since her DXA shows osteopenia

B. Kyphoplasty to reduce her risk of adjacent level fracture

C. Teriparatide for 18 to 24 months followed by antiresorptive therapy

D. Oral alendronate for 5 years followed by a drug holiday

Answer: C) Teriparatide for 18 to 24 months followed by antiresorptive therapy

This patient has the diagnosis of osteoporosis based on a low-trauma fracture[2] and has a very high risk for future fracture; thus, pharmacologic therapy is indicated (thus, Answer A is incorrect). There has been controversy surrounding the use of kyphoplasty (Answer B) for painful vertebral fractures. A recent American Society for Bone and Mineral Research task force advocated against routine use of vertebral augmentation for vertebral fractures based on a review of multiple trials focusing on 1-year outcomes that showed no differences in pain and disability.[10] However, the VAPOUR trial showed vertebroplasty to be superior to placebo for pain reduction in patients with fractures of less than 6 weeks duration. There was particular benefit for patients with severely painful fractures requiring high doses of pain medication and/or hospitalization (where length of stay was reduced in the treatment arm).[11] However, vertebral augmentation would not be expected to reduce the rate of adjacent level fracture. In fact, there have been concerns for an increased risk of adjacent level fracture, but at this point, this risk remains unclear.[10]

As far as the best pharmacologic option, an 18-month randomized head-to-head trial in 414 patients comparing teriparatide with alendronate in patients with glucocorticoid-induced osteoporosis showed larger gains in spine BMD (7.2% vs 3.4%), as well as lower rates of vertebral compression fracture (0.6% vs 6.1%) in the teriparatide-treated group.[12] Although oral alendronate (Answer D) is a reasonable choice if teriparatide is not financially viable, is contraindicated, or is otherwise not desired by the patient, the strongest data for secondary fracture prevention in this scenario would be for teriparatide (Answer C). Although the American College of Rheumatology guidelines would advocate for first-line alendronate based on cost, other guidelines from Europe would advocate for first-line teriparatide in a high-risk patient.[13]

Case 2

A 70-year-old man presents after treatment with denosumab for 8 years, with gains in bone density and no fractures. His estimated glomerular filtration rate is 60 mL/min per 1.73 m². DXA now shows bone mineral density in the osteopenia range. He requests to stop treatment and wants to know what medications will give him the best chance at avoiding bone loss.

Which of the following is the best advice?

A. Stop denosumab; it is time for a drug holiday since denosumab will provide lasting protection

B. Give 5 mg intravenous zoledronic acid when his next injection is due (ie, 6 months after the last denosumab dose)

C. Start oral alendronate when his next injection is due

D. Explain that this has not been studied and there is no other option than to remain on denosumab for life

Answer: C) Start oral alendronate when his next injection is due

There has been much recent discussion of how and when to stop/bridge of denosumab if needed/desired. First, it must be emphasized that there is *no role for a drug holiday* with denosumab (thus, Answer A is incorrect). After stopping denosumab, the treatment effect will be rapidly lost if another agent is not started. The properties

of bisphosphonates are unique in that they are slowly released from the bone, providing continuing protection for an uncertain period (but not forever) after administration is stopped.[1] This does not exist for any other osteoporosis therapy. Stopping denosumab can lead to rapid rise in bone turnover markers, rapid decrease in BMD, return of fracture risk to baseline, and possible increase in the risk of multiple vertebral fractures.[14] However, some patients treated with denosumab may reach a treatment target at which fracture risk has reached an acceptable level and modification of the treatment plan could be considered. Recent data suggest that improvement in hip T-score on denosumab to a level of about −2.0 to −1.5 is associated with maximum reduction of fracture risk.[15] As to how to bridge to another therapy, recent data/case reports can help guide our thinking, but no guidelines exist to counsel patients who do not want to commit to lifelong denosumab (thus, Answer D is incorrect). Giving intravenous zoledronic acid (Answer B) is a very attractive option with its antifracture benefits and ease of administration; however, data have raised concern about the optimal timing. Administering zoledronic acid at 6 months (ie, right when the next shot of denosumab is due), when reviewed in a small case series, did not appear to protect the patient fully from bone loss.[16] Thus far, the data suggest that administration of oral alendronate (Answer C) gives the best ongoing protection.[17] The most recent Endocrine Society guidelines suggest that denosumab be followed with an antiresorptive agent, although which one and the optimal timing of treatment are uncertain.[1]

Case 3

A 73-year-old woman has osteoporosis. She has a history of breast cancer with lumpectomy and radiation followed by treatment with an aromatase inhibitor. She wants to know about romosozumab because she is worried about adverse effects of bisphosphonates and teriparatide.

Which of the following statements is true?

A. There were no cases of osteonecrosis of the jaw or atypical femoral fractures in any of the romosozumab trials

B. There is a boxed warning against using romosozumab in anyone who has had a myocardial infarction in the preceding 12 months

C. Romosozumab should not be given to patients at high risk for osteosarcoma

D. Sclerostin acts to increase bone formation via the Wnt pathway

Answer: B) There is a boxed warning against using romosozumab in anyone who has had a myocardial infarction in the preceding 12 months

Romosozumab is a humanized monoclonal antibody to sclerostin, a cytokine expressed by osteocytes. Sclerostin reduces osteoblastic bone formation by binding to LRP5/6, inhibiting Wnt signaling and stimulating bone resorption, in part by up-regulating RANKL, a stimulator of osteoclast formation, activity, and survival. Romosozumab was approved by the US FDA in April 2019 for treatment of postmenopausal women with osteoporosis who are at high risk of fracture. The mechanism of action is novel: by inhibiting sclerostin, it has a dual action of stimulating bone formation and reducing bone resorption. Bone formation is *increased* when sclerostin is inhibited (thus, Answer D is incorrect). The phase 3 Fracture Study in Postmenopausal Women with Osteoporosis (FRAME) trial examined romosozumab for 12 months followed by denosumab for 12 months vs placebo for 12 months followed by denosumab for 12 months in 7180 postmenopausal women.[18] In the first year, the romosozumab group had a 73% reduction in vertebral fracture incidence but had no significant differences in nonvertebral fractures. Another phase 3 trial, Active-Controlled Fracture Study in Postmenopausal Women with Osteoporosis at High Risk (ARCH), compared romosozumab to alendronate for a year followed by a year of alendronate in both groups.[19] This group of

4093 postmenopausal women was at higher risk of fracture and older than the FRAME group. At 12 months, there were vertebral fractures in 4.0% of the romosozumab group and 6.1% of the alendronate group (a relative risk reduction of 37%). Nonvertebral fractures were not different at 1 year. At the end of the second year, the risk of nonvertebral fractures and hip fractures was lower in the romosozumab to alendronate group than the alendronate to alendronate group. However, there was a numerically increased risk of cardiovascular events in the romosozumab group with (50/2014) 2.5% in the first year compared with 38/2014 (1.9%) in the alendronate group. There is no clear biological plausibility for a possible increase in cardiovascular events with romosozumab and no established causality, although the presence of sclerostin in blood vessels and vascular smooth muscle is a possible factor.[20] It has also been postulated that alendronate may provide cardiovascular protection, but this is not clear from other studies. Due to the ARCH data, there is a boxed warning that romosozumab may increase the risk of myocardial infarction, stroke, and cardiovascular death and should not be initiated in patients who have had a myocardial infarction or stroke within the preceding year (Answer B). The package label also advises to "monitor for signs and symptoms of myocardial infarction and stroke and instruct patients to seek prompt medical attention if symptoms occur," but there are no guidelines as to how to do so. Since there is no evidence of increased risk of osteosarcoma with sclerostin inhibition in rats or humans, there is no warning against its use in patients previously receiving radiation therapy or otherwise at high risk of osteosarcoma (thus, Answer C is incorrect). Atypical femoral fractures and osteonecrosis of the jaw were reported during both the FRAME and ARCH studies, thought to be related to the antiresorptive action (thus, Answer A is incorrect). Romosozumab is given subcutaneously by a health care professional once monthly for 12 months and should be followed up with an additional osteoporosis treatment to maintain or enhance its effects.

References

1. Eastell R, Rosen CJ, Black DM, Cheung AM, Murad MH, Shoback D. Pharmacological management of osteoporosis in postmenopausal women: an Endocrine Society clinical practice guideline. *J Clin Endocrinol Metab.* 2019;104(5):1595-1622. PMID: 30907953

2. Cosman F, de Beur SJ, LeBoff MS, et al; National Osteoporosis Foundation. Clinician's guide to prevention and treatment of osteoporosis. *Osteoporos Int.* 2014;25(10):2359-2381. PMID: 25182228

3. Camacho PM, Petak SM, Binkley N, et al. American Association of Clinical Endocrinologists and American College of Endocrinology clinical practice guidelines for the diagnosis and treatment of postmenopausal osteoporosis - 2016--executive summary. *Endocr Pract.* 2016;22(9):1111-1118. PMID: 27643923

4. Qaseem A, Forciea MA, McLean RM, Denberg TD; Clinical Guidelines Committee of the American College of Physicians. Treatment of low bone density or osteoporosis to prevent fractures in men and women: a clinical practice guideline update from the American College of Physicians. *Ann Intern Med.* 2017;166(11):818-839. PMID: 28492856

5. Dowd R, Recker RR, Heaney RP. Study subjects and ordinary patients. *Osteoporos Int.* 2000;11(6):533-536. PMID: 10982170

6. Miller PD. Underdiagnosis and undertreatment of osteoporosis: the battle to be won. *J Clin Endocrinol Metab.* 2016;101(3):852-859. PMID: 26909798

7. Khosla S, Shane E. A crisis in the treatment of osteoporosis. *J Bone Miner Res.* 2016;31(8):1485-1487. PMID: 27335158

8. Khosla S, Cauley JA, Compston J, et al. Addressing the crisis in the treatment of osteoporosis: a path forward. *J Bone Miner Res.* 2017;32(3):424-430. PMID: 28099754

9. Lewiecki EM, Boyle JF, Arora S, Bouchonville MF 2nd, Chafey DH. Telementoring: a novel approach to reducing the osteoporosis treatment gap. *Osteoporos Int.* 2017;28(1):407-411. PMID: 27439373

10. Ebeling PR, Akesson K, Bauer DC, et al. The efficacy and safety of vertebral augmentation: a second ASBMR Task Force report. *J Bone Miner Res.* 2019;34(1):3-21. PMID: 30677181

11. Clark W, Bird P, Gonski P, et al. Safety and efficacy of vertebroplasty for acute painful osteoporotic fractures (VAPOUR): a multicentre, randomised, double-blind, placebo-controlled trial. *Lancet.* 2016;388(10052):1408-1416. PMID: 27544377

12. Saag KG, Shane E, Boonen S, et al. Teriparatide or alendronate in glucocorticoid-induced osteoporosis. *N Engl J Med.* 2007;357(20):2028-2039. PMID: 18003959

13. Rothman MS, Olenginski TP, Stanciu I, Krohn K, Lewiecki EM. Lessons learned with Bone Health TeleECHO: making treatment decisions when guidelines conflict. *Osteoporos Int.* 2019;30(12):2401-2406. PMID: 31471665

14. Anastasilakis AD, Polyzos SA, Makras P, Aubry-Rozier B, Kaouri S, Lamy O. Clinical features of 24 patients with rebound-associated vertebral fractures after denosumab discontinuation: systematic review and additional cases. *J Bone Miner Res.* 2017;32(6):1291-1296. PMID: 28240371

15. Ferrari S, Libanati C, Lin CJF, et al. Relationship between bone mineral density T-score and nonvertebral fracture risk over 10 years of denosumab treatment. *J Bone Miner Res.* 2019;34(6):1033-1040. PMID: 30919997

16. Reid IR, Horne AM, Mihov B, Gamble GD. Bone loss after denosumab: only partial protection with zoledronate. *Calcif Tissue Int.* 2017;101(4):371-374. PMID: 28500448

17. Freemantle N, Satram-Hoang S, Tang ET, et al; DAPS Investigators. Final results of the DAPS (Denosumab Adherence Preference Satisfaction) study: a 24-month, randomized, crossover comparison with alendronate in postmenopausal women. *Osteoporos Int.* 2012;23(1):317-326. PMID: 21927922

18. Cosman F, Crittenden DB, Adachi JD, et al. Romosozumab treatment in postmenopausal women with osteoporosis. *N Engl J Med.* 2016;375(16):1532-1543. PMID: 27641143

19. Saag KG, Petersen J, Brandi ML, et al. Romosozumab or alendronate for fracture prevention in women with osteoporosis. *N Engl J Med.* 2017;377(15):1417-1427. PMID: 28892457

20. Rosen CJ. Romosozumab - promising or practice changing? *N Engl J Med.* 2017;377(15):1479-1480. PMID: 28892459

What Is the Ideal Vitamin D Level and Dosage for All Circumstances?

Ghada El-Hajj Fuleihan, MD, MPH. American University of Beirut, Beirut, Lebanon; E-mail: gf01@aub.edu.lb

Learning Objectives

As a result of participating in this session, learners should be able to:

- Describe the clinical manifestations of hypovitaminosis D.

- Explain differences in vitamin D assays and the impact on practice.

- Determine efficacy of vitamin D supplementation across the lifetime.

- Determine a desirable serum 25-hydroxyvitamin D range based on major musculoskeletal outcomes.

- Discuss evidence regarding the putative non-skeletal benefits of vitamin D supplementation.

- Underscore knowledge gaps and future directions.

Main Conclusions

- Vitamin D, 400 IU daily, prevents rickets in infants.

- Modest dosages of 400 to 600 IU daily are safe in children, adolescents, and adults. Such dosages prevent secondary hyperparathyroidism (in case of fluctuations in vitamin D nutritional status).

- Vitamin D probably reduces the risk of preeclampsia (± calcium), gestational diabetes, low neonatal birth weight (<2500 g), and severe postpartum bleeding.

- There is no benefit of vitamin D supplementation on fractures or falls in ambulatory adults younger than 65 years.

- There is no clear benefit of vitamin D in combination with calcium on fractures or falls in ambulatory adults younger than 65 years.

- Vitamin D has positive effects on musculoskeletal health in populations at high risk.

- Vitamin D combined with calcium reduces the risk of hip fractures and all fractures in institutionalized individuals (likely to have low 25-hydroxyvitamin D and secondary hyperparathyroidism).

- The above apply to vitamin D–replete, low-risk, western populations.

- Vitamin D, at dosages exceeding 2000 IU daily, has no beneficial effect on nonclassic outcomes.

- Routine measurement of serum 25-hydroxyvitamin D is not indicated in the general population.

- Hypercalcemia and hypercalciuria are unlikely to occur at dosages of up to 2000 IU daily.

- Evidence gaps exist regarding children, pregnant women, and community-dwelling elderly individuals with low vitamin D.

- Individual patient meta-analyses and randomized controlled trials are needed to shed light on areas of unclear evidence.

Significance of the Clinical Problem

Background

Normal Physiology

Vitamin D, a steroid hormone that controls more than several hundreds of genes, amounting to around 3% of mouse and human genomes, impacts a wide range of molecular and cellular functions.[1] It is a pre-hormone derived from diet or skin (sun exposure) whose active metabolite, 1,25-dihydroxyvitamin D (1,25[OH]$_2$D), has a critical role in calcium and mineral homeostasis, bone modeling, and remodeling. The dietary intake is usually low, as few food items contain or are fortified with vitamin D; therefore, synthesis in the skin is the main source of vitamin D. The vitamin D metabolic pathway consists of 3 major steps mediated by hydroxylases (*Figure*).[1] It starts in the skin, where ultraviolet B radiation initiates conversion of 7-dehydrocholesterol (pre-vitamin D$_3$) to cholecalciferol or D$_3$, which is biologically inactive, and undergoes 2 hydroxylation steps before the active 1α-25-dihydroxyvitamin D$_3$ 1,25(OH)$_2$D$_3$ is formed. The vitamin D–binding protein also called GC, has a major role in the transport of D metabolites, including vitamin D to the liver, 25-hydroxyvitamin D (25-OHD) to the kidneys and other organs, and 1,25(OH)$_2$D to target tissues. Several cytochrome P450 (CYP) enzymes are reported as human hepatic vitamin D 25-hydroxylases (25-hydroxylase [CYP2R1], 1-hydroxylase [CYP27B1], 24-hydroxylase [CYP24A1]) (*Figure*).[2,3] As cellular concentrations of 1,25(OH)$_2$D$_3$ increase, it activates the cytoplasmic vitamin D receptor and turns on a number of genes the receptor transcribes. Of the circulating vitamin D metabolites, serum 25-OHD is the most abundant, has the longest half-life (2-3 weeks), and reflects both skin synthesis and dietary intake. It is the metabolite of interest relating vitamin D nutritional status to outcomes.

Genetic Polymorphisms and Environmental Predictors of Serum 25-OHD Levels

Polymorphisms in key genes of the vitamin D pathway (*CYP2R1, CYP27B1, CYP24A1,* and 7-dehydrocholesterol reductase *DHCR7*), the vitamin D–binding protein, and the vitamin D receptor—even when combined—only explain less than 5% of variations in 25-OHD levels. Conversely, environmental and lifestyle factors account for more substantial variations, estimated up to 50%, in vitamin D status or serum 25-OHD levels, amounting to 3 to 15 ng/mL (7.5-37.4 nmol/L). Consistent predictors of low 25-OHD levels are extremes of age, gender, pregnancy in Middle East, UVB/sun exposure, season, pollution, clothing style, high BMI, lower socioeconomic status, skin pigmentation, race, and ethnicity.[2] *CYP2R1* was initially considered to be constitutively expressed and therefore the concentration of serum 25-OHD was thought to be substrate dependent. Recent studies reveal that *CYP2R1* is under tight control of metabolic signals.[3] Indeed, obesity, type 1 and type 2 diabetes

Figure. Vitamin D Metabolic Pathway

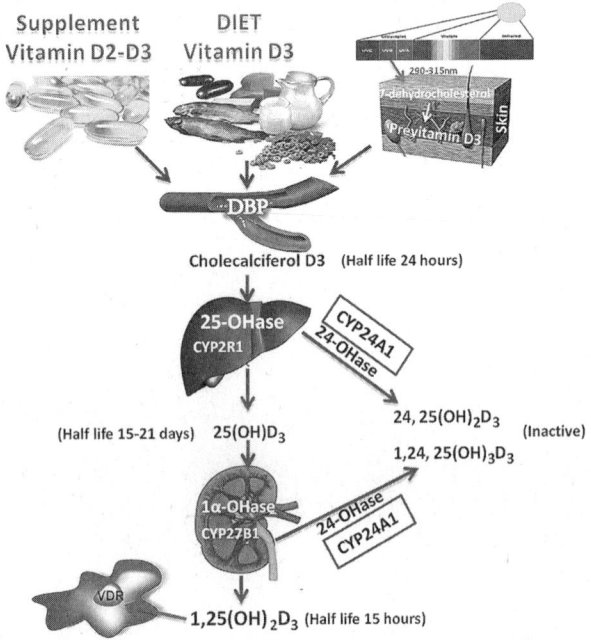

mellitus, fasting, and glucocorticoid therapy are associated with lower serum 25-OHD levels. Compared with nonobese mice, obese mice fed a high-fat diet have been shown to have lower levels of *CYP2R1* mRNA protein expression. Variations in *CYP2R1* expression may explain the variability in serum 25-OHD levels in patients with similar lifestyles, as well as the wide variability observed in response of serum 25-OHD levels to similar vitamin D dosage regimens.[3]

Overview

The implementation of vitamin D supplementation for all infants and small children largely eliminated nutritional rickets in Europe and North America.[4] Nutritional rickets, from simple vitamin D deficiency, or combined calcium and vitamin D deficiency, however, persists in Asian countries and in the Middle East, while calcium deficiency rickets dominates in many African and some Asian countries. Refugees, immigrants, and persons with a darker skin complexion are at risk for this disease. Reported rates for rickets vary between 1% and 25% (Mongolia) worldwide; however, such estimates are derived from older studies that were, for the most part, not population-based studies.[3] The prevalence of severe vitamin D deficiency across the globe (levels less than 10-12 ng/mL [25-30 nmol/L]) in these high risk groups is estimated at 7%.[4-7] Osteomalacia, the adult equivalent of rickets, also persists in these high-risk populations/regions. The vitamin D community unanimously supported an action plan to prepare a dedicated memorandum to ask the World Health Organization to approve and implement an action plan "to eradicate nutritional rickets by 2030" (23rd Vitamin D Workshop, New York, May 2019). This would align with other World Health Organization action plans to correct micronutrient deficiencies in the world.[3]

Milder deficiency (hypovitaminosis D or vitamin D insufficiency) is more prevalent worldwide. A systematic review of 195 studies involving more than 168,000 participants from 44 countries revealed considerable variation in mean 25-OHD values. Around 37% of studies reported mean values below 20 ng/mL (<50 nmol/L), with proportions being higher in the Middle East and Asia.[8]

Barriers to Optimal Practice

Major organizations and societies have developed guidelines for recommended desirable 25-OHD levels and age-specific vitamin D dosages. Their implementation and applicability across age groups and populations are variable for the following reasons:

- Poor recognition of the problem, as hypovitaminosis D is in large part a subclinical disease.
- Multitude of guidelines with contradicting recommendations.
- Knowledge gaps in various age groups (children, pregnant women, community-dwelling adults).
- Concerns regarding safety and fear of cardiovascular diseases.

Strategies for Diagnosis, Therapy, and/or Management
Diagnosis

Nutritional rickets presents with the classic phenotype of musculoskeletal manifestations. Once the infant starts crawling and walking, bowing, fractures, and knock knees become apparent.[4] X-rays reveal fraying of the metaphyses and cupping of the epiphyseal plates.[4,7] Osteomalacia in adults presents with long bone pain, proximal myopathy, bowing, and pseudofractures or Looser zone radiographically.[9] Severe cases can present as cardiomyopathy. The classic biochemical profile of both conditions includes low levels of calcium, phosphate, and 25-OHD (below 10-12 ng/mL [25-30 nmol/L]). If levels are higher, then rickets is exclusively due to calcium deficiency or combined calcium and vitamin D insufficiency. Permanent consequences include hypomineralized teeth and stunted growth in children. Bone histomorphometry is the gold standard to confirm the diagnosis, and double tetracycline labeling reveals unmineralized osteoid bone and increased mineralization lag time. Radiologic studies allow for early diagnosis and scoring of the disease severity (Thatcher score, 4).

While it is universally agreed that prevention and treatment of rickets and osteomalacia are clearly indicated, the approach to vitamin D insufficiency (12-20 ng/mL [30-50 nmol/L]) is quite variable. In most cases, vitamin D insufficiency may have no deleterious impact on health, while in others it could present initially as subclinical disease, progressing from no to subtle biochemical abnormalities. Serious potential concerns are silent adverse outcomes on maternal-neonatal health, bone mass in infants and adolescents, and chronic outcomes such as secondary hyperparathyroidism and fractures (including hip fractures in elderly high-risk individuals). Therefore, examination of the evidence for treatment efficacy and adequate supplementation is indicated. Relating the desirable serum 25-OHD level to outcomes and recommended dosages has been quite challenging because of the scarce evidence relating 25-OHD to outcomes and the wide variability in achieved 25-OHD levels with identical dosages.[10-13]

Management Strategies/ Vitamin D Guidelines

The Endocrine Society, the Institute of Medicine, and many organizations and societies have developed guidelines.[14-18] The Endocrine Society and Institute of Medicine guidelines are based on an extensive review of the literature, but their applicability across age groups and populations worldwide are still debated. They use similar predefined outcomes of mineral metabolism, yet reach differing conclusions in terms of the desirable 25-OHD level, set at 30 ng/mL (75 nmol/L) by the Endocrine Society and 20 ng/mL (50 nmol/L) by the Institute of

Medicine. They also differ in recommended dosages to achieve these levels, varying between 600 and 800 IU for the Institute of Medicine and between 600 and 2000 IU for the Endocrine Society.[17,18] The differences in desirable 25-OHD levels derived by the Institute of Medicine and the Endocrine Society may only in part be explained by different target populations they addressed: the general public (Institute of Medicine) vs individuals at high risk (Endocrine Society). We have provided a detailed synthesis of the approach used by these organizations, and the basis for their recommendations by outcome of interest.[2] Finally, while most, if not all, current vitamin D guidelines consider age, gender, and reproductive status, none has factored in any of the other modulators of vitamin D into their recommendations for desirable levels, with the exception of the Australian guidelines that take season into account.[15] Obese patients require higher dosages.[19]

Impact of Assay Variation on Management Strategies

Although serum 25-OHD is the best index of nutritional vitamin D status, its measurement to define desirable vitamin D levels is limited by large variations incurred by the various methodologies used to date. Such variations by far exceed the differences in desirable 25-OHD levels defined by the Institute of Medicine and the Endocrine Society. DEQAS (Vitamin D External Quality Assessment Scheme, http://www.deqas.org) is an international quality assurance program that evaluates performance of various 25-OHD assays, including the older radioimmunoassays, platform automated assays, liquid chromatography, and the gold standard liquid chromatography/tandem mass spectrometry. Each quarter, DEQAS sends 5 unknown 25-OHD samples to more than 1100 laboratories partaking in its quality assurance program. These unknown samples are run by participating laboratories based on their specific method and the results are mailed back to DEQAS. Once all results are received, DEQAS generates a quarterly general report with details on method-specific mean 25-OHD values obtained for each method separately and specifies the National Institute of Standards and Technology target value for each unknown sample. We had previously reported that serum values measured in parallel with 2 assays could vary between –38 to +19 ng/mL, a bias that was independent of the serum 25-OHD level.[2] The implications of such wide variability on the interpretation of results from trials and the relevance and applicability of guidelines and recommendations, at the public health or individual level, are substantial. Mandatory requirement for vitamin D quality assurance protocols in all clinical laboratories and cross-calibration to a universal NIST standard (National Institute of Standards and Technology) are pressing priorities.

Should We Screen by Measuring Serum 25-OHD Levels?

The Institute of Medicine defines a desirable 25-OHD level to be 20 ng/mL (50 nmol/L), and the Endocrine Society defines a desirable level to be 30 ng/mL (75 nmol/L). Desirable levels by other organizations fall, for the most part, in between these 2 cutoff values. All guidelines concur that screening for vitamin D deficiency is not recommended for the general population and should be reserved for high-risk individuals. High risk is defined slightly differently by the various organizations.[2,5] Measuring serum 25-OHD does not fulfill the World Health Organization criteria for a screening test.

Treatment of Symptomatic Patients

Prevention and Treatment of Rickets

Nutritional rickets is treated with calcium and vitamin D, and dosages are modified according to patient age and adherence. High dosages of 1000 to 6000 IU daily for 3 months followed by 400 to 600 IU daily are preferred to intermittent therapy, but both can heal rickets.

Treatment of Osteomalacia

Several regimens are used and all can heal osteomalacia effectively. A widely used regimen consists of giving 50,000 IU weekly for 6 to 8 weeks followed by 800 IU daily maintenance therapy.

Treatment of Asymptomatic Individuals

The treatment of asymptomatic individuals is described in *Tables 1* and *2*. These recommendations apply to Caucasian populations.

Clinical Case Vignettes

Case 1

A 51-year-old woman presents in a wheelchair with a 1-year history of low back pain, hip and pelvic pain upon walking, difficulty getting up from a chair, and inability to climb stairs. The pain and weakness have been progressive over the past year, interfering with daily activities, until few weeks before admission when she became completely homebound. She does not like dairy products, spends little time outdoors, and uses a concealed clothing style. She has had no diarrhea, no bowel surgery, and no intake of anticonvulsant agents. She had total thyroidectomy 20 years ago for multinodular goiter.

On physical examination, she appears healthy and is in no distress. Her BMI is 31 kg/m^2. She has diffuse musculoskeletal tenderness, tenderness over the shins, waddling gait, and muscular weakness. She is unable to stand from a sitting position. Deep tendon reflexes are +4. Chvostek and Trousseau signs are both positive.

Laboratory test results (sample drawn at admission):

    Calcium = 6.9 mg/dL (8.5-10.5 mg/dL)
        (SI: 1.7 mmol/L [2.1-2.6 mmol/L])
    Phosphate = 2.2 mg/dL (2.9-5.2 mg/dL)
        (SI: 0.7 mmol/L [0.9-1.7 mmol/L])
    Alkaline phosphatase = 820 U/L (35-120 U/L)
        (SI: 13.7 μkat/L [0.6-2.0 μkat/L])
    Albumin = 3.8 g/dL (3.6-5.3 g/dL) (SI: 38 g/L
        [36-53 g/L])

Creatinine = 0.9 mg/dL (0.6-1.2 mg/dL)
  (SI: 79.6 μmol/L [53.0-106.1 μmol/L])
Urinary calcium = 30 mg/24 h (0-250 mg/24 h)
  (SI: 0.75 mmol/d [0-6.3 mmol/d])
Urinary phosphate = 770 mg/24 h (400-1300 mg/24 h)
  (SI: 248.7 mmol/d [129.2-419.9 mmol/d])
Urinary creatinine = 1.4 g/24 h (0.6-2.0 g/24 h)
  (SI: 12.4 mmol/d [5.3-17.7 mmol/d])
25-OHD = <2 ng/mL (desirable >20 ng/mL, not to
  exceed 60 ng/mL) (SI: <5 nmol/L [>50 nmol/L,
  not to exceed 150 nmol/L])
PTH = 250 pg/mL (8-76 pg/mL) (SI: 250 ng/L
  [8-76 ng/L])

D-xylose test is negative, stool test for Sudan stain is negative, assessment for endomysial and transaminase antibodies is negative, and intestinal biopsy shows no flattening of the villi. X-ray of the pelvis shows a generalized decrease in bone density and bilateral pseudofractures (Looser zones) in the pelvic rami. Bone mineral density T-scores are –2.6 in the spine and –2.4 in the hip (NHANES).

Table 1. Recommended Vitamin D Dosages in Children By Organization

		Desirable 25-OHD = 20 ng/mL (50 nmol/L) Institute of Medicine Recommendations			Desirable 25-OHD = 30 ng/mL (75 nmol/L) Endocrine Society Recommendations	
Age Group	AI	EAR	RDA	Upper Limit	Daily Requirement	Upper Limit
Infants						
0-6 months	400 IU			1000 IU	400-1000 IU	2000 IU
6-12 months	400 IU			1500 IU	400-1000 IU	2000 IU
Children						
1-3 years		400 IU	600 IU	2500 IU	600-1000 IU	4000 IU
4-8 years		400 IU	600 IU	3000 IU	600-1000 IU	4000 IU
9-13 years		400 IU	600 IU	4000 IU	600-1000 IU	4000 IU
14-18 years		400 IU	600 IU	4000 IU	600-1000 IU	4000 IU

Abbreviations: AI, adequate intake; EAR, estimated average requirement; RDA, recommended dietary allowance. AI is the amount of a nutrient that will meet an individual's daily requirements. It is used when an RDA cannot be determined. EAR is the intake level for a nutrient at which the needs of 50% of the population are met. RDA is the intake at which 97.5% of the population needs are met.

Table 2. Recommended Vitamin D Dosages in Adults By Organization

	Institute of Medicine Recommendations			Endocrine Society Recommendations (for patients at risk for vitamin D deficiency)	
Life Stage Group	EAR	RDA	Upper Limit	Daily	Upper Limit
Adults					
19-30 years	400 IU	600 IU	4000 IU	1500-2000 IU	10,000 IU
31-50 years	400 IU	600 IU	4000 IU	1500-2000 IU	10,000 IU
51-70 years	400 IU	600 IU	4000 IU	1500-2000 IU	10,000 IU
>70 years	400 IU	600 IU	4000 IU	1500-2000 IU	10,000 IU

Abbreviations: EAR, estimated average requirement; RDA, recommended dietary allowance. EAR is the intake level for a nutrient at which the needs of 50% of the population are met. RDA is the intake at which 97.5% of the population needs are met.

Question 1: Which of the following is this patient's most likely diagnosis?

A. Obesity

B. Malabsorption

C. Nutritional osteomalacia

D. X-linked hypophosphatemic rickets

E. Hypoparathyroidism

Answer: C) Nutritional osteomalacia

Question 2: Does this patient have osteoporosis?

A. Yes

B. No

Answer: B) No

Question 3: In addition to daily calcium, which of the following treatments would you recommend?

A. Vitamin D at 1000 IU daily

B. Vitamin D at 50,000 IU daily

C. Vitamin D at 50,000 IU weekly for several weeks followed by 600 to 1000 IU daily

D. Stoss therapy, 600,000 IU once now and every 6 to 12 months

Answer: C) Vitamin D at 50,000 IU weekly for several weeks followed by 600 to 1000 IU daily

Question 4: When do you expect normalization of her serum PTH and alkaline phosphatase after treatment?

A. Days

B. Weeks

C. Months

D. Years

E. Never

Answer: C) Months

Question 5: How do you expect her bone mineral density will be affected after replacement with calcium and vitamin D?

A. No change

B. Decrease

C. Increase by 3% to 5% at the spine and 1% to 2% at the hip

D. Substantial increments with normalization

Answer: D) Substantial increments with normalization

This vignette is based on a real case report.[9] The patient has the classic clinical, biochemical, radiologic, and densitometric presentation of osteomalacia. This condition, almost eradicated in western populations due to vitamin D supplementation, is still prevalent in immigrants and certain populations (Middle East, India, Asia). She was treated with calcium and vitamin D, 50,000 IU weekly for 1.5 years. Her symptoms resolved and she was able to walk within few days. Serum calcium and phosphate normalized within days, PTH and alkaline phosphatase took more than a year.[9] DXA does not distinguish osteomalacia from osteoporosis. She experienced substantial increments in bone mineral density within 4 months, both at the spine and hip, with steady increments thereafter. Her T-score normalized completely by 14 months. Such changes reflect healing of osteomalacia and not cure of osteoporosis.

Case 2

A 32-year-old woman comes to clinic for routine check-up and advice. She is otherwise healthy and takes no medication. She does consume any vitamin D–fortified food, uses sunscreen, and does not sit in the sun. She has 2 children (ages 10 years and 5 years) and is planning another pregnancy soon. Her son's friend had an arm fracture after falling off a swing. She would like your advice regarding vitamin D supplementation dosages/regimens for her and family members.

Question 1: Are there differences between the following regimens given as daily (1500 IU daily), weekly (10,500 IU weekly), or monthly (45,000 IU daily) in adults?

A. Yes

B. No

Answer: B) No

Question 2: Are vitamin D_3 based supplements superior to D_2 supplements in terms of efficacy?

A. Yes

B. No

C. Unclear

Answer: A) Yes

Question 3: What is the recommended total daily intake of vitamin D during pregnancy?

A. 100 IU daily

B. 600 IU daily

C. 5000 IU daily

D. 10,000 IU daily

Answer: B) 600 IU daily

Question 4: Does vitamin D supplementation during pregnancy decrease the risk of pregnancy-associated complications, such as preeclampsia, gestational diabetes, and cesarean delivery rates?

A. Yes

B. Possibly

C. No

Answer: B) Possibly

Question 5: Does vitamin D supplementation during pregnancy improve neonatal outcomes such as birth height or neonatal bone mineral content?

A. Yes

B. Possibly

C. No

Answer: B) Possibly

Question 6: This patient plans to breastfeed her third child and would like to know the recommended dosage of vitamin D to prevent rickets in her newborn. The universally recommended dosage in breastfed infants is which of the following?

A. 200 IU daily

B. 400 IU daily

C. 600 IU daily

D. 1000 IU daily

Answer: C) 600 IU daily

Question 7: What is the recommended total daily recommended vitamin D intake for the 5-year-old and 10-year-old going into adolescence?

A. 400-600 IU daily

B. 800 IU daily

C. 2500 IU daily

D. 4000 IU daily

E. None of the above

Answer: A) 400-600 IU daily

Question 8: Does vitamin D supplementation decrease the risk of fracture in apparently healthy children?

A. Yes

B. No

C. No data

Answer: C) No data

Prevention of rickets in infants is through early supplementation with 400 IU daily in infancy to be increased to 600 IU daily after age 1 year. While the efficacy of vitamin D treatment in infants and children suffering from rickets is unequivocal, the effect of supplementation in improving bone mineral in apparently healthy children and adolescents is yet to be determined.[2] A meta-analysis of 6 randomized controlled trials with a total of 884 healthy adolescents, mostly girls (mean age 10 to 13 years), on vitamin D supplementation at dosages of 132 IU to 400 IU daily (one study included a 2000 IU daily arm) had no statistically significant effects on total body bone mineral content or on bone mineral density of the hip or forearm.[20] There was a trend to a small effect on lumbar spine bone mineral density. The investigators concluded that it is unlikely that vitamin D supplements are beneficial to bone mineral density in children and adolescents with normal mean serum 25-OHD levels. The planned subgroup analyses suggest that vitamin D supplementation of deficient children and adolescents could result in clinically useful beneficial effect on lumbar spine bone mineral content and total body in a subgroup of children with lower serum 25-OHD levels.[20] One of the trials compared placebo, low-dosage treatment (200 IU daily), and high-dosage treatment (2000 IU daily), on bone density at 1 year in adolescent girls, with a mean baseline 25-OHD level of 14 ng/mL (35 nmol/L). Lean mass increased significantly in both treatment groups, and bone area and total hip bone mineral density increased in the high-dosage group.[21] To date, recommended dosages range from various organizations vary between 600 to 2000 IU daily depending on organization and region, and dosage would probably depend on ethnicity, latitude, and lifestyle (*Table 1*).[14] An ongoing individual patient meta-analysis should shed light on the efficacy of vitamin D on bone mineral density in apparently healthy children and adolescents, at a critical time of bone mass accretion.[22] There are no data on fractures.

The most recent Cochrane systematic review included 30 trials (n = 7033) and revealed that vitamin D probably reduces the risk of preeclampsia (same for calcium/vitamin D), gestational diabetes, and the risk of having a baby with a birth weight less than 2500 g compared with no intervention or placebo. High-quality research is needed, especially in high-risk populations/ethnic groups. To date, the Institute of Medicine recommends a recommended daily allowance of 600 IU of vitamin D daily, and the Endocrine Society recommends 1500 to 2000 IU daily. The World Health Organization 2012 vitamin D guidelines in pregnancy recommend against routine vitamin D supplementation.[2,23,24] One umbrella review had previously reported a consistent effect of maternal vitamin D supplementation on neonatal birth weight, whether considering observational studies or randomized controlled trials.[25]

Case 3

A 70-year-old woman presents to the osteoporosis clinic for advice. She is active and has a healthy diet. She has no personal history of fracture, but her mother had a hip fracture at age 75 years. FRAX estimates her risks of major osteoporotic fracture and hip fracture (with bone mineral density) to be below the country-specific intervention threshold. She has a history of osteoarthritis. She takes calcium, 1000 mg daily, and vitamin D, 600 IU daily, prescribed by her rheumatologist. However, she was told by her primary care physician at her last check-up to discontinue her calcium and vitamin D supplementation because of concerns of an increased risk of cardiovascular events.

Question 1: Does vitamin D administered with calcium decrease the risk of hip fracture in community-dwelling individuals?

A. Yes

B. No

C. No evidence available

Answer: B) No

Question 2: Does vitamin D co-administered with calcium increase the risk of cardiovascular events?

A. Yes

B. No

C. Possibly

Answer: B) No

Vitamin D combined with calcium reduces the risk of hip fracture by 16% to 33% and of any fracture by 5% to 19%,[14] while the effect of vitamin D supplementation on falls is less inconsistent. The effect on fractures is only demonstrated when combining trials in community-dwelling and institutionalized individuals and is potentially driven by data from institutionalized individuals in 3 large systematic reviews and meta-analyses.[15] The best evidence is from a Cochrane meta-analysis,[26] but for all 3 meta-analyses, the evidence is limited by major shortcomings and heterogeneity, including the population studied, dosages, and types of vitamin D used. The impact of routine supplementation on musculoskeletal outcomes in community-dwelling individuals remains unclear. Recommended dosages vary between 600 to 2000 IU daily (*Table 2*). There is no evidence that higher dosages are beneficial in any of the outcomes studies. Intermittent high dosages could be harmful, increasing fall risk.

Despite the long, staggering list of observational studies relating low 25-OHD levels to chronic diseases, several randomized controlled trials conducted in adults (VITAL [n = 25,871; 2000 IU daily; median follow-up 5.3 years], D2D [n = 2435; prediabetes; 3.3 years; 4 000 IU daily; median 2.5 years], ViDA [n = 5110; 50-84 years; bolus 200,000 IU then 100,000 monthly; median 3.3 years]) reveal no beneficial effect of vitamin D compared with placebo on the incidence of cardiovascular events, invasive cancer, diabetes, falls, and nonvertebral fractures.[27-30] There is also no evidence that vitamin D increases the risk of cardiovascular events or blood vessel calcification in elderly patients. Mean 25-OHD levels at study entry were 20 ng/mL or greater (>50 nmol/L) in all 3 trials.

The dosages recommended in both tables have been shown to be safe. Higher dosages do not incur superior efficacy and may actually have an adverse effect on health outcomes.[31-34] Mild hypercalcemia was reported in 3% and 9% of patients receiving 4000 and 10,000 IU daily in the D2D and Calgary studies, respectively.[28,34] The mean 25-OHD levels were 28 and 32 ng/mL at entry and reached 54 and 80 ng/mL in these 2 trials, respectively. Dosages greater than 1000 IU daily may be needed in patients with low baseline levels; dosages greater than 2000 IU daily are rarely necessary.

References

1. Bouillon R, Marcocci C, Carmeliet G, et al. Skeletal and extraskeletal actions of vitamin D: current evidence and outstanding questions. *Endocr Rev.* 2019;40(4):1109-1151. PMID: 30321335

2. Fuleihan Gel-H, Bouillon R, Clarke B, et al. Serum 25-hydroxyvitamin D levels: variability, knowledge gaps, and the concept of a desirable range. *J Bone Miner Res.* 2015;30(7):1119-1133. PMID: 25952470

3. Bouillon R, Bikle D. Vitamin D metabolism revised: fall of dogmas. *J Bone Miner Res.* 2019;34(11):1985-1992. PMID: 31589774

4. Bouillon R, Antonio L. Nutritional rickets: historic overview and plan for worldwide eradication. *J Steroid Biochem Mol Biol.* 2019;198:105563. PMID: 31809867

5. Zhang W, Stoecklin E, Eggersdorfer M. A glimpse of vitamin D status in mainland China. *Nutrition.* 2013;29(7-8):953-957. PMID: 23594582

6. Arabi A, El Rassi R, El-Hajj Fuleihan G. Hypovitaminosis D in developing countries-prevalence, risk factors and outcomes. *Nat Rev Endocrinol.* 2010;6(10):550-561. PMID: 20852586

7. Chakhtoura M, Rahme M, Chamoun N, El-Hajj Fuleihan G. Vitamin D in the Middle East and North Africa. *Bone Rep.* 2018;8:135-146. PMID: 29955632

8. Hilger J, Friedel A, Herr R, et al. A systematic review of vitamin D status in populations worldwide. *Br J Nutr.* 2014;111(1):23-45. PMID: 23930771

9. Al-Ali H, Fuleihan GE. Nutritional osteomalacia: substantial clinical improvement and gain in bone density posttherapy. *J Clin Densitom.* 2000;3(1):97-101. PMID: 10745306

10. Cashman KD, Fitzgerald AP, Kiely M, Seamans KM. A systematic review and meta-regression analysis of the vitamin D intake-serum 25-hydroxyvitamin D relationship to inform European recommendations. *Br J Nutr.* 2011;106(11):1638-1648. PMID: 22000709

11. Gallagher JC, Sai A, Templin T 2nd, Smith L. Dose response to vitamin D supplementation in postmenopausal women: a randomized trial [published correction appears in *Ann Intern Med.* 2012;156(9):672]. *Ann Intern Med.* 2012;156(6):425-437. PMID: 22431675

12. Zhao LJ, Zhou Y, Bu F, et al. Factors predicting vitamin D response variation in non-Hispanic white postmenopausal women. *J Clin Endocrinol Metab.* 2012;97(8):2699-2705. PMID: 22585090

13. Waterhouse M, Tran B, Armstrong BK, et al. Environmental, personal, and genetic determinants of response to vitamin D supplementation in older adults. *J Clin Endocrinol Metab.* 2014;99(7):E1332-E1340. PMID: 24694335

14. Bouillon R. Comparative analysis of nutritional guidelines for vitamin D. *Nat Rev Endocrinol.* 2017;13(8):466-479. PMID: 28387318

15. Chakhtoura M, Chamoun N, Rahme M, Fuleihan GE. Impact of vitamin D supplementation on falls and fractures-a critical appraisal of the quality of the evidence and an overview of the available guidelines. *Bone.* 2020;131:115112. PMID: 31676406

16. Institute of Medicine Committee to Review Dietary Reference Intakes for Vitamin D and Calcium. Dietary reference intake for calcium and vitamin D. Washington, DC: National Academies Press. Available at: http://www.nal. usda.gov/fnic/DRI/DRI_Calcium_Vitamin_D/FullReport.pdf

17. Holick MF, Binkley NC, Bischoff-Ferrari HA, et al; Endocrine Society. Evaluation, treatment, and prevention of vitamin D deficiency: an Endocrine Society clinical practice guideline [published correction appears in *J Clin Endocrinol Metab.* 2011;96(12):3908]. *J Clin Endocrinol Metab.* 2011;96(7):1911-1930. PMID: 21646368

18. Lips KD, Cashman C, Lamberg-Allardt C, et al. Current vitamin D status in European and Middle East countries and strategies to prevent vitamin D deficiency: a position statement of the European Calcified Tissue Society. *Eur J Endocrinol.* 2019;180(4):23-54. PMID: 30721133

19. Bassatne A, Chakhtoura M, Saad R, Fuleihan GE. Vitamin D supplementation in obesity and during weight loss: a review of randomized controlled trials. *Metabolism.* 2019;92:193-205. PMID: 30615949

20. Winzenberg T, Powell S, Shaw KA, Jones G. Effects of vitamin D supplementation on bone density in healthy children: systematic review and meta-analysis. *BMJ.* 2011;342:c7254. PMID: 21266418

21. El-Hajj Fuleihan G, Nabulsi M, Tamim H, et al. Effect of vitamin D replacement on musculoskeletal parameters in school children: a randomized controlled trial. *J Clin Endocrinol Metab.* 2006;91(2):405-412. PMID: 16278262

22. Winzenberg T, Lamberg-Allardt C, El-Hajj Fuleihan G, et al. Does vitamin D supplementation improve bone density in vitamin D-deficient children? Protocol for an individual patient data meta-analysis. *BMJ Open.* 2018;8(1):e019584. PMID: 29362271

23. Palacios C, Kostiuk LK, Pena-Rosas JP. Vitamin D supplementation for women during pregnancy. *Cochrane Database Syst Rev.* 2019;7:CD008873. PMID: 31348529

24. Harvey NC, Holroyd C, Ntani G, et al. Vitamin D supplementation in pregnancy: a systematic review. *Health Technol Assess.* 2014;18(45):1-190. PMID: 25025896

25. Theodoratou E, Tzoulaki I, Zgaga L, Ioannidis JP. Vitamin D and multiple health outcomes: umbrella review of systematic reviews and meta-analyses of observational studies and randomised trials. *BMJ.* 2014;348:g2035. PMID: 24690624

26. Avenell A, Mak JC, O'Connell D. Vitamin D and vitamin D analogues for preventing fractures in post-menopausal women and older men. *Cochrane Database Syst Rev.* 2014;(4):CD000227. PMID: 24729336

27. Scragg R. The vitamin D assessment (ViDA) study - design and main findings. *J Steroid Biochem Mol Biol.* 2019;198:105562. PMID: 31809866

28. Pittas AG, Dawson-Hughes B, Sheehan P, et al. Vitamin D supplementation and prevention of type 2 diabetes. *N Engl J Med.* 2019;381(6):520-530. PMID: 31173679

29. Manson JE, Cook NR, Lee IM, et al. Vitamin D supplements and prevention of cancer and cardiovascular disease. *N Engl J Med.* 2019;380(1):33-44. PMID: 30415629

30. Bouillon R. Vitamin D and cardiovascular disorders. *Osteoporos Int.* 2019;30(11):2167-2181. PMID: 31402402

31. Maalouf J, Nabulsi M, Vieth R, et al. Short- and long-term safety of weekly high-dose vitamin D3 supplementation in school children. *J Clin Endocrinol Metab.* 2008;93(7):2693-2701. PMID: 18445674

32. Gallagher JC, Smith LM, Yalamanchili V. Incidence of hypercalciuria and hypercalcemia during vitamin D and calcium supplementation in older women. *Menopause.* 2014;21(11):1173-1180. PMID: 24937025

33. Bouillon R. Safety of high dose vitamin D supplementation. *J Clin Endocrinol Metab* [Epub ahead of print] PMID: 31858106

34. Billington EO, Burt LA, Rose MS, et al. Safety of high dose vitamin D supplementation: secondary analysis of a randomized controlled trial. *J Clin Endocrinol Metab* [Epub ahead of print] PMID: 31746327

Stopping Bone-Active Medications

Ian R. Reid, MD. Department of Medicine, University of Auckland, New Zealand; E-mail: i.reid@auckland.ac.nz

Learning Objectives

As a result of participating in this session, learners should be able to:

- Describe the different patterns of offset of the various classes of osteoporosis drugs.

- Develop strategies for coping with offset of the various classes of osteoporosis drugs.

Main Conclusions

Suggested drug discontinuation strategies are as follows:

- **Oral Bisphosphonate** If a drug holiday is judged to be indicated, 6 months is usually appropriate for risedronate and 12 to 24 months for alendronate.

- **Zoledronate** Zoledronate is usually given at intervals of 1 to 2 years. Clinicians often increase the dose interval in patients on long-term treatment to 2 to 4 years. Other clinicians give 3 to 6 doses at annual intervals, then have a 3-year gap.

- **Anabolics (teriparatide, abaloparatide, romosozumab)** Bone mineral density (BMD) gains during treatment are lost in the months following cessation. Therefore, for each of these agents, it is important to lock in the BMD gains with the use of an antiresorptive agent (bisphosphonate or denosumab) at the time of anabolic withdrawal.

- **Denosumab** In the months following cessation of denosumab, bone resorption climbs rapidly to substantially exceed the pretreatment levels, and all the BMD gained is lost by 1 year. Up to 15% of patients stopping long-term denosumab experience vertebral fractures, so transition to another antiresorptive agent should always occur. Oral or intravenous bisphosphonates appear to be adequate in patients who have received denosumab for only a few years. In patients who have been treated for more than 5 years, prevention of rebound bone loss appears to be more difficult, so more intensive bisphosphonate therapy may be required with close monitoring of bone resorption markers and BMD. Patients starting denosumab should be told of this phenomenon, so they know that they must not delay injections or discontinue them without transition to a bisphosphonate.

Significance of the Clinical Problem

Osteoporosis is a chronic degenerative condition that usually requires lifelong management. However, treatment will not necessarily be continuous since it is now common to provide drug holidays (particularly when using bisphosphonates) to reduce the risk of atypical femoral fractures. Also, patients sometimes wish to discontinue medications for personal reasons or because of adverse effects. Bisphosphonates bind tightly to bone mineral and continue to exert antiresorptive effects for months to years after their discontinuation. The FLEX study showed residual antifracture efficacy for up to 5 years after a 5-year treatment period with alendronate.[1] Zoledronate inhibits bone resorption for more than 5 years,[2] so annual dosing is unnecessary in most circumstances. Anabolics are typically used for periods of 1 to 2 years. Therefore, it is necessary to understand that different drugs have different rates of offset, and some demonstrate a rebound phenomenon whereby there is excessive bone loss that can result in multiple vertebral fractures. This has been most clearly demonstrated with denosumab.[3] Up to 15% of patients stopping long-term denosumab experience vertebral fractures, and multiple fractures are seen in 10%.[4] This is a potentially catastrophic outcome that must be anticipated by patient counseling at the time of treatment initiation and vigorously prevented by transition to bisphosphonates if denosumab is stopped.

Barriers to Optimal Practice

- Failure to anticipate drug offset when initiating an osteoporosis treatment and thus to have an a priori plan.

- Failure to discuss drug offset with patients, so they are aware of the dangers of discontinuing medication.

Strategies for Diagnosis, Therapy, and/or Management

In most areas of medicine, physicians and their patients assume that medications only act for as long as they are taken. For bone, this has been less clear. Certainly, bone turnover markers show rapid responses to starting and stopping some interventions, but BMD always responds slowly. Also, we have grown accustomed to using bisphosphonates, the principal bone medications, and have accepted their very long duration of action without regarding it as being unique to this group of medications. Now that the pharmacology of bone is becoming more diverse, it is important to recognize differences in rates of offset of the various medications now available.

Bisphosphonates

Bisphosphonates have a very high affinity for bone mineral, to which they bind and remain bound for some years. Their inhibition of bone resorption is not quite so long-lived, and it varies among agents according to their affinity for bone mineral. Thus, zoledronate has the longest duration of action, whereas the effects of risedronate and ibandronate are more transient. Duration of effect is also dosage dependent.

Several studies of rates of offset of antiresorptive activity have been published. McClung et al demonstrated that the effects of alendronate on both bone turnover and BMD lasted considerably longer than those of estrogen.[5] The FLEX study assessed multiple endpoints in women already treated before the trial with alendronate for 5 years, who were then randomly assigned to continue on full-dosage alendronate, half-dosage alendronate (equivalent to 70 mg every 2 weeks), or placebo.[1] Nonvertebral fractures were not different in those randomly assigned to either dosage of alendronate or placebo, although in women entering FLEX with femoral neck T-scores less than –2.5, there were fewer fractures in those on alendronate. For the FLEX cohort as a whole, clinical vertebral fractures were reduced by about one-half in those who continued to take alendronate. This study has been very influential, creating the T-score threshold of –2.5 for determining whether ongoing therapy is indicated. Its other important message, often overlooked, is that after 5 years treatment, the dosage of alendronate can be reduced by one-half without loss of efficacy. It should be remembered that there was continuing prevention of clinical vertebral fractures in those who stayed on treatment for 10 years.

Studies of risedronate demonstrate a more rapid offset of bone turnover suppression, within 12 months of drug discontinuation. Within this period, femoral neck BMD also returned to baseline, in contrast to either alendronate or zoledronate.[6] Despite the transience of effect, in the first year after risedronate discontinuation new vertebral fractures were reduced by about one-half.

Zoledronate has the highest affinity for bone mineral, and it is also the most potent bisphosphonate in terms of its inhibition of the target enzyme in the mevalonate pathway. When given in the conventional intravenous dose of 5 mg, its inhibition of bone turnover lasts for more than 5 years after a single dose, and hip BMD is still 2% above baseline at that time point.[2] Extensions to the pivotal phase 3 trial demonstrated residual antifracture efficacy after the drug had been discontinued, but optimal fracture prevention was seen in those who continued treatment annually for 6 years. A post hoc analysis of the phase 3 trials found that among women who received only 1 injection of trial medication, fracture prevention over 3 years was similar to that observed in those receiving 3 doses of either zoledronate or placebo. This provides some evidence that the long duration of the effects of this drug on bone turnover and BMD might also be reflected in longevity of antifracture effects. The recent trial of 18-month dosing of zoledronate also showed substantial fracture prevention and provides further evidence for this.[7]

Denosumab

The issue of offset of action of osteoporosis medications has come to the forefront with the increasing use of denosumab, a monoclonal antibody directed against RANKL. It suppresses bone turnover by about 90% for a period of 6 months after each subcutaneous injection. The phase 2 trial program demonstrated that offset after the first missed dose is dramatic, with bone resorption rising to about 50% above pretreatment levels within months of drug discontinuation.[3] Most of the bone gained during treatment is lost in the first 6 months after drug discontinuation and BMD is back to baseline at 12 months. In 2016, case reports and case series describing multiple vertebral fractures following denosumab discontinuation began to appear and now represent a substantial literature. Analysis

of patients discontinuing from the 3-year FREEDOM study did not suggest that vertebral fractures were any more common than in those participants discontinuing placebo. However, in the FREEDOM extension study, where denosumab use was up to 10 years in duration, 15% of women discontinuing the drug developed vertebral fractures in the following months, and in 10% of discontinuing participants, there were multiple vertebral fractures. This is a major cause for concern, since multiple vertebral fractures are likely to lead to height loss, spinal deformity, and long-term morbidity. Also, observational studies suggest that more than half of patients treated for osteoporosis discontinue their medications within 2 years of initiation. Thus, it is likely that many patients treated with denosumab receive no benefit from this intervention if they stop it without transitioning to some other antiresorptive agent. Indeed, if they sustain multiple vertebral fractures, they are likely to be significantly worse off than if they had never started the medication.

This problem has led to a number of observational studies assessing the effectiveness of transitioning from denosumab to other antiresorptive agents. After 1 year of denosumab treatment, transitioning to oral alendronate appears to provide good prevention of bone boss.[8] Similarly, some studies have demonstrated satisfactory outcomes from giving zoledronate at the time of denosumab discontinuation,[9] but after long-term denosumab treatment, zoledronate is only partially effective in preventing subsequent bone loss.[10] When denosumab treatment has continued for more than 5 years, it appears that more intensive therapy is necessary to maximize BMD preservation. Following bone resorption markers such as serum CTX may be an aid in optimizing post-denosumab bone preservation.

Anabolics

Bone loss resumes following discontinuation of teriparatide. One year after conclusion of a 1-year treatment course, spine BMD is still several percent above baseline, but hip BMD is only about

0.5% above baseline. Therefore, the convention is to transition to a bisphosphonate, which achieves continued positive trajectories in bone density. Similarly, transition to denosumab results in significant further gains in bone density.[11]

Romosozumab is a monoclonal antibody directed against the osteocyte protein, sclerostin. This has both anabolic and antiresorptive effects and results in substantial increases in BMD. Its discontinuation is followed by substantial BMD loss over the first year off treatment, and bone resorption markers show a rebound similar to that following denosumab.[12] However, if patients transition to denosumab or to alendronate, positive changes in BMD are observed and fracture rates remain low.[13,14]

Strategies for treatment discontinuation are described in the Main Conclusions section. In addition to those specific measures, it is critically important to counsel patients about the offset characteristics of osteoporosis drugs when they are first being prescribed, so that this can be incorporated into the decision to embark upon a particular therapeutic strategy. Just as patients starting β-adrenergic blockers for ischemic heart disease are warned not to discontinue their medications without medical consultation, the same warning must be provided to those starting nonbisphosphonate osteoporosis drugs, particularly denosumab.

Clinical Case Vignettes

Case 1

A patient has been receiving denosumab injections every 6 months for 5 years, and she has been fracture-free during that time. Her current hip T-score is –2.2.

Which of the following is the best recommendation?

A. Continuation of current therapy

B. A 1-year drug holiday

C. Permanent cessation of treatment

D. Transition to a bisphosphonate

Answer: A or D) Continuation of current therapy or transition to a bisphosphonate

Either continuing current therapy (Answer A) or transitioning to a bisphosphonate (Answer D) would be acceptable answers. Cessation of therapy, whether temporary or permanent (Answers B and C), would expose her to risk of rebound vertebral fractures. Whether she needs to remain on osteoporosis treatment cannot be determined from the history provided. Her fracture risk could be high, despite her T-score, if she were elderly or had an extensive history of fractures. However, if she were fracture-free and in her 50s, transitioning her regimen to a bisphosphonate and then weaning therapy would seem the appropriate course.

Case 2

A patient has been taking alendronate for 5 years, and she has been fracture-free during that time. Her current hip T-score is –2.2.

Which of the following is the best recommendation?

A. Continuation of current therapy

B. A 1-year drug holiday

C. A 5-year drug holiday

D. Permanent cessation of treatment

E. Transition to an intravenous bisphosphonate

Answer: B or C) A 1-year drug holiday or a 5-year drug holiday

The preferred responses are a 1-year drug holiday (Answer B) or a 5-year drug holiday (Answer C). Continuing therapy in the next year (Answer A) is probably not necessary in light of her current BMD and recent fracture history. The FLEX study does indicate, however, that after 5 years of treatment, the alendronate dosage can be halved (eg, to 70 mg every 2 weeks) without loss of efficacy. A 1-year drug holiday would be sensible to reduce the small risk of atypical femoral fractures. The FLEX study indicates that a 5-year drug holiday will not increase her risk of nonvertebral fractures, but there may be a rise in the incidence of clinical vertebral fractures. If there was a reasonable indication for the initiation of alendronate in the first place, then permanent cessation of treatment (Answer D) is likely to be inappropriate. She could transition to an intravenous bisphosphonate (Answer E) if she finds that more convenient, but there is no other specific indication to do so, since her clinical course receiving oral alendronate appears to have been satisfactory.

References

1. Black DM, Schwartz AV, Ensrud KE, et al; FLEX Research Group. Effects of continuing or stopping alendronate after 5 years of treatment: the Fracture Intervention Trial Long-Term Extension (FLEX): a randomized trial. *JAMA*. 2006;296(24):2927-2938. PMID: 17190893

2. Grey A, Bolland MJ, Horne A, Mihov B, Gamble G, Reid IR. Duration of antiresorptive activity of zoledronate in postmenopausal women with osteopenia: a randomized, controlled multidose trial. *CMAJ*. 2017;189(36):E1130-E1136. PMID: 28893975

3. Bone HG, Bolognese MA, Yuen CK, et al. Effects of denosumab treatment and discontinuation on bone mineral density and bone turnover markers in postmenopausal women with low bone mass. *J Clin Endocrinol Metab*. 2011;96(4):972-980. PMID: 21289258

4. Cummings SR, Ferrari S, Eastell R, et al. Vertebral fractures after discontinuation of denosumab: a post hoc analysis of the randomized placebo-controlled FREEDOM trial and its extension. *J Bone Miner Res*. 2018;33(2):190-198. PMID: 29105841

5. McClung MR, Wasnich RD, Hosking DJ, et al; Early Postmenopausal Intervention Cohort Study. Prevention of postmenopausal bone loss: six-year results from the Early postmenopausal Intervention Cohort Study. *J Clin Endocrinol Metab*. 2004;89(10):4879-4885. PMID: 15472179

6. Kim TY, Bauer DC, McNabb BL, et al. Comparison of BMD changes and bone formation marker levels 3 years after bisphosphonate discontinuation: FLEX and HORIZON-PFT Extension I Trials. *J Bone Miner Res*. 2019;34(5):810-816. PMID: 30536713

7. Reid IR, Horne AM, Mihov B, et al. Fracture prevention with zoledronate in older women with osteopenia. *N Engl J Med*. 2018;379(25):2407-2416. PMID: 30575489

8. Freemantle N, Satram-Hoang S, Tang ET, et al; DAPS Investigators. Final results of the DAPS (Denosumab Adherence Preference Satisfaction) study: a 24-month, randomized, crossover comparison with alendronate in postmenopausal women. *Osteoporos Int*. 2012;23(1):317-326. PMID: 21927922

9. Horne AM, Mihov B, Reid IR. Effect of zoledronate on bone loss after romosozumab/denosumab: 2-year follow-up. *Calcif Tissue Int*. 2019;105(1):107-108. PMID: 31087124

10. Reid IR, Horne AM, Mihov B, Gamble GD. Bone loss after denosumab: only partial protection with zoledronate. *Calcif Tissue Int*. 2017;101(4):371-374. PMID: 28500448

11. Leder BZ, Tsai JN, Uihlein AV, et al. Denosumab and teriparatide transitions in postmenopausal osteoporosis (the DATA-Switch study): extension of a randomised controlled trial. *Lancet*. 2015;386(999):1147-1155. PMID: 26144908

12. McClung MR, Brown JP, Diez-Perez A, et al. Effects of 24 months of treatment with romosozumab followed by 12 months of denosumab or placebo in postmenopausal women with low bone mineral density: a randomized, double-blind, phase 2, parallel group study. *J Bone Miner Res*. 2018;33(8):1397-1406. PMID: 29694685

13. Cosman F, Crittenden DB, Adachi JD, et al. Romosozumab treatment in postmenopausal women with osteoporosis. *N Engl J Med*. 2016;375(16):1532-1543. PMID: 27641143

14. Saag KG, Petersen J, Brandi ML, et al. Romosozumab or alendronate for fracture prevention in women with osteoporosis. *N Engl J Med*. 2017;377(15):1417-1427. PMID: 28892457

Modern Management of the Patient With Paget Disease

Thomas J. Weber, MD. Division of Endocrinology, Metabolism and Nutrition, Duke University Medical Center, Durham, NC; E-mail: thomas.weber2@dm.duke.edu

Learning Objectives

As a result of participating in this session, learners should be able to:

- Explain the best current approach to the biochemical and radiographic diagnosis of Paget disease of bone (PDB).

- Explain the best therapeutic approach for painful PDB.

- Describe current controversies regarding the management of asymptomatic PDB and specific disease-related complications.

Main Conclusions

PDB is the second most common metabolic bone disease after osteoporosis. This condition is typically identified through routine laboratory testing, based on elevated serum alkaline phosphatase, or identified incidentally on radiographs that are obtained for another indication. PDB most often involves one site (mono-ostotic) or is less commonly multicentric (polyostotic), with the most common sites of involvement being the pelvis, femur, spine, skull, and tibia. Most patients with PDB are asymptomatic; the most common symptom is bone pain, which is generally contingent on site of involvement and effect on local structures. Painful PDB is responsive to treatment with bisphosphonates, with a greater and more sustained effect conferred by intravenous than oral therapy. In addition, patients with recent onset of symptoms due to PDB are more likely to respond to treatment than those with a longer duration of symptoms. On the basis of available evidence, it is important to note that more advanced complications of PDB, such as fractures, skeletal deformities, need for orthopedic interventions, or hearing loss, may or may not benefit from specific pharmacologic or surgical interventions.

Significance of the Clinical Problem

PDB is a common metabolic bone disorder that affects approximately 2% to 3% of individuals older than 55 years in the United States, although the incidence of the disease may be declining for unclear reasons. Most patients are identified incidentally because of an elevated alkaline phosphatase measurement or characteristic findings on radiology studies obtained for other indications, but a substantial number of affected patients present with bone pain. Additionally, patients may develop skeletal deformity, fractures, or neurologic sequelae related to encroaching effects of pagetic lesions, such as cranial nerve palsies or hearing loss. Limited plain radiographic studies (anteroposterior abdomen and pelvis, bilateral tibia, and skull) are recommended for initial radiologic confirmation in patients with asymptomatic PDB who have elevated alkaline phosphatase, although whole-body bone scintigraphy is recommended for confirmation of diagnosis and/or characterization of the extent of disease involvement. While bisphosphonates are proven to reduce bone pain in patients with PDB, treatment appears to be more effective in patients with a more proximate onset of symptoms. Importantly, there is insufficient evidence of other disease benefit (ie, prevention of deformity, fractures, orthopedic surgery, hearing loss) with bisphosphonates or other pharmacologic/nonpharmacologic interventions, such that expectant management and treatment of patients with PDB who have bone pain is currently advised.

Barriers to Optimal Practice

- PDB may be underrecognized in patients with an alkaline phosphatase level within but at the upper limit of the normal range, in which case measurement of bone-specific alkaline phosphatase and/or other bone biomarkers (P1NP, C-telopeptide) may be helpful.

- Biochemical relapse (ie, increase in alkaline phosphatase above the normal range) does not necessarily predict clinical relapse (ie, recurrence of bone pain), thereby presenting a challenge in the long-term management of patients with PDB.

- Although somewhat intuitive, bisphosphonate treatment of patients with PDB has not been proven to reduce the risk for orthopedic and neurologic outcomes.

Strategies for Diagnosis, Therapy, and/or Management
Prevalence and Pathogenesis

PDB is the second most prevalent metabolic bone disease after osteoporosis, affecting approximately 1% of adults older than 50 years in the United Kingdom and approximately 2% to 3% of adults older than 55 years in the United States.[1,2] The incidence of the disease varies significantly, however, by geography and ethnicity/race, with a much greater prevalence in persons of Anglo-Saxon or European heritage than in persons of Asian or African ancestry. The disease is more common in males than in females (~1.4:1), and it

roughly doubles in incidence for each decade after age 50 years.[1] Interestingly, the disease prevalence appears to be declining, as does the degree and severity of the disease,[3,4] although the reasons for this are unclear.

PDB may be sporadic or familial, with evidence that up to 30% of affected patients have a positive family history of the disorder. Within the United States, studies suggest that a first-degree relative of a patient with PDB is 7 times more likely to develop the disease than someone with an unaffected relative.[1] The most frequent pathogenic variant linked to PDB is in the sequestosome 1 gene (SQSTM1), which encodes a ubiquitin-binding protein important for cellular signaling events in osteoclast activation. Patients with the SQSTM1 pathogenic variant appear to have more severe disease at an earlier age of onset.[5] In the New England cohort of patients with PDB, pathogenic variants in SQSTM1 accounted for 21% of cases, resulting in early-onset disease and spinal stenosis in exclusively male patients.[6] There is also evidence of an environmental contribution to PDB, based on earlier animal and human studies suggesting that paramyxovirus infections such as measles may precipitate osteoclast activation and transformation, although studies to date have not been conclusive.

The initial lesion in PDB, which may be solitary (mono-ostotic) or multicentric (polyostotic), is lytic in nature and due to increased number and activity of osteoclasts. Subsequently, osteoblasts are recruited to the skeletal site, resulting in accelerated bone formation that results in woven or immature bone that is incompletely remodeled and subsequently infiltrated by excessive fibrous connective tissue and blood vessel deposition. The result of this process is an enlarged, hypervascular and structurally inferior skeletal site. Over time, hypercellularity typically diminishes, resulting in slower skeletal turnover and "burned out" sclerotic pagetic lesions.

Clinical Presentation

Most patients with PDB are asymptomatic and are identified through an incidentally identified elevated alkaline phosphatase level on routine chemistry testing or by radiologic studies performed for other indications. Patients with symptomatic PDB generally have localized bone pain at the site of pagetic involvement that may occur with movement or at rest, although the mechanism of pain is poorly understood. Bone deformities, particularly when involving the lower limbs, can exacerbate mechanical stress on joints and accelerate the development and progression of osteoarthritis. Less commonly, bony enlargement from PDB may cause symptomatic compression of adjacent structures resulting in cranial nerve palsies and hearing loss, among other symptoms. There is also evidence that hearing loss can be significant and subclinical, although screening with a specific tool may be helpful in identifying affected patients.[7,8] Rarely, hydrocephalus or spinal stenosis may result from basilar invagination of the skull and vertebral involvement, respectively. Fractures may also occur through pagetic bone, particularly in the long bones at sites of lytic involvement. Hypervascularity of affected bone may exacerbate bleeding risk with orthopedic procedures that involve pagetic sites and has been associated, rarely, with high-output cardiac failure. Very rarely, malignant transformation to osteosarcoma (<1%) or giant-cell tumor development occurs. Despite the risk, albeit rare, for osteosarcoma, there is no evidence for premature mortality in patients with PDB.[9]

Diagnosis

An elevated total alkaline phosphatase concentration is a hallmark of PDB, although it may not be consistent with the diagnosis in some patients. Specifically, total alkaline phosphatase reflects both skeletal and hepatic activity, such that a low hepatic fraction may result in a normal total alkaline phosphatase value. Additionally, the degree of skeletal involvement and activity may not be sufficient to raise total alkaline phosphatase.

In some patients, it may be useful to assess markers of bone resorption, including C- and N-terminal telopeptides of collagen (CTX and NTX), as well as markers of bone formation, namely procollagen type 1 N-terminal propeptide, to confirm elevated skeletal turnover due to PDB and provide baseline data to evaluate therapeutic response.[10]

As noted above, PDB is often suspected by radiologic studies (plain x-ray or CT) performed for other indications. If initially suspected because of biochemical findings, a plain radiograph of a suspected skeletal site based on clinical signs or symptoms is reasonable. In patients without localizing complaints, a limited x-ray survey of the skull and facial bones, abdomen (which includes the pelvis and proximal femurs), and tibia is recommended given the high prevalence of involvement of these sites. In the absence of plain radiographic involvement, whole-body bone scintigraphy is recommended based on its superior sensitivity for detecting PDB compared with the sensitivity of plain x-rays, although whole-body bone scintigraphy may be negative at sites of inactive PDB. Whole-body bone scintigraphy is recommended as well, in addition to targeted radiographs, as a means to fully and accurately define the extent of metabolically active disease in patients with PDB.[11]

Therapeutic Management

Based on the accelerated bone turnover that underlies the pathobiology of PDB, bisphosphonates would be an expected appropriate therapeutic agent. However, although PDB may result in several clinically significant adverse outcomes, existing evidence for bisphosphonate use is robust only for reduction in skeletal pain. A Cochrane meta-analysis of existing randomized, placebo-controlled trials confirmed that bisphosphonate treatment is more than 3 times more likely than placebo to eliminate bone pain in PDB (31% vs 9% [relative risk (RR) = 3.42; 95% confidence interval (CI), 1.31-8.90]) and twice as likely to reduce pain compared with placebo (RR, 1.97; 95% CI, 1.29-3.01), with a number needed to treat of only 5 patients to show significant benefit (95% CI, 2-15).[12] There is also evidence that patients with a shorter disease duration are more likely to respond to treatment.[13]

Regarding specific bisphosphonates, there is randomized controlled trial evidence that zoledronic acid, 5 mg intravenously, is superior to risedronate, 30 mg orally for 2 months, in relieving bone pain (RR, 1.36; 95% CI, 1.06-1.74).[14] Patients treated with zoledronic acid are also less likely than those treated with risedronate to experience clinical relapse (recurrence of bone pain) (9.2% vs 25.2%), although lack of biochemical relapse (increase in alkaline phosphatase level) was not helpful in defining which patients were at risk of clinical relapse when treated with zoledronic acid. There are limited comparative data on other oral and parenteral bisphosphonates in PDB. Low level evidence indicates that calcitonin may improve bone pain in patients with PDB, although it may be considered when bisphosphonate use is contraindicated. Finally, denosumab is not recommended for PDB because of insufficient evidence.

The apparent distinct nature between biochemical and clinical relapse in patients treated with zoledronic acid vs risedronate does call into question a "treat to target" approach of normalizing alkaline phosphatase in PDB. Consequently, the PRISM and PRISM-EZ trials sought to determine whether symptomatic or intensive treatment with bisphosphonates was more effective in the short- and long-term management of PDB. The PRISM trial revealed that intensive bisphosphonate treatment did not reduce bone pain, fractures, or need for orthopedic surgery compared with symptom-driven treatment in patients with PDB over an average of 3 years.[15] Furthermore, long-term normalization of alkaline phosphatase over more than 7 years did not improve bone pain, improve quality of life, or reduce the need for orthopedic procedures, and it may actually be associated with a higher fracture risk.[16] It is important to note that these patients were older (mean age 76 years) and had longstanding disease (~12 years since diagnosis),

such that these findings may not necessarily apply to younger patients who are identified earlier in the disease course.

There is insufficient evidence that bisphosphonate treatment prevents hearing loss, bone deformity, or progression of associated neurologic symptoms or osteoarthritis. Nonetheless, patients with skull/spinal involvement or those undergoing major orthopedic surgery that is proximate to areas of pagetic involvement have historically been considered candidates for treatment based on concerns about neurologic or hemorrhagic complications, respectively, the lack of definitive evidence for benefit notwithstanding. As noted above, patients with PDB are at risk for orthopedic complications of their disease, including fractures and requirement for joint replacement, although there is insufficient evidence to support a benefit of intensive pharmacologic therapy on these outcomes, as well as inadequate evidence to support a specific type of surgical intervention. Nonetheless, hip or knee arthroplasty is recommended in patients in whom medical therapy is inadequate. Although only a conditional recommendation, osteotomy may also be considered for correction of bone deformity.

Clinical Case Vignettes

Case 1

A 64-year-old man is referred for evaluation after a recent abnormal abdominal and pelvic CT scan, which he recently underwent for evaluation of left lower abdominal pain of 2 months' duration. He has no obvious abdominal or pelvic findings to explain his pain, although there is fairly extensive cortical and trabecular thickening involving the right iliac and right superior and inferior pubic rami. The patient has no pain, stiffness, or numbness in these areas. His medical history is noncontributory, and family history is negative for "bone disease."

On physical examination, he has no tenderness to palpation over the right lateral or posterior hip. Right hip passive range of motion is normal without elicited pain. Weber and Rinne tests of hearing are normal.

Laboratory test results:

> Alkaline phosphatase = 114 U/L (24-110 U/L)
> (SI: 1.90 µkat/L [0.40-1.84 µkat/L])
> AST, normal
> AST, normal
> Total bilirubin, normal
> 25-Hydroxyvitamin D, normal

On the basis of this patient's clinical presentation, which of the following is the best next step in his management?

A. Zoledronic acid, 5 mg intravenously

B. Alendronate, 40 mg daily for 6 months

C. Technetium ^{99}Tc whole-body bone scintigraphy

D. Fasting serum C-telopeptide measurement

E. Reassurance, as no additional workup or treatment is indicated

Answer: C) Technetium ^{99}Tc whole-body bone scintigraphy

This patient has biochemical and radiographic evidence for PDB, although he is currently asymptomatic. On the basis of this information and current evidence, there is not an indication to treat him with pharmacologic therapy, including bisphosphonates. However, he may have multifocal disease that includes the spine, which could position him as a candidate for treatment because of concerns regarding disease progression and possible neurologic complications. Given this, whole-body bone scanning with technetium ^{99}Tc (Answer C) is indicated. Treatment with an oral or intravenous bisphosphonate (Answers A and B) is not appropriate without the results of the bone scan. Measurement of bone turnover with C-telopeptide (Answer D) is not needed to support the diagnosis of PDB in this patient, and it also has limited utility in predicting or confirming response to pharmacologic therapy. Finally, reassurance (Answer E) should not be given to this patient until the extent of disease is established.

Case 2

A 52-year-old man presents with a 2-year history of gradually worsening left posterior-lateral hip pain. He describes gradual onset of the pain without antecedent trauma or injury. He describes the pain as deep and dull and exacerbated by weight bearing. He has also developed left groin pain within the past 6 months that is worse with movement. He has known degenerative disc and spine disease involving the lumbar spine, although his pain has not responded to oral nonsteroidal antiinflammatory agents, steroid dose-packs, gabapentin, or epidural steroid injections. His medical history is notable for osteoarthritis of both knees and shoulders. He does not smoke cigarettes or drink alcohol. Family history is negative for osteoporosis or other bone disorders.

On physical examination, there is mild tenderness to palpation of the left posterior hip/pelvic region. Passive range of motion of the left hip is also restricted due to elicited pain. The oropharynx is normal to inspection.

Laboratory test results:

> Calcium, normal
> Creatinine, normal
> 25-Hydroxyvitamin D, normal
> Alkaline phosphatase = 114 U/L (24-110 U/L)
> (SI: 1.90 µkat/L [0.40-1.84 µkat/L])
> Bone-specific alkaline phosphatase = 33 µg/L
> (0-20 µg/L [males])

Plain radiograph of the pelvis shows thickening and sclerosis of the left iliac wing cortex extending inferiorly to the medial aspect of the acetabular wall and inferior pubic ramus. Subsequent technetium ^{99}Tc whole-body bone scan shows diffusely increased tracer activity involving most of the left hemipelvis, including the acetabulum, inferior pubic ramus, superior pubic ramus, ischium, and iliac wing, which correlates with the areas of cortical thickening and bony sclerosis on the pelvic radiograph.

On the basis of this patient's clinical presentation, which of the following is the best next step in his management?

A. Zoledronic acid, 5 mg intravenously

B. Risedronate, 30 mg daily for 2 months

C. Calcitonin, 100 units subcutaneously 3 times weekly

D. Fasting serum C-telopeptide measurement

E. Denosumab, 60 mg subcutaneously every 6 months

Answer: A) Zoledronic acid, 5 mg intravenously

This patient has unequivocal evidence for active and symptomatic PDB based on biochemical findings, plain radiographs, and nuclear imaging. Given the available evidence and the relatively recent onset of symptoms, he is an appropriate candidate for pharmacologic therapy. Zoledronic acid intravenously (Answer A) is superior to oral risedronate (Answer B) based on a head-to-head comparison and is the best treatment for this patient. Calcitonin (Answer C) has limited benefit based on available evidence. Denosumab (Answer E) may have benefit in giant-cell tumors in the context of PDB because of its potent antiresorptive effect, but it is not approved specifically for either indication. In addition, the potential consequences of the robust off effect of the drug, as is seen in patients with osteoporosis, is unknown in patients with PDB. As in the first case, measurement of bone turnover (Answer D) has limited utility in either the diagnosis or therapeutic management of this patient.

Case 3

A 60-year-old woman is referred for evaluation of osteoporosis. She has a history of risedronate use (2 years), but she stopped it secondary to unacceptable gastroesophageal reflux symptoms. She is presently on raloxifene, 60 mg daily, which she has taken for 4 years, and she has evidence of stable bone mineral density on therapy, with estimated 10-year risks of hip and major osteoporotic fractures of 1.0% and 12%, respectively.

In the course of her workup, she exhibits a mild elevation of alkaline phosphatase of 133 U/L (25-125 U/L) (SI: 2.22 μkat/L [0.42-2.09 μkat/L]), with a repeated measurement (different assay) of 102 U/L (24-110 U/L) (SI: 1.70 μkat/L [0.40-1.84 μkat/L]). Bone-specific alkaline phosphatase is measured and found to be elevated at 29 μg/L (<22 μg/L [postmenopausal women]). Plain radiographs of the abdomen, pelvis, and bilateral tibia are negative, but subsequent technetium ^{99}Tc whole-body bone scan shows mild, diffuse uptake throughout the calvarium. Plain radiograph of the skull shows mild thickening of the calvarium. Upon relaying this result to the patient, she states that she has no headaches or subjective hearing loss, reporting that her hearing is much better than her husband's.

On the basis of this patient's clinical presentation, which of the following is the best next step in her management?

A. Zoledronic acid, 5 mg intravenously

B. Alendronate, 40 mg daily for 6 months

C. Audiometry testing

D. Fasting serum procollagen type 1 N-terminal propeptide measurement

E. CT of the skull

Answer: C) Audiometry testing

This patient has evidence for PDB with skull involvement that is asymptomatic. Despite this, and not necessarily contingent on skull involvement, the incidence of hearing impairment in patients with PDB is significantly higher than in the general population.[5] Given this, audiometry testing (Answer C) is indicated to determine whether hearing loss is present and whether she would potentially benefit from hearing aids or other assistive technology. There is evidence for a benefit from screening for hearing loss in patients with PDB (Hearing Handicap Inventory for the Elderly-Screening), which also has established utility in elderly patients (without PDB).[6] There is no evidence to date that treatment with bisphosphonates (Answers A and B) slows or reverses hearing loss in patients with PDB. Finally, additional diagnostic studies of bone turnover (Answer D) and imaging (Answer E) are unlikely to provide additional clinical guidance for this patient.

References

1. van Staa TP, Selby P, Leufkens HG, Lyles K, Sprafka JM, Cooper C. Incidence and natural history of Paget's disease of bone in England and Wales. *J Bone Miner Res.* 2002;17(3):465-471. PMID: 11878305

2. Altman RD, Bloch DA, Hochberg MC, Murphy WA. Prevalence of pelvic Paget's disease of bone in the United States. *J Bone Miner Res.* 2000;15(3):461-465. PMID: 10750560

3. 3: Corral-Gudino L, Borao-Cengotita-Bengoa M, Del Pino-Montes J. Epidemiology of Paget's disease of bone: a systematic review and meta-analysis of secular changes. *Bone.* 2013;55(2):347-352. PMID: 23643679

4. Corral-Gudino L, García-Aparicio J, Sánchez-González MD, et al. Secular changes in Paget's disease: contrasting changes in the number of new referrals and in disease severity in two neighboring regions of Spain. *Osteoporos Int.* 2013;24(2):443-450. PMID: 22395312

5. Visconti MR, Langston AL, Alonso N, et al. Mutations of *SQSTM1* are associated with severity and clinical outcome in paget disease of bone. *J Bone Miner Res.* 2010;25(11):2368-2373. PMID: 20499339

6. Seton M, Hansen M, Solomon DH. The implications of the sequestosome 1 mutation P392L in patients with Paget's disease in a United States cohort. *Calcif Tissue Int.* 2016;98(5):489-496. PMID: 26713335

7. Amilibia Cabeza E, Holgado Pérez S, Pérez Grau M, et al. Hearing in Paget›s disease of bone. *Acta Otorrinolaringol Esp.* 2019;70(2):89-96. PMID: 29880223

8. Young CA, Fraser WD, Mackenzie IJ. Detection of hearing impairment and handicap in Paget's disease of bone using a simple scoring system: a case control study. *Bone.* 2007;40(1):189-193. PMID: 16962839

9. Wermers RA, Tiegs RD, Atkinson EJ, Achenbach SJ, Melton LJ 3rd. Morbidity and mortality associated with Paget's disease of bone: a population-based study. *J Bone Miner Res.* 2008;23(6):819-825. PMID: 18269308

10. Singer FR, Bone HG 3rd, Hosking DJ, et al; Endocrine Society. Paget's disease of bone: an Endocrine Society clinical practice guideline. *J Clin Endocrinol Metab.* 2014;99(12):4408-4422. PMID: 25406796

11. Ralston SH, Corral-Gudino L, Cooper C, et al. Diagnosis and management of Paget's disease of bone in adults: a clinical guideline. *J Bone Miner Res.* 2019;34(4):579-604. PMID: 30803025

12. Corral-Gudino L, Tan AJ, Del Pino-Montes J, Ralston SH. Bisphosphonates for Paget's disease of bone in adults. *Cochrane Database Syst Rev.* 2017;12:CD004956. PMID: 29192423

13. Tan A, Ralston SH. Clinical presentation of Paget's disease: evaluation of a contemporary cohort and systematic review. *Calcif Tissue Int.* 2014;95(5):385-392. PMID: 25160936

14. Reid IR, Miller P, Lyles K, et al. Comparison of a single infusion of zoledronic acid with risedronate for Paget's disease. *N Engl J Med.* 2005;353(9):898-908. PMID: 16135834

15. Langston AL, Campbell MK, Fraser WD, MacLennan GS, Selby PL, Ralston SH; PRISM Trial Group. Randomized trial of intensive bisphosphonate treatment versus symptomatic management in Paget's disease of bone. *J Bone Miner Res.* 2010;25(1):20-31. PMID: 19580457

16. Tan A, Goodman K, Walker A, et al; PRISM-EZ Trial Group. Long-term randomized trial of intensive versus symptomatic management in Paget's disease of bone: the PRISM-EZ study. *J Bone Miner Res.* 2017;32(6):1165-1173. PMID: 28176386

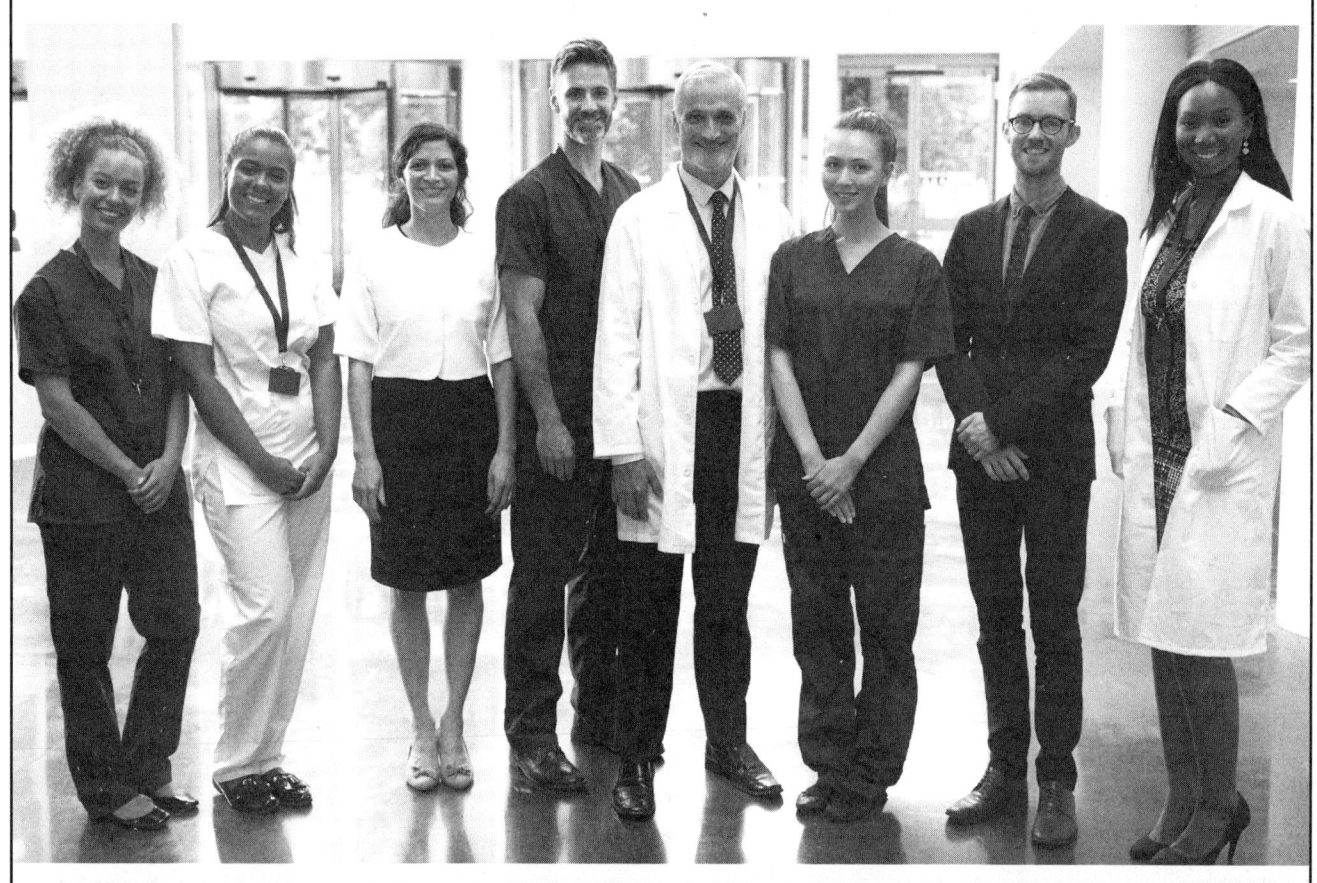

DIABETES MELLITUS AND GLUCOSE METABOLISM

Closing the Loop With Pump and Sensor Communication in Diabetes Mellitus: How to Digest Data and Develop Treatment Recommendations During a Clinic Visit

Steven D. Wittlin, MD. University of Rochester School of Medicine and Dentistry, Rochester, NY; E-mail: steven_wittlin@urmc.rochester.edu

Learning Objectives

As a result of participating in this session, learners should be able to:

- Select a sensor-pump system.
- Interpret pump-sensor downloads in the office or clinic.

Main Conclusions

Use of sensors, smart pumps, and hybrid closed-loop pumps has improved diabetes control. With the use of hybrid closed-loop pumps, despite the improvement in glycemic control, regulating postmeal glucose concentrations is still a challenge. Counting carbohydrates facilitates bolus calculation, but it is an imperfect and unsatisfactory tool when patients eat a mixed meal. Metrics have been developed to assess diabetes control that aid in making adjustments to regimens and interpreting pump downloads.

Significance of the Clinical Problem

In 1993, the DCCT (Diabetes Control and Complications Trial) demonstrated that reducing hemoglobin A_{1c} resulted in a reduced rate of microvascular diabetes complications. However, "intensive" diabetes control resulted in a tripling of the occurrence of severe hypoglycemia.[1] To address this, improvements in insulin pump therapy, and especially real-time continuous glucose monitoring (RT-CGM), have enabled intensification of control while reducing hypoglycemia.[2] There is now integration of RT-CGM with pumps and algorithms, allowing for the development of sensor-augmented pump therapy and its evolution into varying degrees of "closing-the-loop" and hybrid closed-loop systems.[3-5]

This technology has presented the clinician with new challenges, such as (1) correlating hemoglobin A_{1c} and the multitude of data points provided by new sensors, (2) assessing accuracy of sensors vs fingerstick blood glucose measurements, (3) interpreting RT-CGM data, (4) selecting an appropriate system for a given patient, (5) trouble-shooting various data and systems, and

(6) handling downloads of data in an efficient way during a busy clinic visit. This session attempts to address many of these issues.

Barriers to Optimal Practice

- Logistics of office download and interpretation of data from pump/CGM and closed-loop systems.
- Rapid changes in available technology with slow changes in insurance coverage.
- Cost of new diabetes technologies.
- Need for expertise in using the growing number of and changing diabetes technologies.

Strategies for Therapy and Management

Real-Time Continuous Glucose Monitors (Sensors)

RT-CGMs currently available in United States are presented below.

DexCom

- Current iteration: G6

Pros

- Factory calibrated
- Mean absolute relative difference (MARD) <10%
- Sensor life = 10 days
- No need for fingerstick confirmation
- High and low alerts
- Alerts identified individuals

Cons

- Patient must insert every 10 days
- Study confirming no need for calibration had multiple exclusions
- Needle introducer
- "Running out of sites"

- Possible skin/site problems
- "Compression lows"
- Not too close to infusion site

Medtronic

- Current iteration: Guardian 3

Pros

- Alerts
- MARD <10%
- Alerts identified individuals
- Sensor life = 7 days
- Excellent download display
- Has its own "pump partner"

Cons

- Patient must insert every 7 days
- Needle introducer
- "Running out of sites"
- Possible skin/site problems
- Requires calibration

Eversense (Senseonics): Wired-Enzyme Technology

Pros

- Accurate: MARD <10%
- Sensor life = 3 months United States; 6 months European Union
- Implanted, does not use up skin sites
- Improved adherence/use (it is implanted)
- Alerts including vibratory directly
- Alerts identified individuals
- No needle

Cons

- Minor office procedure (time)
- Needs calibration

- Removal of implanted device
- No "pump partner"

Freestyle Libre: Flash Technology

Pros

- Easy to use
- Less expensive
- Accurate: MARD <10%-15%
- Factory calibrated
- Sensor life = 14 days

Cons

- US version does not have alerts (as of 1/17/20)
- Requires patient to actively interrogate sensor for result, raising adherence issues
- Does not notify another person (Flash CGM)
- No current US "pump partners"
- Needle implantation

Choosing a Sensor

If the patient has no hypoglycemia unawareness and/or type 2 diabetes:

- All 4 sensors work; Libre may be easier, less costly, and at least as accurate as fingerstick measurements and is factory calibrated, thus reducing calibration error

If the patient has hypoglycemia unawareness/severe hypoglycemia:

- Not Libre (no alerts)
- Remaining 3 all work; if calibration error is an issue, DexCom has an advantage

If the patient has hypoglycemia unawareness/severe hypoglycemia and a pump or desire for a pump:

- Eversense does not have a "pump partner" at present, so would not use if threshold suspend or hybrid closed loop are desired
- If Medtronic System (vide infra) is desired, then Guardian 3
- If desire Tandem System (vide infra) is desired, then DexCom
- NB: Omnipod may partner with DexCom in the future

So When Eversense?[6]

- Body image issues/athletics
- Adherence to sensor issues
- Patient issues:
  - Such as hearing, seeing
  - Patient preference
- "Running out of sites"
- Needle phobia

Clearly, choosing a sensor requires a conversation between the provider as a guide and the patient. Insurance coverage plays a role. For example, at the time of this writing, Medicare is only "covering" Freestyle Libre and Dexcom.

Selecting a Pump

Again, patient preference is paramount. Below are several considerations:

- If a sensor-augmented system or closed-loop system will be used, the sensor may dictate choice of pump
- *Omnipod* is "tubeless" but has a smaller reservoir; it requires a PDM (Personal Diabetes Manager)
- *Medtronic* has its own sensor
  - Longest time on market

- □ Has a meter that directly communicates with the pump

- *Tandem* has a sensor partner

  - □ Can do software updates without getting a new pump

  - □ Touch screen system

Sensor–Pump Interactions: Toward "Closing the Loop"

Closed-loop systems involve 3 basic elements:

1. Pump
2. Sensor
3. Controller (an algorithm)

The sophistication of these systems has progressed over the past 2 decades:

- *Low-glucose (threshold) suspend systems:* the pump shuts off if a low glucose value is used

- *Predictive low glucose suspend:* the algorithm turns the pump off if low value is impending

- *Hybrid closed-loop systems:* the algorithm corrects the glucose toward a target/target range; the patient still determines meal boluses

  - □ Medtronic 670 G[7]

  - □ Control-IQ (Tandem and DexCom): automated correction bolus[8]

  - □ In France, Diabeloop (DBL G1)

- *DIY Systems (Do-It-Yourself):* not FDA approved; success appears user-related

Successful Meal Bolus

- Ensure the basal rate(s) is/are correct

- Appropriate mode (eg, regular vs square-wave vs "combo bolus") (see below)

- Timing: late boluses can result in both early hyperglycemia and late hypoglycemia

- Type of insulin

- Food content:

  - □ Traditional: insulin-to-carbohydrate ratio

  - □ Bell et al and others have shown a significant effect of fat and protein on glucose levels, resulting in a blunted early glucose peak and a late rise in glucose; there is no proven formula for this adjustment[9]

- Bolus calculators prevent insulin "stacking"

Special Situations

- Exercise

- Pregnancy

- Hospitalization

Reading a Sensor/Pump Download

An international consortium and others have created an Ambulatory Glucose Profile involving metrics for assessing diabetes control when using RT-CGM.[10] The standardized metrics for clinical care (2019) are as follows (recommendations in parentheses):

1. Number of days worn (14 days)
2. Percentage of time CGM active (70%)
3. Mean glucose
4. Glucose management indicator
5. Glycemic variability (<36%)
6. Time above range >250 mg/dL (>13.9 mmol/L)
7. Time above range 181-250 mg/dL (10.0-13.9 mmol/L)
8. Time in range
9. Time below range: 54-69 mg/dL (3.0-3.8 mmol/L)
10. Time below range <54 mg/dL (<3.0 mmol/L)

Usual Target Recommendations

- Time in range >70%

- Time below range <4%

- Time above range <25%

For older patients, looser time in range and time above range are appropriate to avoid time below range. Pregnancy targets for time in range are 63 to 140 mg/dL (3.5-7.8 mmol/L).

Regarding Time in Range[11]

Fourteen days suffice to correlate well with hemoglobin A_{1c}.

Advantages of Time in Range

- It responds faster to interventions than does hemoglobin A_{1c}

- It reflects glycemic variability

- It is unaffected by factors that affect hemoglobin A_{1c} (eg, red-cell half-life)

- It correlates with microvascular complications

- The relative measurement error of time in range is approximately 4%; for hemoglobin A_{1c} approximately 5%

Using Time in Range

- If there is a lack of concordance between time in range and hemoglobin A_{1c}

  □ One needs to assess for any interferences in hemoglobin A_{1c}

  □ One might reset hemoglobin A_{1c} target

  □ It may reflect a recent change in glycemic control

- CGM values are only as good as the "gold-standard" to which the CGM is calibrated

Glucose Management Indicator[12]

Glucose management indicator (GMI) is a new term for estimating hemoglobin A_{1c} from CGM readings—mainly to avoid confusion.

The formula for GMI is as follows:

GMI (%) =3.31+0.02392 × mean CGM glucose (mg/dL)

Each change of 25 mg/dL results in a GMI increase of ~0.6%.

Using GMI

- If GMI is lower than hemoglobin A_{1c}, consider:

  □ Avoiding hypoglycemia

  □ Perhaps increasing hemoglobin A_{1c} target

- If GMI is higher than hemoglobin A_{1c}, consider:

  □ Addressing hyperglycemia

  □ Perhaps lowering hemoglobin A_{1c} target

Clinical Case Vignettes

Case 1

A 35-year-old woman with type 2 diabetes and a history of hearing loss (and a mother with hearing loss) comes to see you. She is 5 months pregnant. She has had persistently elevated fasting blood glucose levels (~110 mg/dL [6.1 mmol/L]). She is prescribed 12 units NPH insulin at bedtime. She took metformin before pregnancy. She is now wearing a Freestyle Libre Sensor. Her sensor download is shown (*see images*).

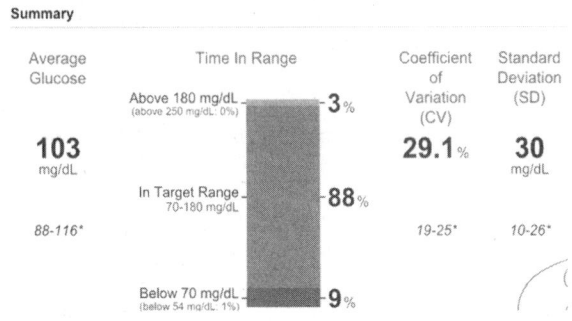

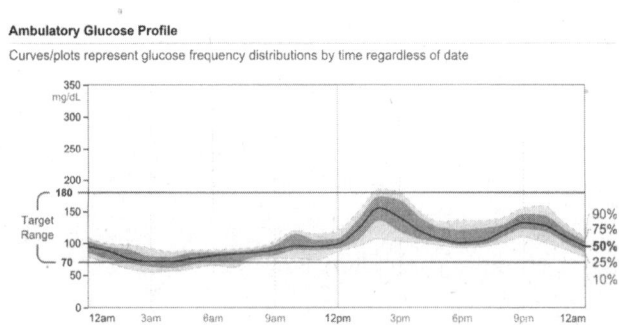

Which of the following is the best next step?

A. Continue the regimen; her time in range is 88%

B. Reduce her dosage of NPH; her time below range is 9%

C. Move her NPH insulin to the morning

D. Re-introduce metformin

Answer: C) Move her NPH insulin to the morning

The target glucose range for pregnancy is 63 to 140 mg/dL (3.5-7.8 mmol/L). Thus, her postlunch blood glucose values are elevated. Moving her NPH insulin to the morning (Answer C) is therefore the best next step. Her overnight glucose levels are on the low side, but still within target range. Adding metformin might decrease the overnight glucose values even further.

Case 2

A 46-year-old man has had type 1 diabetes for 30 years. His hemoglobin A_{1c} level is 8.1% (65 mmol/mol). He has had frequent high and low blood glucose values. He uses a 670G hybrid closed-loop pump. He does not understand why his glucose values are so variable on a closed-loop system. The image below shows 6 days of data from his download.

Which of the following is the most likely explanation?

A. Inaccurate carbohydrate counting

B. High-fat meals

C. Inappropriate insulin-to-carbohydrate ratio

D. Late meal boluses

Answer: D) Late meal boluses

As the figure illustrates, the blood glucose levels start to rise BEFORE the meal bolus delivery. Because of the delay, there is inadequate insulin early after meals and excess insulin in the later postprandial period, resulting in late hypoglycemia. Thus, late meal boluses (Answer D) is the most likely explanation.

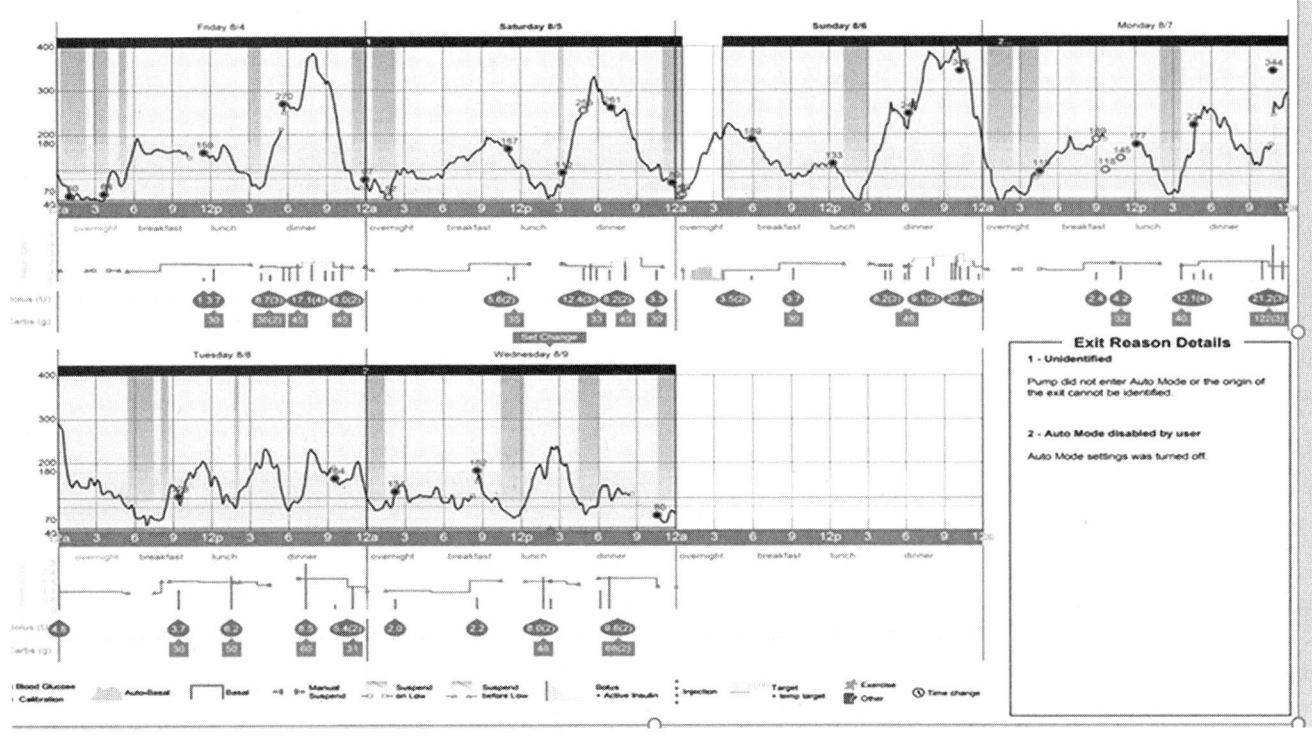

References

1. Hypoglycemia in the Diabetes Control and Complications Trial. The Diabetes Control and Complications Trial Research Group. *Diabetes.* 1997;46(2):271-286. PMID: 9000705

2. Juvenile Research Foundation Continuous Glucose Monitoring Study Group, Tamborlane WV, Beck RW, et al. Continuous glucose monitoring and intensive treatment of type 1 diabetes. *N Engl J Med.* 2008;359(14):1464-1476. PMID: 18779236

3. Roy RW, Bergenstal RM, Laffel LM, Pickup JC. Advances in technology for management of type 1 diabetes. *Lancet.* 2019;394(10205):1265-1273. PMID: 31533908

4. Kovatchev B. A century of diabetes technology: signals, models, and artificial pancrease control. *Trends Endocrinol Metab.* 2019;30(7):432-442. PMID: 31151733

5. Tauschmann M, Hovorka R. *Nat Rev Endocrinol.* 2018;14(8):464-475. PMID: 29946127

6. Deiss D, Szadkowska A, Gordon D, et al. Clinical practice recommendations on the routine use of Eversense, the first long-term implantable continuous glucose monitoring system. *Diabetes Technol Ther.* 2019;21(5):254-264. PMID: 31021180

7. Garg SK, Weinzimer SA, Tamborlane WV, et al. Glucose outcomes with the in-home use of a hybrid closed-loop insulin delivery system in adolescents and adults with type 1 diabetes. *Diabetes Technol Ther.* 2017;19(3):155-163. PMID: 28134564

8. Brown SA, Kovatchev BP, Raghinaru D, et al; iDCL Trial Research Group. Six-month randomized, multicenter trial of closed-loop control in type 1 diabetes. *N Engl J Med.* 2019;381(18):1707-1717. PMID: 31618560

9. Bell KJ, Fio CZ, Twigg S, et al. Amount and type of dietary fat, postprandial glycemia, and insulin requirements in type 1 diabetes: a randomized within-subject trial. *Diabetes Care.* 2020;43(1):59-66. PMID: 31455688

10. Battelino T, Danne T, Bergenstal RM, et al. Clinical targets for continuous glucose monitoring data interpretation: recommendations from the International Consensus on Time in Range. *Diabetes Care.* 2019;42(8):1593-1603. PMID: 31177185

11. Beck RW, Bergenstal RM, Cheng P, et al. The relationships between time in range, hyperglycemia metrics, and HbA1c. *J Diabetes Sci Technol.* 2019;13(4):614-626. PMID: 30636519

12. Bergenstal RM, Beck RW, Close KL, et al. Glucose management indicator (GMI): a new term for estimating A1C from continuous glucose monitoring. *Diabetes Care.* 2018;41:2275-2280. 30224348

Practical Approaches to the Genetic Diagnosis and Management of Patients With Diabetes Mellitus

Rochelle N. Naylor, MD. Departments of Pediatrics and Medicine, Section of Adult and Pediatric Endocrinology, Diabetes and Metabolism, University of Chicago, Chicago, IL; E-mail: rnaylor@bsd.uchicago.edu

Learning Objectives

As a result of participating in this session, learners should be able to:

- Identify the clinical and laboratory features that suggest a diagnosis of monogenic diabetes.

- Describe features and appropriate management for the most common forms of monogenic diabetes.

Main Conclusions

While monogenic diabetes represents an uncommon form of diabetes, accurate diagnosis through genetic testing directs treatment and management and identifies affected and at-risk family members. Several clinical and laboratory features can help identify a patient highly likely to have monogenic diabetes, who should be referred for genetic testing. These include negative pancreatic autoantibodies and continued endogenous insulin production more than 3 years after diabetes diagnosis. The most common forms of monogenic diabetes have gene-directed therapies that may improve glycemic control and outcomes. This includes sulfonylureas for K-ATP channel–related neonatal diabetes, relapsed 6q24 neonatal diabetes, HNF1A-MODY, and HNF4A-MODY. GCK-MODY does not need treatment outside of pregnancy. In pregnancies affected by GCK-MODY, treatment is based on fetal genotype. HNF1B-MODY most often requires insulin therapy, but accurate diagnosis can allow for surveillance and management of the renal and other extra-pancreatic features that are a common manifestation of heterozygous *HNF1B* pathogenic variants. Clinicians must consider monogenic diabetes at initial diabetes classification to ensure timely diagnosis and appropriate treatment to improve diabetes outcomes.

Significance of the Clinical Problem

Monogenic diabetes, due to single gene pathogenic variants or chromosomal abnormalities, accounts for approximately 2% of young-onset diabetes. The main phenotypes are neonatal diabetes, which can be permanent or transient, and maturity-onset diabetes of the young (MODY). The vast majority of monogenic diabetes cases are misdiagnosed as type 1 or type 2 diabetes. Studies estimate that more than 80% of cases go undiagnosed or are misdiagnosed for many years.[1,2] Misdiagnosis of MODY leads to improper and unnecessary treatment. Misdiagnosis increases health care expenditures due to unnecessary treatment or inappropriate medications, including intensive insulin therapy. Patients with MODY are also exposed to adverse medication effects as a result of improper management.[2]

While there is considerable clinical overlap between monogenic diabetes and both type 1 and type 2 diabetes, there are clinical and laboratory features that can help providers identify patients who may have monogenic diabetes. Several studies have demonstrated the usefulness of biomarkers to identify patients who should undergo genetic testing for monogenic diabetes.[3-5] Additionally, there is a MODY probability calculator that uses clinical information to assess the probability of a patient having MODY.[6] Cost-effectiveness analyses suggest that genetic testing for monogenic diabetes in appropriate populations can be cost-saving.[7-9] Genetic diagnosis of certain forms of monogenic diabetes is clinically actionable, allowing therapy selection based on the genetic cause, often with decreased burden of treatment and stable or improved glycemia. Proband diagnosis also aids in earlier diagnosis and correct classification of diabetes in family members.

Barriers to Optimal Practice

- Significant overlap between type 1 and type 2 diabetes precludes definitive diagnosis of monogenic diabetes solely on a clinical basis. Providers may be unaware of the clinical features that should prompt consideration of a monogenic diabetes diagnosis.

- Navigating the process for genetic testing to confirm monogenic diabetes can be time- and labor-intensive for providers. Moreover, genetic testing reports may be difficult to interpret.

- Providers may be unaware of the benefits of gene-targeted therapy in certain forms of monogenic diabetes.

- Providers may be unaware of the extra-pancreatic features and complication risks in certain forms of monogenic diabetes.

Strategies for Diagnosis, Therapy, and/or Management

Several clinical features can raise suspicion for monogenic diabetes. Diabetes diagnosis in patients younger than 6 months nearly always implies a monogenic cause. MODY is an autosomal dominant condition and thus is typically characterized by a strong family history of diabetes over several generations. While obesity does not preclude monogenic diabetes, nonobese, young-onset, non–insulin-dependent diabetes, particularly with a positive family history, is highly likely to be monogenic in nature.

Laboratory testing can also help to identify patients likely to have monogenic diabetes, with published studies showing the utility of using biomarkers to identify individuals for genetic testing.[3-5] "Type 1 diabetes" with absence of pancreatic autoantibodies or continued endogenous insulin production, as measured by serum or urine C-peptide, several years after diabetes diagnosis should raise suspicion for monogenic diabetes.[10,11] Studies in "type 2 diabetes" have used anthropometric data (BMI, absence of metabolic syndrome) and high-sensitivity C-reactive protein levels to discriminate likely type 2 diabetes from possible HNF1A-MODY.[12] A prediction model for MODY, known as the MODY calculator, based on clinical features and hemoglobin A_{1c}, was developed and validated in a United Kingdom population and is available without charge.[6]

Genetic testing for monogenic diabetes is available in numerous certified clinical laboratories. All individuals diagnosed with diabetes under 6 months of age should undergo comprehensive genetic testing using next-generation sequencing strategies. It is reasonable to consider testing in those diagnosed between 6 and 12 months of age, although rates of neonatal diabetes are markedly decreased compared with rates in individuals diagnosed before 6 months of age. In contrast, MODY lacks a single clinical criterion to identify patients who should have genetic testing, and screening the entire diabetes population for MODY is not economically feasible. Thus, it is important to target genetic testing to high-risk populations, using biomarkers as described above. Interpretation of genetic testing reports can be confusing and lead to erroneous diagnosis of monogenic diabetes when a variant of uncertain significance is detected. Consultation with experts in monogenic diabetes is advised for any uncertainty after genetic testing.

Genetic diagnosis of certain forms of monogenic diabetes is clinically actionable, allowing therapy selection based on the genetic cause. Permanent neonatal diabetes owing to pathogenic variants in *KCNJ11* or *ABCC8*, the genes encoding the ATP-sensitive potassium channel in the β cell, respond to high-dosage sulfonylureas with excellent glycemic control and improvement in neurologic outcomes. Those with transient neonatal diabetes often have relapse of diabetes in adolescence or early adulthood. Relapse of transient neonatal diabetes due to 6q24 abnormalities can be treated with low doses of sulfonylureas.[13]

GCK-MODY is characterized by stable mildly elevated blood glucose due to a glucose-sensing defect. Mild hyperglycemia is present at birth but often diagnosed incidentally, such as during a routine exam or while investigating another medical complaint. *GCK* pathogenic variants cause mild, regulated hyperglycemia, so treatment is not needed outside of pregnancy. Studies have shown that discontinuation of therapy in GCK-MODY does not alter hemoglobin A_{1c}. There is very minimal deterioration of glucose tolerance over the long term due to decreased insulin sensitivity with insulin secretion remaining stable, as also occurs in the nondiabetic population with age. At this level of glycemic control, diabetes-related complications are rare. In pregnancies of women with GCK-MODY, the risk of fetal macrosomia is based on whether the fetus inherits the heterozygous *GCK* pathogenic variants from the mother. Insulin therapy is recommended only when the fetus is known or suspected to not carry a *GCK* pathogenic variant, based on fetal abdominal circumference rising disproportionally above the 75th percentile on second trimester scans.[14]

Other forms of MODY (HNF1A-MODY, HNF4A-MODY, and HNF1B-MODY) are typically diagnosed in adolescence or early adulthood (before age 35 years, and often under 25 years). HNF1A-MODY and HNF4A-MODY exhibit a marked sensitivity to sulfonylureas, which bypass the major β-cell defect. A number of studies have demonstrated equal or improved control as compared with insulin therapy.[15,16] The majority of people with HNF1B-MODY require insulin therapy. Heterozygous *HNF1B* pathogenic variants cause a spectrum of abnormalities that can be assessed for and managed once an accurate diagnosis is made. Heterozygous *HNF1B* pathogenic variants are the most common cause of developmental renal disease, which often manifests as cysts but single kidneys and renal hypoplasia may also occur. Renal function is often impaired. Additional features include pancreatic hypoplasia that may include subclinical exocrine pancreas dysfunction, genital tract abnormalities, abnormal liver function, magnesium wasting, and hyperuricemia and gout.[17]

Clinical Case Vignettes
Case 1

A 32-year-old woman with a known diagnosis of GCK-MODY is currently on no treatment. She plans to conceive this year and is asking for guidance on management of GCK-MODY during pregnancy.

Based on current recommendations and studies in GCK-MODY, which of the following should you tell her regarding insulin therapy?

A. Early initiation of insulin therapy will reduce fetal macrosomia and has not been associated with adverse effects

B. Initiation of insulin therapy should be based on second-trimester maternal glycemia

C. Initiation of insulin therapy should be based on second-trimester fetal growth

D. Fetal genotype should be assessed by amniocentesis or chorionic villus sampling to guide decisions on insulin therapy

E. Insulin therapy is not needed in pregnancies affected by GCK-MODY

Answer: C) Initiation of insulin therapy should be based on second-trimester fetal growth

With the exception of pregnancy, treatment is not effective and not recommended in GCK-MODY. In pregnancies of women with GCK-MODY, the risk of fetal macrosomia is based on whether the fetus inherits the heterozygous *GCK* pathogenic variant from the mother. If the fetus carries a heterozygous *GCK* pathogenic variant, it will sense mother's mildly elevated blood glucose levels as normal and grow normally. If the fetus does not carry the heterozygous *GCK* pathogenic variant, it is at risk for macrosomia.

While there is some debate in the literature, the largest consensus on management of GCK-MODY in pregnancy is to base therapy on known or suspected fetal genotype. Amniocentesis or chorionic villus sampling for the sole purpose of assessing fetal genotype for a heterozygous *GCK* pathogenic variant (Answer D) is not recommended due to the risk of pregnancy loss. For most cases where fetal genotype is not known, it can be inferred based on second-trimester fetal growth on ultrasonography. Current recommendations advise to consider insulin therapy if fetal abdominal circumference is rising disproportionally above the 75th percentile (Answer C) and to induce labor at 38 weeks.

Women with GCK-MODY may experience hypoglycemia, including severe hypoglycemia, when treated with insulin during pregnancy. Additionally, there is a theoretical risk of growth restriction in GCK-MODY affected fetuses whose mothers receive insulin therapy. In cases where insulin is given for known or suspected unaffected fetuses, the effect on birthweight is limited due to the difficulty in altering maternal glycemia (thus, Answer A is incorrect).

Case 2

A 26-year-old man has been referred to you for a recent genetic diagnosis of HNF1A-MODY. Monogenic diabetes was suspected due to his ability to miss basal insulin and continued C-peptide production. He was initially misdiagnosed with type 1 diabetes 6 years ago and is on insulin therapy. He has no additional significant medical history, including no known complications of diabetes. He is currently receiving insulin glargine, 8 units daily, and takes 1 to 2 units of insulin aspart with meals. On physical examination, his weight is 176 lb (80 kg), and height is 74 in (188 cm) (BMI = 22.6 kg/m²). Vital signs are normal and examination findings are unremarkable. His hemoglobin A_{1c} value is 7.2% (55 mmol/mol).

In addition to monitoring blood glucose closely via glucose meter, which of the following is the best plan for transitioning him to sulfonylurea therapy?

A. Continue insulin at his current dosages and start glyburide ½ of the 1.25 mg tablet daily

B. Discontinue meal-time insulin and start glyburide ½ of the 1.25 mg tablet daily

C. Discontinue basal insulin and start glyburide ½ of the 1.25 mg tablet daily

D. Stop all insulin and start glyburide ½ of the 1.25 mg tablet daily

Answer: D) Stop all insulin and start glyburide ½ of the 1.25 mg tablet daily

There are several things to consider when transitioning to sulfonylurea therapy, including current treatment (insulin vs noninsulin glucose-lowering therapy), duration of diabetes, and weight (presence or absence of obesity). Patients should have evidence of ongoing endogenous insulin production. For those who are on insulin therapy, this can be inferred from subreplacement doses or the ability to miss insulin, and can be confirmed via measurement of C-peptide. Successful transfer off insulin is more likely in patients younger than 40 years who have had a diabetes duration less than 20 years. Normal-weight patients are also more likely to successfully transition off insulin.

Patients with HNF1A-MODY are often very sensitive to low dosages of sulfonylureas; starting with one-half tablet of the lowest dose and titrating up to achieve adequate glycemic control is advised. Those who are on oral or other noninsulin therapy or who are on subreplacement doses of insulin can be transitioned directly to low-dosage sulfonylureas. For patients on replacement doses of insulin or who have a long duration of diabetes (>20 years), basal insulin can be decreased by half and bolus insulin discontinued upon starting a low-dosage sulfonylurea. Basal insulin should be decreased as the sulfonylurea dose is titrated up.

In this vignette, positive C-peptide indicates that the patient continues to make insulin. Additionally, he is on subreplacement doses of insulin (0.14-0.18 units per kg daily). He is young, normal weight, and has a short diabetes duration. Thus, he is very likely to successfully transition to sulfonylurea therapy (Answer D).

References

1. Shields BM, Hicks S, Shepherd MH, Colclough K, Hattersley AT, Ellard S. Maturity-onset diabetes of the young (MODY): how many cases are we missing? *Diabetologia.* 2010;53(12):2504-2508. PMID: 20499044

2. Carmody D, Naylor RN, Bell CD, et al. GCK-MODY in the US National Monogenic Diabetes Registry: frequently misdiagnosed and unnecessarily treated. *Acta Diabetol.* 2016;53(5):703-708. PMID: 27106716

3. Pihoker C, Gilliam LK, Ellard S, et al; SEARCH for Diabetes in Youth Study Group. Prevalence, characteristics and clinical diagnosis of maturity onset diabetes of the young due to mutations in HNF1A, HNF4A, and glucokinase: results from the SEARCH for Diabetes in Youth. *J Clin Endocrinol Metab.* 2013;98(10):4055-4062. PMID: 23771925

4. Shepherd M, Shields B, Hammersley S, et al; UNITED Team. Systematic population screening, using biomarkers and genetic testing, identifies 2.5% of the U.K. pediatric diabetes population with monogenic diabetes. *Diabetes Care.* 2016;39(11):1879-1888. PMID: 27271189

5. Shields BM, Shepherd M, Hudson M, et al; UNITED study team. Population-based assessment of a biomarker-based screening pathway to aid diagnosis of monogenic diabetes in young-onset atients. *Diabetes Care.* 2017;40(8):1017-1025. PMID: 28701371

6. Shields BM, McDonald TJ, Ellard S, Campbell MJ, Hyde C, Hattersley AT. The development and validation of a clinical prediction model to determine the probability of MODY in patients with young-onset diabetes. *Diabetologia.* 2012;55(5):1265-1272. PMID: 22218698

7. Greeley SAW, John PM, Winn AN, et al. The cost-effectiveness of personalized genetic medicine: the case of genetic testing in neonatal diabetes. *Diabetes Care.* 2011;34(3):622-627. PMID: 21273495

8. Johnson SR, Carter HE, Leo P, et al. Cost-effectiveness analysis of routine screening using massively parallel sequencing for maturity-onset diabetes of the young in a pediatric diabetes cohort: reduced health system costs and improved patient quality of life. *Diabetes Care.* 2019;42(1):69-76. PMID: 30523035

9. Goodsmith MS, Skandari MR, Huang ES, Naylor RN. The impact of biomarker screening and cascade genetic testing on the cost-effectiveness of MODY genetic testing. *Diabetes Care.* 2019;42(12):2247-2255. PMID: 31558549

10. McDonald TJ, Colclough K, Brown R, et al. Islet autoantibodies can discriminate maturity-onset diabetes of the young (MODY) from type 1 diabetes. *Diabet Med.* 2011;28(9):1028-1033. PMID: 21395678

11. Besser REJ, Shepherd MH, McDonald TJ, et al. Urinary C-peptide creatinine ratio is a practical outpatient tool for identifying hepatocyte nuclear factor 1-{alpha}/hepatocyte nuclear factor 4-{alpha} maturity-onset diabetes of the young from long-duration type 1 diabetes. *Diabetes Care.* 2011;34(2):286-291. PMID: 21270186

12. Thanabalasingham G, Shah N, Vaxillaire M, et al. A large multi-centre European study validates high-sensitivity C-reactive protein (hsCRP) as a clinical biomarker for the diagnosis of diabetes subtypes. *Diabetologia.* 2011;54(11):2801-2810. PMID: 21814873

13. Hattersley AT, Patel KA. Precision diabetes: learning from monogenic diabetes. *Diabetologia.* 2017;60(5):769-777. PMID: 28314945

14. Chakera AJ, Steele AM, Gloyn AL, et al. Recognition and management of individuals with hyperglycemia because of a heterozygous glucokinase mutation. *Diabetes Care.* 2015;38(7):1383-1392. PMID: 26106223

15. Shepherd M, Shields B, Ellard S, Rubio-Cabezas O, Hattersley AT. A genetic diagnosis of HNF1A diabetes alters treatment and improves glycaemic control in the majority of insulin-treated patients. *Diabet Med.* 2009;26(4):437-441. PMID: 19388975

16. Bacon S, Kyithar MP, Rizvi SR, et al. Successful maintenance on sulphonylurea therapy and low diabetes complications rates in a HNF1A-MODY cohort. *Diabet Med.* 2016;33(7):976-984. PMID: 26479152

17. Clissold RL, Hamilton AJ, Hattersley AT, Ellard S, Bingham C. HNF1B-associated renal and extra-renal disease-an expanding clinical spectrum. *Nat Rev Nephrol.* 2015;11(2):102-112. PMID: 25536396

Using Clinical Trial Results to Optimize Patient Care: Cardiovascular Outcomes in Patients With Type 2 Diabetes Mellitus Treated With GLP-1 Receptor Agonists and SGLT-2 Inhibitors

Jennifer B. Green, MD. Department of Medicine, Division of Endocrinology, Duke University Medical Center, Durham, NC; E-mail: jennifer.green@duke.edu

Learning Objectives

As a result of participating in this session, learners should be able to:

- Identify patients with type 2 diabetes mellitus (T2DM) who have indications for GLP-1 receptor agonist or SGLT-2 inhibitor therapy to reduce the risk of cardio-renal complications.

- Plan for modifications in already complex regimens of care to permit incorporation of SGLT-2 inhibitors or GLP-1 receptor agonists.

Main Conclusions

Patients with T2DM are at high risk for major cardio-renal complications. When used in addition to traditional modalities of cardiovascular risk reduction, numerous agents in the GLP-1 receptor agonist and SGLT-2 inhibitor classes have been shown to significantly reduce rates of important adverse outcomes in patients with T2DM and atherosclerotic cardiovascular disease (ASCVD) or multiple ASCVD risk factors. Findings from the outcomes trials conducted thus far suggest that several GLP-1 receptor agonists primarily reduce the risk of atherosclerotic type complications and progression of albuminuria, while SGLT-2 inhibitors consistently reduce the risks of heart failure and important renal outcomes. Trials of SGLT-2 inhibitor therapy in patients with diabetes and chronic kidney disease and in patients with heart failure with reduced ejection fraction with or without diabetes, have shown significant outcomes benefit in those patient populations as well. These newer agents should be preferentially used in patients at high risk for cardio-renal complications, including those with established major comorbidities, likely irrespective of the need for additional glucose lowering or preexisting antihyperglycemic therapy. In patients who have already achieved an individually appropriate degree of glycemic control, alteration of background antihyperglycemic therapy may be indicated to reduce the risk of hypoglycemia and/or mitigate regimen expense. In addition, anticipatory modification of diuretic or other antihypertensive therapy may be needed to avoid significant volume depletion or hypotension with the addition of an SGLT-2 inhibitor.

Significance of the Clinical Problem

Although rates of morbidity and mortality in persons with diabetes have decreased over time, individuals with diabetes still have an approximately 2-fold excess risk of cardiovascular outcomes (including coronary heart disease, stroke, and vascular death) compared with outcomes of persons without diabetes.[1,2] This excess risk of vascular events in persons with diabetes appears higher in younger individuals and in women, and in those with a longer duration of diabetes and established microvascular complications such as kidney disease. In addition, diabetes increases the risk of heart failure by up to 5-fold, and diabetes is strongly associated with adverse outcomes in patients with heart failure, particularly heart failure with reduced ejection fraction.[3,4] Intensive multifactorial therapy to manage cardiovascular risk factors is effective in reducing the risk of vascular events in patients with T2DM.[5] However, progress in the control of traditional cardiovascular risk factors is slowing. It is estimated that 33% to 49% of patients still do not meet recommended targets for the management of hemoglobin A_{1c}, blood pressure, or lipids. In fact, only 14% meet targets for glycemic and blood pressure control and lipid management and do not smoke cigarettes.[6]

Findings from many recent large outcomes trials designed to assess the cardiovascular effects of newer classes of diabetes medications have further altered recommendations for the care of persons with T2DM. Numerous agents in the GLP-1 receptor agonist and SGLT-2 inhibitor classes reduce the risk of important cardiovascular and renal complications when included as part of usual care in patients with T2DM and established ASCVD or multiple risk factors for ASCVD.[4,7]

Thus, preferential use of these medications is recommended for such patients, and may help to address the residual cardiovascular risk that still affects those with diabetes. However, implementation of these therapies has thus far been quite limited, particularly in the populations of patients most likely to derive an outcomes benefit.[8] There are many potential barriers to provider implementation of these guideline-based practices into diabetes care, including lack of familiarity with the rapidly emerging body of cardiovascular outcomes trials data. In addition, concerns about potential adverse effects of newer drug classes and how they may best fit into existing complex medication regimens may pose additional obstacles to optimization of care.

Barriers to Optimal Practice

- Complexity of emerging data from cardiovascular outcomes trials and understanding applicability to individual at-risk patients.
- Difficulty in assessing the balance of overall benefits and risks with use of newer antihyperglycemic agents in patients with diabetes-related comorbidities.
- Challenges in introducing newer, beneficial antihyperglycemic agents into an already complex medication regimen.

Strategies for Diagnosis, Therapy, and/or Management

In 2008, the US FDA issued a guidance recommending thorough evaluation of all new diabetes therapies for cardiovascular safety. Since that time, numerous cardiovascular outcomes trials of drugs in the DPP-4 inhibitor, GLP-1 receptor agonist, and SGLT-2 inhibitor classes have been completed. Most of these trials were designed to assess the cardiovascular impact of a particular new diabetes medication compared with placebo when added to the otherwise usual care of patients with T2DM. These trials primarily enrolled patients with established ASCVD (including coronary, cerebrovascular, or peripheral vascular disease) or patients who were otherwise at high risk for major adverse cardiovascular events (MACE) such as cardiovascular death, myocardial infarction, and stroke. The findings of these trials, including the effects of the studied medications on risks of MACE and hospitalization for heart failure, are summarized in the tables (*Table 1* and *Table 2*).

Cardiovascular Effects of Newer Medication Classes

DPP-4 Inhibitors

Trials of the DPP-4 inhibitor medications completed thus far have consistently demonstrated a neutral effect of these drugs on rates of MACE. Most of the DPP-4 inhibitors have also had a neutral effect on rates of hospitalization for heart failure. However, the SAVOR TIMI-53 trial of saxagliptin therapy unexpectedly found an increase in hospitalization for heart failure in patients assigned to that medication when compared with placebo. This increase in risk has not been explained or reproduced in other trials, but it should be carefully considered when managing patients with diabetes and existing heart failure or

Table 1. Effects of Newer Diabetes Medications: Major Adverse Cardiovascular Events

Drug Class	SAVOR-TMI-53 saxagliptin	EXAMINE alogliptin	TECOS sitagliptin	CARMELINA linagliptin	
DPP-4 inhibitor	Neutral	Neutral	Neutral	Neutral	
	LEADER linagliptin	ELIXA lixisenatide	SUSTAIN-6 semaglutide injection	EXSCEL exenatide once weekly	REWIND dulaglutide
GLP-1 receptor agonist	Beneficial	Neutral	Beneficial	Neutral	Beneficial
	EMPA-REG empagliflozin	CANVAS canagliflozin	DECLARE dapagliflozin		
SLGT-2 inhibitor	Beneficial	Beneficial	Neutral*		

MACE = Major Adverse Cardiovascular Events: CV death, MI, stroke
*One of two primary composite endpoints

Table 2. Effects of Newer Diabetes Medications: Heart Failure

Drug Class	SAVOR-TMI-53 saxagliptin	EXAMINE alogliptin	TECOS sitagliptin	CARMELINA linagliptin	
DPP-4 inhibitor	Increased Risk	Neutral	Neutral	Neutral	
	LEADER linagliptin	ELIXA lixisenatide	SUSTAIN-6 semaglutide injection	EXSCEL exenatide once weekly	REWIND dulaglutide
GLP-1 receptor agonist	Neutral	Neutral	Neutral	Neutral	Neutral
	EMPA-REG empagliflozin	CANVAS canagliflozin	DECLARE dapagliflozin	DAPA HF* dapagliflozin	
SLGT-2 inhibitor	Beneficial	Beneficial	Beneficial	Beneficial	

All trials listed other than DAPA-HF enrolled patients with type 2 diabetes and established atherosclerotic CV disease, or multiple risk factors for the same. HF endpoints in most trials were hospitalizations due to heart failure. *DAPA-HF enrolled patients with HFrEF with or without diabetes. Primary outcome was worsening HF event or cardiovascular death (worsening HF event = unplanned HF hospitalization or an urgent heart failure visit requiring intravenous therapy).

high heart failure risk. DPP-4 inhibitors, although largely found to be safe from a cardiovascular perspective, should not be used to reduce cardiovascular risk in patients with T2DM.

GLP-1 Receptor Agonists

The GLP-1 receptor agonist class is quite diverse with respect to molecular structure, duration of action, and potency. Thus, it is perhaps unsurprising that the findings from cardiovascular outcomes trials of these medications have differed. These trials have shown that liraglutide, semaglutide, and dulaglutide all reduce the risk of MACE when compared with placebo in patients with T2DM at high risk for such events. Of note, the REWIND trial of dulaglutide also enrolled patients at high risk, but in contrast to the other cardiovascular outcomes trials, most of the patients included had not had a prior cardiovascular event. A MACE benefit was also seen in the cardiovascular outcomes trial of albiglutide; however, that medication is no longer available for use. As shown in the summary table, the trials of GLP-1 receptor agonists have found a neutral effect of these agents on rates of heart failure hospitalization. Of these agents, thus far in the United States liraglutide is indicated to reduce the risk of MACE in adults with T2DM and established ASCVD.

SGLT-2 Inhibitors

Trials of agents in the SGLT-2 inhibitor class have had more consistent outcomes results. The cardiovascular outcomes trials of empagliflozin and canagliflozin demonstrated a significant reduction in MACE with use of those agents. The DECLARE trial did not find a reduction in MACE risk with dapagliflozin; however, a second primary heart failure outcome in that trial was significantly reduced with active therapy compared with placebo. All of the completed cardiovascular outcomes trials of SGLT-2 inhibitors have shown a significant reduction in heart failure outcomes with use of those agents. Most recently, the DAPA heart failure trial evaluated the effects of dapagliflozin in patients with heart failure with reduced ejection fraction, with or without

diabetes.[9] In that trial, dapagliflozin therapy significantly reduced the risk of worsening heart failure or death from cardiovascular causes compared with placebo.

In the United States, empagliflozin is indicated to reduce the risk of cardiovascular death in adult patients with T2DM and established ASCVD; canagliflozin is indicated to reduce the risk of MACE in the same population; and dapagliflozin is indicated to reduce the risk of hospitalization for heart failure in adults with T2DM and established ASCVD or multiple cardiovascular risk factors.

Renal Effects of GLP-1 Receptor Agonists and SGLT-2 Inhibitors

Although not the primary outcomes of interest, the effects of the newer drug classes on a variety of renal outcomes were also analyzed in most of the cardiovascular outcomes trials completed to date. Meta-analyses of these data suggest that the renal outcomes benefit noted in the trials of GLP-1 receptor agonists were primarily attributable to a reduction in macroalbuminuria, while SGLT-2 inhibitors were found to reduce the risks of worsening estimated glomerular filtration rate, end-stage kidney disease, or death due to renal causes.[10] The CREDENCE trial has since specifically evaluated the effects of SGLT-2 inhibitors in patients with T2DM and albuminuric chronic kidney disease.[11] In that trial, canagliflozin, 100 mg daily, significantly reduced the risk of kidney failure and cardiovascular events at 2.62 years compared with placebo. As a result, canagliflozin is now also indicated to reduce the risk of end-stage kidney disease, doubling of serum creatinine, cardiovascular death, and hospitalization for heart failure in adults with T2DM and diabetic nephropathy with albuminuria and an estimated glomerular filtration rate of 30 mL/min per 1.73 m^2 or higher.

GLP-1 Receptor Agonists and SGLT-2 Inhibitors Outcomes Summary

Meta-analyses of the cardiovascular outcomes trials data suggest the following summary of drug class effects:

1. Both GLP-1 receptor agonists and SGLT-2 inhibitors decrease risk of MACE in patients with established ASCVD.

   a. In REWIND, the GLP-1 receptor agonist dulaglutide reduced risk of MACE in patients without a prior cardiovascular event.

2. SGLT-2 inhibitors reduce hospitalization for heart failure and progression of kidney disease in patients with established ASCVD or who are at high cardiovascular risk.[10,12]

The cardiovascular benefits of GLP-1 receptor agonist therapy may be due to beneficial antiatherogenic effects of the medications mediated by improvements in cardiovascular risk factors such as weight and blood pressure. The mechanisms of benefit provided by SGLT-2 inhibitors are likely different and may be in part attributable to favorable hemodynamic and other effects induced by glycosuria and natriuresis. The cardiovascular benefits identified in the cardiovascular outcomes trials do not appear attributable to or dependent on glucose lowering.

In applying this information to clinical practice, it is important to recognize the variable outcomes noted in cardiovascular outcomes trials of the individual diabetes medications. Current diabetes care guidelines note that drugs with proven outcomes benefit should be specifically selected when used to reduce cardiovascular risk in patients with T2DM.[4,7] Some guidelines suggest preferential use of GLP-1 receptor agonists in patients with ASCVD, with SGLT-2 inhibitors as a second choice if GLP-1 receptor agonist therapy is not feasible or tolerated. However, there are no head-to-head trials comparing the effects of the 2 drug classes in this patient population; thus, choice of a proven agent from either class is reasonable, based on individual patient characteristics and preferences. SGLT-2 inhibitors also appear particularly effective in improving outcomes in patients with T2DM and chronic kidney disease or heart failure with reduced ejection fraction.

Therapeutic Issues

GLP-1 Receptor Agonists

The agents in this class with demonstrated cardiovascular outcomes benefit are delivered via subcutaneous injection. Primary contraindications to use of these medications include a personal or family history of medullary thyroid cancer or multiple endocrine neoplasia type 2. Other potential contraindications include history of pancreatitis or bariatric surgery. Worsening of retinopathy has been noted with semaglutide use. These agents may cause nausea and vomiting, particularly with dose initiation or up-titration. Cautious dosage adjustment may be prudent.

SGLT-2 Inhibitors

These agents have a diuretic effect that may cause volume depletion or hypotension. Increased urinary glucose excretion increases the risk of genital mycotic infections, particularly in women, and some SGLT-2 inhibitor users have experienced Fournier gangrene. Good genitourinary/perineal hygiene should be encouraged. An increased amputation risk was seen with canagliflozin therapy in the CANVAS trial, but not in CREDENCE, which implemented a rigorous strategy of foot care. Diabetic ketoacidosis with lower than expected blood glucose elevation may occur with use of any SGLT-2 inhibitor. Thus, the drug should be discontinued during significant illness, dehydration, major procedures, or hospitalization.

Strategies for Incorporation of Cardioprotective Diabetes Medications

Patients with T2DM and high cardiovascular risk are often already taking highly complex regimens of medication. This may make the addition of new agents with cardiovascular outcomes benefit particularly challenging. In addition to the above therapeutic concerns, the patient's degree of glycemic control and risk of hypoglycemia should be considered before adding either a GLP-1 receptor agonist or SGLT-2 inhibitor. In addition, if an SGLT-2 inhibitor is chosen, the patient's blood pressure and volume status should be carefully assessed.[13] Adjustments to baseline medications should be considered as outlined in the *Figure*.

Figure. Addition of Cardioprotective Diabetes Medication

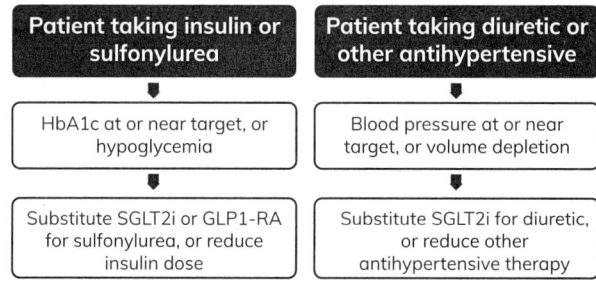

Clinical Case Vignettes

Case 1

A 76-year-old woman with T2DM complicated by hyperlipidemia, hypertension, and coronary artery disease requiring stent placement is seen for evaluation. Her current medications include aspirin, clopidogrel, lisinopril, hydrochlorothiazide, and atorvastatin. Her BMI is 33 kg/m²; blood pressure is 124/80 mm Hg; and she appears euvolemic. Her hemoglobin A_{1c} level is 7.2% (55 mmol/mol) and estimated glomerular filtration rate is 56 mL/min per 1.73 m².

Which of the following change(s) to her medication regimen would be recommended at this time?

A. No change

B. Start metformin

C. Start empagliflozin

D. Discontinue hydrochlorothiazide

Answer: C and D) Start empagliflozin and discontinue hydrochlorothiazide

This patient with T2DM has established ASCVD and indications for a medication to reduce her risk of future cardiovascular events (thus, Answer A is incorrect). She is currently on no medications to manage glycemia and has a hemoglobin A_{1c} level only slightly above 7% (53 mmol/mol). Although the cardiovascular outcomes trials of newer medications enrolled patients who were often using metformin (Answer B) as background therapy, there is no evidence to suggest that the beneficial effects of SGLT-2 inhibitors or GLP-1 receptor agonists are restricted to metformin users, or to patients who have hemoglobin A_{1c} values above a certain threshold. Although some guidelines still suggest that metformin therapy should always be included as initial therapy for T2DM, metformin has no demonstrated efficacy in the reduction of cardiovascular risk in patients with established ASCVD. Thus, the initiation of empagliflozin (Answer C) would be the preferred next step for this patient. Should additional glucose lowering be needed in the future, metformin could be added to empagliflozin therapy. As this older patient is essentially normotensive on a regimen that includes the diuretic hydrochlorothiazide, that medication should be discontinued (Answer D) when empagliflozin is started, and the patient's volume status and blood pressure should be reassessed at follow-up. A GLP-1 receptor agonist might also be a reasonable consideration for this patient to reduce her risk of future MACE.

Case 2

A 57-year-old man with T2DM, peripheral vascular disease, coronary artery disease, chronic kidney disease, obesity, hyperlipidemia, and hypertension presents for evaluation. His current medications include sitagliptin; insulin glargine, 10 units once daily; aspirin; losartan; furosemide; and rosuvastatin. His BMI is 40 kg/m², and blood pressure is 144/86 mm Hg. His hemoglobin A_{1c} level is 8.4% (68 mmol/mol), and estimated glomerular filtration rate is 28 mL/min per 1.73 m². He has had no problems with hypoglycemia on his current regimen.

Which of the following change(s) to his medication regimen would be recommended at this time?

A. No change

B. Add empagliflozin

C. Add lixisenatide

D. Add liraglutide

E. Substitute liraglutide for sitagliptin

Answer: E) Substitute liraglutide for sitagliptin

This patient with T2DM and multiple manifestations of ASCVD has indications for a medication to further reduce his risk of cardiovascular events (thus, Answer A is incorrect). His hemoglobin A$_{1c}$ is not well controlled, even in light of his established comorbidities. He is on a low insulin dosage but has not had issues with hypoglycemia. He is also taking the DPP-4 inhibitor sitagliptin, which does not increase, but also does not reduce, his risk of cardiovascular events. Empagliflozin (Answer B) is not currently the correct choice for this patient given his low estimated glomerular filtration rate, as this medication is at present only indicated for use in patients with an estimated glomerular filtration rate of 45 mL/min per 1.73 m^2 or higher. Although canagliflozin may be considered for use in patients with lower estimated glomerular filtration rate values, this patient's current estimated glomerular filtration rate is too low for use of that drug as well. Therefore, introduction of a GLP-1 receptor agonist would be an appropriate choice. Lixisenatide (Answer C) was not found to reduce cardiovascular risk in the ELIXA trial, so liraglutide is the appropriate choice for this patient. Careful use with slow up-titration and monitoring for tolerability is needed in patients with significantly impaired renal function. This patient's sitagliptin should be discontinued when liraglutide is started, as combined use of a GLP-1 receptor agonist and a DPP-4 inhibitor is not recommended (thus, Answer E is correct and Answer D is incorrect). In addition, as both medications may be expensive, this will minimize the cost associated with his diabetes care regimen.

References

1. Rawshani A, Rawshani A, Franzen S, et al. Mortality and cardiovascular disease in type 1 and type 2 diabetes. *N Engl J Med.* 2017;376(15):1407-1418. PMID: 28402770

2. Emerging Risk Factors Collaboration, Sarwar N, Gao P, et al. Diabetes mellitus, fasting blood glucose concentration, and risk of vascular disease: a collaborative meta-analysis of 102 prospective studies. *Lancet.* 2010;375(9733):2215-2222. PMID: 20609967

3. Ghosh RK, Ghosh GC, Gupta M, et al. Sodium glucose co-transporter 2 inhibitors and heart failure. *Am J Cardiol.* 2019;124(11):1790-1796. PMID: 31627834

4. Cosentino F, Grant PJ, Aboyans V, et al; ESC Scientific Document Group. 2019 ESC guidelines on diabetes, pre-diabetes, and cardiovascular diseases developed in collaboration with the EASD. *Eur Heart J.* 2019;pii:ehz486. PMID: 31497854

5. Gaede P, Vedel P, Larsen N, Jensen GV, Parving HH, Pedersen O. Multifactorial intervention and cardiovascular disease in patients with type 2 diabetes. *N Engl J Med.* 2003;348(5):383-393. PMID: 12556541

6. American Diabetes Association. Standards of medical care in diabetes. 1. Promoting health and reducing disparities in populations. *Diabetes Care.* 2017;40(Suppl 1):S6-S10. PMID: 27979888

7. American Diabetes Association. Cardiovascular disease and risk management: standards of medical care in diabetes-2019. *Diabetes Care.* 2019;42(Suppl 1):S103-S123. PMID: 30559236

8. McCoy R, Dykhoff H, Sangaralingham L, Ross JS, Karaca-Mandic P, Montori VM, Shah ND. Adoption of new glucose-lowering medications in the U.S.-the case of SGLT2 inhibitors: nationwide cohort study. *Diab Technol Ther.* 2019;21(12);702-712. PMID: 31418588

9. McMurray JJV, Solomon SD, Inzucchi SE, et al; DAPA-HF Trial Committees and Investigators. Dapagliflozin in patients with heart failure and reduced ejection fraction. *N Engl J Med.* 2019;381(21):1995-2008. PMID: 31535829

10. Zelniker TA, Wiviott SD, Raz I, et al. Comparison of the effects of glucagon-like peptide receptor agonists and sodium-glucose cotransporter 2 inhibitors for prevention of major adverse cardiovascular and renal outcomes in type 2 diabetes mellitus. *Circulation.* 2019;139(17):2022-2031. PMID: 30786725

11. Perkovic V, Jardine MJ, Neal B, et al; CREDENCE Trial Investigators. Canagliflozin and renal outcomes in type 2 diabetes and nephropathy. *N Engl J Med.* 2019;380(24):2295-2306. PMID: 30990260

12. Zelniker TA, Wiviott SD, Raz I, et al. SGLT2 inhibitors for primary and secondary prevention of cardiovascular and renal outcomes in type 2 diabetes: a systematic review and meta-analysis of cardiovascular outcome trials. *Lancet.* 2019;393(10166):31-39. PMID: 30424892

13. Gomez-Peralta F, Abreu C, Lecube A, et al. Practical approach to initiating SGLT2 inhibitors in type 2 Diabetes. *Diabetes Ther.* 2017;8(5):953-962. PMID: 28721687

Pharmacologic Approaches to the Patient With Nonalcoholic Fatty Liver Disease

Diana Barb, MD. Department of Medicine, Division of Endocrinology, Diabetes, and Metabolism, University of Florida, Gainesville, FL; E-mail: diana.barb@medicine.ufl.edu

Learning Objectives

As a result of participating in this session, learners should be able to:

- Recognize burden of disease and how to diagnose nonalcoholic fatty liver disease (NAFLD) and nonalcoholic steatohepatitis (NASH).

- Describe optimal management of patients with type 2 diabetes mellitus (T2DM) and NAFLD.

- Describe current therapeutic targets for treating NAFLD.

Main Conclusions

- NAFLD is one of the silent, often unrecognized complications of obesity and T2DM. It is important to identify patients with NAFLD at risk for disease progression.

- Patients with diabetes are considered a high-risk population for this condition and should be screened for the presence of NAFLD and NASH even if concentrations of plasma aminotransferases are normal. The presence of NASH in a patient with T2DM should prompt early treatment with lifestyle intervention and use of therapies proven to be effective in randomized controlled trials.

- Treatment of NAFLD should also include aggressive cardiovascular risk factor management (ie, obesity, dyslipidemia, hypertension, and glycemic control).

- There are currently no FDA-approved pharmacologic therapies for NAFLD or NASH. However, pioglitazone should be considered first-line therapy in patients with NASH confirmed on liver biopsy and in patients with diabetes and NAFLD/NASH. Vitamin E demonstrated efficacy in patients without diabetes but not for the treatment of NASH in patients with T2DM. GLP-1 receptor agonists promote weight loss and are promising new agents for NASH that are undergoing testing. SGLT-2 inhibitors also reduce hepatic steatosis, but their ability to reverse steatohepatitis has not been explored.

- Recent progress in understanding the pathophysiology of NASH has led to the development of a number of novel pharmacological agents that are in ongoing clinical trials in an effort to develop safe and effective treatments.

- Finally, endocrinologists should become more involved in the management of NAFLD/NASH given the significant overlap of NASH with obesity and diabetes and the many clinical implications of the disease.

Significance of the Clinical Problem

Despite remarkable progress in understanding the pathogenesis of NAFLD/NASH and subsequently, in developing medications to target the disease, currently there are no pharmacologic agents approved specifically for this condition. Treatment of NAFLD/NASH should include aggressive management of hyperglycemia and cardiovascular risk factors. Agents tested with some success in patients with NASH without T2DM include pioglitazone, liraglutide, and vitamin E. In patients with T2DM and NASH, pioglitazone and liraglutide have been shown to significantly improve liver histology on repeat liver biopsy. This session focuses on available antidiabetes drugs that could potentially be useful for management of NAFLD/NASH. Many new molecules targeting metabolic pathways, inflammation, or oxidative stress and fibrosis are being studied, and understanding of the complex pathophysiology of NASH provides a rationale in the future for using combination of drugs to treat this condition.

NAFLD is the most common chronic liver disease in developed countries. Its prevalence depends on the population studied and diagnostic methodology used. In a recent meta-analysis, the global prevalence of NAFLD was estimated to be 25% in the general population[1] and up to approximately 56% in patients with T2DM.[2] However, due to a lack of reliable noninvasive diagnostic tests, this prevalence of NAFLD is likely underestimated.[1,3] When using a more sensitive and specific imaging method, such as proton magnetic resonance spectroscopy (^{1}H-MRS), the prevalence of NAFLD in the general population has been reported to be as high as 34% and even up to 70% in overweight or obese adults with T2DM.[4,5] NAFLD can progress from simple steatosis to its more severe form, known as NASH, and is characterized by the presence of inflammation and hepatocyte injury (ballooning and hepatocyte necroinflammation). It can lead to cirrhosis and hepatocellular carcinoma.[3] The global prevalence of NASH is estimated to be 3.5%,[1] but this is likely grossly underestimated, as it is currently the second leading cause of liver transplantation in the United States.[3,6] More importantly, NAFLD and NASH carry a high risk of diabetes and cardiovascular disease.[3] The prevalence of diabetes is increased across fibrosis stages in NASH anywhere from 21% in mild to moderate fibrosis stages and up to 50% in NASH cirrhosis.[7] Conversely, and by mechanisms that are still incompletely understood, patients with T2DM are susceptible to more severe forms of NAFLD, have a 2- to 4-fold higher risk of progression from NAFLD to NASH, and a higher prevalence of cirrhosis and hepatocellular carcinoma due to NASH.[8,9] Presence of diabetes promotes NASH, and is one of the important factors associated with advanced fibrosis.[3] Prevalence of NASH in persons with T2DM is estimated at 37%, or 10-fold higher than in the general population in a recent meta-analysis,[2] with advanced fibrosis in up to 17%.[2] It is important to recognize that about half of obese patients with T2DM and normal concentrations of plasma aminotransferases (AST/ALT levels ≤40 IU/L [≤0.67 μkat/L]) may have NAFLD and about 28% may have NASH on liver biopsy.[10]

Why should endocrinologists care about NAFLD? Despite being the most common cause of liver disease in patients with T2DM and estimated to be the number one reason for liver transplantation by 2020, NAFLD/NASH is frequently overlooked and commonly undiagnosed. Only a few affected patients receive a diagnosis of NASH or are ever treated in clinic. The disease carries a greater cardiovascular risk and unfortunately, when it progresses to fibrosis, it can lead to cirrhosis, liver failure, hepatocellular carcinoma, and premature death. Although traditionally viewed as a disease of hepatologists, NAFLD should become a major concern for endocrinologists and those caring for patients with obesity and T2DM. This session will focus on available treatment options for patients with NAFLD and/or NASH.

Barriers to Optimal Practice

- Patients and clinicians rarely think of NAFLD/NASH as a potentially serious medical condition.

- The diagnosis of NAFLD and NASH is often missed due to a reliance on low-sensitivity diagnostic tests (ie, plasma aminotransferase measurements or liver ultrasonography); transient elastography and ^{1}H-MRS are not being routinely used in clinical practice.

- Definite diagnosis of NASH involves liver biopsy, which has many limitations and it is rarely pursued by providers, even in patients who are at high risk of NASH. There is a need for better noninvasive tests in clinical practice.

- More specific screening and treatment recommendations are needed for patients with NAFLD and T2DM, and there is a need for more pharmacologic agents with proven efficacy and favorable weight profile.

- Common "barriers" to using pioglitazone more often in patients with NASH include unawareness about its efficacy (>50% have NASH resolution with pioglitazone), lack of familiarity with prescribing the drug, and misinformation about weight gain or the risk of other adverse effects with its use.

Strategies for Diagnosis, Therapy, and/or Management
Diagnosis of NAFLD and NASH

The cornerstone of medical management of NAFLD and NASH remains early diagnosis and intervention, as treatment success is less likely in advanced stages of fibrosis.[5] The diagnosis of NAFLD[6,11] is based on the following: (1) presence of hepatic steatosis in addition to (2) lack of significant alcohol consumption (defined as ongoing or recent alcohol consumption of >21 units/week for men and >14 units/week for women), and (3) exclusion of other liver diseases. Hepatic steatosis is usually seen on radiologic imaging (ie, liver ultrasonography, control attenuation parameters, and CT or by the gold standard technique ^{1}H-MRS) and is defined as liver fat content above 5.56% when measured by ^{1}H-MRS. In patients with T2DM, diagnosis should not solely rely on elevated plasma liver aminotransferases as up to 50% of patients with normal ALT levels (<40 U/L [<0.67 μkat/L]) may have NAFLD. If available, vibration-controlled transient elastography or magnetic resonance elastography can also be used to determine the severity (stage) of fibrosis.

Noninvasive algorithms based on metabolic and anthropometric parameters could be used in clinical practice to identify patients at risk for NAFLD (ie, fatty liver index) and advanced fibrosis (ie, NAFLD fibrosis score, FIB-4 index, AST-to-platelet ratio index, and many others). However, these are usually less sensitive and specific than the "gold standard" of liver biopsy.[4] Therefore, current guidelines[6] advise that liver biopsy is the only way to diagnose NASH and that noninvasive techniques have not yet been fully validated for the diagnosis of this condition.[4] In the future, as better noninvasive diagnostic techniques develop, it will become likely to shift toward noninvasive measures and not rely on liver biopsy before treatment initiation for NASH.

Although liver biopsy remains the gold standard for diagnosis of NASH, it has multiple caveats: it is invasive, subject to interpretation errors, and difficult to apply to large populations.[6,8] Definite NASH is determined on low- to medium-power microscopy based on the presence of at least grade 1 in each of the following 3 components: (1) steatosis (5%-33% of parenchyma is involved or grade 1, >33%-66% for grade 2, and >66% for grade 3), (2) lobular inflammation (<2 foci are present per 200× field for grade 1, 2 to 4 foci for grade 2, and >4 foci per 200× field are present for grade 3) and hepatocellular ballooning (few balloons cells are present per high-power field for grade 1 and many ballooning cells present for grade 2). NAFLD Activity Score is the sum of scores of steatosis (0-3), lobular inflammation (0-3), and hepatocellular ballooning (0-2).

Selecting Candidates for Liver Biopsy

In clinical practice, physicians have to decide whom to screen for advanced fibrosis and when to recommend liver biopsy. Patients with high risk of having NASH include those who are older (>45 years), have higher BMI, have T2DM, and have an AST-to-ALT ratio of 1 or greater. Patients with T2DM are at increased risk for more severe forms of NASH, and this has been recently acknowledged by the American Diabetes Association in the 2019 Standard of Care guidelines, recommending that "patients with T2DM or prediabetes and elevated liver enzymes or fatty liver on ultrasonography should be evaluated for the presence of NASH and liver fibrosis" (Recommendation 4.14, page S40). There is no further guidance on how to evaluate for NASH or who should be considered for a liver biopsy. One simple algorithm that could be applied in clinical practice is to screen patients with obesity and/or T2DM and elevated liver enzymes, after ruling out other causes for liver disease, to assess for fibrosis. Another important category is patients with normal liver enzymes and a history of longstanding uncontrolled diabetes (10 plus years in duration) or high triglycerides. Assessment of fibrosis can be estimated by applying a fibrosis biomarker panel and/or if available, magnetic resonance elastography or vibration-controlled transient elastography, which is a simple and noninvasive test (similar to ultrasonography), validated to measure liver fat and estimate for the presence of fibrosis. Patients with high or intermediate risk for fibrosis may need referral to hepatology for a liver biopsy. Bril and Cusi[4] propose an algorithm for management of patients with NAFLD and T2DM.

Strategies for Therapy and Management of NAFLD and NASH

Current guidelines advise that patients with biopsy-proven NASH should receive pharmacological treatment along with lifestyle intervention.[6] It is also important to recognize that NAFLD—through increased lipotoxicity and glucotoxicity—carries an increased cardiovascular disease risk,[4] and treatment of NAFLD should include aggressive cardiovascular risk-factor management (ie, weight, lipids, blood pressure, and treatment of hyperglycemia). Statins are safe to use in patients with NAFLD/NASH even if liver enzymes are elevated, and should be used as first-line therapy for lipid lowering.[5] In a few small randomized controlled trials, statins improved steatosis; however, there was no significant change in inflammation or fibrosis.[12] Fibrates and fish oil can be added as second-line therapy when indicated for treatment of dyslipidemia (ie, elevated triglycerides and low HDL cholesterol); however, they do not have direct effects on steatohepatitis.[4,5]

Presently, there are no FDA-approved agents with a specific indication for the treatment of NASH. The *Table* summarizes current pharmacologic approaches under evaluation in patients with NAFLD and NASH and their metabolic effects and histologic effects, when available, in randomized controlled trials. The endpoints usually evaluated in pharmacotherapy randomized controlled clinical trials are improvement in liver histology (each histologic component [ie, steatosis, inflammation, ballooning, and fibrosis]), ≥2-point improvement in NAFLD Activity Score, and/or NASH resolution without worsening of fibrosis and improvement in liver fibrosis of 1 or more stages with no worsening of steatohepatitis, with the last 2 being endorsed by the FDA. Other imaging endpoints are improvement in liver fat by ¹H-MRS, or liver proton density fat fraction and/or improvement in fibrosis by magnetic resonance elastography.

Although many agents show significant reduction in steatosis (either by histology or imaging [*Table*]), it should be noted that only treatment with pioglitazone (30 or 45 mg daily);[13-15] vitamin E, 800 IU daily;[14] and liraglutide, 1.8 mg daily[16] resulted in a significant proportion of patients achieving resolution of NASH when compared with placebo. The proportions

Table. Therapeutic Agents Under Evaluation for the Management of NAFLD and NASH and Their Effects on Liver Steatosis, Inflammation, and Fibrosis in Clinical Trials

Class	Drug	Metabolic effect	Effects on			Ref
			Steatosis	Inflammation	Fibrosis	
Biguanides	Metfomin	↓ Hepatic glucose output	↓[H, I]	↔	↔	24
PPAR agonists						
PPARγ (TZD's)	Pioglitazone	↑ Adipose, hepatic and muscle insulin sensitivity	↓[H, I]	↓	↓	13,14,15
PPARα/γ	Saroglitazar*	↓ Lipids and ↑ insulin sensitivity	↓[I]	N/A	N/A	38
PPARα/δ	Elafibranor*	↓ Hepatic lipogenesis	↓[I]	↔	↔	37
PPARα/γ/δ	Lanifibranor*	↓ Hepatic lipogenesis and ↑ Insulin sensitivity	Phase 2 RCT ongoing			N/A
DPP-4 inhibitors	Sitagliptin	↑ Endogenous level of GLP-1	↓↔[H, I]	↔	↔	25,26,27
	Vildagliptin		↓[I]	N/A	N/A	28
GLP-1 receptor agonists	Exenatide	↑ Glucose-dependent insulin secretion	↓[I]	N/A	N/A	22
	Liraglutide	↓ Gastric emptying and appetite	↓[H, I]	↓	↓	16,22,23
	Semaglutide*	↓ Body weight	Phase 2 RCT ongoing			N/A
SGLT-2 inhibitors	Canagliflozin	↓ Renal glucose reabsortion	↓[I]	N/A	N/A	29
	Empagliflozin	↓ Body weight	↓[I]	N/A	N/A	32,33
	Ipragliflozin	↑ Hepatic insulin sensitivity	↓[I]	N/A	N/A	31
	Dapagliflozin		↓[I]	N/A	N/A	34
Antioxidants	Vitamin E	↓ Lipid peroxidation	↓[H, I]	↓	↔	14,17,18
		↓ Repletion of glutathione				
		↓ Cytokine production				
Lipid-lowering drugs	Fish Oil	↓ VLDL-triglyceride and Apo B production	↔[H, I]	↔	↔	4,5,12
	Fibrates	↓ Hepatic secretion of VLDL	↔[I]	↔	↔	
	Statins	↓ Cholesterol biosynthesis by HMG CoA reductase	↔[H, I]	↔	↔	
PDE inhibitors	Pentoxiphiline	↓ TNFα	↓[H, I]	↓	↔	5
FXR receptor agonist*	Obeticholic acid*	↑ Hepatic insulin sensitivity	↓[H, I]	↓	↓	35, 36
		↓ Hepatic gluconeogenesis				
FGF21 analogue	BMS-986036*	↑ Hepatic insulin sensitivity and promote weight loss	↓[I]	N/A	N/A	40
FGF19 analogue	NGM-282*	↑ Insulin sensitivity, weight loss ↓ Bile acid synthesis	↓[I]	N/A	N/A	41

Abbreviations: H, NAFLD assessed by histology; I, NAFLD assessed by imaging (ultrasonography, CT, ¹H-MRS, or liver proton density fat fraction); PDE, phosphodiesterase inhibitor; PPAR, peroxisome proliferator–activated receptors
* Investigational

achieving NASH resolution reported in clinical trials are approximately 51% with pioglitazone, 39% with liraglutide, and 36% with vitamin E (*Figure*). The placebo subtracted treatment differences were: 32% for pioglitazone,[13] 30% for liraglutide,[16] 15% for vitamin E,[14] and less than 10% with other drugs.

Figure. Proportion of Patients Achieving Resolution of NASH (Drug vs Placebo) for Pharmacologic Agents Assessed in Randomized Controlled Trials

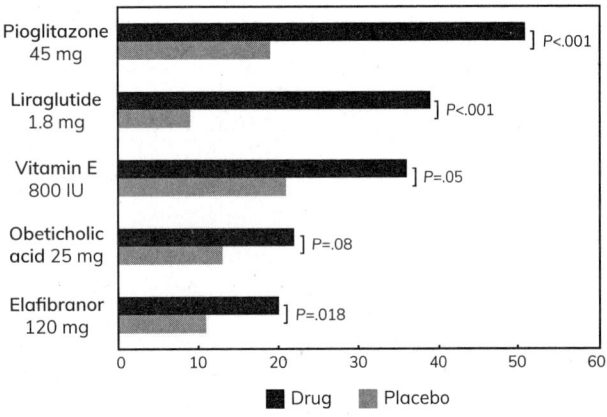

Data are presented from the references: pioglitazone trials;[13,15] liraglutide (LEAN trial);[16] vitamin E (PIVENS trial);[14] obeticholic acid (OCA) (FLINT trial);[35] and elafibranor (GOLDEN505 trial).[37]

Pioglitazone

Pioglitazone is a thiazolidinedione that modulates the transcription factor peroxisome proliferator–activated receptor γ (PPAR-γ) (and to a lesser extent PPAR-α) and affects positively insulin sensitivity in adipose tissue, liver, and skeletal muscle, resulting in improved glucose and lipid metabolism and redistribution of excess ectopic triglyceride accumulation from the liver (and other tissues) to a "metabolically healthier" adipose tissue. Pioglitazone has also been shown to decrease cardiovascular- and stroke-related mortality.[5] Belfort et al reported improvement in hepatic steatosis and necroinflammation with a reduction in score of 2 or greater after 6 months of treatment in 55 patients with biopsy-proven NASH and prediabetes or T2DM.[15] The reduction in steatosis and necroinflammation were proportionally higher in the pioglitazone arm vs the placebo group: 43% vs 0% for steatosis and 46% vs 14% for necroinflammation. The NAFLD Activity Score improved in 73% of patients with pioglitazone versus 24% on placebo with a trend for less fibrosis (but not statistically significant in this study). A longer-term study in 101 patients with prediabetes or T2DM and NASH also showed robust improvement in insulin sensitivity, as well as in histology on sequential liver biopsies at 18 and 36 months and confirmed the safety and efficacy of pioglitazone in this setting.[13] More patients in the pioglitazone group (58%) achieved the primary outcome of a 2-point reduction or greater in NAFLD Activity Score (in 2 categories) without worsening of fibrosis compared with the placebo group (17%). When the same analysis was limited to patients with definite NASH at baseline, 67% achieved the primary outcome with pioglitazone vs 17% with placebo (treatment difference of 50% points). In this trial (as shown in the *Figure*), 51% of patients in the pioglitazone arm had NASH resolution (a secondary outcome) vs 19% in the placebo group, with a placebo subtracted treatment difference of 32% points (confidence interval, 13%-51%; *P*<.001).[13] This histologic improvement was closely correlated with improvement in adipose tissue insulin resistance and increased adiponectin level.[13] In patients with NASH but without T2DM, positive but less striking results were also reported, possibly because a lower dosage of pioglitazone was used in these studies or because of differences in the populations studied.[14,19] In the study by Cusi et al, a mean reduction in fibrosis stage was significant only for pioglitazone at the higher dosage of 45 mg daily.[13] Belfort et al also reported a trend for changes in fibrosis compared with baseline, and Aithal et al reported a reduction in fibrosis in patients without diabetes treated with pioglitazone, 30 mg daily.[15,19] Concerns related to pioglitazone use remain: weight gain of approximately 3 kg on average, most likely related to expansion of body fat and less often from fluid retention, peripheral edema, congestive heart failure when treatment is initated in a patient with unknown diastolic disfunction or history of heart failure, and bone loss, especially in women.[5,20] The association between pioglitazone and bladder cancer remains controversial, and was negative in a long-term study.[21] In conclusion, pioglitazone leads to resolution of NASH (>50%) in patients with and without T2DM, and long-term (3-year) data show improvement in NAFLD Activity Score in two-thirds of patients (75%). Given safety and efficacy shown by pioglitazone in nonalcoholic steatohepatitis, combined with its proven cardiovascular benefit and relatively low cost, pioglitazone should be a first-line treatment in patients with confirmed NASH on liver biopsy and in patients with diabetes and NAFLD, and could be used empirically in patients with T2DM and elevated liver enzymes when other causes of liver disease are excluded.

Vitamin E

Vitamin E is an antioxidant and has been evaluated in 2 randomized controlled trials with reported liver histology outcomes in adults.[14,17] In the PIVENS trial, adults with biopsy-proven NASH without diabetes received vitamin E at a dosage of 800 IU daily vs placebo for 96 weeks.[14] Vitamin E treatment led to a higher proportion of patients achieving the primary histologic endpoint of improvement in NAFLD Activity Score of 2 or more grades, with no worsening of fibrosis (43% vs 19%; $P = .001$).[14] However, resolution of NASH only reached borderline statistical significance (36% with vitamin E vs 21% with placebo; $P = .05$), an endpoint reached in the same study by pioglitazone (47% with pioglitazone vs placebo; $P = .001$). A recent randomized controlled trial in patients with T2DM randomly assigned to receive placebo, vitamin E alone, or vitamin E plus pioglitazone, showed that vitamin E alone did not significantly change the primary histologic outcome of 2-point or greater reduction in NAFLD Activity Score (31% vs 19%; $P = .26$). However, in the treatment arm with vitamin E alone, more patients achieved NASH resolution (33% vs 12%; $P = .04$) when compared with placebo,[17] and this improvement was similar to what was reported in the PIVENS trial in patients without diabetes, with an overall placebo

subtracted treatment effect of 21% to 24%.[14] The resolution of NASH reported in the combination arm (vitamin E plus pioglitazone) was 43% vs 12% in the placebo group ($P = .005$)[17] and similar to, not superior to, pioglitazone alone (51% vs 19% in the placebo group) in a different randomized controlled trial reported by the same investigators.[13] Again, in the study by Bril and Cusi, only steatosis assessed by histology improved with vitamin E alone ($P = .018$); no improvement in inflammation ($P = .018$), ballooning ($P = .022$), or fibrosis scores were observed.[17] These findings will have to be reproduced in a larger trial in patients with T2DM in order to establish whether there is a potential role for vitamin E alone or in combination with pioglitazone in patients with T2DM. Finally, in a pediatric population with NASH, vitamin E did not significantly improve histology.[18] In line with these findings, the 2018 guidance from the American Association for the Study of Liver Diseases states that "until further evidence supporting its effectiveness become available, vitamin E is not recommend treating NASH in diabetic patients."[6] Vitamin E has not been studied in patients with liver cirrhosis. Long-term safety concerns of vitamin E administration include increased risk for the development of hemorrhagic stroke and potentially prostate cancer.[5]

GLP-1 Receptor Agonists

In 25 patients with T2DM and NAFLD, exenatide (n = 19) and liraglutide (n = 6) showed 42% reduction in liver fat assessed by ^{1}H-MRS.[22] A meta-analysis of the LEAD program also reported positive results with liraglutide improving liver enzymes and showing a positive trend for hepatic steatosis by CT after 26 weeks of treatment.[23] In the LEAN trial, liraglutide 1.8 mg daily, given for 48 weeks showed improvement in histology in 52 patients with biopsy-proven NASH.[16] Resolution of NASH occurred in 39% of patients treated with liraglutide compared with 9% of patients in the placebo group, and fewer patients on liraglutide experienced worsening of fibrosis.[16] These effects on the liver are related to significant reduction of body weight and improved glycemic control in patients with T2DM (about one-third), as well as improved insulin sensitivity.[16] The relatively high rates of resolution of NASH, despite nonsignificant changes in individual histologic scores, may be a result of the small study size, with only 45 patients having paired biopsies. Certainly, larger studies with liraglutide and other GLP-1 receptor agonists are needed to establish their future role in the treatment of NASH. A large phase 2 clinical trial evaluating the efficacy of semaglutide (daily administration) on histologic endpoints (with paired biopsy) in patients with NASH and advanced fibrosis is currently ongoing. Novel GLP-1 and glucagon receptor agonists are also in development and may be promising in the future by inducing weight loss of at least 10%. In general, GLP-1 receptor agonists are well tolerated and the gastrointestinal adverse effects can be minimized with careful titration. Risk of pancreatitis and pancreatic cancer with long-term use of these agents remains to be determined. Current guidelines state that it is premature to recommend GLP-1 receptor agonists for treatment of patients with NAFLD or NASH, but hopefully this will change in the future.[6]

Other Antidiabetes Drugs

The effects of other antidiabetes drugs on NASH histologic outcomes are summarized in the *Table*. Although metformin remains first-line therapy for the management of hyperglycemia in T2DM and may reduce liver fat, it is not effective for the treatment of steatohepatitis, as it does not significantly impact resolution of NASH or fibrosis.[24] It is considered neutral by current guidelines.

Sitagliptin was evaluated in small studies with imaging and histology. In patients with NAFLD and T2DM or prediabetes (n = 50), sitagliptin was no better than placebo in reducing liver fat as assessed by MRI- proton density fat fraction[25] or in improving liver fibrosis in patients with biopsy-proved NASH (n = 12) after 24 weeks of treatment.[26] In an open-labeled study of 50 patients with NASH and paired liver biopsies after 1 year treatment, sitagliptin improved NAFLD activity score, steatosis, and ballooning.[27] Treatment with vildagliptin for 6 months also showed a modest

decrease hepatic steatosis (from 7.3% to 5.3% measured by ^{1}H-MRS; normal being ≤5.5%).[28]

Finally, significant interest has recently been given to SGLT-2 inhibitors because of recent evidence on reduction in cardiovascular mortality with these agents. Specifically, in NAFLD, our group showed that treatment with canagliflozin, 300 mg daily, improved hepatic insulin sensitivity and showed a trend to decrease intrahepatic triglyceride measured by proton magnetic resonance spectroscopy compared with placebo (−6.9% vs −3.8%, respectively, although this did not reach statistical significance), with the reduction in intrahepatic triglyceride depending on the magnitude of weight loss, which was greater and more often with the SGLT-2 inhibitor.[29] Positive results with a decrease in liver fat were observed with luseogliflozin,[30] ipragliflozin,[31] empagliflozin,[32,33] and dapagliflozin.[34] Of note, there are no randomized controlled trials assessing the effect of SGLT-2 inhibitors on liver histology. The favorable weight profile and beneficial effects on reduction in liver fat make these agents an attractive second- or third-line treatment and could possibly be used in combination with pioglitazone. In general, SGLT-2 inhibitors are well tolerated and potential risks, such as volume depletion due to osmotic diuresis, genital mycotic and urinary tract infections, bone loss, and euglycemic diabetes ketoacidosis must be carefully monitored and avoided by educating patients and providers.

A number of investigational drugs are currently being pursued for an indication in NASH. A few of them are briefly reviewed in this session. The efficacy of obeticholic acid, a synthetic farnesoid X receptor agonist, was studied in patients with NASH in a multicenter randomized controlled trial (FLINT) by Tetri and colleagues.[35] Although treatment with obeticholic acid, 25 mg daily, improved steatosis, hepatocellular ballooning, and lobular inflammation in 46% vs 21% of patients on placebo ($P = .0002$), and reduced fibrosis in 35% vs 19% of patients on placebo ($P = .004$), disappointingly, resolution of NASH was not achieved in a substantial proportion of patients (only 22% of patients treated with obeticholic acid vs 13% in the placebo group; $P = .08$). Results from a large phase 3 multicenter study (REGENERATE) in a primary intent-to-treat population (n = 931) with stage 2 and 3 fibrosis, randomly assigned 1:1:1 to receive obeticholic acid, 25 mg (n = 308), obeticholic acid, 10 mg (n = 312), or placebo (n = 311) once daily over 18 months[36] just became available. Once-daily obeticholic acid, 25 mg, met the primary endpoint of fibrosis improvement (≥1 stage) with no worsening of NASH in 23.1% of patients compared with 11.9% of patients in the placebo group ($P = .0002$). However, the study did not meet the NASH resolution primary endpoint at the 18-month interim analysis.[36] Common adverse effects reported included pruritus (one-third of patients), increased LDL cholesterol, and decreased HDL cholesterol, which raises concerns regarding long-term risk for cardiovascular safety and the use of this agent in the future.

Elafibranor (GFT505), a dual agonist of PPAR-α and PPAR-δ, with positive effects on lipid glucose metabolism, has been evaluated in the GOLDEN 505 randomized controlled trial at 2 dosages (80 mg daily [n = 93] and 120 mg daily [n = 91]) against placebo (n = 92) for 52 weeks in patients with biopsy-proven NASH.[37] Elafibranor failed to meet the primary endpoint of resolution of NASH and showed histologic benefit in patients with a higher NAFLD Activity Score (≥4) at the higher dosage of 120 mg compared with placebo (20% vs 11% NASH resolution; $P = .018$ [see Figure]). A larger phase 3 trial (RESOLVE-IT) is currently evaluating elafibranor vs placebo in patients with biopsy-confirmed NASH and NAFLD Activity Score of 4 or higher and fibrosis.

Saroglitazar is PPAR-α and PPAR-γ agonist that is currently approved in India and Mexico for treatment of dyslipidemia and hypertriglyceridemia in T2DM that is uncontrolled by statins. A phase 2 randomized controlled trial in NASH is currently ongoing. In 221 patients with T2DM and NAFLD, 24 weeks of treatment with saroglitazar, 4 mg daily, significantly improved liver enzymes and elastography findings along with lipids and glycemia.[38]

MSDC-0602K, a second-generation oral insulin sensitizer designed to selectively modulate the mitochondrial pyruvate carrier while minimizing direct PPAR-γ activation, was studied in the 12-month EMMINENCE trial.[39] Results were reported in a late-breaking oral abstract at the liver meeting this year. In the trial, 402 patients with biopsy-confirmed NASH (NAFLD Activity Score ≥4 and fibrosis score F1-F3) were randomly assigned to daily oral doses of MSDC-0602K (62.5 mg daily, 125 mg daily, or 250 mg daily) or placebo. Treatment with MSDC-0602K improved insulin sensitivity and liver enzyme levels and showed a dose-dependent trend toward improvement in liver histopathology, which did not, however, reach statistical significance, for the primary histologic outcome at any dosage. In a post hoc analysis, NASH resolution with 2-point or greater reduction in NAFLD Activity Score was only significant with a higher dosage of the drug (250 mg daily) (26.7% vs 13.8% in the placebo group; $P = .026$). There was no reported edema, but weight gain of 2.3% was reported with the higher dosage.[39] A phase 3 trial may be planned with a higher dosage in the future.

BMS-986036, a pegylated recombinant FGF21 analogue, was evaluated in one randomized controlled trial in 74 patients with NASH at 2 dosages (10 mg daily and 20 mg weekly) vs placebo (randomized 1:1:1).[40] After 16 weeks, liver fat by MRI proton density fat fraction decreased by 6.8% with the 10 mg daily dosage and by 5.2% with the 20 mg weekly dosage vs 1.3% in placebo (both $P<.01$). NGM282, a novel variant of FGF19, was evaluated in a phase 2 randomized controlled trial (n = 82) at 2 dosages (3 mg daily and 6 mg daily for 12 weeks vs placebo) in patients with NAFLD with baseline liver fat by MRI proton density fat fraction ≥8%.[41] NGM282 decreased ALT (43% and 45% with 3 mg daily and 6 mg daily dosage, respectively) and liver fat by more than 5% in 79% of participants, with 34% achieving normal liver fat (mean reduction in liver fat was −9.7% and −11.9% with 3 mg daily and 6 mg daily dosage, respectively).

Many other new compounds targeting metabolic homeostasis, oxidative stress, inflammation apoptosis, or fibrosis, not discussed here, are being evaluated with some undergoing phase 2B/3 randomized controlled trials.

In conclusion, it is important to screen patients with prediabetes and diabetes and identify those at risk for developing NASH-induced liver fibrosis. Patients should be offered effective therapies, including lifestyle changes and weight loss, and medications currently available to treat diabetes and proven to be effective in NASH (ie, pioglitazone and liraglutide).

Clinical Case Vignettes

Case

A 69-year-old man with history of T2DM presents with right upper-quadrant discomfort. He is overall healthy except for longstanding T2DM (>10 years), hypertension, and dyslipidemia. He takes metformin, 1000 mg twice daily; lisinopril, 40 mg daily; atorvastatin, 40 mg daily; and aspirin, 81 mg daily. His family history is notable for T2DM in his mother and sister and prostate cancer in his father. Liver ultrasonography ordered by his primary care physician to evaluate the right upper-quadrant discomfort shows hepatic steatosis. Physical examination findings are normal except for a BMI of 35.0 kg/m^2.

Laboratory test results:

Fasting glucose = 127 mg/dL (70-99 mg/dL)
   (SI: 7.0 mmol/L [3.9-5.5 mmol/L])
Hemoglobin A$_{1c}$ = 7.5% (4.0%-5.6%)
   (58 mmol/mol [20-38 mmol/mol])
ALT = 52 U/L (7-40 U/L)
   (SI: 0.87 μkat/L [0.12-0.67 μkat/L])
AST = 39 U/L (7-40 U/L)
   (SI: 0.65 μkat/L [0.12-0.67 μkat/L])
Albumin = 3.5 g/dL (3.4-5.4 g/dL)
   (SI: 35 g/L [34-54 g/L])
Platelet count = 132 × 10^3/μL (150-450 × 10^3/μL)
   (SI: 132 × 10^9/L [150-450 × 10^9/L])
LDL cholesterol = 10 mg/dL (<100 mg/dL [optimal])
   (SI: 2.85 mmol/L [<2.59 mmol/L])
HDL cholesterol = 40 mg/dL (>60 mg/dL [optimal])
   (SI: 1.04 mmol/L [>1.55 mmol/L])
Triglycerides = 290 mg/dL (<150 mg/dL [optimal])
   (SI: 3.28 mmol/L [<1.70 mmol/L])

Which of the following assessments is/ are indicated to further evaluate the etiology of transaminitis in this patient?

A. Review CAGE questionnaire
B. Order viral and autoimmune hepatitis serologies
C. Review current medications
D. Review herbal supplements
E. All of the above

Answer: E) All of the above

The diagnosis of NAFLD requires exclusion of other competing causes that could lead to elevation of liver enzymes and fatty infiltration of the liver.[6] Since accumulation of intrahepatic triglycerides can be due to alcoholic liver disease, excessive alcohol use must be ruled out. Significant alcohol consumption is defined as ongoing or recent alcohol consumption of greater than 21 units per week for men and greater than 14 units per week for women. In addition, other liver diseases that should be investigated include chronic viral hepatitis, hemochromatosis, α1-antitrypsin deficiency, Wilson disease, and autoimmune hepatitis. Medications that can cause hepatic steatosis should also be excluded such as corticosteroids, methotrexate, amiodarone, and hormone replacement with estrogens. Thus, pursuing all of the assessments listed (Answer E) is correct.

Case (Continued)

You discuss the laboratory findings with the patient and inform him that he has a fatty liver.

Which of the following statements regarding why NAFLD is associated with a 2- to 3-fold risk of developing hyperglycemia and T2DM is correct?

A. Individuals with NAFLD are more insulin resistant at the level of muscle, liver, and adipose tissue than individuals without NAFLD, even if they are lean and without diabetes
B. In NAFLD, insulin resistance is present in the muscle and liver but not in adipose tissue

C. In NAFLD, insulin resistance is present in the liver and adipose tissue but not in muscle

D. Nonobese individuals are not insulin resistant and rarely develop NAFLD

E. Obese individuals with diabetes without NAFLD are usually insulin sensitive (about 30% of all patients with diabetes)

Answer: A) Individuals with NAFLD are more insulin resistant at the level of muscle, liver, and adipose tissue than individuals without NAFLD, even if they are lean and without diabetes

As reviewed by Gastaldelli et al,[42] individuals with NAFLD are more insulin resistant than those without NAFLD, even if they are lean and without diabetes (Answer A). In patients with NAFLD, the insulin resistance is present at the level of muscle, liver, and adipose tissue, and as a direct consequence, hepatic glucose production and adipose tissue lipolysis are increased (less suppressed by insulin), thus resulting in higher fasting glucose and free fatty acid concentrations. This leads to increased risk of T2DM in these patients. Bril et al[11] have shown that liver insulin resistance, assessed as suppression of endogenous glucose production during a hyperinsulinemic euglycemic insulin clamp, already develops with intrahepatic triglyceride accumulation of only 2% to 3% and that this progressively worsens at higher levels of accumulation. However, nonobese individuals can also be insulin resistant, and particularly if they have T2DM, they are often insulin resistant and develop NAFLD.[43] Individuals with diabetes without NAFLD are usually not insulin sensitive (about 30% of all patients with diabetes), but they have less insulin resistance and a more favorable metabolic profile.

Case (Continued)

You use the Fibrosis-4 (FIB-4) calculator to estimate this patient's risk of having liver fibrosis.

Which of the following is your conclusion?

A. The FIB-4 cannot be calculated in this patient

B. He has a very low risk of liver fibrosis, so no additional workup is needed

C. He has a low to moderate risk of liver fibrosis, so no additional workup is needed

D. He has a moderate to high risk of liver fibrosis, so additional workup and referral to hepatology are needed

E. If positive (>2.67), the FIB-4 is unreliable to rule advanced liver fibrosis in patients with diabetes

Answer: D) He has a moderate to high risk of liver fibrosis, so additional workup and referral to hepatology are needed

Calculating FIB-4 can help clinicians in the management of NASH by ruling out those at the highest risk of having advanced liver fibrosis and can be easily computed with available clinical and routine laboratory information such as age, AST, ALT, and platelet count.[44] Several websites offer calculators to assess the risk of having liver fibrosis. Examples of such sites are https://www.hepatitisc.uw.edu/page/clinical-calculators/fib-4 or https://www.mdcalc.com/fibrosis-4-fib-4-index-liver-fibrosis. The calculated FIB-4 in this case is 2.87, which indicates a moderate to high risk of liver fibrosis, so additional workup is and referral to hepatology are needed (Answer D).

NASH is associated with liver damage in the form of hepatocellular injury with hepatocyte ballooning/necrosis and predominantly lobular inflammation. Hepatic fibrosis has 4 stages based on its severity: stage F0 (no fibrosis), mild (stage F1), moderate (stage F2, with zone 3 sinusoidal fibrosis plus periportal fibrosis), or severe with bridging fibrosis (stage 3) or cirrhosis (stage 4). Moderate to severe fibrosis (F2-F3) has been linked to higher mortality.[1,2] Advanced liver fibrosis and cirrhosis occur more often in obesity, but in particular, in patients with T2DM.[6] NAFLD is also associated with a 2- to 3-fold increased risk of diabetes and of cardiovascular disease. FIB-4 has proven useful in identifying patients at high risk of advanced fibrosis (≥F3) fibrosis.[4,45] Noninvasive plasma tests are not as good to diagnose early stages of fibrosis, but they have been useful for the diagnosis of advanced disease (≥F3). In other words, they are best used to rule out severe disease (good specificity/negative predictive value), but they have poor sensitivity (positive predictive value) to diagnose or monitor the disease.

Case (Continued)

You order elastography to further evaluate NAFLD. This shows CAP (controlled attenuation parameter) of 300 dB/m and VCTE (vibration-controlled transient elastography) of 10 kPa. You advise that liver biopsy is indicated based on above results and that additional therapy to improve both his diabetes and NAFLD should be considered.

What second-line therapy after metformin for management of hyperglycemia has been shown to result in a significant proportion of patients achieving resolution of NASH when compared with placebo?

A. Liraglutide

B. Dulaglutide

C. Empagliflozin

D. Sitagliptin

E. Pioglitazone

Answer: A and E) Liraglutide and pioglitazone

In the LEAN trial, liraglutide, 1.8 mg daily, given for 48 weeks showed improvement in histology in 52 patients with biopsy-proven NASH.[16] Resolution of NASH occurred in 39% of patients with liraglutide compared with 9% of patients in the placebo group, and fewer patients on liraglutide experienced worsening of fibrosis. Kuchay et al[32] and others[33] have showed reduction in liver fat with empagliflozin and other SGLT-2 inhibitors; however, there are no studies reporting on NASH histologic outcomes. The effects of DPP-4 inhibitors on NAFLD are modest and variable, but with an overall neutral impact on histology (see *Table*). In patients with prediabetes or T2DM, Belfort et al[15] reported

improvement with a reduction in score of 2 or greater in hepatic steatosis and necroinflammation in the pioglitazone arm vs patients in the placebo group after 6 months of treatment in 55 patients with biopsy-proven NASH. In a longer-term randomized controlled trial, Cusi et al[13] showed that more patients in the pioglitazone group (58%) achieved the primary outcome of a 2 or more point reduction in NAFLD Activity Score than in the placebo group (17%). Resolution of NASH, a secondary outcome in this trial, occurred in 51% of pioglitazone-treated patients vs in 19% of those receiving placebo (treatment difference of 32% points $P<.001$).

Case (Continued)

The patient is concerned about continuing atorvastatin in the setting of elevated liver enzymes. Which of the following should be recommended?

A. He should continue atorvastatin because of increased cardiovascular disease risk from T2DM and NAFLD

B. He should stop atorvastatin since you are discussing starting pioglitazone and there is potential for drug interaction

C. He should continue atorvastatin due to known effects of statins to improve NASH and reduce fibrosis in clinical studies

D. He should stop atorvastatin because his liver enzymes are elevated and statins have no effect on liver histology

Answer: A) He should continue atorvastatin because of increased cardiovascular disease risk from T2DM and NAFLD

Statins are safe to use in patients with T2DM and NASH.[12,46] Given the high cardiovascular risk profile in these patients, statin therapy should be standard of care. Most prospective studies with 10 or more patients evaluating statin effects on liver histology in NASH failed to show significant histologic improvement (or change in aminotransferase levels) when compared with placebo. In the placebo arm of the pioglitazone trial by Cusi,[12] there were no significant changes in liver histology observed in patients with NASH newly started on a statin.

Case (Continued)

The patient is hesitant to start either pioglitazone or liraglutide and wants to know if you would recommend treatment with vitamin E. Regarding the use of vitamin E in patients with T2DM and NASH, which of the following statements is INCORRECT?

A. Vitamin E at a dosage of 800 IU daily should be recommended given the known benefit of vitamin E in NASH reported in the PIVENS trial

B. Current guidelines do not recommend vitamin E for treatment of NASH in patients with T2DM

C. Current guidelines recommend vitamin E for treatment of NASH in patients without T2DM

D. Vitamin E may increase overall mortality and risk of prostate cancer in men

Answer: A) Vitamin E at a dosage of 800 IU daily should be recommended given the known benefit of vitamin E in NASH reported in the PIVENS trial

The findings from the PIVENS trial included adults with biopsy-proven NASH without T2DM.[14] Vitamin E treatment led to a higher proportion of patients achieving the primary histologic endpoint of improvement in 2 or more points in NAFLD Activity Score, with no worsening of fibrosis (43% vs 19%; $P = .001$). However, resolution of NASH only reached borderline statistical significance, an endpoint reached in the same study by pioglitazone (47% with pioglitazone vs placebo [$P = .001$] and 36% with vitamin E vs 21% with placebo [$P = .05$]). A recent randomized controlled trial in patients with T2DM showed that vitamin E alone did not significantly change the primary histologic outcome in patients with NASH and T2DM.[17] In line with these findings, 2018 guidance from the American Association for the Study of Liver Diseases states that, "until further evidence supporting its effectiveness become available, vitamin E is not recommend treating NASH in diabetic patients."[6] Caution should be taken when prescribing vitamin E, as recent data suggest that it may increase overall mortality and risk of prostate cancer in men.

References

1. Younossi Z, Anstee QM, Marietti M, et al. Global burden of NAFLD and NASH: trends, predictions, risk factors and prevention. *Nat Rev Gastroenterol Hepatol.* 2018;15(1):11-20. PMID: 28930295

2. Younossi ZM, Golabi P, de Avila L, et al. The global epidemiology of NAFLD and NASH in patients with type 2 diabetes: A systematic review and meta-analysis. *J Hepatol.* 2019;71(4):793-801. PMID: 31279902

3. Stefan N, Häring HU, Cusi K. Non-alcoholic fatty liver disease: causes, diagnosis, cardiometabolic consequences, and treatment strategies. *Lancet Diabetes Endocrinol.* 2019;7(4):313-324. PMID: 30174213

4. Bril F, Cusi K. Management of nonalcoholic fatty liver disease in patients with type 2 diabetes: a call to action. *Diabetes Care.* 2017;40(3):419-430. PMID: 28223446

5. Barb D, Portillo-Sanchez P, Cusi K. Pharmacological management of nonalcoholic fatty liver disease. *Metabolism.* 2016;65(8):1183-1195. PMID: 27301803

6. Chalasani N, Younossi Z, Lavine JE, et al. The diagnosis and management of nonalcoholic fatty liver disease: practice guidance from the American Association for the Study of Liver Diseases. *Hepatology.* 2018;67:328-357. PMID: 28714183

7. Neuschwander-Tetri BA, Clark JM, Bass NM, et al; NASH Clinical Research Network. Clinical, laboratory and histological associations in adults with nonalcoholic fatty liver disease. *Hepatology.* 2010;52(3):913-924. PMID: 20648476

8. Bril F, Cusi K. Nonalcoholic fatty liver disease: the new complication of type 2 diabetes mellitus. *Endocrinol Metab Clin North Am.* 2016;45(4):765-781. PMID: 27823604

9. Cusi K. Treatment of patients with type 2 diabetes and non-alcoholic fatty liver disease: current approaches and future directions. *Diabetologia.* 2016;59(6):1112-1120. PMID: 27101131

10. Portillo-Sanchez P, Bril F, Maximos M, et al. High prevalence of nonalcoholic fatty liver disease in patients with type 2 diabetes mellitus and normal plasma aminotransferase levels. *J Clin Endocrinol Metab.* 2015;100(6):2231-2238. PMID: 25885947

11. Bril F, Barb D, Portillo-Sanchez P, et al. Metabolic and histological implications of intrahepatic triglyceride content in nonalcoholic fatty liver disease. *Hepatology.* 2017;65(4):1132-1144. PMID: 27981615

12. Barb D, Cusi K. Reply to "statins and non-alcoholic steatohepatitis." *Metabolism.* 2017;66:e3-e5. PMID: 278655560

13. Cusi K, Orsak B, Bril F, et al. Long-term pioglitazone treatment for patients with nonalcoholic steatohepatitis and prediabetes or type 2 diabetes mellitus: a randomized trial. *Ann Intern Med.* 2016;165(5):305-315. PMID: 27322798

14. Sanyal AJ, Chalasani N, Kowdley KV, et al; NASH CRN. Pioglitazone, vitamin E, or placebo for nonalcoholic steatohepatitis. *N Engl J Med.* 2010;362(18):1675-1685. PMID: 20427778

15. Belfort R, Harrison SA, Brown K, et al. A placebo-controlled trial of pioglitazone in subjects with nonalcoholic steatohepatitis. *N Engl J Med.* 2006;355(22):2297-2307. PMID: 17135584

16. Armstrong MJ, Gaunt P, Aithal GP, et al; LEAN trial team. Liraglutide safety and efficacy in patients with non-alcoholic steatohepatitis (LEAN): a multicentre, double-blind, randomised, placebo-controlled phase 2 study. *Lancet.* 2016;387(10019):679-690. PMID: 26608256

17. Bril F, Biernacki D, Kalavalapalli S, et al. Role of vitamin E for nonalcoholic steatohepatitis in patients with type 2 diabetes: a randomized controlled trial. *Diabetes Care.* 2019;42(8):1481-1488. PMID: 31332029

18. Lavine JE, Schwimmer JB, Van Natta ML, et al; Nonalcoholic Steatohepatitis Clinical Research Network. Effect of vitamin E or metformin for treatment of nonalcoholic fatty liver disease in children and adolescents: the TONIC randomized controlled trial. *JAMA.* 2011;305(16):1659-1668. PMID: 21521847

19. Aithal GP, Thomas JA, Kaye PV, et al. Randomized, placebo-controlled trial of pioglitazone in nondiabetic subjects with nonalcoholic steatohepatitis. *Gastroenterology.* 2008;135(4):1176-1184. PMID: 18718471

20. Portillo-Sanchez P, Bril F, Lomonaco R, et al. Effect of pioglitazone on bone mineral density in patients with nonalcoholic steatohepatitis: a 36-month clinical trial. *J Diabetes.* 2019;11(3):223-231. PMID: 30073778

21. Lewis JD, Habel LA, Quesenberry CP, et al. Pioglitazone use and risk of bladder cancer and other common cancers in persons with diabetes. *JAMA.* 2015;314(3):265-277. PMID: 26197187

22. Cuthbertson DJ, Irwin A, Gardner CJ, et al. Improved glycaemia correlates with liver fat reduction in obese, type 2 diabetes, patients given glucagon-like peptide-1 (GLP-1) receptor agonists. *PLoS One.* 2012;7(12):e50117. PMID: 23236362

23. Armstrong MJ, Houlihan DD, Rowe IA, et al. Safety and efficacy of liraglutide in patients with type 2 diabetes and elevated liver enzymes: individual patient data meta-analysis of the LEAD program. *Aliment Pharmacol Ther.* 2013;37(2):234-242. PMID: 23163663

24. Loomba R, Lutchman G, Kleiner DE, et al. Clinical trial: pilot study of metformin for the treatment of non-alcoholic steatohepatitis. *Aliment Pharmacol Ther.* 2009;29(2):172-182. PMID: 18945255

25. Cui J, Philo L, Nguyen P, et al. Sitagliptin vs. placebo for non-alcoholic fatty liver disease: a randomized controlled trial. *J Hepatol.* 2016;65(2):369-376. PMID: 27151177

26. Joy TR, McKenzie CA, Tirona RG, et al. Sitagliptin in patients with non-alcoholic steatohepatitis: a randomized, placebo-controlled trial. *World J Gastroenterol.* 2017;23(1):141-150. PMID: 28104990

27. Alam S, Ghosh J, Mustafa G, Kamal M, Ahmad N. Effect of sitagliptin on hepatic histological activity and fibrosis of nonalcoholic steatohepatitis patients: a 1-year randomized control trial. *Hepat Med.* 2018;10:23-31. PMID: 29740221

28. Macauley M, Hollingsworth KG, Smith FE, et al. Effect of vildagliptin on hepatic steatosis. *J Clin Endocrinol Metab.* 2015;100(4):1578-1585. PMID: 25664602

29. Cusi K, Bril F, Barb D, et al. Effect of canagliflozin treatment on hepatic triglyceride content and glucose metabolism in patients with type 2 diabetes. *Diabetes Obes Metab* [Epub ahead of print] PMID: 30447037

30. Shibuya T, Fushimi N, Kawai M, et al. Luseogliflozin improves liver fat deposition compared to metformin type 2 diabetes patients with non-alcoholic fatty liver disease: a prospective randomized controlled pilot study. *Diabetes Obes Metab.* 2018;20(2):438-442. PMID: 28719078

31. Ito D, Shimizu S, Inoue K, et al. Comparison of ipragliflozin and pioglitazone effects on nonalcoholic fatty liver disease in patients with type 2 diabetes: a randomized, 24-week, open-label, active-controlled trial. *Diabetes Care.* 2017;40(10):1364-1372. PMID: 28751548

32. Kuchay MS, Krishan S, Mishra SK, et al. Effect of empagliflozin on liver fat in patients with type 2 diabetes and nonalcoholic fatty liver disease: a randomized controlled trial (E-LIFT Trial). *Diabetes Care.* 2018;41(8):1801-1808. PMID: 29895557

33. Kahl S, Gancheva S, Strassburger K, et al. Empagliflozin effectively lowers liver fat content in well-controlled type 2 diabetes: a randomized, double-blind, phase 4, placebo-controlled trial. *Diabetes Care.* 2020;43(2):298-305. PMID: 31540903

34. Latva-Rasku A, Honka MJ, Kullberg J, et al. The SGLT2 inhibitor dapagliflozin reduces liver fat but does not affect tissue Insulin sensitivity: a randomized, double-blind, placebo-controlled study with 8-week treatment in type 2 diabetes patients. *Diabetes Care.* 2019;42(5):931-937. PMID: 30885955

35. Neuschwander-Tetri BA, Loomba R, Sanyal AJ, et al; NASH Clinical Research Network. Farnesoid X nuclear receptor ligand obeticholic acid for non-cirrhotic, non-alcoholic steatohepatitis (FLINT): a multicentre, randomised, placebo-controlled trial [published correction appears in *Lancet.* 2015;385(9972):946]. *Lancet.* 2015;385(9972):956-965. PMID: 25468160

36. Ratziu V, Sanyal AJ, Loomba R, et al. REGENERATE: design of a pivotal, randomised, phase 3 study evaluating the safety and efficacy of obeticholic acid in patients with fibrosis due to nonalcoholic steatohepatitis. *Contemp Clin Trials.* 2019;84:105803. PMID: 31260793

37. Ratziu V, Harrison SA, Francque S, et al; GOLDEN-505 Investigator Study Group. Elafibranor, an agonist of the peroxisome proliferator-activated receptor-α and -δ, induces resolution of nonalcoholic steatohepatitis without fibrosis worsening. *Gastroenterology.* 2016;150(5):1147-1159. PMID: 26874076

38. Joshi S, Ruby S, Saboo B, Chawla R, Bhandari S. Saroglitazar in non-alcoholic fatty liver disease. Abstract presented at: American Association of Clinical Endocrinologists 25th Annual Scientific & Clinical Congress; May 25-29, 2016; Orlando, FL.

39. Harrison SA. LO1: Results of MSDC-0602K in a large phase 2b NASH study demonstrate improvement in markers of insulin resistance, glucose metabolism, serum aminotransferases, non-invasive markers of NASH and histopathology. Presented at: Liver Meeting; November 2019; Boston, MA.

40. Sanyal A, Charles ED, Neuschwander-Tetri B, et al. BMS-986036 (pegylated FGF21) in patients with non-alcoholic steatohepatitis: a phase 2 study. *J Hepatol.* 2017;66(1):S89-S90.

41. Harrison SA, Rinella ME, Abdelmalek MF, et al. NGM282 for treatment of non-alcoholic steatohepatitis: a multicenter, randomized, double-blind, placebo-controlled, phase 2 trial. *Lancet.* 2018;391(10126):1174-1185. PMID: 29519502

42. Gastaldelli A, Cusi K. From NASH to diabetes and from diabetes to NASH: mechanisms and treatment options. *JHEP Reports.* 2019;1(4):312-328.

43. Lomonaco R, Bril F, Portillo-Sanchez P, et al. Metabolic impact of nonalcoholic steatohepatitis in obese patients with type 2 diabetes. *Diabetes Care.* 2016;39(4):632-638. PMID: 26861926

44. Sterling RK, Lissen E, Clumeck N, et al; APRICOT Clinical Investigators. Development of a simple noninvasive index to predict significant fibrosis patients with HIV/HCV coinfection. *Hepatology.* 2006;43(6):1317-1325. PMID: 16729309

45. Castera L, Friedrich-Rust M, Loomba R. Noninvasive assessment of liver disease in patients with nonalcoholic fatty liver disease. *Gastroenterology.* 2019;156(5):1264-1281. PMID: 30660725

46. Bril F, Portillo Sanchez P, Lomonaco R, et al. Liver safety of statins in prediabetes or T2DM and nonalcoholic steatohepatitis: post hoc analysis of a randomized trial. *J Clin Endocrinol Metab.* 2017;102(8):2950-2961. PMID: 28575232

Type 1 Diabetes Mellitus: From Preconception to Postpartum

Elizabeth O. Buschur, MD. Division of Endocrinology, Diabetes, and Metabolism, Ohio State University Wexner Medical Center, Columbus, OH; E-mail: Elizabeth.Buschur@osumc.edu

Learning Objectives

As a result of participating in this session, learners should be able to:

- Describe goals of preconception care for women with type 1 diabetes mellitus (T1DM).

- Recognize changes in insulin sensitivity and therefore insulin requirements during pregnancy in women with T1DM.

- Explain typical necessary changes in insulin dosing in the postpartum period.

Main Conclusions

Women with T1DM can have healthy pregnancies with preparation and multidisciplinary care. For several months prior to and during pregnancy, glucose levels should be as close to normal as possible for optimal health of the mother and fetus. The goal hemoglobin A_{1c} level before conception is less than 6.5% (<48 mmol/mol) and during pregnancy it is less than 6.0% (<42 mmol/mol) with avoidance of hypoglycemia.[1] In planning for conception, women with diabetes should work with their diabetes team to prepare for pregnancy. However, up to 50% of pregnancies in women with diabetes are unplanned.[2] Therefore, it is recommended to begin preconception counseling in early puberty and continue throughout the reproductive years. Women with hyperglycemia at the time of conception and in the first trimester during organogenesis have a much higher risk of having a baby with a congenital anomaly. During pregnancy, glycemic goals are as follows: fasting glucose less than 95 mg/dL (<5.3 mmol/L), postprandial glucose less than 140 mg/dL (<7.8 mmol/L) at 1 hour after the start of the meal and less than 120 mg/dL (<6.7 mmol/L) 2 hours after the start of a meal.[1,3] During pregnancy, insulin sensitivity and therefore insulin requirements change dramatically. Due to increases in insulin sensitivity, women with T1DM are at risk for hypoglycemia, especially in the first trimester of pregnancy. Insulin requirements increase significantly during the second half of pregnancy, as women require 2 to 3 times preconception insulin dosing at the time of delivery. Postpartum, insulin requirements plummet to preconception requirement levels and maybe even lower for women who are breastfeeding.

Significance of the Clinical Problem

The prevalence of all types of diabetes in pregnancy, including gestational diabetes and preexisting T1DM and T2DM, has been increasing worldwide. Pregestational T1DM and T2DM have been estimated to affect 1% to 2% of all pregnancies.[4] Uncontrolled hyperglycemia at the time of conception and in early pregnancy increases the risk of spontaneous abortion and congenital anomalies. In addition, suboptimal glycemic control throughout pregnancy increases the risk of spontaneous abortion, congenital anomalies, preeclampsia, fetal demise/loss, and macrosomia and often results in operative delivery, neonatal hypoglycemia, and neonatal hyperbilirubinemia.[1,3,5] Maternal hyperglycemia may increase the risk of preterm delivery, which can lead to neonatal intensive care stays and increased duration of hospitalization for infants. Furthermore, diabetes during pregnancy may increase the risk of obesity and T2DM in offspring of mothers with diabetes.[1] Hemoglobin A_{1c} levels less than 6.5% (<48 mmol/mol) before conception are associated with the lowest risk of congenital anomalies, including anencephaly, microcephaly, cardiac defects, and caudal regression.[1,3]

During pregnancy, women with T1DM should try to achieve a goal hemoglobin A_{1c} level less than 6.0% (<42 mmol/mol) with minimization of hypoglycemia. Women with T1DM should have a dilated retinal exam before pregnancy or in the first trimester and should have serial exams during pregnancy every trimester and postpartum as recommended by an ophthalmologist. Before pregnancy, women should have nephropathy screening with assessment of the urine albumin-to-creatinine ratio and measurement of serum creatinine. Women with diabetic nephropathy have an increased risk of poor perinatal outcomes and potential progression of nephropathy during pregnancy.

Insulin requirements change during pregnancy, and this should be reviewed with pregnant women to expect certain changes in insulin dosing. In early pregnancy, insulin sensitivity is increased, resulting in lower glucose levels and the need for reduced insulin dosing. This can increase the risk of hypoglycemia in the first trimester. It is imperative that pregnant women with T1DM have unexpired glucagon kits.

Continuous subcutaneous insulin infusion (CSII) pumps and continuous glucose monitoring (CGM) may be beneficial in women planning pregnancy, as well as during pregnancy and the postpartum period. Symptoms of hypoglycemia may change during pregnancy, and patients may lose symptoms they previously had with hypoglycemia. This can quickly become dangerous for the mother and fetus if not detected. CGM may help with recognition of hypoglycemia earlier than it would be detected by symptoms alone.

Barriers to Optimal Practice

- Unplanned pregnancies: up to 45% of pregnancies in women with T1DM are unplanned.[2]

- Late presentation when pregnant: some women with T1DM present for prenatal care after organogenesis is complete, leading to an increase in congenital anomalies among women with hyperglycemia at conception and during the first trimester.

- Access to care: women with T1DM may have difficulty finding providers to care for diabetes during pregnancy or have difficulty with the cost of health care visits.

Strategies for Diagnosis, Therapy, and/or Management
Preconception

Preconception counseling should begin at puberty and continue throughout the reproductive years. Women should be counseled on the risks of hyperglycemia during pregnancy, the need to start a prenatal vitamin including folic acid at least 3 months before anticipated conception, and choice of contraceptive options if pregnancy is not desired. Glycemic targets before and during pregnancy should be discussed, with a goal hemoglobin A_{1c} level less than 6.5% (<48 mmol/mol) before pregnancy and less than 6.0% (<42 mmol/mol) during pregnancy[1,2] if able to achieve with minimal hypoglycemia. Hemoglobin A_{1c} values are proportionally associated with congenital anomalies in multiple studies.[3] A hemoglobin A_{1c} value at the upper end of the normal range (5.0%-6.0%) (31-42 mmol/mol) has been shown to have a rate of anomalies similar to the background rate of congenital anomalies in pregnant women without diabetes.[3] Older studies have shown up to 25% risk of major congenital anomaly in women with a hemoglobin A_{1c} level greater than

10% (>86 mmol/mol) in the first trimester of pregnancy.[3]

Medications should be reviewed and those deemed unsafe for pregnancy should be discontinued, especially statins, ACE inhibitors, and/or angiotensin-receptor blockers. Preconception blood pressure goals are less than 130/80 mm Hg. Referral for a dilated retinal examination is recommended for any woman with T1DM planning pregnancy. Repeated exams during each trimester and during the first year postpartum are recommended based on severity of any baseline retinopathy or as suggested by an ophthalmologist. Women who are overweight or obese should lose weight before attempting conception.[5] Women planning pregnancy should have the following laboratory evaluation completed before conception: TSH and TPO antibody status (if not known), serum creatinine, estimated glomerular filtration rate, urine albumin-to-creatinine ratio, and hemoglobin A_{1c}.[5] Women with T1DM and a history of risk factors for coronary artery disease should have screening studies for coronary artery disease or should see a cardiologist if they have known coronary artery disease for discussion of risks during pregnancy.[5]

During Pregnancy

Once pregnancy is confirmed, a woman with T1DM should inform her endocrinologist immediately and work closely with her diabetes team throughout pregnancy. Weekly, if not more frequent, glucose review should occur. Referral to a multidisciplinary diabetes-in-pregnancy clinic with maternal-fetal medicine specialists, endocrinologists, dieticians, sonographers, social workers, and diabetes educators should be done if possible. Women should be counseled about typical insulin requirement changes during pregnancy and the need for frequent (weekly or more often) review of glucose data. Weekly adjustments in insulin dosing are common with increases, especially after 18 weeks' gestation.[6] According to the American College of Obstetrics and Gynecology,[3] the American Diabetes Association,[1] and the Endocrine Society,[5] glycemic targets are stricter than in nonpregnant adults (*Table*). It is recommended that women test their glucose fasting, before meals, and 1 or 2 hours after meals (measured from the first bite of food intake), as well as at bedtime. Glucose monitoring overnight may be recommended if there are any concerns for hypoglycemia. Insulin resistance can increase early in pregnancy requiring increases in insulin dosing; some women require a doubling of insulin requirements at delivery compared with prepregnancy doses. A nadir in insulin requirements is typically met around gestational weeks 9 to 10. However, between weeks 9 to 16, insulin resistance decreases and insulin doses must be reduced to prevent hypoglycemia. Some women may discover they are pregnant around this timeframe with evaluation for unexplained hypoglycemia. Women and their families should be trained on hypoglycemia recognition and management, including having an unexpired glucagon kit in the home and wearing a medical alert ID. Diabetic ketoacidosis may occur at lower glucose levels in women with T1DM than in nonpregnant women. Therefore, women with T1DM should be counseled to have ketone testing supplies and to check ketones with any glucose value greater than 200 mg/dL (>11.1 mmol/L) or any signs or symptoms of nausea, vomiting, or abdominal pain.[3]

Table. Glycemic Targets in Pregnancy[3,6]

Time of Day	Glucose Target
Fasting	<95 mg/dL (<5.3 mmol/L)
1-hour postprandial	<140 mg/dL (<7.8 mmol/L)
2-hour postprandial	<120 mg/dL (<6.7 mmol/L)

Insulin is the only recommended pharmacologic treatment for T1DM. Multiple insulin types are safe to use in pregnancy, and none of the available human insulins that have been studied have been shown to cross the placenta.[3] Historically, NPH and regular insulin were most frequently used in pregnancy. However, rapid-acting lispro and aspart better achieve glycemic control, especially postprandial targets, compared with regular insulin. Glulisine, degludec, and aspart have not been specifically studied in pregnancy, and there are no clear reports of any abnormality caused by their use in pregnancy.[7,8] Regular concentrated U500 insulin may be used for women who have severe insulin resistance, typically requiring more than 200 to 300 units total daily. Basal insulin NPH and detemir are both pregnancy category B. Glargine is considered pregnancy category C and there are some concerns given its increased affinity to the IGF-1 receptor and the potential to have detrimental effects when used in pregnancy. However, a meta-analysis of more than 300 pregnant women with T1DM showed no difference in maternal or neonatal outcomes between NPH and glargine.[9]

Advancements in diabetes technology, including CSII and CGM, may be beneficial in women before, during, and after pregnancy. CSII may be beneficial for women planning pregnancy and during pregnancy for several reasons, including the ability to administer small, precise insulin doses (fractions of a unit if needed), suspend insulin delivery if needed for impending hypoglycemia, and dose insulin very accurately taking into consideration active insulin time. CGM may help women identify glycemic trends at different times and with varying food choices or activities, allowing them to change insulin doses as needed to achieve euglycemia. Furthermore, insulin pumps and CGM can be downloaded remotely by the patient to share with her diabetes team between office visits. Some CGM devices allow real-time glucose values to be seen and some have alerts to inform a woman of impending hypoglycemia or hyperglycemia. Some CGM systems allow users to share the data with a loved one, which can also be very helpful, especially for women with nocturnal hypoglycemia or hypoglycemia unawareness. It is important to note that some diabetes technology is not approved for use during pregnancy and is used off label in this setting. Therefore, a pregnant woman should discuss her diabetes technology with her provider during pregnancy.

One study of CGM use in pregnancy (CONCEPTT) found an improvement in neonatal outcomes with only slight reduction in hemoglobin A1c compared with values in patients using fingerstick glucose testing alone.[10,11] In the group of pregnant women using CGM, the offspring had less neonatal hypoglycemia and were less likely to be large for gestational age or to require neonatal intensive care unit admission.[10] In contrast, a second study showed lower rates of preeclampsia in pregnant women using intermittent CGM, but did not show a difference in macrosomia.[12] Several semi-closed loop automated insulin pumps whose insulin delivery is adjusted based on sensor glucose reading are now on the market, although they have not been approved for use in pregnancy. One small study of 16 women suggested lower rates of hypoglycemia in pregnant women using the closed-loop system compared with those using sensor-augmented pump therapy.[13] For women using CGM, metrics besides hemoglobin A_{1c} and fingerstick glucose tests can be used, including time in range, time below range, and time above range.[14] Recommendations from the International Consensus on Time in Range recommend increasing time in range quickly and safely in pregnancy, with the goal glucose sensor range being 63 to 140 mg/dL (3.5-7.8 mmol/L) with greater than 70% of time in range, less than 25% of time above range (>140 mg/dL [>7.8 mmol/L]), less than 4% of time below 63 mg/dL (<3.5 mmol/L), and less than 1% of time below 54 mg/dL (<3 mmol/L).[14] Data from CONCEPTT and Swedish data show that CGM measures are associated with neonatal risks. For instance, a 5% to 7% greater time in range during the second and third trimesters has been associated with lower risk of being large for gestational age, macrosomia, shoulder dystocia, neonatal hypoglycemia, and neonatal intensive care unit stay.[14] More research is needed in the area of CGM and closed-loop systems in pregnancy. Furthermore, there are increasing numbers of patients using do-it-yourself closed-loop systems that have not been studied in pregnancy.

For women with a history of retinopathy (especially proliferative retinopathy), pregnancy can result in progression of retinopathy, especially with rapid improvement in glycemic control.[15] Women are recommended to have a dilated retinal exam before or during early pregnancy and then each trimester and postpartum or as recommended by an ophthalmologist. Women with T1DM should have regular thyroid screening during pregnancy and postpartum with serum TSH measurement each trimester and postpartum given the increased risk of coexistent autoimmune thyroid disease. A baseline 24-hour urine protein assessment is recommended early in pregnancy and should be repeated with any concerns for gestational hypertension or preeclampsia during pregnancy.

Women with a history of nephropathy have increased risk of poor perinatal outcomes, including intrauterine growth restriction, being small for gestational age, preterm birth, cesarean delivery, and preeclampsia.[16,17] Furthermore, women with T1DM and underlying nephropathy may have progression of nephropathy during pregnancy.[16,17] Women with T1DM are at increased risk for preeclampsia. This risk is heightened for women with known nephropathy, hypertension, and/or suboptimal glycemic control with approximately 15% to 20% of women with T1DM without nephropathy experiencing preeclampsia and approximately 50% of women with T1DM complicated by nephropathy developing preeclampsia.[3] Preeclampsia can significantly affect maternal and neonatal health with the potential need for preterm delivery and resultant adverse neonatal outcomes and urgent delivery requiring cesarean delivery.[1] The US Preventative Services Task Force recommends that women at high risk for preeclampsia take aspirin, 60 to 150 mg daily (typically a baby aspirin), after 12 weeks' gestation.[1,18]

Tight glycemic control is recommended during pregnancy for maternal and fetal health. Mean glucose levels during pregnancy should be approximately 100 mg/dL (5.6 mmol/L) to reduce maternal and fetal risks.[1,3,5] Hemoglobin A_{1c} is not always the best marker for glycemic control, especially during pregnancy when there are more rapid physiologic changes in red blood cell turnover causing hemoglobin A_{1c} levels to decrease during normal pregnancy.[19] Preconception and in the first trimester during organogenesis, near-normal glucose levels reduce the risk of congenital anomalies. However, later in pregnancy in the second and third trimesters, adverse outcomes, including being large for gestational age, preterm delivery, and preeclampsia, are reduced in women with a hemoglobin A_{1c} level less than 6.0% (<42 mmol/mol).

During labor and delivery, blood glucose targets are 72 to 126 mg/dL (3.99-6.99 mmol/L) according to the Endocrine Society Clinical practice guideline.[5] Hyperglycemia during labor and delivery increases the risk of neonatal hypoglycemia, fetal distress, heart rate abnormalities, and the need for neonatal intensive care unit stay. Recommendations for how to achieve tight glycemic control during labor and delivery are up to the practitioner. Regular insulin infusion is often used to achieve glucose targets and minimize neonatal hypoglycemia. Women on CSII pumps who are achieving glucose targets may continue their pump during labor and delivery pending discussion between the provider and patient. However, if hyperglycemia ensues, switching to intravenous insulin therapy is recommended.

Postpartum

Women with T1DM in pregnancy have reduced insulin requirements immediately following delivery of the placenta. Within the first few days to 2 weeks of delivery, women typically require about one-third less insulin than before pregnancy.[1,6] This can be further reduced with breastfeeding. Breastfeeding should be encouraged for all women with diabetes given the immense benefits to the infant for nutrition and immunity and potential long-term metabolic effects for the infant and the mother, including optimal changes in weight and risk for obesity.[1] Women with T1DM who experience hypoglycemia with breastfeeding should be encouraged to have a small snack before or during breastfeeding, consider insulin reduction as needed, and discuss with their diabetes provider any necessary changes to their insulin regimen. Women should be counseled on postpartum contraception options and optimal planning for any subsequent pregnancies if desired.

Clinical Case Vignettes

Case 1

A 27-year-old woman (G0) with a 21-year history of T1DM is planning on trying to conceive and asks for advice. She is on an insulin pump with CGM, and her hemoglobin A_{1c} level is 7.9% (63 mmol/mol). She has no known complications of diabetes and is up to date on retinal examinations and urine albumin testing.

Which of the following is the best advice?

A. Start trying to conceive today

B. Start a prenatal vitamin and start trying to conceive today

C. Do not try to conceive, as her risk of complications is too high given her 21-year duration of diabetes

D. Try to optimize glycemic control with a preconception goal hemoglobin A_{1c} less than 6.5% (<48 mmol/mol)

E. Meet with a diabetes educator, if interested, and review downloaded insulin pump and CGM data to see if any changes can be made to optimize glycemic control

Answer: D and E) Try to optimize glycemic control with a preconception goal hemoglobin A_{1c} less than 6.5% (<48 mmol/mol) and meet with a diabetes educator, if interested, and review downloaded insulin pump and CGM data to see if any changes can be made to optimize glycemic control

The recommended hemoglobin A_{1c} goals are as follows: before pregnancy less than 6.5% (<48 mmol/mol) and during pregnancy less than 6.0% (<42 mmol/mol). This patient should start

a prenatal vitamin and work toward improving her glycemic control until her hemoglobin A_{1c} level is less than 6.5% (<48 mmol/mol) if possible without frequent hypoglycemia and use adequate contraceptive options until that hemoglobin A_{1c} goal is achieved (Answer D). Offering to have her meet with a nutritionist and/or certified diabetes educator to optimize current diabetes management and reviewing her pump and CGM downloads to help her achieve her goal hemoglobin A_{1c} level (Answer E) would be useful. Trying to conceive now (Answers A and B) would not be recommended, as her glycemic control is above target for preconception, and this can pose a risk to the fetus in terms of miscarriage, congenital anomalies, etc, and later in pregnancy can pose a risk to both the fetus and the mother. Advising against pregnancy altogether (Answer C) is incorrect, as she has no known complications of diabetes and many women with T1DM have healthy, safe pregnancies with planning and optimal glucose control.

Case 2

A 30-year-old woman (G2P1001) with a 16-year history of T1DM presents to clinic at 9 weeks' gestation. She is on insulin pump therapy and uses CGM. She is having nausea and vomiting and giving boluses after her meals to reduce the risk of hypoglycemia. She notes overnight hypoglycemia around 1 AM to 3 AM with a recent glucose value of 28 mg/dL (1.6 mmol/L) at 2:30 AM while asleep. Her last meal and insulin bolus were at 7 PM. She was woken by her CGM alarm and able to treat her hypoglycemia independently, but she is fearful of increasing frequency of hypoglycemia. She asks for advice about hypoglycemia prevention. Her pump settings are listed:

Basal rates:

> 12 AM = 0.9
> 4 AM = 1.1
> 8 AM = 1

Insulin-to-carbohydrate ratios are 1 unit per 10 g of carbohydrates throughout the day with a sensitivity factor of 70 mg/dL, a target glucose value of 100 mg/dL (5.6 mmol/L), and active insulin time of 3 hours.

Which of the following should be recommended to prevent hypoglycemia?

A. Reduce 11 PM and 12 AM basal rates by at least 20% to 30%

B. Set a temporary basal rate reduction of 75% every night before going to bed for 12 hours

C. Set an alarm at 1 AM to check glucose nightly

D. Ensure she has an active glucagon prescription

Answer: A) Reduce 11 PM and 12 AM basal rates by at least 20% to 30%

The best strategy would be to reduce her overnight basal rates approximately 2 hours before the hypoglycemia is occurring (Answer A). This can help prevent hypoglycemia. The other options are reasonable additional steps. Having an active glucagon prescription (Answer D) is recommended but will not address her current frequency and severity of hypoglycemia. Setting an alarm prior to the onset of anticipated hypoglycemia (Answer C) is an option, but reducing her insulin preceding the hypoglycemia is a better choice. Setting a temporary basal rate (Answer B) is an option; however, this is labor intensive for the patient to do every night, making her prone to possibly forgetting. Also, she most likely does not need a 25% basal rate reduction for 12 hours starting at bedtime, as this may lead to fasting hyperglycemia.

Case 3

A 28-year-old woman (G1P0) with T1DM is currently at 30 weeks' gestation and has significant hyperglycemia following meals. She is on a multiple daily dose insulin regimen with detemir twice daily and lispro with meals dosed with an insulin-to-carbohydrate ratio of 1 unit per 5 g carbohydrates and 1 unit per 50 mg/dL (2.8 mmol/L) glucose correction for glucose values over 100 mg/dL (>5.6 mmol/L). Her fasting glucose levels are at goal with 2-hour postprandial glucose values in the range of 180 to 190 mg/dL (10.0-10.5 mmol/L) most days.

Which of the following should be recommended to reduce her hyperglycemia?

A. Increase activity such as walking after meals

B. Increase the evening detemir dose by 25%

C. Change the insulin-to-carbohydrate ratio for lispro dosing to 1 unit per 8 g of carbohydrates with meals and snacks

D. Change the insulin-to-carbohydrate ratio for lispro dosing to 1 unit per 3 g of carbohydrates with meals and snacks

Answer: D) Change the insulin-to-carbohydrate ratio for lispro dosing to 1 unit per 3 g of carbohydrates with meals and snacks

This woman is in her third trimester of pregnancy, and maternal hyperglycemia at this stage of pregnancy can increase the risk for macrosomia and neonatal hyperglycemia at birth. While increasing exercise (Answer A) may help with mild hyperglycemia, this would not be enough given her degree of postprandial glucose elevations. Her fasting glucose values are at goal, so her basal insulin dose, especially at night, seems appropriate. Thus, increasing the evening detemir dose by 25% (Answer B) is incorrect. The best approach would be to adjust her insulin-to-carbohydrate ratio to a more aggressive level—moving from 1 unit per 5 g of carbohydrates to 1 unit per 3 g of carbohydrates (Answer D) to provide more insulin with meals (rather than reducing the dose with a move to 1 unit per 8 g of carbohydrates [Answer C]). The timing of insulin boluses should also be discussed, and she should be advised to give lispro at least 10 to 15 minutes before the start of a meal if her glucose concentration is in the 100s mg/dL (5.5 mmol/L), and even 20 to 25 minutes before the start of a meal in the third trimester or with higher premeal glucose levels.

References

1. American Diabetes Association. 14. Management of diabetes in pregnancy: standards of medical care in diabetes-2019. *Diabetes Care.* 2019;42(Suppl 1):S165-S172. PMID: 30559240

2. ACOG Committee Opinion No. 762: prepregnancy counseling. *Obstet Gynecol.* 2019;133(1):e78-e89. PMID: 30575679

3. ACOG Practice Bulletin No. 201: pregestational diabetes mellitus. *Obstet Gynecol.* 2018;132(6):e228-e248. PMID: 30461693

4. Peterson C, Grosse SD, Li R, et al. Preventable health and cost burden of adverse birth outcomes associated with pregestational diabetes in the United States. *Am J Obstet Gynecol.* 2015;212(1):74 e1-e9. PMID: 25439811

5. Blumer I, Hader E, Hadden DR, et al. Diabetes and pregnancy: an Endocrine Society clinical practice guideline. *J Clin Endocrinol Metab.* 2013;98(11):4227-4249. PMID: 24194617

6. Garcia-Patterson A, Gich I, Amini SB, Catalano PM, de Leiva A, Corcoy R. Insulin requirements throughout pregnancy in women with type 1 diabetes mellitus: three changes of direction. *Diabetologia.* 2010;53(3):446-451. PMID: 20013109

7. Doder Z, Vanechanos D, Oster M, Landgraf W, Lin S. Insulin glulisine in pregnancy - experience from clinical trials and post-marketing surveillance. *Eur Endocrinol.* 2015;11(1):17-20. PMID: 29632561

8. Bacon S, Feig DS. Glucose targets and insulin choice in pregnancy: what has changed in the last decade? *Curr Diab Rep.* 2018;18(10):77. PMID: 30116911

9. Lepercq J, Lin J, Hall GC, et al. Meta-analysis of maternal and neonatal outcomes associated with the use of insulin glargine versus NPH insulin during pregnancy. *Obstet Gynecol Int.* 2012;2012:649070. PMID: 22685467

10. Feig DS, Donovan LE, Corcoy R, et al; CONCEPTT Collaborative Group. Continuous glucose monitoring in pregnant women with type 1 diabetes (CONCEPTT): a multicentre international randomised controlled trial. *Lancet.* 2017;390(10110):2347-2359. PMID: 28923465

11. Feig DS, Murphy HR. Continuous glucose monitoring in pregnant women with type 1 diabetes: benefits for mothers, using pumps or pens, and their babies. *Diabet Med.* 2018;35(4):430-435. PMID: 29352491

12. Voormolen DN, DeVries JH, Sanson RME, et al. Continuous glucose monitoring during diabetic pregnancy (GlucoMOMS): a multicentre randomized controlled trial. *Diabetes Obes Metab.* 2018;20(8):1894-1902. PMID: 29603547

13. Stewart ZA, Wilinska ME, Hartnell S, et al. Day-and-night closed-loop insulin delivery in a broad population of pregnant women with type 1 diabetes: a randomized controlled crossover trial. *Diabetes Care.* 2018;41(7):1391-1399. PMID: 29535135

14. Battelino T, Danne T, Bergenstal RM, et al. Clinical targets for continuous glucose monitoring data interpretation: recommendations from the International Consensus on Time in Range. *Diabetes Care.* 2019;42(8):1593-1603. PMID: 31177185

15. Chew EY, Mills JL, Metzger BE, et al. Metabolic control and progression of retinopathy. The Diabetes in Early Pregnancy Study. National Institute of Child Health and Human Development Diabetes in Early Pregnancy Study. *Diabetes Care.* 1995;18(5):631-637. PMID: 8586000

16. Vestgaard M, Sommer MC, Ringholm L, Damm P, Mathiesen ER. Prediction of preeclampsia in type 1 diabetes in early pregnancy by clinical predictors: a systematic review. *J Matern Fetal Neonatal Med.* 2018;31(14):1933-1939. PMID: 28574296

17. Zhang JJ, Ma XX, Hao L, Liu LJ, Lv JC, Zhang H et al. A systematic review and meta-analysis of outcomes of pregnancy in CKD and CKD outcomes in pregnancy. *Clin J Am Soc Nephrol.* 2015;10(11):1964-1978. PMID: 26487769

18. LeFevre ML; U.S. Preventive Services Task Force. Force, low-dose aspirin use for the prevention of morbidity and mortality from preeclampsia: U.S. Preventive Services Task Force recommendation statement. *Ann Intern Med.* 2014;161(11):819-826. PMID: 25200125

19. Nielsen LR, Ekbom P, Damm P, et al. HbA1c levels are significantly lower in early and late pregnancy. *Diabetes Care.* 2004;27(5):1200-1201. PMID: 15111545

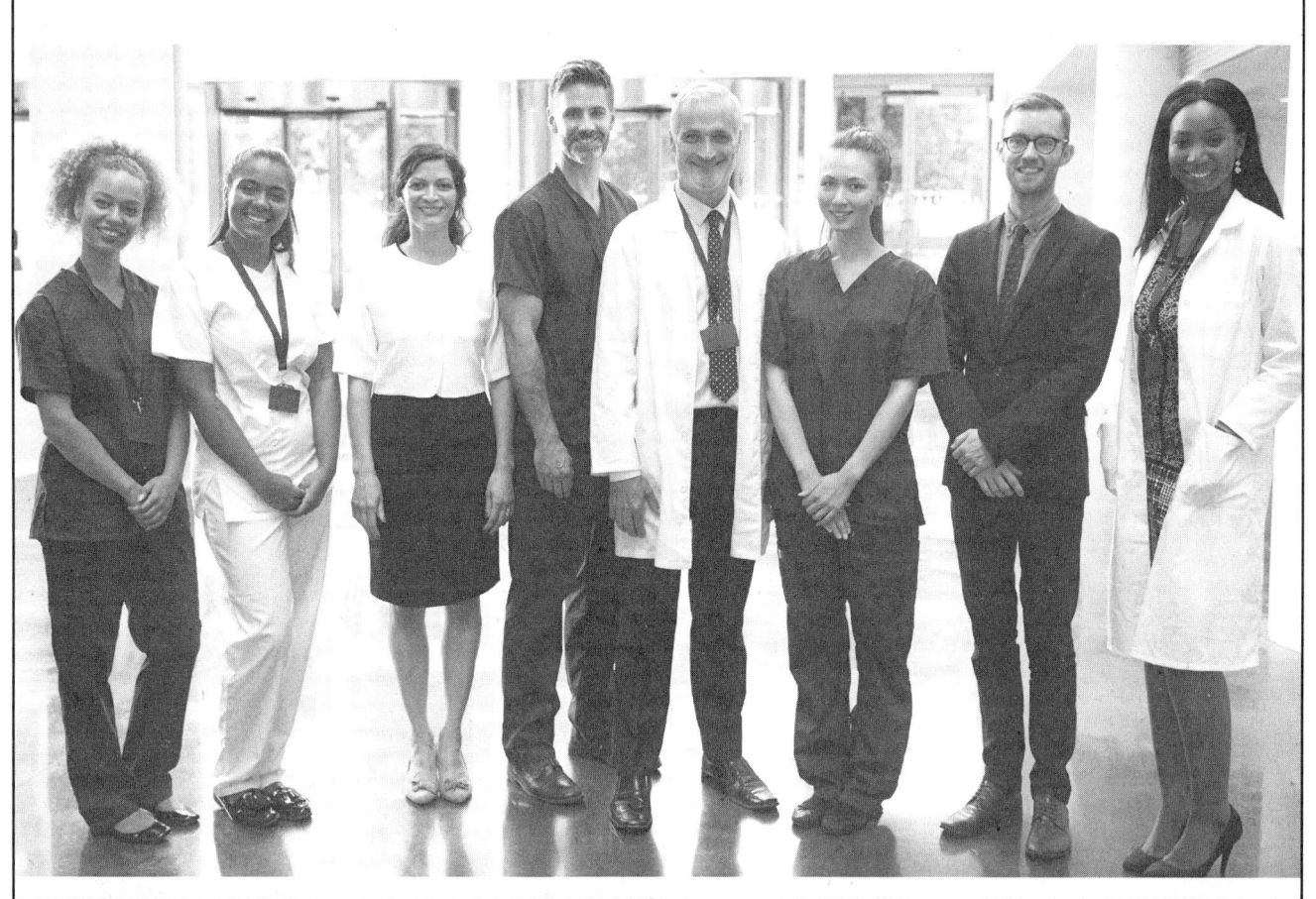

NEUROENDOCRINOLOGY AND PITUITARY

Pseudoacromegaly Syndromes

Marta Korbonits, MD, PhD. Department of Endocrinology, Barts and the London School of Medicine, Queen Mary University of London, London, United Kingdom; E-mail: m.korbonits@qmul.ac.uk

Pedro Marques, MD. Department of Endocrinology, Barts and the London School of Medicine, Queen Mary University of London, London, United Kingdom; E-mail: p.marques@qmul.ac.uk

Learning Objectives

As a result of participating in this session, learners should be able to:

- Recognize the possibility that patients may have a pseudoacromegaly condition.

- Differentiate among manifestations aiding clinical and biochemical diagnosis.

- Explain genetic causes and molecular mechanisms of the disease.

Main Conclusions

- There are conditions that can mimic some features of acromegaly or pituitary gigantism.

- Awareness of these rare conditions will help the differential diagnosis in patients with acromegaloid features but no GH excess.

- Most pseudoacromegaly conditions have a genetic origin, so referral for genetic consultation is recommended if endocrine causes have been ruled out.

Significance of the Clinical Problem

Acromegaly-related physical abnormalities are usually distinctive at clinical examination, which should lead to the prompt assessment of the GH/IGF-1 axis. However, some conditions can mimic acromegaly (at least for less trained eyes) but have no associated GH/IGF-1 anomalies: these conditions are collectively termed pseudoacromegaly.[1] Overlapping features can include acromegaloid facies and acral enlargement, prognathism, visceromegaly, hypertension, fatigue, headaches, arthralgias, paresthesia, hyperhidrosis, oily odorous skin, hypertrichosis, hyperpigmentation, and low-pitched voice.

Apart from hyperinsulinemia, pseudoacromegaly states are rare conditions, and general physicians and endocrinologists rarely encounter them. Affected patients are often seen by pediatricians or specialists in other disciplines and are referred to endocrinology for differential diagnosis. Pseudoacromegaly covers a heterogeneous range of diseases where 1 or 2 features may be reminiscent of acromegaly, but the overall picture suggests a different diagnosis. Examples include Sotos syndrome, pachydermoperiostosis, hyperinsulinemia, non–islet-cell tumor-induced hypoglycemia syndrome, and even drug adverse effects such as prolonged use of phenytoin and minoxidil.

Barriers to Optimal Practice

Because pseudoacromegaly conditions are rare, most physicians have no experience with these diseases, thus hindering diagnosis. We have reported a case in which a patient was referred to endocrinology on 4 different occasions over 40 years, from age 10 to 50 years, by the time the correct diagnosis was made.[2] There is a need to increase awareness of this entity and the associated rare, usually genetic, disorders.

Strategies for Diagnosis, Therapy, and/or Management

The differential diagnosis of pseudoacromegaly can be challenging due to the long list of sometimes overlapping and rare conditions. Key facial features (the overall "gestalt") may characterize Sotos syndrome. Distinctive forehead skin folds and joint abnormalities assist in the diagnosis of pachydermoperiostosis. Severe hypoglycemia is typical in persons with IGF-2–secreting tumors, while generalized infant-onset hypertrichosis indicates Cantú syndrome.

To systematically review these conditions, the main features can be assigned to 3 categories: (1) primarily acromegaloid features with tall, normal, or short stature; (2) primarily tall stature; and (3) biochemical abnormalities suggestive of high GH or IGF-1 levels. In addition to acromegaloid features and accelerated growth, parameters such as dysmorphism, proportionate/disproportionate growth, pubertal anomalies, and intellectual disability can help in the differential diagnosis.

Acromegaloid Features

Acromegaloid features with rapid growth in childhood are typical of several overgrowth syndromes[3] such as Sotos syndrome, Weaver syndrome, Beckwith-Wiedemann syndrome, and Tatton-Brown syndrome and are often associated with a typical gestalt and mental retardation. Marfanoid syndromes such as Marfan and Loeys-Dietz syndromes, are not usually associated with delayed development, while fragile X syndrome is. Endocrine or metabolic syndromes such as severe insulin resistance, IGF-2–related hypoglycemia, Berardinelli-Seip congenital generalized lipodystrophy, and even untreated primary hypothyroidism can be associated with acromegaloid clinical features. Phenytoin can induce some acromegaloid features. Longstanding minoxidil treatment, via its stimulating activity on the ATP potassium channel, produces symptoms similar to those observed in Cantú syndrome, acromegaloid skin changes, and hypertrichosis. Osteopetrosis can also produce bony changes mimicking acromegaly. The differential diagnostic algorithm is shown in *Figure 1*.

Tall Stature

Tall stature is most often due to constitutive tall stature, while endocrine conditions such as hyperthyroidism, congenital adrenal hyperplasia, accelerated puberty in a child, or delayed puberty, and familial glucocorticoid resistance can also result in advanced height. Some skeletal disease can produce extreme tall stature. The differential diagnostic algorithm is shown in *Figure 2*.

Biochemical Alterations

There are 2 physiological states where both GH and IGF-1 are elevated: pregnancy and adolescence. The complex interplay of pituitary and placental GH, increased levels of IGF-binding protein cleaving proteases, and elevated estradiol and IGF-2 result in a unique metabolic scenario promoting fetal growth. In early pregnancy, there is a slight drop in IGF-1 followed by 2 to 3 times increased IGF-1 peaking at the 37th week of pregnancy. GH axis evaluation is challenging in adolescence. GH levels are increased, particularly at the peak of pubertal growth, and often do not fully suppress during an oral glucose tolerance test. GH nadir after oral glucose tolerance testing is gender- and pubertal stage-specific. GH nadir is highest in Tanner stage 2 to 3 girls (1.57 ng/mL [1.57 µg/L]) and lower in other pubertal stages (0.64 ng/mL [0.64 µg/L]) or for boys (0.5 ng/mL [0.5 µg/L]). Serum IGF-1 correlates better with pubertal stage than chronological age. Delayed or accelerated puberty can result in a mismatch between the measured hormone level and the chronological IGF-1 reference range. Evaluation of adolescents and young women can be further complicated by the commonly seen increased pituitary volume in this setting.

Figure 1. Differential Diagnostic Algorithm of Acromegaloid Features

Conditions with hypertrichosis/ hirsutism
Berardinelli-Seip congenital generalized lipodystrophy
Cantú sy.
Coffin-Siris sy.
Cornelia de Lange sy.
Drugs: Minoxidil; Phenytoin
Gorlin-Chaudhry-Moss sy.
Fryns sy.
Insulin-mediated pseudoacromegaly
Kabuki sy.
Marshall-Smith sy.
Nicolaides-Baraitser sy.

Acromegaloid facies

GH/IGF-1 excess — YES → Acromegaly / Pituitary gigantism
IGF-2 excess — YES → Non-islet cell tumor-induced hypoglycemia
NO

Accelerated growth / tall stature | **Normal growth / normal stature** | **Growth retardation / short stature**

Intellectual disability (YES / NO) | Intellectual disability (YES / NO) | Intellectual disability (YES / NO)

Accelerated growth / tall stature — Intellectual disability YES:
Proportionate overgrowth
Berardinelli-Seip congenital lipodystrophy
EED-related sy.
Malan sy.
Marshall-Smith sy.
Microduplications 15q26
Microduplications 17q13.3
Perlman sy.
Phelan-McDermid sy.
SETD2-related sy.
Simpson-Golabi-Behmel sy.
Sotos sy.
Tatton-Brown-Rahman sy.
Weaver sy.
X-tetrasomy

Disproportionate overgrowth
α-mannosidosis
β-mannosidosis
CLOVES sy.
Fragile X sy.
MCAP sy.

Accelerated growth / tall stature — Intellectual disability NO:
Proportionate overgrowth
Beckwith-Wiedmann sy.
Chromosome 11 inversion
HMGA2 rearrangements-related overgrowth

Disproportionate overgrowth
Beals sy.
Loeys-Dietz sy.
Marfan sy.
Proteus sy.

Normal growth / normal stature — Intellectual disability YES:
Acral enlargement
FG sy. type 1
Lujan sy.
Microdeletions 12q24.31
Pallister-Killian sy.
X-linked Ohdo sy.

Hand non-acromegaloid deformities /joint laxity
Coffin-Siris sy.
Mabry sy.
Shprintzen-Goldberg sy.

Normal hands
Fryns sy.

Normal growth / normal stature — Intellectual disability NO:
Acral enlargement
Cantú sy.
Insulin-mediated pseudoacromegaly
Minoxidil
Primary hypothyroidism

Hand non-acromegaloid deformities /joint laxity
Klippel-Trenaunay sy.
Pachydermoperiostosis

Normal hands
Ascher sy.
Anti-retrovirals
Barraquer-Simons sy.
Fabry disease
Oculo-facial-cardio-dental sy.
Phenytoin

Growth retardation / short stature — Intellectual disability YES:
Hand non-acromegaloid deformities /joint laxity
Börjeson-Forssman-Lehmann sy.
Coffin-Lowry sy.
Cornelia de Lange sy.
Kabuki sy.
Nicolaides-Baraitser sy.
SETD5-related sy.
Williams sy.

Normal hands
CHOPS sy.
Microdeletions 17p13.3

Growth retardation / short stature — Intellectual disability NO:
Hand non-acromegaloid deformities /joint laxity
Gorlin-Chaudhry-Moss sy.
Sclerosteosis

Normal hands
Osteopetrosis

There is only one known disease condition in which both high GH and IGF-1 can be seen without the patient having clinical acromegaly: the recently described IGSF1 deficiency syndrome.[4]

Discrepant GH and/or IGF-1 levels can be detected in several conditions (*Table*) and considering these diagnoses will help to interpret unusual biochemical results.

Clinical Case Vignettes

Case 1

A 26-year-old man with tall stature is referred to endocrinology for possible gigantism. The patient is significantly taller than his midparental height, has had painful joints since age 6 years, and has had excessive sweating since age 15 years.

On physical examination, he has enlarged hands and feet with wide wrists and ankles that have lost their contour, furrowing of the forehead skin, and clubbing of fingers and toes. His body habitus is lean rather than the bulky habitus typical of patients with acromegaly.

Although all are reasonable options, which of the following is the best step to help in the diagnosis?

A. Take a family history, including questions regarding consanguinity

B. Perform baseline pituitary function tests

C. Refer for a genetic consultation

D. Measure urinary prostaglandin E2

Answer: D) Measure urinary prostaglandin E2

The key clinical diagnostic clue in this case is the clubbing, with additional clues being furrowing of forehead, profuse sweating, young-onset joint pain, and skinny body habitus—these

Figure 2. Differential Diagnostic Algorithm of Tall Stature

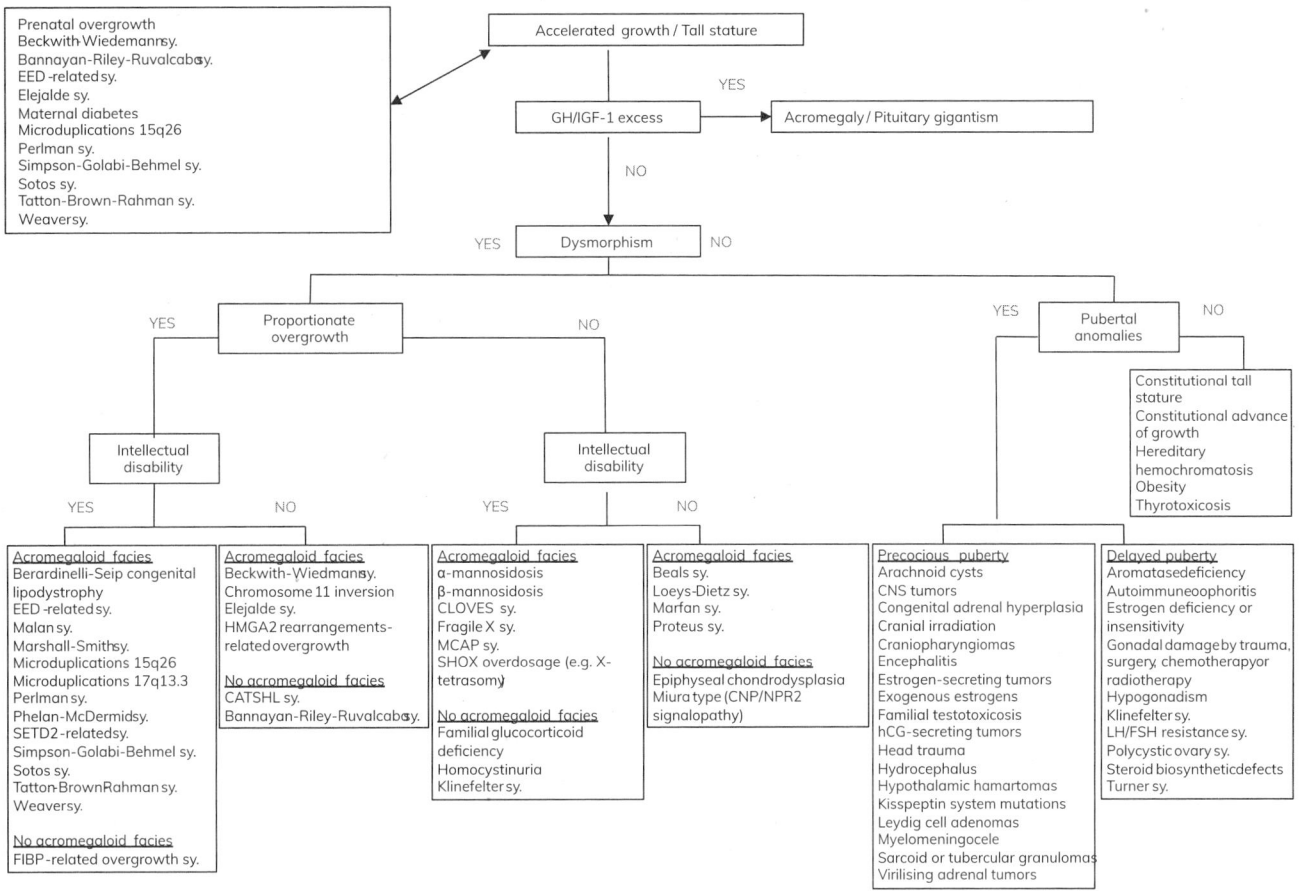

Table. Conditions Associated With Discrepant GH and/or IGF-1 Levels

Normal GH and High IGF-1	High GH and Normal or Low IGF-1
• Adolescence	• Adolescence
• Pregnancy	• Pregnancy
• Increased tissue responsiveness to GH (eg, genotype D3 of the GH receptor)	• Diabetes mellitus
• Supraphysiologic testosterone levels	• Obesity
• Early or mild acromegaly	• Malnutrition
• "Burnt out acromegaly"	• Eating disorders
• Early postoperative period of acromegaly	• Cystic fibrosis
• GH cutoff too high	• Renal failure
• IGF-1 cutoff too low	• Liver disease
• Technical issues with biochemical assays	• Hypothyroidism
	• Oral estrogen treatment
	• "Burnt out acromegaly"
	• GH cutoff too low
	• IGF-1 cutoff too high
	• Technical issues with biochemical assays

are all characteristics of patients with pachydermoperiostosis. The tall stature could be a red herring; although striking in this case, it is not typically described with pachydermoperiostosis. Measuring baseline pituitary hormones (Answer B) can help rule out acromegaly. This disease is due abnormally high prostaglandin E2 (PGE2) levels in the blood either caused by defective uptake into the lung (biallelic pathogenic variants in the transporter *SLCO2A1* gene) where PGE2 is degraded, or due to defective enzymatic clearing of PGE2 caused by biallelic pathogenic variants in the *HPGD* gene (15-hydroxyprostaglandin-dehydrogenase). A positive family history and the presence of consanguinity (Answer A) would support the diagnosis. Clinical features include clubbing, joint problems, and pachydermia. Arthralgia is present in 40% of cases, with synovial effusions, periosteal changes, acroosteolysis, and ligaments/interosseous membranes ossifications. There are some phenotypic differences between the 2 subtypes. Genetic consultation (Answer C) could facilitate identifying the disease-causing pathogenic variants. There is male preponderance, hypocellular myelofibrosis, and more prominent cutis verticis gyrata in patients with *SLCO2A1* pathogenic variants, while younger onset of disease is more characteristic of patients with *HPGD* pathogenic variants. In patients with *HPGD* pathogenic variants, there is elevated urinary PGE2 (Answer D), with low/undetectable PGE2 metabolites, while in patients with *SLCO2A1* pathogenic variants, both PGE2 and its metabolites are high in the urine.

The patient in this vignette has homozygous frameshift mutations in the *HPGD* gene, and his younger brother is also affected. The most obvious differential diagnosis for clubbing includes lung disease, and the mechanism is probably linked, as lung is the primary site for PGE2 degradation. Cutis verticis gyrata can be seen in acromegaly, severe hyperinsulinemia, amyloidosis, hypothyroidism, and Noonan syndrome, etc.

Case 2

A female patient is referred due to prominent acromegaloid facial features with course skin, thickened fingers, and wide-spread hirsutism. There is a family history of infant-onset generalized hirsutism in 5 members (2 males, 3 females) of this 3-generational family and pericardial effusions in 1 member.

Which of the following is the best approach to this patient?

A. Measure GH and IGF-1
B. Measure gonadal hormones
C. Type clinical features into Google

Answer: C) Type clinical features into Google

This is a challenging diagnosis of a multisystem disorder. This patient has hypertrichotic osteochondrodysplasia or Cantú syndrome. Previously used names include acromegaloid facial appearance syndrome or hypertrichosis acromegaloid facial features syndrome. There is a long list of possible manifestations,[5] which probably explains the various names. The most prominent manifestation is the generalized hypertrichosis, in addition to the coarse facial features, bulbous nose, thick lips, long philtrum, macroglossia, epicanthic folds, cardiomegaly, patent ductus arteriosus, pericardial effusions, broad ribs, hyperextensibility of joints, wrinkled skin, macrosomia at birth, and recurrent infections. The disease is caused by activating pathogenic variants in the *ABCC9* gene (sulfonylurea receptor 2) or, rarely, its partner the *KCNJ8* gene (coding for Kir6.1), resulting in overactive ATP-sensitive potassium channels. While these receptors are present in skeletal and heart muscle, probably explaining the heart phenotype, the mechanism leading to the abnormal skin changes and hirsutism is unclear. A unique phenocopy of this disease is seen in patients with prolonged use of minoxidil, as minoxidil activates this potassium channel and is of course used to induce hair growth. In this vignette, the coarse facial features and thickened fingers raise the possibility of acromegaly (Answer

A). Hypertrichosis in a female patient raises the possibility of androgen excess (Answer B).

Case 3

A 4-year-old girl is referred because of extreme tall stature (SD +5). There is no family history of tall stature or pituitary disease.

Which of the following should be included in the differential diagnosis?

A. X-linked acrogigantism
B. McCune-Albright syndrome
C. Pathogenic variants in the *AIP* gene
D. Neurofibromatosis type 1
E. Carney complex
F. Multiple endocrine neoplasia type 1 or 4
G. Congenital adrenal hyperplasia
H. Skeletal disease (Marfan syndrome, Loeys-Dietz syndrome, epiphyseal chondrodysplasia, Miura type, and homocystinuria)
I. Overgrowth syndromes (Sotos syndrome, Weaver syndrome, Tatton-Brown syndrome)

Answer: H) Skeletal disease (epiphyseal chondrodysplasia, Miura type)

To explore the diagnosis, the following questions could be asked:

- Does the patient have features compatible with GH excess, such as acromegaloid body habitus, increased appetite, sweating, vision problems, and headache?

- What was the patient's birthweight?

- Is there evidence of mental retardation or central nervous system abnormalities?

- Does the patient have signs of early puberty, skin lesions, or bony abnormalities?

- Are there biochemical features of abnormal gonadal and adrenal hormones?

- Is there a family history of tall stature or gigantism?

- What do the patient's toes look like?

The differential diagnosis of tall stature is broad and we refer to excellent reviews.[6] This patient has extreme tall stature at a young age. Of the endocrine causes, the only abnormality resulting in this degree of SD in height is X-linked acrogigantism (Answer A), characterized by infant-onset acromegaly. Overgrowth syndromes can cause tall stature in early childhood, although such individuals often have normal adult height due to advanced bone age. Marfan syndrome can be associated with rapid growth in small children. For Miura type epiphyseal chondrodysplasia, the length of the toes could be diagnostic—a striking feature, although not described in every case.[7]

If pituitary gigantism is suspected, serum GH, IGF-1, and prolactin measurement, as well as pituitary MRI, would help to establish the diagnosis. Almost 80% of patients with X-linked acrogigantism are female. Normal birth weight with rapid growth under the age of 1 year is typical. Associated clinical features include coarse facial features, widened hands and feet, increased appetite, and increased BMI. X-linked acrogigantism is due to duplication of the orphan receptor *GPR101* gene and results in excess of GH/IGF-1 and usually prolactin due to pituitary hyperplasia or a tumor. The genetic diagnosis can be confirmed by a comparative genomic hybridization array, although a small duplication may not be detected by this technique. Droplet digital polymerase chain reaction or targeted array could be used if comparative genomic hybridization array is negative. In male patients, mosaicism is associated with the disease; therefore, ideally, DNA extracted from pituitary tissue can identify the *GPR101* duplication. For overgrowth syndromes, clinical phenotyping is key, followed by targeted gene sequencing or overgrowth gene panel testing to verify the genetic diagnosis.

Epiphyseal chondrodysplasia, Miura type is caused by the upregulation of the natriuretic peptide C (abbreviated either as NPC or CNP) pathway. NPC lacks natriuretic functions and via activation natriuretic peptide receptor type 2 (NPR2), it stimulates endochondral bone growth, promoting synthesis of cartilage matrix and stimulating chondrocyte differentiation and proliferation. The most striking and practically pathognomonic feature is the significantly extended halluces. Long hands and feet, arachnodactyly, camptodactyly, clinodactyly, syndactyly, feet deformities, tibia and femur bowing, unstable slipped capital femoral epiphysis, scoliosis, hyperlordosis, dorsal dysmorphism, multiple hernias, wide vertebral canal, and low bone mineral density can be present. Genetic testing includes searching for activating pathogenic variants in the NPC receptor *NPR2* gene, upregulation/duplication of the gene coding for NPC (*NPR1*), or loss-of-function pathogenic variants in the scavenger receptor *NPR3* gene.[8] Biochemical assessment of serum NTproCNP can be useful. In the setting of NPC duplication/upregulation, NTproCNP levels are high, while in the setting of activating *NPR2* pathogenic variants and loss-of-function *NPR3* pathogenic variants, NTproCNP levels are low. cGMP, the second messenger downstream of *NPR2*, is elevated in all 3 cases.

Marfan syndrome is due to pathogenic variants in the fibrillin-1 gene (*FBN1*). Altered fibrillin-1 leads to upregulation of the TGFβ pathway. Clinical features include tall stature, which could be comparable to that observed in acromegalic gigantism,[9] and typically disproportionately long extremities for trunk size (dolichostenomelia) leading to an increased arm span-to-height ratio and lower-to-upper segment ratio. Pectus carinatum or excavatum, scoliosis, pes planus or cavus, and long fingers are common.

Skeletal manifestations can be present in young children and progress in periods of rapid growth. Facial features include narrow and long face, enophthalmos, downslanting palpebral fissures, malar hypoplasia, and micro/retrognathia, although prognathism may be present in 30% of patients. Myopia is the most common ocular finding, but ectopia lentis is the hallmark feature seen in nearly 60% of cases. Patients should be evaluated for cardiovascular features such as dilation of the aorta, predisposition to aortic rupture, enlarged pulmonary artery, and mitral valve prolapse. The Ghent criteria could be used for diagnosis. Marfan-like syndromes include Beals syndrome due to pathogenic variants in the fibrillin-2 gene (*FBN2*) and Loeys-Dietz syndrome due to pathogenic variants in genes part of the TGFβ-pathway (*SMAD2, SMAD3, TGFB2, TGFB3, TGFBR1, TGFBR2*).

Does the patient have features compatible with GH excess, such as acromegaloid body habitus, increased appetite, sweating, vision problems, or headache?
One could consider early-onset GH excess, X-linked acrogigantism, or possibly McCune-Albright syndrome.

What was the patient's birthweight?
Increased birth weight would be compatible with overgrowth syndromes or some Miura type abnormalities.

Is there evidence of mental retardation or central nervous system abnormalities?
This would suggest overgrowth syndromes, possibly fragile X syndrome.

Does the patient have signs of early puberty with skin lesions and bony abnormalities?
This would suggest McCune-Albright syndrome.

Are there biochemical features of abnormal gonadal and adrenal hormones?
This would suggest congenital adrenal hyperplasia.

Is there a family history of tall stature or gigantism?
This could be present in several diseases, such as skeletal disorders, X-linked acrogigantism, AIP pathogenic variants.

What do the patient's toes look like?
Extra-long halluces could be diagnostic for diseases affecting the natriuretic peptide C pathway.

References

1. Marques P, Korbonits M. Pseudoacromegaly. *Front Neuroendocrinol.* 2019;52:113-143. PMID: 30448536

2. Dahlqvist P, Spencer R, Marques P, et al. Pseudoacromegaly: a differential diagnostic problem for acromegaly with a genetic solution. *J Endocr Soc.* 2017;1(8):1104-1109. PMID: 29264563

3. Kamien B, Ronan A, Poke G, et al. A clinical review of generalized overgrowth syndromes in the era of massively parallel sequencing. *Mol Syndromol.* 2018;9(2):70-82. PMID: 29593474

4. Sun Y, Bak B, Schoenmakers N, et al. Loss-of-function mutations in IGSF1 cause an X-linked syndrome of central hypothyroidism and testicular enlargement. *Nat Genet.* 2012;44(12):1375-1381. PMID: 23143598

5. Marques P, Spencer R, Morrison PJ, et al. Cantu syndrome with coexisting familial pituitary adenoma. *Endocrine.* 2018;59(3):677-684. PMID: 29327300

6. Albuquerque EVA, Scalco RC, Jorge AAL. Management of endocrine disease: diagnostic and therapeutic approach of tall stature. *Eur J Endocrinol.* 2017;176(6):R339-R353. PMID: 28274950

7. Hannema SE, van Duyvenvoorde HA, Premsler T, et al. An activating mutation in the kinase homology domain of the natriuretic peptide receptor-2 causes extremely tall stature without skeletal deformities. *J Clin Endocrinolo Metab.* 2013;98(12):E1988-E1998. PMID: 24057292

8. Boudin E, de Jong TR, Prickett TCR, et al. Bi-allelic loss-of-function mutations in the NPR-C receptor result in enhanced growth and connective tissue abnormalities. *Am J Hum Genet.* 2018;103(2):288-295. PMID: 30032985

9. Marques P, Collier D, Barkan A, Korbonits M. Coexisting pituitary and non-pituitary gigantism in the same family. *Clin Endocrinol (Oxf).* 2018;89(6):887-888. PMID: 30223298

Prevention and Management of Carcinoid Crisis

Electron Kebebew, MD. Stanford University, Stanford, CA; E-mail: kebebew@stanford.edu

Learning Objectives

As a result of participating in this session, learners should be able to:

- Recognize the symptoms and signs of carcinoid syndrome and crisis.

- Identify risk factors for carcinoid crisis.

- Treat carcinoid crisis.

Main Conclusions

The clinical hallmarks of classic carcinoid syndrome include episodic flushing, diarrhea, cardiac valvular disease, and, less frequently, bronchospasm. Most patients with classic carcinoid syndrome have metastatic small bowel carcinoid. Extraintestinal carcinoids can cause the syndrome in the absence of metastatic disease, because the substances that they secrete gain direct access to the central venous circulation. Carcinoid crisis is defined as a severe episode of flushing, hypotension, tachyarrhythmia, confusion, and respiratory distress. Some patients with functioning gastric or bronchial carcinoids have clinical and biochemical variations from the classic carcinoid syndrome. It is very important to understand the biochemical and pathophysiological link between the carcinoid tumor and the carcinoid syndrome, because the physician may be easily misled into thinking the patient has isolated functional problems rather than a syndrome caused by a tumor. Risk factors for or precipitating events for carcinoid crisis include, most common to least common, the presence of carcinoid heart disease, anesthesia or surgery, interventional therapy, radionuclide therapy, examination, medication (eg, serotonergic drugs such as clomipramine and amitriptyline), and biopsy. Carcinoid crisis can also occur spontaneously. The treatment for carcinoid crisis and syndrome includes somatostatin analogues, histamine-receptor blockers, vasopressin or phenylephrine for significant hypotension, and α-adrenergic and β-adrenergic receptor blockers for hypertension.

Significance of the Clinical Problem

The family of neuroendocrine tumors consists of a spectrum of neoplasms that can arise from the diffuse endocrine system throughout the body. The incidence of neuroendocrine tumors (commonly referred to carcinoid) is increasing, so many health care providers will encounter patients with neuroendocrine tumors.[1,2] The carcinoid tumor, a member of this fascinating family of tumors, is characterized by its ability to uptake (or synthesize), store, and release a variety of biogenic amines, polypeptides, and prostaglandins.[3-4] Although carcinoid tumors have been reported in essentially all tissues, the overwhelming majority of these neoplasms originate in the gastrointestinal tract. Most carcinoid tumors have a relatively slow-growing, indolent natural history, but sometimes they can behave in a highly malignant fashion, exhibiting metastatic behavior, most often to the liver and lungs.

The early symptoms of carcinoid tumor are nonspecific and may include abdominal pain, diarrhea, intermittent intestinal obstruction, and gastrointestinal bleeding. These often vague and generalized signs and symptoms produce a delay in diagnosis in many patients. Although symptoms may be caused by mechanical effects of the tumors, symptoms of carcinoid tumors are also caused by the effects of amine and neuropeptide substances secreted into the gastrointestinal tract or the systemic circulation. The effects of these chemicals, collectively referred to as the carcinoid syndrome, are diverse and include cutaneous flushing, diarrhea, carcinoid heart disease, bronchoconstriction, hypotension, hypertension, and pellagra. Carcinoid crisis occurs with worsening of all of these symptoms and can result in cardiovascular collapse and death if not recognized and treated early. The cornerstone of avoiding carcinoid crisis is identifying at-risk patients and ensuring rapid and effective treatment.

Barriers to Optimal Practice

- Carcinoid syndrome and crisis symptoms may be nonspecific.

- There is a great deal of heterogeneity regarding the clinical definition of carcinoid crisis for assessing treatment effectiveness.

- The role of prophylactic somatostatin analogues in the treatment of carcinoid crisis is unclear.

Strategies for Diagnosis, Therapy, and/or Management

Classic carcinoid syndrome does not develop until a tumor has metastasized to the liver and/or lung, and the hormonal products released by the tumor reach the central venous circulation in substantial concentrations. Some patients with functioning gastric or bronchial carcinoids have clinical and biochemical variations from the classic syndrome, as this tumor can directly drain into the central venous circulation without the metabolites from the tumor being metabolized by the liver.

The incidence of classic carcinoid syndrome, which is characterized by flushing, diarrhea, abdominal cramping, and, less often, wheezing, heart-valve dysfunction, and pellagra, varies depending on the study population. While studies that include patients with localized and incidental tumors report the frequency of carcinoid syndrome to be about 10% to 18%, the prevalence may be as high as 50% among patients with advanced and metastatic disease. The syndrome results from synergistic interactions between biochemical substances secreted by the tumor, and it is often observed in patients with metastatic disease or when the primary tumor site allows the secreted amines to escape enteral hepatic circulation. The presence of carcinoid syndrome is associated with poor survival.

In 1954, Pernow and Waldenstrom demonstrated presence of serotonin in the blood and urine of 2 patients with carcinoid tumor during an attack of flushing. Originally, the whole spectrum of symptoms was thought to be related to the production and secretion of serotonin by the tumor and its metastases; however, since that time, a number of hormonal substances contributing to the signs and symptoms of carcinoid syndrome have been described, and the syndrome itself has been more fully characterized. Carcinoid tumors produce and secrete a great variety of bioactive compounds, including serotonin, histamine, bradykinin, tachykinin, motilin, substance P, kallikrein, prostaglandins, catecholamines, and in some cases ACTH. Although the contribution of each of these mediators is not yet completely understood, some of them, including serotonin, histamine, tachykinins, and kallikrein, are thought to have a major role in the development of the clinical picture of carcinoid syndrome and crisis.

Clinical Presentation of Classic Carcinoid Syndrome

Carcinoid syndrome, the hormonal manifestation of carcinoid tumors, is generally characterized by flushing, diarrhea, and, less commonly, wheezing, heart-valve dysfunction, and pellagra (*Table 1*).

The frequency of carcinoid syndrome correlates with the extent of the metastatic carcinoid disease, and it can be as low as 10% in localized cases, but it can occur in 40% to 50% of patients with more advanced disease. The presence of carcinoid syndrome is associated with poor survival. Not all patients with carcinoid tumors develop carcinoid syndrome. Symptoms develop when the secretory products released from the tumors gain direct access to the systemic circulation, bypassing metabolism in the liver. The conditions in which such a bypass may develop include the presence of liver and lung metastases draining directly into the caval circulation, retroperitoneal disease with drainage into paravertebral veins, or primary sites of disease outside the gastrointestinal tract. In up to 90% of patients, the development of carcinoid syndrome is associated with metastatic tumors originating in the midgut. In contrast, bronchial carcinoid tumors are associated with carcinoid syndrome in approximately 10% of cases, and nearly all hindgut tumors are hormonally silent. As many as 40 different substances have been identified in various carcinoid tumors.[4] Some of these tumor products are responsible for the carcinoid syndrome, but the relative contributions of each and specificity of any for particular components of the syndrome are yet unknown (*Table 2*). Thus, the diagnosis of carcinoid syndrome and crisis is clinical based on the symptoms and signs.

Table 1. Common Symptoms in Patients With Carcinoid Syndrome: Frequency and Association With Secreted Compounds

Symptoms	Putative Substances	Frequency, %
Flushing	Histamine, tachykinins, kallikrein, bradykinin	>90
Diarrhea	Serotonin, substance P, motilin, prostaglandins	70-85
Cardiac valvular disease	Serotonin, 5-hydroxyindoleacetic acid, neurokinin A, substance P	~40-60
Telangiectasias	Serotonin, bradykinin, prostaglandins	25
Bronchospasm	Serotonin, bradykinin	15-19
Pellagra (dermatitis, diarrhea, dementia)	Niacin deficiency due to excess tryptophan metabolism	5-7

Table 2. Association of Carcinoid Syndrome With Carcinoid Tumor Localization and Secreted Compounds

Site of Tumor	Localization	Secreted Substances	Carcinoid Syndrome
Foregut	Bronchus	5-hydroxytryptophan, histamine, peptide hormones, ACTH (bronchial, thymus)	Atypical, rarely Cushing syndrome
	Thymus		
	Stomach		
	Duodenum		
Midgut	Jejunum	Serotonin, peptide hormones, prostaglandins	Classic
	Ileum		
	Appendix		
	Ascending colon		
Hindgut	Transverse colon	Variable peptide hormones	Rare
	Descending colon		
	Sigmoid colon		
	Rectum		

Some patients with functioning gastric or bronchial carcinoids have clinical and biochemical variations from the classic carcinoid syndrome.

Gastric Variant Syndrome

Gastric carcinoid tumors have 2 important biochemical features, which may explain at least in part the pathophysiologic basis of variant gastric carcinoid syndrome. First, gastric carcinoids are usually unable to convert the dietary tryptophan into serotonin, because they are frequently deficient in the enzyme aromatic L-amino acid decarboxylase. Serotonin has been increasingly implicated in the pathophysiology of diarrhea and carcinoid heart disease. As a consequence, the diarrhea and cardiac lesions, which are common features of classic midgut carcinoid syndrome, are unusual in the gastric variant of the syndrome. Second, gastric carcinoids can produce large amounts of histamine, which has been shown to have primary role in the atypical flushing and pruritus associated with these tumors. In patients with the gastric carcinoid variant, the flushes may be patchy, sharply demarcated, serpiginous, and cherry red; they are also intensely pruritic.

Bronchial Carcinoid Variant Syndrome

Bronchial carcinoids produce less serotonin than do midgut carcinoids, accounting for a lower rate of carcinoid syndrome. Although carcinoid syndrome is encountered only rarely among patients with localized bronchial carcinoids (majority of typical carcinoids), it can be present in more than 80% of patients with liver metastases. The symptoms of bronchial carcinoid syndrome may be atypical, with episodes of severe and prolonged flushing, lasting hours to days. Other related manifestations include disorientation, anxiety, tremor, lacrimation, salivation, hypotension, tachycardia, diarrhea, asthma, and edema. Approximately 1% to 2% of bronchial carcinoids (both typical and atypical) are associated with Cushing syndrome due to ectopic production of ACTH.

Carcinoid Crisis

Some patients with carcinoid tumors develop carcinoid crisis, a life-threatening form of carcinoid syndrome, characterized by profound flushing, diarrhea, arrhythmias, extreme changes in blood pressure, bronchospasm, and altered mental status.[1-3] This medical emergency may occur spontaneously, after palpation of the tumor, or during anesthesia, surgery, or chemotherapy. It has been hypothesized that these precipitating events may stimulate release of an overwhelming amount of bioactive compounds by the tumor, leading to a multisystem functional collapse refractory to fluid resuscitation and administration of vasopressors. A great deal of precaution is needed prior to surgery, embolization, or chemotherapy, because carcinoid crisis may be precipitated by anesthesia with intraoperative complications occurring in 2% to greater than 50% of patients. Octreotide should be available for intraoperative use or given preemptively, especially in patients with extensive tumor load.[5] During carcinoid crisis, an initial bolus dose of 50 mg intravenously with further increments as required can be successful in reversing the condition. In addition, histamine-receptor blockers may be useful in reducing histamine release from gastric carcinoid tumors. Close hemodynamic monitoring may be required for patients with carcinoid heart disease, who are at risk of developing arrhythmias and extreme changes in blood pressure. Regional anesthesia and specific pharmacologic agents such as morphine, suxamethonium, β-adrenergic blockers, tubocurarine, halothane, and atracurium should be avoided. Additional supportive treatment in patients with a carcinoid crisis includes vasopressin or phenylephrine for significant hypotension and α-adrenergic and β-adrenergic receptor blockers for hypertension and tachyarrhythmias.

Clinical Case Vignettes

Case 1

A 68-year-old woman with flushing is found to have an ileal neuroendocrine tumor (carcinoid) with regional involved lymph nodes and liver metastasis (*see image*). Her 5-hydroxyindoleacetic acid level is elevated.

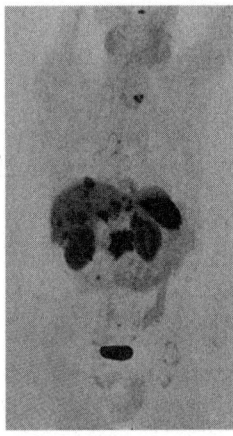

⁶⁸Gallium DOTATATE imaging showing small bowel neuroendocrine tumor, mesenteric lymph node disease, and liver metastasis.

Her risk of having a carcinoid crisis at the time of her operation is which of the following?

A. None existent

B. Very low

C. 100%

D. Intermediate

Answer: D) Intermediate

This patient has carcinoid symptoms and a large tumor burden and will be having general anesthesia, so she is at intermediate risk (Answer D) of developing a carcinoid crisis. Some providers give patients an octreotide drip (50-500 mcg/h) to prevent a carcinoid crisis during an operation, but it is unclear if this reduces the risk of a carcinoid crisis. Answers A and B are incorrect because the patient has significant burden of disease and already has carcinoid symptoms. Answer C is incorrect because not all patients with carcinoid symptoms will have a carcinoid crisis during procedures.

Case 2

A 54-year-old man is having cryoablation of liver neuroendocrine tumor metastases from an ileal neuroendocrine tumor (carcinoid). During the procedure he develops flushing and becomes hypotensive (70/30 mm Hg) and develops bronchospasm.

Which of the following should be administered as the most appropriate management for this patient?

A. β-adrenergic blockers

B. Octreotide bolus with continuous infusion, antihistamine, and vasopressin

C. An antihistamine

D. A blood transfusion

E. Phentolamine

Answer: B) Octreotide bolus with continuous infusion, antihistamine, and vasopressin

This patient has classic signs of carcinoid crisis that is best managed with octreotide bolus and drip, vasopressin for hypotension, and antihistamine (Answer B), as some neuroendocrine tumors may secrete histamine. The patient has hypotension, and β-adrenergic blockers (Answer A) would make it worse. An antihistamine (Answer C) would only block the effect of histamine and would not treat the hypotension. A blood transfusion (Answer D) is incorrect, as the patient is not having active bleeding. Phentolamine (Answer E) is incorrect, as it would further lower the patient's blood pressure.

References

1. Howe JR, Cardona K, Fraker DL, et al. The surgical management of small bowel neuroendocrine tumors: consensus guidelines of the North American Neuroendocrine Tumor Society. *Pancreas.* 2017;46(6):715-731. PMID: 28609357

2. Larouche V, Akirov A, Alshehri S, Ezzat S. Management of small bowel neuroendocrine tumors. *Cancers (Basel).* 2019;11(9). Pii:E1395. PMID: 31540509

3. Tapia Rico G, Li M, Pavlakis N, Cehic G, Price TJ. Prevention and management of carcinoid crises in patients with high-risk neuroendocrine tumours undergoing peptide receptor radionuclide therapy (PRRT): literature review and case series from two Australian tertiary medical institutions. *Cancer Treat Rev.* 2018;66:1-6. PMID: 29602040

4. Fottner C, Ferrata M, Weber MM. Hormone secreting gastro-entero-pancreatic neuroendocrine neoplasias (GEP-NEN): when to consider, how to diagnose? *Rev Endocr Metab Disord.* 2017;18(4):393-410. PMID: 29256148

5. Borna RM, Jahr JS, Kmiecik S, Mancuso KF, Kaye AD. Pharmacology of octreotide: clinical implications for anesthesiologists and associated risks. *Anesthesiol Clin.* 2017;35(2):327-339. PMID: 28526153

Surveillance and Management of Long-Term Complications of Acromegaly

Robert D. Murray, MBBS, MD. Leeds Centre for Diabetes and Endocrinology, St James's University Hospital, Leeds, United Kingdom; E-mail: robertmurray@nhs.net

Learning Objectives

As a result of participating in this session, learners should be able to:

- Recognize the long-term complications of GH and IGF-1 hypersecretion.

- Undertake a structured surveillance program for patients with acromegaly to identify complications.

- Explain the importance of timely control of GH and IGF-1 in reducing long-term complications.

- Recognize those complications that still require addressing and mitigate their impact.

Main Conclusions

In addition to an increase in mortality, patients with acromegaly have significant and diverse morbidity reflecting the widespread expression of the GH and IGF-1 receptor in multiple organ systems. Morbidity includes hypopituitarism, hypertension, diabetes mellitus, dyslipidemia, cardiovascular disease, obstructive sleep apnea, arthropathy, vertebral fractures, carpal tunnel syndrome, malignancy, and impaired quality of life. Patients require holistic assessment at time of diagnosis, with surveillance for complications repeated after interventions to normalize GH and IGF-1 levels and at least annually thereafter. Control of GH and IGF-1 levels can resolve or improve most complications. Biochemical control has less impact, however, on impaired quality of life and arthropathy, which remain areas for improvement in management.

Significance of the Clinical Problem

Acromegaly is the clinical syndrome resulting from chronic excessive GH and IGF-1 secretion. In almost all cases, the cause is a GH-secreting adenoma. As a result of the low incidence (3 to 4 cases/10^6 per year) and nonspecific presentation early in the disease process, diagnosis is frequently delayed. In the vast majority of individuals, the initial management is selective hypophyseal adenomectomy. Postoperative remission rates for microadenomas in specialist centers approach 90%. However, remission rates are significantly less for macroadenomas, particularly when there is notable invasion of the cavernous sinus. In these latter cases, remission rates even in specialist centers are less than 50%. Most somatotroph adenomas are macroadenomas, and therefore overall remission rates postoperatively are in the range of 42% to 65%.[1] In patients with persistent disease following surgery, somatostatin analogue therapy is generally favored as second-line management. Long-acting somatostatin analogue therapy leads to control of both GH and IGF-1 in 30% to 40% of patients not in remission following surgery.[2] Therefore, combined use of surgery and somatostatin analogue therapy leads to overall biochemical remission rates of around 70%. Approximately 30% of patients still require further therapy to achieve optimal disease control. It is clear, therefore, that remission in a significant proportion of patients requires multimodality therapy (surgery, radiation therapy, and medical therapy) and takes time to achieve.[3]

Almost all tissues express the GH and IGF-1 receptor, so there is the potential for adverse effects of excess secretion on multiple tissues and biological systems. Acromegaly is associated with increased mortality, which can be normalized by control of GH and IGF-1 secretion.[4,5] There is, in addition, a notable associated long-term morbidity, including hypopituitarism, hypertension, diabetes mellitus, dyslipidemia, cardiovascular disease, obstructive sleep apnea, arthropathy, vertebral fractures, carpal tunnel syndrome, malignancy, and impaired quality of life.[6,7] Furthermore, interventions used to achieve biochemical remission are not themselves without potential early and late sequelae. Complications of surgery generally occur early, whereas those associated with radiation therapy (hypopituitarism, second malignancies, vascular disease) usually take a number of years to be realized. Adverse events relating to medical therapy are specific to the medication used and add further complexity to long-term monitoring of patients with acromegaly.

With the plethora of long-term complications of acromegaly, affected individuals require prolonged follow-up and surveillance. Early recognition and aggressive management of complications is essential, although management strategies to reduce the frequency of long-term complications remain the ultimate goal. For a few outcomes (arthropathy, quality of life), management has had less of an impact and future research is needed.[8,9]

Barriers to Optimal Practice

- Due to the low prevalence of acromegaly, the diagnosis is frequently delayed by 8 to 10 years, leading to potentially irreversible changes in tissues by the time of diagnosis.

- Rapid control of GH and IGF-1 excess is not always achievable, and many patients require multimodality therapy to meet biochemical targets.

Strategies for Diagnosis, Therapy, and/or Management

In the long-term, multimodality therapy achieves biochemical control of acromegaly in almost all individuals. Patients, however, achieve disease control at different time points during their therapeutic journey. For example, surgery can lead to immediate biochemical remission, whereas in patients who receive radiation therapy for persistent disease, control of biochemical markers of disease activity can take many years to be realized. Furthermore, a number of individuals must remain on long-term medical therapy to maintain biochemical control either as secondary therapy after unsuccessful pituitary surgery or while awaiting the effects of radiation therapy. Given the heterogeneity in treatment regimens and degree of biochemical control, most specialist pituitary centers are likely to undertake surveillance on patients with biochemical remission, GH/IGF-1 dichotomy, and mild biochemical disease activity achieved after variable treatment duration.

Baseline assessment of many putative complications should be done at the time of presentation due to their impact on initial management. Of most importance at diagnosis is assessment and management of ACTH deficiency, hypertension, diabetes mellitus, cardiac function, and obstructive sleep apnea. Once acceptable GH and IGF-1 levels are achieved, surveillance for morbidity in most individuals is undertaken annually, with more frequent visits when intervention to manage morbidity is uncovered. Central to surveillance for long-term complications is a thorough history and listening to patient concerns, followed by blood pressure measurement and relevant laboratory tests and imaging. A structured surveillance program must be personalized and should consider:

- Hypopituitarism
- Blood pressure
- Vascular risk factors (lipid profile and glucose intolerance)
- Obstructive sleep apnea
- Echocardiography
- Colonoscopy
- Bone densitometry
- Spinal x-rays
- Joint x-rays/ultrasonography
- Thyroid ultrasonography
- Quality of life

Not all of these screening tests require regular repetition, and others potentially only performed should the patient have symptoms or signs. Whether, and when, surveillance regimens could be discontinued or simplified needs consideration. This may be particularly relevant in elderly patients, very long-term survivors, and those who achieve remission immediately following primary pituitary surgery. Individualization of screening is essential; however, all aspects should be considered at the patient's follow-up visits.

Control of GH and IGF-1 reduces the severity, or prevalence, of most complications observed, and therefore biochemical control should be pursued rapidly and aggressively.[6,7] Exceptions to this rule may be sleep apnea, arthropathy, and quality of life.[8,9,10] Following biochemical control, management of most complications of acromegaly is not dissimilar to that of the same conditions when present within the general population. Management of many of the complications requires multidisciplinary care, frequently coordinated by the endocrinologist.

Clinical Case Vignettes

Case 1

A 34-year-old man with acromegaly (GH = 24 ng/mL [24 µg/L]; IGF-1 = 2.3 times the upper normal limit) undergoes transsphenoidal adenomectomy for a microadenoma and achieves postoperative control of GH and IGF-1.

Which of the following complications is most likely to improve?

A. Diabetes mellitus
B. Arthropathy
C. Vertebral fractures
D. Sleep apnea

Answer: A) Diabetes mellitus

Biochemical control of acromegaly fails to prevent progression of premature degenerative arthropathy (Answer B), which correlates most closely to GH and IGF-1 levels at presentation. The incidence of vertebral fractures (Answer C) does appear to slow with biochemical control; however, the incidence remains greater than expected. Data on sleep apnea (Answer D) are variable, although most studies fail to show resolution of sleep apnea with biochemical control of acromegaly. This most likely reflects that the soft-tissue changes observed in patients with acromegaly frequently remain after achieving biochemical control. The excess GH secretion that defines acromegaly antagonizes insulin action, leading to glucose intolerance and diabetes. With the fall in GH levels, insulin resistance and glucose tolerance improve in almost all patients, with resolution of diabetes in a number of individuals (thus, Answer A is correct).

Case 2

A 46-year-old woman with a GH-secreting adenoma with persistent disease relating to cavernous invasion fails to show GH suppression with first-generation somatostatin analogues. Pasireotide is initiated with successful control of the GH axis, but she develops diabetes mellitus as a complication.

Which of the following would be the best class of medication to help control glucose metabolism?

A. Sulfonylurea

B. Metformin

C. GLP-1 receptor agonist

D. Insulin

Answer: C) GLP-1 receptor agonist

Pasireotide inhibits not only insulin secretion, but also gut hormones including the incretins. As a consequence, GLP-1 receptor agonists (Answer C) and DPP-4 inhibitors appear to be the most appropriate treatment modality for pasireotide-induced diabetes.

Case 3

A 58-year-old man with acromegaly who has had control of GH and IGF-1 for 15 years presents with worsening joint pain and functional limitation.

Which of the following are features of acromegalic arthropathy?

A. Joint space widening

B. Hyperosteophytosis

C. Fissuring of the cartilage

D. Joint space narrowing

E. All of the above

Answer: E) All of the above

All of these are features of acromegalic arthropathy at different stages of the process (Answer E). Acromegalic arthropathy appears to have 2 distinct phases. The initial phase is characterized by an increase in joint space (Answer A) resulting from hypertrophy of the cartilage and ligamentous laxity. At this stage, the arthropathy may have a degree of reversibility. The inherent instability of such joints in the longer term leads to the second phase, characterized by fissuring (Answer C) and degeneration of the cartilage (joint space narrowing) (Answer D), subchondral bone cysts, and bone remodeling (osteophytosis) (Answer B).

References

1. Minniti G, Jaffrain-Rea ML, Esposito V, Santoro A, Tamburrano G, Cantore G. Evolving criteria for post-operative biochemical remission of acromegaly: can we achieve a definitive cure? An audit of surgical results on a large series and a review of the literature. *Endocr Relat Cancer*. 2003;10(4):611-619. PMID: 14713271

2. Murray RD, Melmed S. A critical analysis of clinically available somatostatin analog formulations for therapy of acromegaly. *J Clin Endocrinol Metab*. 2008;93(8):2957-2968. PMID: 18477663

3. Katznelson L, Laws ER Jr, Melmed S, et al; Enodcrine Society. Acromegaly: an Endocrine Society clinical practice guideline. *J Clin Endocrinol Metab*. 2014;99(11):3933-3951. PMID: 25356808

4. Holdaway IM, Bolland MJ, Gamble GD. A meta-analysis of the effect of lowering serum levels of GH and IGF-I on mortality in acromegaly. *Eur J Endocrinol*. 2008;159(2):89-95. PMID: 18524797

5. Orme SM, McNally RJ, Cartwright RA, Belchetz PE. Mortality and cancer incidence in acromegaly: a retrospective cohort study. United Kingdom Acromegaly Study Group. *J Clin Endocrinol Metab*. 1998;83(8):2730-2734. PMID: 9709939

6. Gadelha MR, Kasuki L, Lim DST, Fleseriu M. Systemic complications of acromegaly and the impact of the current treatment landscape: an update. *Endocr Rev*. 2019;40(1):268-332. PMID: 30184064

7. Giustina A, Barkan A, Beckers A, et al. A consensus on the diagnosis and treatment of acromegaly comorbidities: an update. *J Clin Endocrinol Metab* [Epub ahead of print] PMID: 31606735

8. Claessen KM, Ramautar SR, Pereira AM, et al. Increased clinical symptoms of acromegalic arthropathy in patients with long-term disease control: a prospective follow-up study. *Pituitary*. 2014;17(1):44-52. PMID: 23344976

9. Kyriakakis N, Lynch J, Gilbey SG, Webb SM, Murray RD. Impaired quality of life in patients with treated acromegaly despite long-term biochemically stable disease: results from a 5-years prospective study. *Clin Endocrinol (Oxf)*. 2017;86(6):806-815. PMID: 28316090

10. Parolin M, Dassie F, Alessio L, et al. Obstructive sleep apnea in acromegaly and the effect of treatment: a systematic review and meta-analysis. *J Clin Endocrinol Metab* [Epub ahead of print] PMID: 31722411

Dopamine Agonists: Risks, Adverse Effects, Surveillance, and Intervention

Mark E. Molitch, MD. Division of Endocrinology, Metabolism, and Molecular Medicine, Northwestern University Feinberg School of Medicine, Chicago, IL; E-mail: molitch@ northwestern.edu

Learning Objectives

As a result of participating in this session, learners should be able to:

- List at least 3 risks of prescribing cabergoline at high dosages.

- Recognize the consequences of tumor shrinkage by dopamine agonists.

- Explain the risks and benefits of dopamine agonist use in women who become pregnant.

Main Conclusions

Although dopamine agonists have been shown to be highly effective and remain the mainstay of the treatment of patients with prolactinomas, their use does entail some risks and adverse effects. An unusual adverse effect is the development of obsessive-compulsive behavior, such as hypersexuality and gambling. This is usually seen with cabergoline. With either cabergoline or bromocriptine, shrinkage of a large skull-based macroadenoma that invades the sellar floor can result in the leakage of cerebrospinal fluid around the now smaller tumor. Cerebrospinal fluid rhinorrhea can be diagnosed by measuring β2-transferrin in the nasal fluid, and the leak must be repaired to prevent meningitis. About 15% to 20% of patients require larger than standard dosages of cabergoline to normalize prolactin levels, and large dosages may cause cardiac valve abnormalities.

Women who wish to become pregnant while using dopamine agonists have a risk of tumor enlargement—2% of those with microadenomas and 18% of those with macroadenomas. Neither drug has been shown to increase the risk of fetal malformations.

Significance of the Clinical Problem

Prolactinomas are the most common hormone-secreting pituitary tumors.[1] Dopamine agonists remain the treatment mainstay for patients with prolactinomas because of their high degree of efficacy and low adverse effect profiles.[2] Bromocriptine, in use since the mid-1970s, can normalize prolactin levels in 80% to 90% of patients and shrink prolactinomas by more than 50% in about 50% of patients. Cabergoline, in use since the mid-1990s, can achieve these goals in more than 90% of patients. Cabergoline, therefore, is more effective and better tolerated. The common adverse effect of nausea can be lessened by starting with low dosages and gradually increasing over weeks to months, monitoring the prolactin response. About 15% to 20% of patients are resistant to these medications, requiring more than standard dosing to achieve prolactin normalization. Approximately 50% of those resistant to bromocriptine respond to cabergoline. Very high cabergoline dosages have been associated with cardiac valve abnormalities in patients with Parkinson disease, but such valve disease is not found in patients with prolactinomas treated with conventional dosages (≤2 mg weekly). The dosage at which the risk for valve disease increases is not known, and it is recommended that patients taking dosages greater than 2 mg weekly be monitored with echocardiography. Of special concern is the woman with a prolactinoma who wishes to become pregnant. Since the dopamine agonists must be used to allow ovulation, there is some finite period of fetal exposure to the dopamine agonists, but fortunately no adverse consequences to the mother or fetus have been found with such exposure. There is a small risk of tumor enlargement, especially macroadenomas, due to the high estrogen levels present during pregnancy.[2]

Barriers to Optimal Practice

• Adverse effects related to obsessive-compulsive disorders and tumor shrinkage are not well understood.

• The increased risks associated with more than conventional dosages of cabergoline are not well understood.

• Clinicians often do not appreciate the problems associated with dopamine agonist use in women with prolactinomas who become pregnant.

Strategies for Diagnosis, Therapy, and/or Management

The lowest dosages of dopamine agonists that normalize prolactin levels should be used. Clinicians should query their patients and family members about the possible development of obsessive-compulsive behavior.

Increased rhinorrhea can be due to cerebrospinal fluid leakage. Measurement of β2-transferrin in the nasal mucus is diagnostic, paving the way for surgical repair to prevent meningitis.

Endocrinologists should not hesitate to increase dosages of cabergoline beyond 2 mg weekly when needed to control prolactin secretion

and tumor size, but they must recognize the need to perform periodic echocardiography to monitor for cardiac valvular disease and switch to bromocriptine or other modes of therapy if such valve disease develops.

Both bromocriptine and cabergoline are safe for the developing fetus when given to women who wish to become pregnant. Although symptomatic monitoring is sufficient for women with microadenomas because their risk for tumor enlargement is only about 2%, visual field testing each trimester in addition to symptomatic monitoring is necessary for those with macroadenomas, as their risk for tumor enlargement is 18%.

Clinical Case Vignettes
Case 1

A 29-year-old man presents with decreased libido, erectile dysfunction, and headaches. His prolactin concentration is 2904 ng/mL (126.3 nmol/L). MRI shows a 2.4-cm macroadenoma with lateral, intrasellar, and suprasellar extension. His testosterone concentration is borderline-low at 250 ng/dL (8.7 nmol/L), and the rest of his pituitary function is normal. Cabergoline is initiated, and the dosage is gradually increased to 3.5 mg weekly. As a result, his prolactin level normalizes and MRI shows marked tumor size reduction. His libido and erectile function normalize and his headaches disappear. At a recent clinic visit, his wife asks whether his cabergoline dosage could be reduced.

Which of the following adverse effects of cabergoline is she most likely concerned about?

A. Difficulty urinating

B. Hypersexuality

C. Sleep apnea

D. Restless legs

Answer: B) Hypersexuality

Impulse control disorders can be defined as "a failure to resist an impulse, drive, or temptation to perform an act that is harmful to the person or others."[3] Impulse control disorders include, but are not limited to, problem gambling, hypersexuality, compulsive eating, compulsive shopping, and "punding." Punding is characterized by compulsive performance of and fascination with repetitive mechanical tasks; for example, assembling and disassembling household objects or collecting or sorting various items.

The mechanism of action behind impulse control disorders seems to be an interaction between the dopamine agonists and the D_3 receptors in the mesolimbic system, known to be responsible for the processes governing behavior, pleasure, and addiction.[4] Several studies have shown that both cabergoline and bromocriptine can cause compulsive behavior in 15% to 20% of treated patients.[4,5] The effect appears to be somewhat dosage dependent, so lowering the dosage may be helpful in some circumstances. In a recent cross-sectional multicenter study in Turkey of 308 patients with prolactinomas (289 on cabergoline, 19 on bromocriptine), 17% were found to have impulse control disorders (hypersexuality alone 6.5%, pathologic gambling alone 0.6%, compulsive eating alone 2.9%, compulsive shopping 1%, more than 1 impulse control disorder 5.5%). Hypersexuality was more common in men, and compulsive eating was more common in women.[6]

Clinicians should warn patients and their significant others or family members about this potential adverse effect when first prescribing dopamine agonists, but they should also ask about impulse control disorders at subsequent visits. It is important to also ask the spouse, as some impulse control disorders, such as gambling and compulsive shopping, may be hidden from the family.

Case 1 (Continued)

The patient's cabergoline dosage is gradually reduced to 2 mg weekly. His prolactin concentration increases to 45 ng/mL (2.0 nmol/L) after 1 month and then stabilizes with improvement in his hypersexuality. His testosterone concentration, which had increased to 570 ng/dL (19.8 nmol/L), remains in the reference range (400-450 ng/mL [13.9-15.6 nmol/L]). MRI at 6 months shows a 50% reduction in tumor size. During treatment, he has some nasal stuffiness and at 7 months he notices a substantial increase in watery rhinorrhea.

Which of the following is the best next step in his management?

A. Switch to bromocriptine

B. Send nasal fluid for glucose and protein measurements

C. Send nasal fluid for β2-transferrin measurement

D. Start pseudoephedrine

Answer C) Send nasal fluid for β2-transferrin measurement

Cerebrospinal fluid rhinorrhea can occur when there is a large, invasive, skull-based prolactinoma that serves as a "cork" in the base of the skull. When the tumor size is reduced substantially through dopamine agonist use, cerebrospinal fluid can leak around the tumor into the sphenoid sinus and nasal passages. The development of profuse rhinorrhea in this patient suggests that this is what is happening.[7] To distinguish between cerebrospinal fluid and simple nasal mucus, the fluid should be sent to the laboratory for measurement of β2-transferrin (Answer C), which is an asialo-transferrin isoform found only in cerebrospinal fluid, ocular fluids, and perilymph and an accepted marker of cerebrospinal fluid leakage.[8] Measurements of nasal fluid glucose and protein levels (Answer B) are not specific. β-trace protein (prostaglandin D synthase) can also be used to distinguish between cerebrospinal fluid and nasal mucus.

The major concern with such leaks is the risk of meningitis. Although a reduction in cabergoline dosage may cause the tumor to get larger, thus plugging the leak, judging the exact dosage and tumor size change is difficult and not reliable and surgery is the best course once the diagnosis is made. Endonasal, endoscopic surgical repair (urgent, but not emergent) to prevent meningitis generally recommended.[7,9] Use of prophylactic antibiotics pending surgery is controversial. Lumbar drainage is usually not successful.[7,9] Switching to bromocriptine (Answer A) would not help. Pseudoephedrine (Answer D) may decrease nasal congestion but will not affect cerebrospinal fluid leakage.

Case 2

An 18-year-old woman presents with primary amenorrhea but otherwise normal prior growth and development. She has also been experiencing headaches and decreased visual acuity.

On physical examination, her height is 61 in (154.9 cm) and weight is 140 lb (63.6 kg) (BMI = 26.4 kg/m²). Blood pressure is normal. She has galactorrhea with Tanner stage 3 breast and pubic hair development.

Laboratory test results:

    Karyotype, 46,XX
    LH = 3.8 mIU/mL (SI: 3.8 IU/L)
    FSH = <2.0 mIU/mL (SI: <2.0 IU/L)
    Estradiol = 34 pg/mL (SI: 124.8 pmol/L)
    Free T$_4$ = 0.8 mIU/L (0.8-1.8 ng/dL)
        (SI: 10.30 pmol/L [10.30-23.17 pmol/L])
    Cortisol (8 AM) = 14 µg/dL (5-25 µg/dL)
        (SI: 386.2 nmol/L [137.9-689.7 nmol/L])
    Pregnancy test, negative

Her prolactin concentration is 29 ng/mL (1.3 nmol/L). On 1:100 dilution, it is 12,840 ng/mL (558.3 nmol/L). MRI shows a 3.4-cm pituitary adenoma.

Cabergoline is initiated at a dosage of 0.5 mg twice weekly, and the dosage is increased at monthly intervals. On a dosage of 1 mg twice weekly (the package insert maximum), her prolactin concentration is 438 ng/mL (19.0 nmol/L), with some tumor shrinkage but no beginning of menses.

Which of the following is the best next step in this patient's management?

A. Perform transsphenoidal debulking

B. Switch to bromocriptine

C. Increase the cabergoline dosage

D. Perform stereotactic radiosurgery

Answer: C) Increase the cabergoline dosage

Fifteen to twenty percent of patients with prolactinomas do not achieve normal prolactin levels with conventional dosages of cabergoline (≤2 mg weekly).[10,11] For such patients, there are a number of alternatives. Occasionally, patients who do not respond to cabergoline do respond to bromocriptine, but the numbers reported are too low to determine how common this is. Conversely, about 50% of patients who do not respond to bromocriptine do respond to cabergoline. However, most patients who have some response to cabergoline will have a further response if the dosage is increased. Dosage increases should be done in a stepwise fashion, documenting a reduction in prolactin levels with each dosage increase. The major issue with increasing dosage is an increase in adverse drug effects. Studies in patients with Parkinson disease, who may be treated with 3 to 5 mg daily, show that adverse effects are uncommon.[11]

The major concern has been the finding of cardiac valve disease with these high cabergoline dosages in as many as 34% of patients with Parkinson disease, with tricuspid regurgitation being the abnormality. Valve abnormalities are not seen with bromocriptine. It is thought that the cabergoline has action at the serotonin (5-HT) 2B receptors, which are present in valves, thereby activating a variety of mitogenic pathways. This results in a plaquelike process that extends along the leaflet surfaces and chordae tendineae and is similar to the lesions seen in patients with carcinoid syndrome.[12] Almost all echocardiographic studies have not shown an increase in valve abnormalities in hyperprolactinemic patients taking cabergoline compared with control patients when dosages are kept to a maximum of 2 mg weekly.[13] However, given the Parkinson disease data, there clearly is an increased risk with higher dosages, but exactly where that threshold is for increased risk is not known. Because of this, it has been recommended that hyperprolactinemic patients receiving greater than 2 mg weekly of cabergoline have echocardiography performed when that dosage threshold is crossed with then annually thereafter.[10] Limited data in patients with Parkinson disease show that if valve abnormalities develop, one-third have regression and half have lack of further progression of valve disease if the drug is stopped. However, if the drug is continued about 15% have progression of valve abnormalities.

Case 3

A 42-year-old physician who was treated 20 years ago for a 2-cm macroprolactinoma calls with a question. Cabergoline shrunk the prolactinoma, her prolactin levels normalized, and ovulatory menses returned. She had tried going off cabergoline several times over the years without maintaining normal prolactin levels. Now she is 20 weeks pregnant and asks whether she should continue cabergoline. She notes that she feels much better when taking cabergoline than when she does not.

Which of the following is the best next step in this patient's management?

A. Switch cabergoline to bromocriptine and continue throughout pregnancy

B. Continue cabergoline throughout the pregnancy

C. Stop cabergoline now

D. Stop cabergoline now but restart if she starts feeling badly

Answer: C) Stop cabergoline

Neither cabergoline nor bromocriptine should be continued once the pregnancy is diagnosed, so as to limit the exposure of the developing fetus to either drug. The dopamine agonist should be stopped once pregnancy is diagnosed (Answer C).[14,15] When these drugs are stopped within the first few weeks of pregnancy, the frequency of major malformations is not greater than would be expected in the general population, and an elective termination is not justified. The databases establishing such safety are greater for bromocriptine (5000 to 6000) than for cabergoline (900 to 1000),[14] so some clinicians prefer bromocriptine to allow ovulation when women wish to become pregnant. Many clinicians think that the cabergoline database is sufficiently large to feel comfortable with the safety aspect. A concern about stopping the dopamine agonist is the risk of tumor enlargement. The chance of clinically significant tumor growth related to the pregnancy is about 18% for patients with macroadenomas and 2.5% for those with microadenomas.[14] The data regarding safety for using dopamine agonists throughout pregnancy and, in this case, after 20 weeks, are sparse. However, organogenesis is usually complete by 8 weeks' gestation, so no additional malformations would be expected. A recent compilation of the literature does not suggest any late complications either.[14] However, Hurault-Delarue et al reported an increased risk of preterm birth and early pregnancy loss with dopamine agonist use.[16]

References

1. Molitch ME. Diagnosis and treatment of pituitary adenomas. *JAMA.* 2017;317(5):516-524. PMID: 28170483

2. Gillam MP, Molitch MP, Lombardi G, Colao A. Advances in the treatment of prolactinomas. *Endocr Rev.* 2006;27(5):485-534. PMID: 16705142

3. American Psychiatric Association. *Diagnostic and Statistical Manual of Mental Disorders—Text Revision (DSM-IV-TR).* Washington, DC: American Psychiatric Association; 2000.

4. Noronha S, Stokes V, Karavitaki N, Grossman A. Treating prolactinomas with dopamine agonists: always worth the gamble? *Endocrine.* 2016;51(2):205-210. PMID: 26336835

5. Bancos I, Nannenga MR, Bostwick JM, Silber MH, Erickson D, Nippoldt TB. Impulse control disorders in patients with dopamine agonist-treated prolactinomas and nonfunctioning pituitary adenomas: a case-control study. *Clin Endocrinol (Oxf).* 2014;80(6):863-868. PMID: 24274365

6. Dogansen SC, Cikrikcili U, Oruk G, et al. Dopamine agonist-induced impulse control disorders in patients with prolactinoma: a cross-sectional multicenter study. *J Clin Endocrinol Metab.* 2019;104(7):2527-2534. PMID: 30848825

7. Suliman SG, Gurlek A, Byrne JV, et al. Nonsurgical cerebrospinal fluid rhinorrhea in invasive macroprolactinoma: incidence, radiological, and clinicopathological features. *J Clin Endocrinol Metab.* 2007;92(10):3829-3835. PMID: 17623759

8. Warnecke A, Averbeck T, Wurster U, Harmening M, Lenarz T, Stover T. Diagnostic relevance of beta2-transferrin for the detection of cerebrospinal fluid fistulas. *Arch Otolaryngol Head Neck Surg.* 2004;130(10):1178-1184. PMID: 15492165

9. Lam G, Mehta V, Zada G. Spontaneous and medically induced cerebrospinal fluid leakage in the setting of pituitary adenomas: review of the literature. *Neurosurg Focus.* 2012;32(6):E2. PMID: 22655691

10. Molitch ME. Management of medically refractory prolactinoma. *J Neurooncol.* 2014;117(3):421-428. PMID: 24146188

11. Ono M, Miki N, Kawamata T, et al. Prospective study of high-dose cabergoline treatment of prolactinomas in 150 patients. *J Clin Endocrinol Metab.* 2008;93(12):4721-4727. PMID: 18812485

12. Roth BL. Drugs and valvular heart disease. *N Engl J Med.* 2007;356(1):6-9. PMID: 17202450

13. Stiles CE, Tetteh-Wayoe ET, Bestwick J, Steeds RP, Drake WM. A meta-analysis of the prevalence of cardiac valvulopathy in hyperprolactinemic patients treated with cabergoline. *J Clin Endocrinol Metab* 2019;104(2):523-538.

14. Huang W, Molitch ME. Pituitary tumors in pregnancy. *Endocrinol Metab Clin N Am.* 2019;48(3):569-581. PMID: 31345524

15. Glezer A, Bronstein MD. Prolactinomas, cabergoline, and pregnancy. *Endocrine.* 2014;46(1):64-69. PMID: 24985062

16. Hurault-Delarue C, Montastruc JL, Beau AB, Lacroix I, Damase-Michel C. Pregnancy outcome in women exposed to dopamine agonists during pregnancy: a pharmacoepidemiology study in EFEMERIS database. *Arch Gynecol Obstet.* 2014;290(2):263-270. PMID: 24664257

The Patient Who Presents With Hyponatremia

Chris J. Thompson, MBChB, MD, FRCPI, FRCPE, FFSEM RCSI. Medical School, Dublin, Ireland; E-mail: christhompson@beaumont.ie

Stephen G. Ball, MBBS, BSc, PhD, FRCP. Manchester University Foundation Trust and University of Manchester, Manchester, England; E-mail: s.ball@manchester.ac.uk

Learning Objectives

As a result of participating in this session, learners should be able to:

- Explain the etiology of hyponatremia.

- Devise a diagnostic strategy to discover the cause of hyponatremia.

- Initiate therapy that is appropriate to the cause of hyponatremia and to the needs of the patient.

Main Conclusions

Hyponatremia is the most common electrolyte abnormality in clinical practice. Almost every published study has demonstrated that patients with hyponatremia have a worse prognosis, longer hospital stay, and higher standard mortality ratio than patients who are eunatremic. Acute hyponatremia is a medical emergency that is associated with high mortality and requires urgent therapy to prevent cerebral edema and early death. New guidelines have suggested that intravenous boluses of hypertonic (3%) saline should be administered to rapidly elevate plasma sodium by 4 to 6 mEq/L (4-6 mmol/L) in the first 6 hours, and there is emerging evidence that this treatment strategy leads to more rapid normalization of conscious levels than traditional slow intravenous infusion of hypertonic saline.

Chronic hyponatremia is associated with gait abnormalities, falls, and fractures. There is convincing new evidence to indicate that hyponatremia predisposes to osteoporosis, which contributes to the fracture rate. Mortality is increased in the setting of chronic hyponatremia, particularly with hypervolemic and hypovolemic hyponatremia. Establishing the underlying cause of chronic hyponatremia is important, as treatment is specific to the etiology. Glucocorticoid deficiency is often overlooked as a cause of hyponatremia; data suggest that tests for causation of hyponatremia are infrequently performed in routine clinical practice. Treatment of chronic hyponatremia is less urgent, and indeed, rapid overcorrection is associated with the development of catastrophic osmotic demyelination syndrome. Treatment options are varied; guidelines recommend fluid restriction as first-line therapy, with pharmacologic agents, such as vaptans and urea, reserved for symptomatic cases.

Significance of the Clinical Problem

Hyponatremia is the most common electrolyte abnormality seen in clinical practice, and approximately 15% to 20% of patients develop hyponatremia at some stage of hospital admission. Abundant data demonstrate that hyponatremia is associated with increased mortality in almost all clinical scenarios.[1] Although there is some debate about whether the excess mortality reflects the severity of the underlying causative condition, there is gathering evidence to suggest that some of the excess mortality is due to the electrolyte abnormality itself. In other words, hyponatremia confers negative prognosis of itself, rather than simply acting as a biomarker of severe underlying disease. The mortality associated with hypervolemic and hypovolemic hyponatremia is higher than that seen with syndrome of inappropriate antidiuresis (SIAD).

The key to appropriate treatment of hyponatremia is accurate definition of the underlying etiology. However, published data consistently show that the minimum investigations needed to arrive at an accurate diagnosis of hyponatremia are seldom complete. As Table 1 shows, measurement of key diagnostic parameters is poor in routine practice and, in particular, tests for glucocorticoid deficiency are rarely performed.

Acute, symptomatic hyponatremia is a life-threatening condition. Clinicians are often afraid to commit to aggressive treatment with hypertonic saline, because of the fear of inducing the dreadful iatrogenic condition of osmotic demyelination, which manifests as spastic quadriplegia and cranial nerve palsies. However, recent guidelines have stressed the need for intervention to prevent cerebral edema and improve prognosis. In this chapter, the new guidelines and their potential impact on the management of acute symptomatic hyponatremia will be reviewed.

Barriers to Optimal Practice

- Awareness of the impact of hyponatremia, particularly on mortality, is not widely appreciated.

- Hyponatremia is often regarded as a diagnosis in itself, rather than the biochemical manifestation of a wide variety of diseases. As a result, the comprehensive investigations that are essential to establish the cause of hyponatremia are often omitted from the workup.

- Incorrect treatment may then be commenced on the basis of insufficient diagnostic data; glucocorticoid deficiency in particular is often missed.

- Lack of confidence in the management of acute symptomatic hyponatremia may lead to undertreatment and avoidable deaths.

Table 1. Measurement of Diagnostic Parameters in Patients With Hyponatremia

	Studies		
Study Aspects	**Tzoulis and Bouloux** **Clin Med (Lond), 2015[2]**	**Greenberg et al** **Kidney Int, 2015[3]**	**Cuesta et al** **Clin Endocrinol (Oxf), 2016[4]**
Patient diagnosis	All-cause hyponatremia	Syndrome of inappropriate antidiuresis	Euvolemic hyponatremia
Study design	Retrospective Routine practice	Prospective Study patients	Prospective Study patients
No. of patients	139	1524	1323
Inclusion plasma sodium	<128 mEq/L (SI: <128 mmol/L)	<130 mEq/L (SI: <130 mmol/L)	<130 mEq/L (SI: <130 mmol/L)
Urine osmolality measured, % of patients	29%	68%	87%
Urine sodium measured, % of patients	29%	63%	87%
Plasma cortisol measured, % of patients	33%	33%	88%

Strategies for Diagnosis, Therapy, and/or Management

Acute Symptomatic Hyponatremia

In acute hyponatremia (<48 hours), there is no time for cerebral adaptation to take place. As a result, there is an osmotic shift of extracellular water into the brain, which develops cerebral edema and swells. In the confined cavity of the skull, the brain swelling leads to raised intracranial pressure, with the development of neurological symptoms such as headache, nausea, reduced conscious level, and, if severe enough, seizures, coma, and the fatal condition of coning of the brain. Neurological symptoms are very likely to be manifestations of cerebral edema, and flag the condition as potentially fatal, with older published articles reporting greater than 50% mortality.

Newer guidelines have stressed the importance of reversal of hyponatremia in the acute setting[1] and the relatively low risk of inducing osmotic demyelination, if there is certainty that hyponatremia has developed over less than 48 hours. It has been suggested that the aim of treatment of acute symptomatic hyponatremia is rapid elevation in plasma sodium of 4 to 6 mEq/L (4-6 mmol/L), using intravenous boluses of hypertonic saline over the first 6 hours of treatment. The theory is that this elevates the plasma sodium concentration, causing an osmotic shift of water out of the brain and into the circulation, with a consequent reduction of intracranial pressure. Over the subsequent hours, the target elevation of plasma sodium elevation is still 8 to 12 mEq/L (8-12 mmol/L) in 24 hours in total. Practically speaking, the elevation in plasma sodium is front loaded into the first 6 hours, in an attempt to reduce intracranial pressure.

This changed treatment protocol was audited in a paper published this year (*Table 2*).[5] The data showed that bolus therapy was more effective in acutely elevating plasma sodium than traditional low-dose hypertonic saline infusion. The benefit of the bolus system was that the Glasgow Coma Scale assessment of cognitive function returned to normal more rapidly, in line with the faster reversal of hyponatremia. Bolus therapy was associated with a more frequent need to reverse overcorrection with desmopressin or hypotonic fluids, but there were no instances of osmotic demyelination.

Glucocorticoid Deficiency

Primary adrenocortical deficiency is well recognized to cause hyponatremia, associated with hyperkalemia and volume depletion, due to the combination of glucocorticoid and mineralocorticoid deficiency. However, glucocorticoid deficiency, arising from pituitary disease or from suppression of the hypothalamic-pituitary-adrenal axis from immunosuppressive steroids, also presents with hyponatremia. In contrast to primary adrenal failure, however, deficiency of glucocorticoid alone presents with a biochemical pattern indistinguishable from SIAD.

Table 2. Low-Dose Infusion vs Bolus Therapy for Reversal of Hyponatremia[5]

Findings	Low-Dose Infusion	Bolus Therapy	P Value
Nadir plasma sodium	119 mEq/L (SI: 119 mmol/L)	120 mEq/L (SI: 120 mmol/L)	.30
6-hour Δ plasma sodium	3 mEq/L (SI: 3 mmol/L)	6 mEq/L (SI: 6 mmol/L)	<.0001
24-hour Δ plasma sodium	10 mEq/L (SI: 10 mmol/L)	10 mEq/L (SI: 10 mmol/L)	.99
Baseline Glasgow Coma Scale score	12	12	.22
6-hour Glasgow Coma Scale score	13	15	.0006
Intervention for overcorrection	0/28	7/24	.0026
Mortality	4/28	1/24	.36

Patients presenting with glucocorticoid deficiency may therefore be misdiagnosed as having SIAD, with delayed diagnosis of cortisol deficiency. In one prospective study of patients presenting to the hospital with hyponatremia, 4% of those presenting with apparent SIAD had underlying cortisol deficiency,[6] half had new pituitary disease, and half had been on immunosuppressive prednisolone therapy and had developed hypothalamic-pituitary-adrenal axis depression. Similarly, many patients who present with SIAD with neurosurgical emergencies, such as trauma and subarachnoid hemorrhage, have hyponatremia due to acute ACTH/cortisol deficiency.

Chronic Hyponatremia

Chronic hyponatremia is by far the most common presentation seen by clinicians. The key issue is to establish the etiology of hyponatremia, as treatment is etiology specific. Hypovolemic patients are treated with intravenous fluids, hypervolemic patients are treated with diuretic therapy, and euvolemic patients are managed with a variety of agents specifically aimed at reducing plasma water. There are many different algorithms for the differential diagnosis of hyponatremic states, and it is important to acknowledge that none of them take the place of experience and good clinical acumen.

Hypovolemic hyponatremia is most often due to gastrointestinal upsets, causing vomiting and diarrhea, or diuretic therapy. Hypervolemic hyponatremia is seen in end-stage cardiac and hepatic failure. SIAD is strictly defined as euvolemic hyponatremia with an elevated urine sodium concentration (>30 mmol/L) and evidence of inappropriate vasopressin action in the form of elevated urine osmolality (>100 mOsm/kg). Thyroid and adrenal failure, as well as recent diuretic therapy, should be excluded before arriving at a diagnosis of SIAD. Published data show that if the 0900h cortisol concentration is greater than 10.9 µg/dL (>300 nmol/L), a cosyntropin (tetracosactrin) stimulation test is not needed to prove cortisol deficiency in patients with SIAD.

Management of Chronic SIAD

The issue of management of chronic SIAD has been addressed in management guidelines.[1,7] There is a general consensus that fluid restriction is first-line therapy; it is cheap and relatively free from harm, as long as it is not prescribed for a patient with hypovolemic hyponatremia. There are no published data to justify its use, however, and reports from one international multicenter database suggest that it has very marginal benefits compared with no therapy.[2] A number of parameters have been suggested to predict poor response to fluid deprivation, including urine osmolality greater than 500 mOsm/kg at diagnosis and a Furst ratio greater than 1. However, the main difficulty is patient adherence to a level of fluid restriction that will be effective.

A number of second-line therapies are available for the management of SIAD, including vasopressin receptor antagonists (vaptans), urea therapy, and demeclocycline. Only vaptans have an evidence base that includes prospective, randomized, placebo-controlled trials.[8] Vaptans are effective in the management of chronic SIAD, but the cost of therapy is significant and the absence of hard end-point outcomes limits more widespread use. A summary of the comparisons of the various second-line treatments for SIAD is shown in Table 3.

Clinical Case Vignettes
Case 1

A 28-year-old woman is brought to the emergency department with seizures and is unconscious. She recently saw her primary care physician who prescribed a selective serotonin reuptake inhibitor for depression and encouraged her to increase her fluid intake. Her plasma sodium concentration is 115 mEq/L (115 mmol/L), and serum urea nitrogen concentration is 5.0 mg/dL (1.8 mmol/L). She is clinically

Table 3. Comparison of Second-Line Treatments for SIAD

Treatments	Cost	Efficacy	Reliability	Evidence Base	License	Adverse Effects
Fluid restriction	-	+	+	–	N/A	–
Demeclocycline	+	++	+	–	-	++++
Urea	++	+++	++++	Nonrandomized, retrospective	-	+
Frusemide + oral NaCl	+	Anecdotal	++	–	-	+
Vaptans	+++++	+++++	+++++	Prospective, randomized, placebo	✓	+

euvolemic, with a urine sodium concentration of 45 mEq/L (45 mmol/L) and urine osmolality of 482 mOsm/kg. She has another seizure in the emergency department, and the endocrine team is called to review. Brain CT shows loss of cerebral sulci, typical of cerebral edema.

Which of the following statements regarding this patient is true?

A. A random plasma cortisol concentration of 18.5 μg/dL (510 nmol/L) indicates adrenal failure

B. Fluid restriction is the recommended first-line treatment

C. Emergency treatment with hypertonic saline is the treatment of choice

D. The selective serotonin reuptake inhibitor can be safely continued

Answer: C) Emergency treatment with hypertonic saline is the treatment of choice

This is a medical emergency, and treatment should be started with hypertonic saline (Answer C). Fluid restriction (Answer B) would not raise the plasma sodium sufficiently (or quickly enough) to impact this life-threatening situation of cerebral edema. A plasma cortisol concentration less than 10.9 μg/dL (<300 nmol/L) indicates the possibility of adrenal failure (thus, Answer A is incorrect). The selective serotonin reuptake inhibitor is likely to have a caused the SIAD, compounded by excess fluid intake, and should be stopped (thus, Answer D is incorrect). Selective serotonin reuptake inhibitors are a well-recognized cause of SIAD and can produce significant hyponatremia within 2 to 3 weeks of introduction.

Case 2

A 48-year-old man presents with a severe traumatic brain injury following a car crash. Brain CT shows bitemporal fractures, cerebral contusions, and blood in the subarachnoid space. Over the next 3 days, his plasma sodium concentration falls from 143 to 128 mEq/L (143 to 128 mmol/L), with a urine osmolality of 760 mOsm/kg. His 24-hour urine output falls to 900 mL. The patient remains on a ventilator.

Which of the following is correct about this patient's diagnosis?

A. The most likely diagnosis is cerebral salt wasting

B. Primary polydipsia should be considered as a diagnosis

C. SIAD can be discounted as a diagnosis

D. Acute ACTH deficiency should be considered as a diagnosis

Answer: D) Acute ACTH deficiency should be considered as a diagnosis

The elevated urine osmolality indicates that significant vasopressin is present, and SIAD is the most common cause of hyponatremia following traumatic brain injury. A significant proportion of patients who have moderate to severe traumatic brain injury develop acute ACTH/cortisol deficiency (Answer D) and may present with hyponatremia.

Cerebral salt wasting (Answer A) can be discounted in view of the low urine output. Primary polydipsia (Answer B) is not a diagnosis to consider in a ventilated patient, although incorrect intravenous fluid therapy is important to consider. The elevated urine osmolality indicates significant vasopressin is present, and SIAD is the most common cause of hyponatremia following traumatic brain injury. Therefore, it is important to consider this option rather than discount it (Answer C).

Case 3

A 54-year-old man is transferred from another hospital for further management. He has a 15-year history of celiac disease and a 6-month history of weight loss and central abdominal pain. Imaging at the referring center has noted a small bowel mass consistent with lymphoma. On physical examination, he is fully alert and there is moderate bilateral pitting edema to mid-calf. He is clinically euvolemic and euadrenal.

Laboratory test results:

    Plasma sodium = 116 mEq/L (136-142 mEq/L)
        (SI: 116 mmol/L [136-142 mmol/L])
    Serum albumin = 2.2 g/dL (3.5-5.0 g/dL)
        (SI: 22 g/L [35-50 g/L])
    Plasma cortisol (9 AM) = 7.4 µg/dL (5-25 µg/dL)
        (SI: 205 nmol/L [137.9-689.7 nmol/L])
    Urine osmolality = 680 mOsm/kg

Which of the following is the best investigation now?

A. Measure urine protein concentration

B. Perform a cosyntropin-stimulation test

C. Measure urine sodium concentration

D. Perform thyroid function tests

Answer: C) Measure urine sodium concentration

The urine sodium concentration (Answer C) is key in establishing the effective circulating volume of the patient and the etiology of hyponatremia. In this case, hypoalbuminemia from a protein-losing enteropathy has led to effective hypovolemia, confirmed by a urine sodium concentration of 12 mEq/L (12 mmol/L). Physiological vasopressin production can lead to hyponatremia, as baroregulated vasopressin continues even when the plasma sodium concentration is below the threshold for osmoregulated vasopressin release.

A urine protein leak, assessed by measuring the urine protein concentration (Answer A), may be important to consider as a contributor to hypoalbuminemia, but in this context a protein-losing enteropathy is more likely. While a morning cortisol concentration of 7.4 µg/dL (205 nmol/L) does not exclude adrenal insufficiency, it should not increase clinical suspicion in a low probability scenario. Therefore, a cosyntropin-stimulation test (Answer B) is unnecessary. Thyroid function tests (Answer D) rarely contribute useful data in this context. While profound hypothyroidism can lead to reduced free water excretion, thyroid function testing at this stage would not contribute to clinical management.

References

1. Verbalis JG, Goldsmith SR, Greenberg A, et al. Diagnosis, evaluation, and treatment of hyponatremia: expert panel recommendations. *Am J Med*. 2013;126(10 Suppl 1):S1-S42. PMID: 24074529

2. Tzoulis P, Bouloux PM. Inpatient hyponatremia: adequacy of investigation and prevalence of endocrine causes. *Clin Med (Lond)*. 2015;15(1):20-24. PMID: 25650193

3. Greenberg A, Verbalis JG, Amin AN, et al. Current treatment practice and outcomes. Report of the hyponatremia registry. *Kidney Int*. 2015;88(1):167-177. PMID: 25671764

4. Cuesta M, Garrahy A, Slattery D, et al. Mortality rates are lower in SIAD than in hypervolaemic or hypovolaemic hyponatraemia: results of a prospective observational study. *Clin Endocrinol (Oxf)*. 2017;87(4):400-406. PMID: 28574597

5. Garrahy A, Dineen R, Hannon AM, et al. Continuous versus bolus infusion of hypertonic saline in the treatment of symptomatic hyponatremia caused by SIAD. *J Clin Endocrinol Metab*. 2019;104(9):3595-3602. PMID: 30882872

6. Cuesta M, Garrahy A, Slattery D, et al. The contribution of undiagnosed adrenal insufficiency to euvolaemic hyponatraemia; results of a large prospective single-centre study. *Clin Endocrinol (Oxf)*. 2016;85(6):836-844. PMID: 27271953

7. Spasovski G, Vanholder R, Allolio B, et al; Hyponatraemia Guideline Development Group. Clinical practice guidelines on diagnosis and treatment of hyponatraemia. *Eur J Endocrinol*. 2014;170(3):G1-G47. PMID: 24569125

8. Schrier RW, Gross P, Gheorghiade M, et al; SALT Investigators. Tolvaptan, a selective oral vasopressin V2-receptor antagonist for hyponatremia. *N Engl J Med*. 2006;355: 2099-2112

Treatment of Functioning Gonadotroph Pituitary Adenomas

Philippe Chanson, MD. Endocrinology and Reproductive Diseases, Reference Center for Rare Pituitary Diseases, Bicêtre Hospital, and University Paris-Saclay, Le Kremlin-Bicêtre, France; E-mail: philippe.chanson@bct.aphp.fr

Learning Objectives

As a result of participating in this session, learners should be able to:

- Diagnose functioning pituitary gonadotroph adenomas.

- Treat gonadotroph pituitary adenomas.

Main Conclusions

More than 80% of clinically nonfunctioning pituitary adenomas are gonadotroph adenomas. Very rarely, gonadotroph adenomas may be clinically functioning. They preferentially secrete FSH and are thus associated with unusual clinical pictures. In women of reproductive age, such functioning adenomas may induce spontaneous ovarian hyperstimulation syndrome (OHSS) with multiple large ovarian cysts, generally discovered on pelvic ultrasonography performed for menstrual disturbances or abdominal or pelvic pain. In affected men, macroorchidism has been described, while children may present with precocious puberty. Mass effects related to the pituitary adenoma may also occur.

In general, FSH is the gonadotropin that is oversecreted. In the case of OHSS, serum FSH levels are often increased, but they may be in the normal range, while serum LH levels are invariably low (in contrast to the gonadotropin pattern of polycystic ovary syndrome). In most cases of OHSS, estradiol levels are high or very high.

Surgical removal of the pituitary adenoma is the treatment of choice, as it leads to a rapid fall in FSH levels and thus, in case of OHSS, reversal of ovarian hyperstimulation that is rapidly associated with a diminution of estradiol levels and regression of ovarian cysts. Medical treatment is limited to cabergoline, which in some cases has been reported decrease FSH and estradiol levels. However, its effect is generally transient and surgery must not be delayed. GnRH agonists are not recommended, as they may be responsible for pituitary apoplexy.

Significance of the Clinical Problem

Aside from prolactinomas (responsible for hyperprolactinemia), somatotropinomas (acromegaly), corticotropinomas (Cushing disease), and thyrotropinomas (central hyperthyroidism), gonadotropinomas (or gonadotroph adenomas) are generally clinically nonfunctioning and are discovered incidentally or because of mass effects. However, few of them are functioning with excess production of gonadotropins that stimulate the gonads, leading to clinical phenotypes such as OHSS in premenopausal women, macroorchidism in men, and precocious puberty in children.

Barriers to Optimal Practice

Barriers to optimal practice include lack of knowledge about this potential diagnosis due to its rarity and lack of familiarity among physicians, leading to failure to recognize clinical phenotypes associated with gonadotroph adenomas. There are often delays in diagnosis and neurosurgical treatment of functioning gonadotroph adenomas.

Strategies for Diagnosis, Therapy, and/or Management

Background

Clinically nonfunctioning pituitary adenomas include all pituitary adenomas that are not hormonally active and are therefore not associated with clinical syndromes such as amenorrhea or galactorrhea (prolactinomas), acromegaly, Cushing disease, or hyperthyroidism (TSH-secreting adenomas). However, most such nonfunctioning pituitary adenomas, which are "chromophobic" on classic histology, in fact secrete gonadotropins or are actually gonadotroph pituitary adenomas as assessed by immunocytochemistry.[1,2] Very rarely these gonadotroph adenomas are clinically functioning, and the hypersecretion of gonadotropins are responsible for stimulation of the gonads, particularly in women who may develop OHSS. The first case was described in 1995.[3]

Pathology

The cells of gonadotroph adenomas are well delineated, oval or polyhedral, and generally show no signs of secretion (small nuclei without nucleoli).[4] The percentage of cells positive for gonadotropin antibodies ranges from 100% to a few islands, but it is usually low (<20%-30%). Some tumors contain cells positive for β-FSH, β-LH, and α-subunit, while others contain cells that are only positive for β-FSH or, more rarely, β-LH or α-SU. Previously, when less than 5% of the adenomatous cells immunostained positively, the tumor was considered to be a "null cell adenoma." However, thanks to improved knowledge of pituitary cell differentiation and availability of cytogenetic markers, we now know that some null cell adenomas express steroidogenic factor 1 (SF-1), a transcription factor specific to the gonadotroph lineage, implying that they also belong to the gonadotroph family.[5]

Gonadal Hyperstimulation

In the case of gonadotroph adenomas, it remains largely unknown why the gonadotropins are seldom secreted in the bloodstream and, when they are, why they are exceptionally responsible for clinical syndromes related to gonadotropin excess (functioning gonadotroph adenomas) but are much more likely to be associated with hypogonadism. Chromatofocusing analysis has shown that gonadotroph adenomas produce more basic FSH isoforms,[6] which, paradoxically, are considered to be more biologically active. As glycosylation of gonadotropins is essential for their biological activity, hypogonadism may thus be related to decreased biological activity of gonadotropins related to abnormal glycosylation of the isoforms produced by the adenoma.

Epidemiology

The prevalence of pituitary adenomas is 80 to 100 per 100,000 persons, and 15% to 30% of these adenomas are nonfunctioning.[7-9] On immunocytochemistry, greater than 80% of them are gonadotroph. While nonfunctioning gonadotroph adenomas are generally diagnosed during the fifth or sixth decade of life and show a male predominance, functioning gonadotroph adenomas are more often described in women of reproductive age (very rarely in men).[10,11] They represent a minority (3%-13%) of nonfunctioning pituitary adenomas/gonadotroph adenomas.[12,13]

Clinical Presentation

Clinically nonfunctioning gonadotroph adenomas are mostly revealed by mass effect (or incidentally), while functioning gonadotroph adenomas, by definition, present with symptoms and signs of gonad hyperstimulation.

Hyperstimulation Syndromes

Gonadotropin hypersecretion by the adenoma may stimulate the gonads and lead to OHSS in premenopausal women with FSH-secreting tumors, macroorchidism in men, and precocious puberty in children. Spontaneous OHSS is the most typical picture in premenopausal women.[14] Generally identified at time of ovarian ultrasonography performed for menstrual disorders such as amenorrhea, oligomenorrhea, or irregular menses, it can also be revealed after ultrasonography is performed to evaluate abdominal and pelvic pain or bloating. Ultrasonography shows the presence of multiple ovarian cysts, similar to those observed in OHSS in women undertaking assisted reproductive technology using ovulation induction. Ovarian MRI may demonstrate large (>5 cm), multiseptated cysts. Sometimes OHSS is complicated by adnexal torsion.[11] In men, macroorchidism has been described in very few cases.[6,15,16] Isosexual precocious puberty has also very rarely been described in both sexes.[17-20]

Mass Effects

Most functioning gonadotroph adenomas are macroadenomas. As in the case of nonfunctioning gonadotroph pituitary adenomas,[1] mass effects on anatomic structures in the vicinity of the pituitary (headache, optic chiasm compression, occasional compression of cranial nerves III, IV, and VI) and/or on pituitary hormonal function, lead to hypopituitarism. Hypopituitarism can be caused by anterior pituitary compression, pituitary stalk interruption, or hypothalamic involvement. Pituitary stalk compression can also produce hyperprolactinemia by disinhibiting the dopaminergic tone that normally acts at the level of pituitary lactotrophs, causing amenorrhea and galactorrhea, but prolactin serum levels are always below 150 to 200 ng/mL (<6.5-8.7 nmol/L). This distinguishes them from macroprolactinomas, which are associated with much higher prolactin levels, proportional to tumor size.[21]

Pituitary Apoplexy

Pituitary apoplexy can be the presenting feature of gonadotroph adenomas, with severe headaches of sudden onset, meningismus, a variably depressed sensorium, and visual disturbances.[22] Apoplexy may be triggered by stimulation tests or injection of GnRH analogues.

Biochemical Evaluation

Gonadotropin Secretion

Baseline plasma dimeric FSH and/or LH levels are rarely elevated in patients with nonfunctioning pituitary gonadotroph adenomas[23,24] and elevation of free subunit levels (mainly α-LH, more rarely β-LH) is more common but is generally moderate. In patients with functional gonadotroph adenomas, the gonadotropin oversecreted is generally FSH. FSH levels are increased in more than half of OHSS cases due to gonadotroph adenomas, but they can be also in the normal range (in the other half). However, LH levels are invariably low.[10,14,25] This is the opposite gonadotropin pattern of that observed in polycystic ovary syndrome. In most cases of OHSS, estradiol levels are high or very high.[10,14,25] Free α-subunit levels may be increased or normal. In men, FSH levels are also generally increased and LH and testosterone levels are decreased.

The hormonal pattern of increased FSH contrasting with low LH levels and generally low levels of all pituitary hormones in postmenopausal women can help with the preoperative diagnosis of a gonadotroph adenoma.[23]

It was previously recommended to measure the response of gonadotropins and their free subunits to thyrotropin-releasing hormone and GnRH stimulation, but these tests are neither sensitive nor specific for indicating the gonadotroph nature of nonfunctioning pituitary adenomas.[24] Although rare, stimulation tests can also trigger pituitary apoplexy,[22] so they are no longer recommended.[24]

Other Pituitary Hormones

Patients with pituitary macroadenomas, whether discovered fortuitously or revealed by a mass effect, require assessment of secretion of the various pituitary hormones to detect deficiencies that may require preoperative replacement therapy.

Treatment

Surgical Treatment

Surgical removal of the culprit pituitary adenoma is the treatment of choice, as not only it treats the mass effect, but it also rapidly produces a fall in FSH levels and thus, in the case of OHSS, decreases ovarian stimulation, which is associated with rapid diminution of estradiol levels and regression of ovarian cysts, leading to clinical improvement.[14] This is achieved in a few days postoperatively. Pregnancy has been achieved shortly after the operation in a few cases, emphasizing the excellent gonadal outcome after treatment of a functioning gonadotroph adenoma. If necessary, large invasive or even aggressive tumors that cannot be totally surgically removed may be treated by adjuvant radiotherapy or radiosurgery.[26] The occurrence of pituitary apoplexy may also prompt surgical removal of the lesion, particularly if there is visual field and/or acuity impairment or a reduced level of consciousness.

Medical Management

Medical treatment currently available for functional pituitary gonadotroph adenomas is limited to cabergoline, which, in some cases, may decrease FSH and estradiol levels and allow pregnancy.[27,28] However, the effect is generally transient and surgery must not be delayed. GnRH agonists are not recommended, as they may be responsible for pituitary apoplexy.[22,29]

Clinical Case Vignettes

Case 1

A 29-year-old woman has a history of menstrual irregularity thought to be related to polycystic ovary syndrome. A moderate increase in prolactin (40 ng/mL [1.7 nmol/L]) has prompted a pituitary MRI, which shows a 23-mm pituitary macroadenoma without optic chiasm compression or visual field or acuity defects (*see images*).

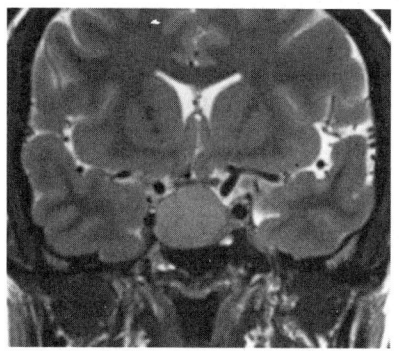

Pituitary MRI. T2-weighted coronal section.

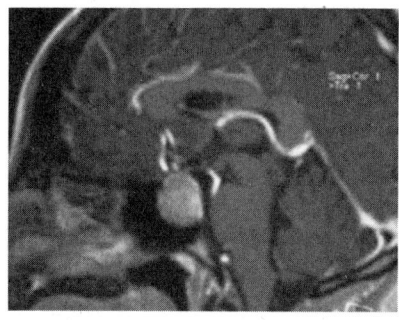

Pituitary MRI. T1-weighted sagittal section.

Surgical resection is planned, but the patient then presents with progressive abdominal and pelvic pain. Pelvic ultrasonography shows multiple ovarian cysts.

Laboratory test results:

Total testosterone = 8.6 ng/dL (8.6-86.5 ng/dL) (SI: 0.3 nmol/L [0.3-3.0 nmol/L])
Estradiol = 3241.6 pg/mL (<163 pg/mL) (SI: 11,900 pmol/L [<600 pmol/L])
LH = <0.1 mIU/mL (0.7-5.6 mIU/mL) (SI: <0.1 IU/L [0.7-5.6 IU/L])
FSH = 11.6 mIU/mL (2.0-10.0 mIU/mL) (SI: 11.6 IU/L (2.0-10.0 IU/L)

Three days after the workup, she is admitted to the hospital for severe acute pelvic pain. Pelvic MRI reveals the presence of large ovarian cysts and suspected right ovarian torsion (*see images*). Bilateral adnexal detorsion is performed laparoscopically, resulting in a favorable outcome.

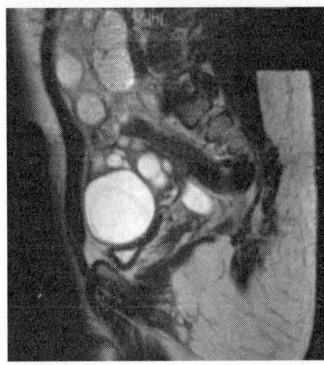

Pelvic MRI. T2-weighted sagittal section.

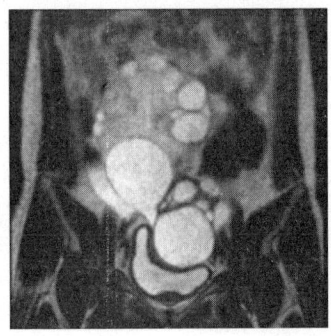

Pelvic MRI. T2-weighted coronal section.

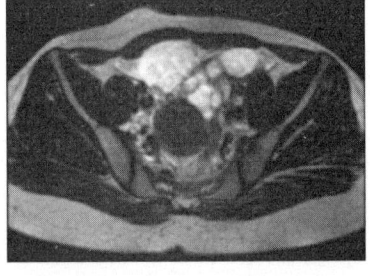

Pelvic MRI. T2-weighted axial section.

Which of the following is this patient's most likely diagnosis?

A. Polycystic ovary syndrome

B. OHSS related to FSH-secreting adenoma

C. McCune-Albright syndrome

D. Ovarian granulosa-cell tumor

Answer: B) OHSS related to FSH-secreting adenoma

While OHSS is a well-known complication of assisted reproductive procedures, particularly with gonadotropin stimulation, spontaneous OHSS is a very unusual occurrence and its presence suggests the diagnosis of an FSH-secreting adenoma (Answer B), particularly when FSH levels are increased. The finding of OHSS should lead to pituitary MRI, even in the absence of pituitary mass effects. MRI allows for the diagnosis of a pituitary adenoma. It is important to remember that the size of the adenoma may be quite variable. With microadenomas, mass effects may not be present at time of diagnosis. Macroadenomas can vary in size and invasion has been described.

Menstrual disturbances, infertility, and multiple ovarian cysts may suggest polycystic ovary syndrome (Answer A). However, multiple follicles in women with polycystic ovary syndrome are much smaller (<10 mm) and the hormonal pattern is quite different in terms of LH and FSH levels (LH is generally increased with an increased LH-to-FSH ratio). Moreover, polycystic ovary syndrome is often associated with hyperandrogenism, but not with such high estradiol levels. Such large ovarian cysts with very high estradiol levels and low testosterone levels may be encountered in patients with McCune-Albright syndrome (Answer C), but these patients generally have a history of precocious puberty and often display other manifestations of the syndrome (café-au-lait skin lesions, fibrous dysplasia, or even acromegaly). Moreover, their gonadotropins are low, suppressed by the very high levels of estrogens autonomously produced by the ovarian cysts (related to the activating gsp mutation). Ovarian granulosa-cell tumors (Answer D) often present at the time of premenopause or early menopause and, if associated with high estradiol levels, also show suppressed levels of gonadotropins.

In this case, treatment with cabergoline was initiated 7 days before pituitary surgery. The patient then underwent endoscopic transsphenoidal removal of the pituitary adenoma. The outcome was excellent. Pathologic

Analyte	Preoperative	Day 3 Postoperative	Reference Ranges
FSH	11.6 mIU/mL (SI: 11.6 IU/L)	1.4 mIU/mL (SI: 1.4 IU/L)	2.0-10.0 mIU/mL (SI: 2.0-10.0 IU/L)
LH	<0.1 mIU/mL (SI: <0.1 IU/L)	0.6 mIU/mL (SI: 0.6 IU/L)	0.7-5.6 mIU/mL (SI: 0.7-5.6 IU/L)
Estradiol	3242 pg/mL (SI: 11,900 pmol/L)	98 pg/mL (SI: 360 pmol/L)	<163 pg/mL (SI: <600 pmol/L)
Prolactin	79.4 ng/mL (SI: 3.5 nmol/L)	5.6 ng/mL (SI: 0.2 nmol/L)	4.8-23.4 ng/mL (0.2-1.0 nmol/L)

examination of the adenoma displayed FSH immunostaining in 40% of the cells and diffuse expression of chromogranin A. Ki67 was positive in 2% of the cells. The course of gonadotropins and estradiol postoperatively is depicted below. After 3 months, her hormonal workup was normal and the ovarian cysts had disappeared. No residual tumor was observed on MRI. Five months later, the patient achieved a spontaneous pregnancy, which was uneventful, and the long-term outcome was favorable.

This case illustrates that OHSS can have severe consequences, which are fortunately rare. In addition to hypovolemia and thromboembolism, OHSS can be complicated by ovarian torsion, as seen in this case, justifying surgical detorsion. This case also illustrates that the treatment of choice is surgery and that it must not be delayed. Correction of the FSH excess allows for rapid resolution of ovarian cysts and pituitary mass effect if present.

Case 2

A 78-year-old man underwent 2 operations for prostate cancer, 7 years and 1 year ago, after which hormonal therapy was decided. A course of antiandrogen treatment (cyproterone acetate 200 mg/day) is started 1 month before the injection of the GnRH agonist. The long-acting GnRH agonist DTrp6-GnRH (triptorelin) (375 mg) is then administered intramuscularly. A few minutes after the injection, the patient complains of increasing retroorbital headache, which is followed 24 hours later by the occurrence of postural dizziness and left partial ophthalmoplegia caused by a third-nerve lesion.

Visual field testing is normal. CT and MRI of the skull disclose the presence of a large pituitary mass with suprasellar extension and lateral invasion of cavernous sinuses, particularly on the left side (*see images*). Cyproterone acetate and GnRH agonist treatments are discontinued.

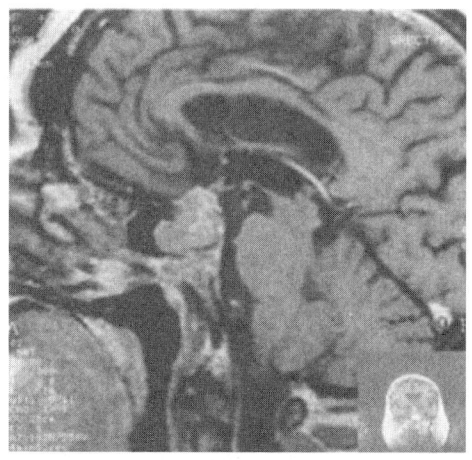 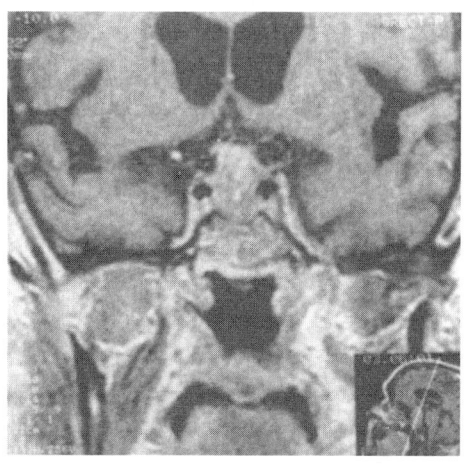

Pituitary MRI. T1-weighted sagittal and coronal sections following administration of gadolinium-DTPA, demonstrating a large, hyperintense pituitary adenoma with suprasellar, infrasellar, and laterosellar extension. Reproduced with permission from Chanson P, Schaison G. Pituitary apoplexy caused by GnRH-agonist treatment revealing gonadotroph adenoma. *J Clin Endocrinol Metab.* 1995;80(7):2267-2268.[29]

In the following days, clinical symptoms progressively improve. Because of the absence of visual field alteration and the spontaneous improvement of ophthalmoplegia, conservative management of the pituitary tumor is pursued. Two months after the interruption of hormonal treatment, hormonal testing shows the following:

> Total testosterone = 47.8 ng/dL (296.8-798.2 ng/dL)
> (SI: 1.66 nmol/L [10.3-27.7 nmol/L])
> LH = 0.16 mIU/mL (2.0-6.0 mIU/mL) (SI: 0.16 IU/L
> [2.0-6.0 IU/L])
> FSH = 9.2 mIU/mL (1.0-5.0 mIU/mL) (SI: 9.2 IU/L
> [1.0-5.0 IU/L])
> Free α-subunit = 2.3 ng/mL (0.20-6.0 ng/mL)

Which of the following proposals concerning this patient is/are the correct one(s)?

A. There is no relationship between the injection of the GnRH analogue and the pituitary mass effect in this patient

B. The injection of GnRH analogue triggered pituitary apoplexy

C. The hormonal pattern in this patient is typical of a gonadotroph adenoma

D. The hormonal pattern in this patient is related to the flair-up effect of GnRH agonist

Answer: B and C) The injection of GnRH analogue triggered pituitary apoplexy and the hormonal pattern in this patient is typical of a gonadotroph adenoma

Pituitary apoplexy, a rare complication of pituitary adenomas, is characterized by sudden headache, vision impairment, and ophthalmoplegia and is often associated with hemorrhagic infarction of the tumor. Usually, pituitary apoplexy occurs spontaneously and may thus reveal the adenoma. However, there have been occasional reports of pituitary apoplexy following administration of a GnRH agonist. In this vignette, the sequence of events strongly suggests a causal relationship between the administration of the GnRH agonist and subsequent apoplexy. While GnRH agonists are known to acutely stimulate both LH and FSH and then to desensitize GnRH receptors and decrease gonadotropin secretion in patients with a normal pituitary gland, they may have a persistent stimulatory effect on tumoral secretion in patients with FSH-secreting pituitary adenomas. Indeed, increased serum FSH levels with low levels of LH and testosterone in a patient with a pituitary macroadenoma who has no evidence of excess secretion of prolactin, GH, ACTH, or TSH is typical of a pituitary gonadotroph adenoma. Whether gonadotroph adenomas are more prone to develop apoplexy when stimulated by a GnRH agonist than other types of adenomas is unknown.

Case 1 and Case 2 have been published.[11,29]

References

1. Chanson P, Lecoq A-L, Raverot G, et al. Physiopathology, diagnosis, and treatment of nonfunctioning pituitary adenomas. In: Casanueva FF, Ghigo E, eds. *Hypothalamic-Pituitary Diseases.* Cham: Springer International Publishing AG, Switzerland; 2018:1-37.

2. Chanson P, Raverot G, Castinetti F, et al; French Endocrinology Society non-functioning pituitary adenoma work-group. Management of clinically non-functioning pituitary adenoma. *Ann Endocrinol (Paris).* 2015;76(3):239-247. PMID: 26072284

3. Djerassi A, Coutifaris C, West VA, et al. Gonadotroph adenoma in a premenopausal woman secreting follicle-stimulating hormone and causing ovarian hyperstimulation. *J Clin Endocrinol Metab.* 1995;80(2):591-594. PMID: 7852525

4. Asa SL. Pituitary adenomas. In: Asa SL, ed. *Tumors of the Pituitary Gland.* Vol Fourth Series Fascicle 15. Washington, DC: Armed Forces Institute of Pathology; 2011:55-172.

5. Nishioka H, Inoshita N, Mete O, et al. The complementary role of transcription factors in the accurate diagnosis of clinically nonfunctioning pituitary adenomas. *Endocr Pathol.* 2015;26(4):349-355. PMID: 2641628

6. Pigny P, Henric B, Lahlou N, et al. A gonadotroph adenoma with a high proportion of basic FSH isohormones by chromatofocusing. *J Clin Endocrinol Metab.* 1996;81(6):2407-2408. PMID: 8964889

7. Raappana A, Koivukangas J, Ebeling T, Pirila T. Incidence of pituitary adenomas in Northern Finland in 1992-2007. *J Clin Endocrinol Metab.* 2010;95(9):4268-4275. PMID: 20534753

8. Daly AF, Rixhon M, Adam C, Dempegioti A, Tichomirowa MA, Beckers A. High prevalence of pituitary adenomas: a cross-sectional study in the province of Liege, Belgium. *J Clin Endocrinol Metab.* 2006;91(12):4769-4775. PMID: 16968795

9. Fernandez A, Karavitaki N, Wass JA. Prevalence of pituitary adenomas: a community-based, cross-sectional study in Banbury (Oxfordshire, UK). *Clin Endocrinol (Oxf).* 2010;72(3):377-382. PMID: 19650784

10. Ntali G, Capatina C, Grossman A, Karavitaki N. Clinical review: functioning gonadotroph adenomas. *J Clin Endocrinol Metab.* 2014;99(12):4423-4433. PMID: 25166722

11. Graillon T, Castinetti F, Chabert-Orsini V, et al. Functioning gonadotroph adenoma with severe ovarian hyperstimulation syndrome: a new emergency

in pituitary adenoma surgery? Surgical considerations and literature review. *Ann Endocrinol (Paris).* 2019;80(2):122-127. PMID: 30825998

12. Caretto A, Lanzi R, Piani C, Molgora M, Mortini P, Losa M. Ovarian hyperstimulation syndrome due to follicle-stimulating hormone-secreting pituitary adenomas. *Pituitary.* 2017;20(5):553-560. PMID: 28676954

13. Kawaguchi T, Ogawa Y, Ito K, Watanabe M, Tominaga T. Follicle-stimulating hormone-secreting pituitary adenoma manifesting as recurrent ovarian cysts in a young woman--latent risk of unidentified ovarian hyperstimulation: a case report. *BMC Res Notes.* 2013;6:408. PMID: 24119690

14. Halupczok J, Kluba-Szyszka A, Bidzinska-Speichert B, Knychalski B. Ovarian hyperstimulation caused by gonadotroph pituitary adenoma--review. *Adv Clin Exp Med.* 2015;24(4):695-703. PMID: 26469116

15. Heseltine D, White MC, Kendall-Taylor P, de Kretser DM, Kelly W. Testicular enlargement and elevated serum inhibin concentrations occur in patients with pituitary macroadenomas secreting follicle-stimulating hormone. *Clin Endocrinol (Oxf).* 1989;31(4):411-423. PMID: 2627747

16. Dahlqvist P, Koskinen LO, Brannstrom T, Hagg E. Testicular enlargement in a patient with a FSH-secreting pituitary adenoma. *Endocrine.* 2010;37(2):289-293. PMID: 20960265

17. Tashiro H, Katabuchi H, Ohtake H, Kaku T, Ushio Y, Okamura H. A follicle-stimulating hormone–secreting gonadotroph adenoma with ovarian enlargement in a 10-year-old girl. *Fertil Steril.* 1999;72(1):158-160. PMID: 10428166

18. Di Rocco C, Maira G, Borrelli P. Pituitary microadenomas in children. *Childs Brain.* 1982;9(3-4):165-178. PMID: 7105883

19. Faggiano M, Criscuolo T, Perrone L, Quarto C, Sinisi AA. Sexual precocity in a boy due to hypersecretion of LH and prolactin by a pituitary adenoma. *Acta Endocrinol (Copenh).* 1983;102(2):167-172. PMID: 6681924

20. Ambrosi B, Bassetti M, Ferrario R, Medri G, Giannattasio G, Faglia G. Precocious puberty in a boy with a PRL-, LH- and FSH-secreting pituitary tumour: hormonal and immunocytochemical studies. 1990;122(5):569-576. PMID: 2112813

21. Chanson P, Maiter D. The epidemiology, diagnosis and treatment of prolactinomas: the old and the new. *Best Pract Res Clin Endocrinol Metab.* 2019;33(2):101290. PMID: 31326373

22. Briet C, Salenave S, Bonneville JF, Laws ER, Chanson P. *Pituitary apoplexy. Endocr Rev.* 2015;36(6):622-645. PMID: 26414232

23. Chanson P, Brochier S. Non-functioning pituitary adenomas. *J Endocrinol Invest.* 2005;28(11 Suppl International):93-99. PMID: 16625856

24. Raverot G, Assie G, Cotton F, et al. Biological and radiological exploration and management of non-functioning pituitary adenoma. *Ann Endocrinol (Paris).* 2015;76(3):201-209. PMID: 26122495

25. Cooper O, Geller JL, Melmed S. Ovarian hyperstimulation syndrome caused by an FSH-secreting pituitary adenoma. *Nat Clin Pract Endocrinol Metab.* 2008;4(4):234-238. PMID: 18268519

26. Chanson P, Dormoy A, Dekkers O. Use of radiotherapy after pituitary surgery for non-functioning pituitary adenomas. *Eur J Endocrinol.* 2019;181(1):D1-D13. PMID: 31048560

27. Knoepfelmacher M, Danilovic DL, Rosa Nasser RH, Mendonca BB. Effectiveness of treating ovarian hyperstimulation syndrome with cabergoline in two patients with gonadotropin-producing pituitary adenomas. *Fertil Steril.* 2006;86(3):719.e15-e18. PMID: 16952513

28. Paoletti AM, Depau GF, Mais V, Guerriero S, Ajossa S, Melis GB. Effectivenesses of cabergoline in reducing follicle-stimulating hormone and prolactin hypersecretion from pituitary macroadenoma in an infertile woman. *Fertil Steril.* 1994;62(4):882-885. PMID: 7926104

29. Chanson P, Schaison G. Pituitary apoplexy caused by GnRH-agonist treatment revealing gonadotroph adenoma. *J Clin Endocrinol Metab.* 1995;80(7):2267-2268. PMID: 7608291

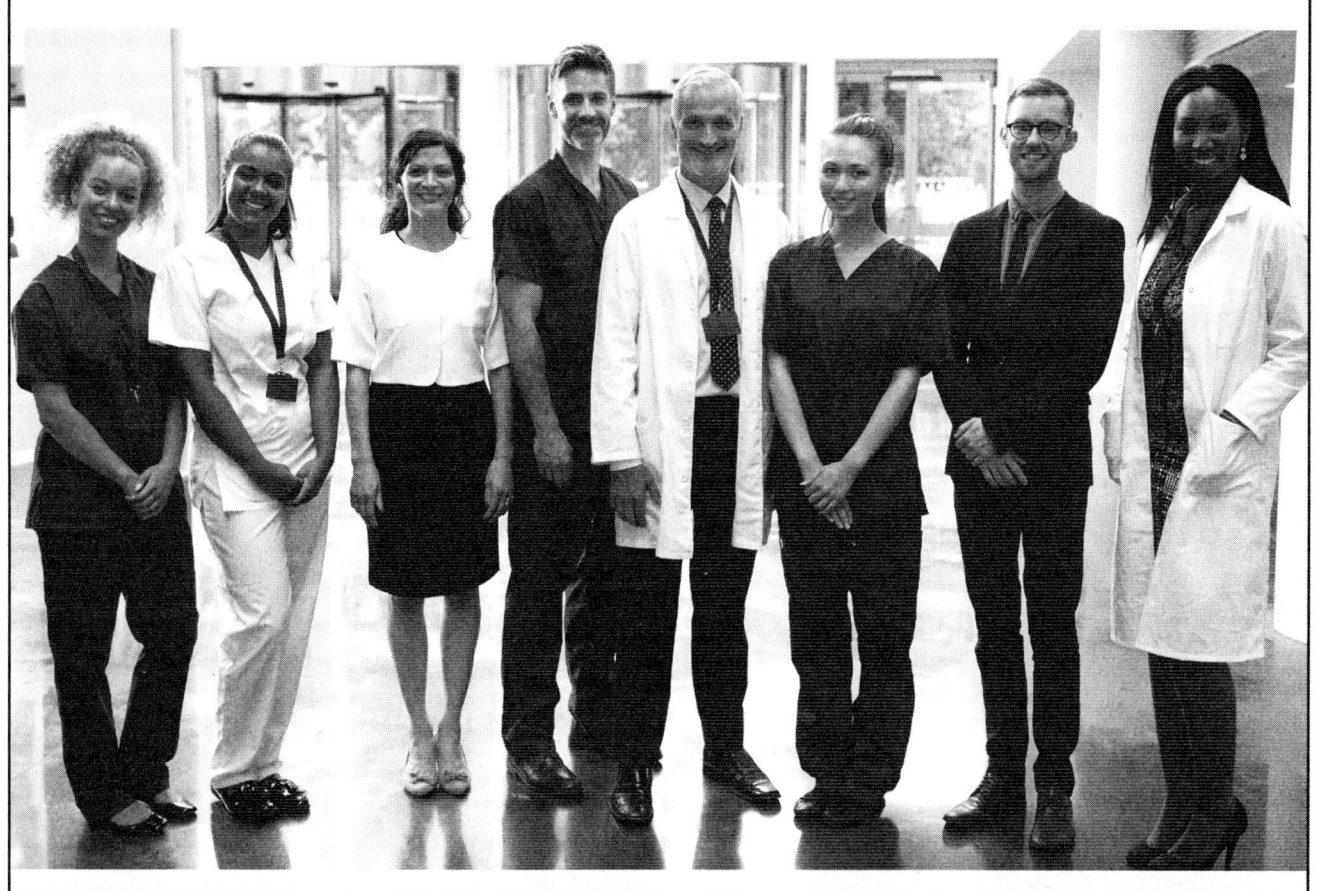

PEDIATRIC
ENDOCRINOLOGY

Management of Pituitary Hormone Replacement Through Transition From Adolescence to Young Adulthood

Mehul T. Dattani, MBBS, DCH, FRCPCH, FRCP, MD. Genetics and Genomic Medicine Programme, UCL GOS Institute of Child Health, London, United Kingdom; E-mail: mdattani@ucl.ac.uk

Learning Objectives

As a result of participating in this session, learners should be able to:

- Describe the dynamic nature of hypopituitarism and adapt to the needs of the young person at all stages, but particularly at the time of adolescence and transition.

- Develop a holistic approach to the management of hypopituitarism at the time of transition.

Main Conclusions

Hypopituitarism is phenotypically a highly variable condition that may encompass a single hormone deficiency or multiple pituitary hormone deficiencies, including both anterior and posterior pituitary hormones. The condition may evolve throughout adolescence and childhood, and hence there is a need for vigilance and regular testing of pituitary function on a lifelong basis. The endocrine morbidity score may be a useful marker, but it is highly variable in these children. Importantly, puberty is highly variable in children with hypopituitarism, and may be normal in timing, delayed, or absent. Paradoxically, in patients with septo-optic dysplasia, it may occur early. Reversibility of pituitary hormone deficits may occur, even in the presence of a structurally abnormal pituitary gland. Nevertheless, MRI remains an extremely useful tool in the management of hypopituitarism. Careful hormone replacement with diligent monitoring of auxology, general well-being, and biochemical profiles is critical to ensuring good outcomes in terms of height, weight, and clinical well-being. Finally, hypopituitarism may be associated with a range of other clinical phenotypes, including morbid obesity, autism, learning difficulties, and visual impairment, necessitating a careful multidisciplinary approach to the problem. A holistic approach involves a pediatric and adult (at transition and thereafter) endocrinologist, ophthalmologist, neurodevelopmental pediatrician, clinical nurse specialist, psychologist, dietitian, and social worker.

Significance of the Clinical Problem

Hypopituitarism is a rare disorder and may be congenital (1 in 4000 to 1 in 10,000 live births) or acquired due to tumors, inflammation, infiltration, infection, etc.[1] Congenital hypopituitarism is a highly variable condition that evolves over time. It may be associated with a range of other abnormalities, including midline forebrain abnormalities (eg, absence of the septum pellucidum and hypoplasia/absence of the corpus callosum), eye abnormalities (eg, optic nerve hypoplasia, coloboma, and microphthalmia/anophthalmia), cleft lip and/or palate, and sensorineural deafness.[2] Rare cases may be associated with holoprosencephaly or other syndromes associated with hypopituitarism. The disorder can have significant morbidity and mortality if undiagnosed and managed suboptimally. Additionally, these children and adolescents often have associated challenging comorbidities such as sleep disturbance, obesity, learning difficulties, behavioral issues, and visual impairment. Optimal management remains a challenge, particularly at the time of transition, when there are complex issues with respect to puberty and fertility, adherence, the need to conform with peers, and the emergence of high-risk behaviors. Few studies have explored the trajectory of these patients through puberty and to adulthood. Hence, data are sparse in terms of optimal management.

What is becoming increasingly clear is that the need for a holistic, multidisciplinary approach is never greater than at puberty. Significant input is required from the clinician and the clinical nurse specialist/nurse practitioner. Challenges around adherence, optimal dosage, behavior, psychology, and emerging independence from parents should be tackled with the help of a range of multidisciplinary professionals. The need for a pause of, for example, GH therapy, before possible retesting needs to be addressed.

Barriers to Optimal Practice

- Lack of resources in terms of time and management from the multidisciplinary team to provide optimal care.

- Lack of engagement from the young person.

- Lack of consensus with respect to optimal management.

Strategies for Diagnosis, Therapy, and/or Management

Introduction

Hypopituitarism may be due to congenital or acquired causes. Congenital hypopituitarism can arise from pathogenic variants in any of the genes involved in pituitary development and has a reported incidence of 1 in 3000 to 4000 births. It is a highly heterogeneous disorder that manifests either as an isolated hormone deficiency, the most common being isolated GH deficiency, or as combined pituitary hormone deficiency when 2 or more pituitary hormones are affected. The clinical features vary in severity and timing of presentation; its onset may be early in the neonatal period or later in life. Congenital hypopituitarism can also be part of a syndrome where abnormalities in extrapituitary structures that share a common embryologic origin with the pituitary gland (eg, eye, midline, and forebrain) occur in addition to pituitary hormone deficiencies. The etiology remains unknown in most patients.[3] Recent data suggest that pathogenic variants in genes implicated in hypothalamic-pituitary development or GH secretion can be identified in approximately 10% of cases.[2,3] Congenital forms of hypopituitarism are rare and account for only 4.5% of hypopituitarism in adults.[4] Acquired hypopituitarism may be due to tumors and their treatment, trauma, inflammation, infiltration, or infection. In the pediatric and adolescent population, intracranial tumors are probably the most frequent cause. In adult cohort studies, suprasellar tumors cause the majority of hypothalamic-pituitary dysfunction (50%-60%).[4,5] Other causes include surgery or radiotherapy, traumatic brain injury, infection, autoimmune processes, infiltration by granulomatous disease, iron overload states, and vascular causes.

Diagnosis

The diagnosis of hypopituitarism is based on a combination of clinical assessment, looking for the presence of not just endocrine-related symptoms and signs (eg, frontal bossing and growth failure, micropenis, and cryptorchidism in males), but also for other features related to the presence of a congenital syndrome or an acquired form such as raised intracranial pressure, auxology (height, weight, BMI and their corresponding standard deviation scores), pubertal assessment, biochemistry, neuroradiology, and possibly genetics. If available, prior growth curves from community screening may indicate the presence of growth failure or rapid weight gain in the months preceding diagnosis. For instance, in patients with craniopharyngiomas, early changes in weight and BMI have been shown to precede the diagnosis of a suprasellar mass by several months and may be predictive of future hypothalamic obesity.[6] The presence of precocious, delayed, or arrested puberty supported by an inappropriately delayed or advanced bone age can also help predict future growth potential and determine if intervention is needed to achieve this.

Confirmation of hypopituitarism is a stepwise process, usually beginning with a baseline pituitary function screen, followed by dynamic pituitary function tests. Normal hormone secretion is dependent on the presence of an intact hypothalamic-pituitary-target gland axis. Dynamic tests aim to stimulate the relevant axis if hormone deficiency is suspected. Basal pituitary hormone screening helps risk-stratify patients who require prioritizing for dynamic testing before definitive treatment, particularly to establish the status of the hypothalamic-pituitary-adrenal and antidiuretic hormone axes in order to avoid the fatal consequences of uncorrected cortisol insufficiency and/or central diabetes insipidus (eg, during surgery). In this situation, early-morning cortisol and ACTH concentrations should be measured, particularly before administration of high-dosage dexamethasone for peritumoral edema. In some cases, dynamic function testing is not required—for instance, a low concentration of free T_4 in the presence of an inappropriately low or normal concentration of TSH is sufficient for the diagnosis of secondary or tertiary hypothyroidism, and an additional thyrotropin-releasing hormone

stimulation test neither distinguishes the 2 nor changes clinical management.[7]

The timing of basal and dynamic function tests may be important. Testing for hypogonadotropic hypogonadism is not useful outside of the mini-puberty (up to age 6 months) and pubertal phases (boys aged >9 years, girls aged >8 years), as the hypothalamic-pituitary-gonadal axis is quiescent outside these periods. In some cases, 24-hour (cortisol) or overnight (GH) hormone profiling to determine spontaneous hormone secretion may be necessary to detect more subtle endocrine deficits that would otherwise appear to be normal based on values obtained from artificial stimulation tests. The interaction between the different hypothalamic-pituitary axes is relevant to interpreting endocrine tests. For instance, cortisol sufficiency is required to permit renal free water clearance via inhibition of antidiuretic hormone secretion, so ACTH deficiency may mask coexistent central diabetes insipidus until glucocorticoid replacement is initiated. If a suprasellar tumor is suspected or has already been confirmed by neuroimaging, additional investigations should also be performed to determine whether the mass is responsible for secreting α-fetoprotein and/or β-hCG (germinomas), prolactin (prolactinomas), GH (somatotropinomas), or ACTH (corticotropinomas). Occasionally, measurement of cerebrospinal fluid α-fetoprotein and β-hCG concentrations may be needed to support the diagnosis of a germinoma. Evidence of tumor secretion of various molecules can help avoid the need for a diagnostic biopsy or unnecessary surgical resection, since such procedures carry significant risks of further damaging the hypothalamic-pituitary axis.

MRI is warranted in all patients with documented hypopituitarism. In a retrospective study of MRI findings and endocrine function in 170 children with or "at risk" for congenital hypopituitarism (optic nerve hypoplasia), holoprosencephaly, or multiple midline systemic defects), the risk of hypopituitarism was 27 times greater in patients with an ectopic posterior pituitary.[8] Anterior pituitary hypoplasia and pituitary stalk agenesis were also significantly associated with hypopituitarism. With respect to the type or severity of hypopituitarism, combined pituitary hormone deficiency was more often associated with an abnormal corpus callosum and stalk abnormalities. Overall, midline forebrain defects were 5.2 times more prevalent in patients with combined pituitary hormone deficiency than in patients with isolated GH deficiency. The results of this study confirm that midline forebrain defects are associated with a higher risk of combined pituitary hormone deficiency, but also suggest that in children at risk of developing hypopituitarism due to the presence of optic nerve hypoplasia and/ or midline brain abnormalities, corpus callosum and pituitary stalk abnormalities are strong predictors of combined pituitary hormone deficiency.

The role of genetics in congenital hypopituitarism remains to be established, and testing is offered on a research basis only. The past decades have witnessed an explosion in our understanding of the development of the anterior pituitary gland and of mechanisms that underlie the diagnosis of GH deficiency and combined pituitary hormone deficiency. However, to date, pathogenic variants have been identified in only a modest proportion of patients.[1-3] It is clear that many genes remain to be identified and the characterization of these genes will further elucidate the pathogenesis of these complex conditions.

Transcription factors encoded by the genes *HESX1*, *PROP1*, *POU1F1*, *LHX3*, *LHX4*, *SOX2*, and *SOX3* are involved in the etiology of combined pituitary hormone deficiency, and they are associated with highly variable phenotypes encompassing isolated GH deficiency, combined pituitary hormone deficiency, or more complex disorders such as septo-optic dysplasia.[2,3] *PROP1* pathogenic variants constitute the most common genetic cause for combined pituitary hormone deficiency, with a poor genotype-phenotype correlation and different pattern of evolution of endocrinopathies. Appropriate genetic testing is an important adjunct to management because understanding the pathophysiologic process

may predict prognosis, improve early diagnosis and management, and assist with counseling the family. Identifying certain pathogenic variants may assist in the differential diagnosis. For example, *PROP1* pathogenic variants are associated with suprasellar masses that undergo spontaneous resolution, and the presence of a *PROP1* pathogenic variant may help to reassure families of the absence of a brain tumor and circumvent the need for surgery. Given the variable penetrance of many dominant pathogenic variants, prenatal diagnosis should not be offered until understanding of the genetic basis of many of these conditions has advanced significantly. Whole exome- and genome-sequencing technologies are currently offered on a research basis and may further improve understanding of the genetic etiology of these conditions.

Evolution of Endocrinopathies

Children with isolated GH deficiency have a significant risk of developing additional pituitary deficiencies.[9] This risk ranges between 5.5% in childhood-onset idiopathic isolated GH deficiency and 35% in adult-onset organic isolated GH deficiency. In a large prospective, multinational study (GeNeSIS), data were analyzed in 5805 pediatric patients with idiopathic isolated GH deficiency. Combined pituitary hormone deficiency developed in 2.0% of the overall cohort and in 5.5% among children followed for a minimum of 3.5 years. The relative frequency of additional deficiencies was TSH > LH/FSH > antidiuretic hormone > ACTH. Median interval from diagnosis of GH deficiency to additional pituitary hormone deficiency was 1.9 years for TSH, 2.4 years for both antidiuretic hormone and ACTH, and 3.3 years for LH/FSH.[10] In 716 pediatric patients from the same database with isolated GH deficiency due to organic causes, there was a higher frequency of combined pituitary hormone deficiency (9.9% in the overall cohort, and 20.7% in the subgroup followed up for a minimum of 3.5 years). The most frequent additional deficiencies were TSH and LH/FSH.[11] In a retrospective study of 83 patients initially diagnosed as having isolated GH deficiency in childhood, 45% developed combined pituitary hormone deficiency after a median follow-up of 5.4 years.[12]

Hypothalamic-pituitary, optic nerve, and midline brain abnormalities predispose to a higher risk of developing additional pituitary deficits (up to 45%-100% in children with pituitary stalk interruption syndrome). Pituitary stalk agenesis as demonstrated on MRI after gadolinium administration and an ectopic posterior pituitary located at the median eminence and hypothalamic level are highly predictive of combined pituitary hormone deficiency. Empty sella, absent/hypoplastic corpus callosum, and optic nerve hypoplasia are also associated with a higher risk of evolution of endocrinopathy. The type and age at occurrence of additional pituitary deficits are highly variable and they cannot be easily predicted based on the etiology, severity, and age at onset of isolated GH deficiency. Importantly, idiopathic isolated GH deficiency without structural hypothalamic-pituitary abnormalities does not exclude the occurrence of additional pituitary deficits. A longer duration of follow-up is associated with a higher risk of additional pituitary deficits, suggesting that hypopituitarism is a dynamic condition where new deficiencies can appear years after the initial diagnosis. Adrenal insufficiency can silently evolve years after the onset of GH deficiency and the start of GH treatment in patients with GH deficiency can unmask central hypothyroidism.

To conclude, current available evidence supports longstanding recommendations for the need, in all patients diagnosed with isolated GH deficiency, of careful and indefinite follow-up for additional pituitary hormone deficiencies, irrespective of the age at presentation, severity, etiology, and reversibility of GH deficiency in adolescence. In patients with an initial diagnosis of isolated GH deficiency, particularly those with an ectopic posterior pituitary or other developmental abnormalities, the clinician should be alert to the risk of the development of combined pituitary hormone deficiency. Similarly, adult guidelines suggest that thyroid and adrenal function should be monitored during GH therapy.

Treatment

The mainstay of treatment is replacement of the appropriate hormones. In both congenital and acquired hypopituitarism, it is crucial to recognize the potential for evolution of endocrine deficits over time, and all patients with documented endocrine dysfunction require lifelong follow-up with appropriate transition into adulthood.

Growth and puberty should be monitored and GH deficiency should be treated with recombinant human GH (rhGH) until linear growth ceases, although there is increasing evidence for continued GH treatment into adulthood due to its possible metabolic effects on body composition and bone mineral density. In most countries, ongoing GH treatment is only indicated in those young people who have been shown to have permanent GH deficiency. Retesting of GH secretion is indicated in those with childhood-onset GH deficiency, usually after the completion of statural growth. Current guidelines suggest that retesting is not required for those with more than 2 pituitary hormone deficiencies, a confirmed genetic pathogenic variant accounting for the hypopituitarism, and/or a specific hypothalamic-pituitary structural defect on MRI with the exception of an ectopic posterior pituitary.[13] The insulin-tolerance test or the GHRH-arginine test are recommended for retesting. Between 25% and 88% of patients reverse their GH secretion at the time of transition. The dosages recommended are variable, but generally lower than those used in childhood, and titration with IGF-1 concentrations is recommended. It has been recommended that GH be continued until full skeletal and muscle maturation has been attained. In tumor survivors, GH therapy in replacement dosages is not associated with an increased risk of recurrence or progression, although some evidence suggests that there may be a small increased risk of second primary neoplasms, but this is not completely clear. Hence, minimum effective dosages for GH replacement should be used, aiming for normal IGF-1 concentrations and an age-appropriate height velocity.

Puberty may be precocious or occur at the normal time in those with hypopituitarism associated with septo-optic dysplasia, but it may be delayed or absent in those with isolated combined pituitary hormone deficiency.[14] Treatment of coexistent precocious puberty with GnRH analogues can help restore adult height if commenced early, but the decision to artificially delay puberty should be decided on an individual basis. Conversely, in the face of coexistent hypogonadotropic hypogonadism, it is not unusual to commence GH supplementation at least 6 months before sex steroid replacement, the timing of which again should be tailored to the individual child. Delaying commencement of the latter beyond the usual pubertal age (~12 years in girls and 14-15 years in boys) is not generally recommended, given the long-term benefits on bone mineral accretion.[15] Precocious puberty does not preclude the evolution of subsequent hypogonadotropic hypogonadism, and children should continue to be monitored carefully after cessation of GnRH analogue therapy to ensure normal pubertal progress. With respect to hypogonadotropic hypogonadism, treatment in males is commonly in the form of testosterone (parenteral, oral, or transdermal). This is induced slowly over the period of approximately 2.5 to 3 years, with careful monitoring of growth, virilization, and trough testosterone concentrations. Longer-acting testosterone preparations may be used once growth has been completed. Monitoring of the full blood count is recommended, given the adverse effect of polycythemia. In females, 17β-estradiol is the preferred option, and is available as gel, transdermal patch, and oral preparation. It has been suggested that the transdermal route is superior to the oral route in terms of bone accrual and uterine growth.[16] Concentrations of genotoxic estrogens (mutagenic metabolites linked to breast carcinogenesis) are lower with the use of transdermal estrogen than with oral estrogen.[17]

The dosage is gradually increased over a period of 24 months or so. A cyclical progestogen is added once breakthrough bleeding occurs. Monitoring growth, secondary sexual characteristics, uterine volume, blood pressure, and bone mineral density is recommended. Pulsatile GnRH treatment or the administration of gonadotropins is recommended for the achievement of spermatogenesis and testicular enlargement in males and ovarian follicular maturation in females.

TSH deficiency is easily replaced with levothyroxine supplementation, with dose titrations being based entirely on free T_4 concentrations and not TSH. Free T_4 concentrations should be maintained in the upper half of the normal range, particularly given the risk of hypothalamic obesity in many forms of hypopituitarism. Before commencing replacement, preexisting ACTH deficiency should be detected to avoid the risk of precipitating a hypocortisolemic crisis.

The diagnosis of ACTH deficiency is challenging during adolescence. Because fatigue is commonly observed in adolescence, this is not a good discriminatory feature in the selection of adolescents for testing. Once the diagnosis is made, replacement doses of hydrocortisone should be given at least 3 times daily and titrated in the growing child and adolescent against trough concentrations using a cortisol day curve. Doses should be doubled or even tripled in the face of illness, with patient education on how and when to administer emergency intramuscular hydrocortisone (doses <1 year, 25 mg; 1-5 years, 25-50 mg; >5 years, 100 mg) and correct hypoglycemia during crises. Input from the endocrine clinical nurse specialist is particularly critical at the time of transition. Discussions around timing of hydrocortisone replacement are critical, as adolescents may stay up late and wake up late. Additionally, empowering adolescents with critical information on how to prevent adrenal crises, as well as addressing lifestyle changes such as drinking alcohol, may save lives. Longer-acting corticosteroids such as prednisolone may provide better control on less frequent dosing once growth is complete.

Management of central diabetes insipidus, particularly in patients with coexisting ACTH deficiency and/or hypothalamic adipsia (eg, in some patients with postsurgical suprasellar tumor), is complex and needs specialist care. Oral desmopressin may be preferred, as it is widely available, is generally well absorbed especially with intercurrent respiratory tract infections, less likely to lead to hyponatremia, and easier to use in patients with visual impairment and physical disability.[18] Untreated patients with an intact thirst axis and free access to fluid are able to maintain euvolemia and eunatremia by adjusting their oral intake appropriately. DDAVP treatment aims to provide the patient with a relatively normal quality of life by reducing the burden of polyuria and polydipsia. Doses should be titrated against trough paired plasma and urine osmolalities, and treatment should ideally be started in the inpatient setting. Treatment should generally err on the side of underdosing, since overdosing DDAVP can result in water intoxication, hyponatremia, and rapid fluid shifts that are difficult to correct safely due to the risk of cerebral edema or even death. Patients with hypothalamic adipsia require a strict fluid intake regimen to maintain euvolemia. Additionally, it is important to remember that certain "recreational" drugs such as MDMA ("Ecstasy") may lead to overdrinking, which could be extremely dangerous in patients on desmopressin.

Management at Transition

Transition presents significant challenges in the management of hypopituitarism. It is defined as the time between the completion of normal puberty and the achievement of peak bone mass.[15] The transition period is a highly complex stage of life, as adolescents complete their secondary education, change lifestyles, demonstrate greater independence from their parents and thereby lose parental supervision, engage in high-risk behaviors, and prepare to move away from their parental homes. As with most conditions, adherence to treatment may be an issue, putting the young person at risk for significant morbidity and mortality. Psychological issues may be a major feature of the disease phenotype, with the adolescent facing the prospect of a lifelong condition requiring ongoing medication. This in turn may lead to isolation. The presence of hypogonadism may raise concerns with respect to future relationships and prospects for fertility. Associated abnormalities such as vision impairment, obesity, and the presence of varying degrees of autism and other complications of the underlying condition may add to difficulties in management.

Transition is also a time for re-evaluation of the endocrinopathy and planning long-term management. Transition clinics with input from pediatric/adolescent endocrinologists, adult endocrinologists, and the endocrinology clinical nurse specialist are critical to the successful transition of patients. In patients with learning disabilities, it is important that "best interest" meetings take place to ensure that a suitable advocate is available to act on behalf of the patient. Appropriate arrangements must be implemented for patients to function as independently as possible. Loss to follow-up by a physician may be associated with the risk of adrenal crisis, a hypothyroid state, reduced bone mineral density, and fatigue with reduced libido.

Clinical Case Vignettes
Case 1

A 5-month-old male infant presents with cryptorchidism and poor growth. His birth weight was 5 lb 0 oz (2260 g) at 35 weeks' gestation, and he required nasogastric feeding. At the age of 1.5 years, he is noted to have a length of 22.8 in (58 cm; -8 SDS) with a growth rate of 2 cm/y. He has excess skin folds. Basal investigations reveal a total T_4 concentration of 2.95 µg/dL (38 nmol/L) with a TSH concentration of 1.0 mIU/L. Levothyroxine is initiated. He has a hypoglycemic convulsion and undergoes a clonidine test, which reveals all GH concentrations to be less than 0.3 ng/mL (<0.3 µg/L). The 8-AM cortisol concentration is 40.1 µg/dL (1105 nmol/L).

GH therapy is initiated at age 2.5 years, and he has an excellent response, with a growth velocity of 20 cm/y. At age 3.5 years, CT reveals a hypoplastic anterior pituitary gland. His early-morning cortisol peak is 11.0 μg/dL (303 nmol/L). At age 6.5 years, hydrocortisone is initiated at a dosage of 12 mg/m² per day in view of a perceived suboptimal cortisol peak on glucagon-stimulation testing (12.1 μg/dL [335 nmol/L] at baseline).

He gains weight rapidly with weight at the 75th percentile and height at the 3rd percentile. At age 12 years, intramuscular testosterone is initiated. Although the testes are palpable, they are thought to be small. Weight gain remains an issue, with height between the 3rd and 10th percentiles and the weight around the 90th percentile. Random cortisol concentrations are elevated.

At age 16.44 years, his near-final height is 60.1 in (152.6 cm) and weight is 152.1 lb (69 kg). Genetic screening confirms the presence of a pathogenic variant in a gene regulating GH secretion. He is then retested off all treatment at 18 years of age, and the results document GH, prolactin, and TSH deficiencies with normal LH (15.1 mIU/mL [15.1 IU/L]), FSH (5.8 mIU/mL [5.8 IU/L]), and peak cortisol of 22.7 μg/dL (627 nmol/L) on insulin-tolerance testing. Hydrocortisone and testosterone treatment are then stopped. MRI confirms a hypoplastic anterior pituitary with a normal stalk and eutopic posterior pituitary.

A mutation/pathogenic variant in which of the following genes most likely accounts for the patient's phenotype?

A. *KAL1*

B. *LHX4*

C. *PROP1*

D. *POU1F1*

E. *GLI2*

Answer: D) POU1F1

The pathogenic variant was a de novo p.R271W in the *POU1F1* gene (Answer D), which is a dominant-negative mutation. The protein encoded

by *POU1F1* is a transcription factor that is implicated in somatotroph, thyrotroph, and lactotroph development. Pathogenic variants are associated with GH, TSH, and prolactin deficiencies, but not ACTH or gonadotropin deficiencies. MRI usually reveals a small anterior pituitary with a normally placed posterior pituitary.

Case 2

An 11-and-2/12-year-old girl presents with short stature (height, –2.5 SDS; weight, –1.69 SDS). Birth weight was 4 lb 1 oz (1875 g) at 32 weeks' gestation (0.47 SDS). Her growth slowed down after 3 years of age. She was evaluated at 8 years of age, and the results of basal investigations were unremarkable. It was thought that she had a probable diagnosis of constitutional growth delay. The growth velocity is 5 cm/y, and she has a bone age delay of 2 years. She is completely prepubertal.

Laboratory test results:

IGF-1 = 53 ng/mL (218-965 ng/mL) (SI: 6.9 nmol/L [28.6-126.4 nmol/L])
Free T$_4$ = 1.05 ng/dL (0.93-1.7 ng/dL) (SI: 13.5 pmol/L [12-22 pmol/L])
LH = <0.7 mIU/mL (SI: <0.7 IU/L)
FSH = 3.7 mIU/mL (SI: 3.7 IU/L)
Celiac screen, negative
Karyotype = 46,XX

Skeletal survey and prepubertal pelvic ultrasonography are normal.

Constitutional delay of growth and puberty is diagnosed, and ethinyl estradiol is initiated at a dosage of 2 mcg daily. She is then lost to follow-up. She stops the estradiol 4 months after being seen in the clinic. She reappears in the clinic a year later, and her growth rate is 3 cm/y. A primed insulin-tolerance test is performed. This reveals a peak GH concentration of 5.6 ng/mL (5.6 μg/L) with a peak cortisol concentration of 33.5 μg/dL (924 nmol/L). The GnRH test reveals a peak LH concentration of 19.4 mIU/mL (19.4 IU/L) and a peak FSH concentration of 3.3 mIU/mL (3.3 IU/L). MRI of the brain and pituitary is performed and reveals a hypoplastic anterior pituitary, an ectopic or undescended posterior pituitary, and an absent pituitary stalk. GH treatment is initiated, and she responds well with a growth velocity of 8 cm/y. At age 15.4 years, she has progressed to breast Tanner stage 4/5, but complains of fatigue.

Which of the following is the best next step?

A. Re-start ethinyl estradiol

B. Check the adequacy of GH dosage

C. Assess her cortisol and thyroid function

D. Investigate for other associated conditions

E. B, C, and D

Answer: E) B, C, and D

With an ectopic posterior pituitary, this patient would most likely have developed other hormone deficiencies. Additionally, if the GH dosage is inadequate, it would need to be increased.

Testing documented the following:

IGF-1 = 128 ng/mL (224-896 ng/mL) (SI: 16.8 nmol/L [29.4-117.4 nmol/L])

Free T_4 = 0.9 ng/dL (0.9-1.7 ng/dL) (SI: 12.1 pmol/L [12-22 pmol/L])

TSH = 3.9 mIU/L (<6 mIU/L)

Peak cortisol on cosyntropin-stimulation testing = 14.5 µg/dL (normal >20 µg/dL) (SI: 401 nmol/L [>550 nmol/L]) with a mean 24-hour cortisol value of 3.9 µg/dL (normal >5.3 µg/dL) (SI: 107 nmol/L [>145 nmol/L]) on 2 hourly profile

Low-dosage hydrocortisone and levothyroxine were started, and the GH dosage was adjusted. She felt better and achieved menarche at 16.1 years with a final height of 61.4 in (156 cm).

References

1. Castinetti F, Reynaud R, Saveanu A, et al. Clinical and genetic aspects of combined pituitary hormone deficiencies [article in French]. *Ann Endocrinol (Paris)*. 2008;69(1):7-17. PMID: 18291347

2. Gregory LC, Dattani MT. The molecular basis of congenital hypopituitarism and related disorders. *J Clin Endocrinol Metab* [Epub ahead of print] PMID: 31702014

3. Fang Q, George AS, Brinkmeier ML, et al. Genetics of combined pituitary hormone deficiency: roadmap into the genome era. *Endocr Rev*. 2016;37(6):636-675. PMID: 27828722

4. Tanriverdi F, Dokmetas HS, Kebapci N, et al. Etiology of hypopituitarism in tertiary care institutions in Turkish population: analysis of 773 patients from Pituitary Study Group database. *Endocrine*. 2014;47(1):198-205. PMID: 24366641

5. Regal M, Paramo C, Sierra SM, Garcia-Mayor RV. Prevalence and incidence of hypopituitarism in an adult Caucasian population in northwestern Spain. *Clin Endocrinol (Oxf)*. 2001;55(6):735-740. PMID: 11895214

6. Muller HL, Emser A, Faldum A, et al. Longitudinal study on growth and body mass index before and after diagnosis of childhood craniopharyngioma. *J Clin Endocrinol Metab*. 2004;89(7):3298-3305. PMID: 165240606

7. Mehta A, Hindmarsh PC, Stanhope RG, Brain CE, Preece MA, Dattani MT. Is the thyrotropin-releasing hormone test necessary in the diagnosis of central hypothyroidism in children. *J Clin Endocrinol Metab*. 2003;88(12):5696-5703. PMID: 14671155

8. Mehta A, Hindmarsh PC, Mehta H, et al. Congenital hypopituitarism: clinical, molecular and neuroradiological correlates. *Clin Endocrinol (Oxf)*. 2009;70(1):96-103. PMID: 19320653

9. Cerbone M, Dattani MT. Progression from isolated growth hormone deficiency to combined pituitary hormone deficiency. *Growth Horm IGF Res*. 2017;37:19-25. PMID: 29107171

10. Blum WF, Deal C, Zimmermann AG, et al. Development of additional pituitary hormone deficiencies in pediatric patients originally diagnosed with idiopathic isolated GH deficiency. *Eur J Endocrinol*. 2014;170(1):13-21. PMID: 24088548

11. Child CJ, Blum WF, Deal C, et al. Development of additional pituitary hormone deficiencies in pediatric patients originally diagnosed with isolated growth hormone deficiency due to organic causes. *Eur J Endocrinol*. 2016;174(5):669-679. PMID: 26888628

12. Otto AP, Franca MM, Correa FA, et al. Frequent development of combined pituitary hormone deficiency in patients initially diagnosed as isolated growth hormone deficiency: a long term follow-up of patients from a single center. *Pituitary*. 2015;18(4):561-567. PMID: 25315032

13. Molitch ME, Clemmons DR, Malozowski S, Merriam GR, Vance ML; Endocrine Society. Evaluation and treatment of adult growth hormone deficiency: an Endocrine Society clinical practice guideline. *J Clin Endocrinol Metab*. 2011;96(6):1587-1609. doi: PMID: 21602453

14. Cerbone M, Guemes M, Wade A, Improda N, Dattani M. Endocrine morbidity in midline brain defects: differences between septo-optic dysplasia and related disorders. *EClinical Medicine*. In press.

15. Sbardella E, Pozza C, Isidori AM, Grossman AB. Endocrinology and adolescence: dealing with transition in young patients with pituitary disorders. *Eur J Endocrinol*. 2019;181(4):R155-R171. PMID: 31370006

16. Nabhan ZM, Dimeglio LA, Qi R, Perkins SM, Eugster EA. Conjugated oral versus transdermal estrogen replacement in girls with Turner syndrome: a pilot comparative study. *J Clin Endocrinol Metab*. 2009;94(6):2009-2014. PMID: 19318455

17. Mauras N, Torres-Santiago L, Santen R, et al. Impact of route of administration on genotoxic oestrogens concentrations using oral vs transdermal oestradiol in girls with Turner syndrome. *Clin Endocrinol (Oxf)*. 2019;90(1):155-161. PMID: 30281805

18. Kalra S, Zargar AH, Jain SM, et al. Diabetes insipidus: the other diabetes. *Indian J Endocrinol Metab*. 2016;20(1):9-21. PMID: 26904464

When to Request Thyroid Ultrasonography in a Child and When to Worry About the Result

Andrew J. Bauer, MD. Department of Pediatrics, Division of Endocrinology and Diabetes, The Thyroid Center, The Children's Hospital of Philadelphia, University of Pennsylvania, Philadelphia, PA; E-mail: bauera@chop.edu

Mary C. Frates, MD. Department of Radiology, Brigham and Women's Hospital and Boston Children's Hospital, Harvard Medical School, Boston, MA; E-mail: mfrates@bwh.harvard.edu

Learning Objectives

As a result of participating in this session, learners should be able to:

- Identify which ultrasonography (US) characteristics predict benign vs malignant disease in pediatric patients.

- Incorporate US data to stratify which patients should undergo FNA and surgery vs surveillance.

Main Conclusions

An increasing number of pediatric patients are referred for the evaluation and management of thyroid nodules and thyroid cancer. Providers involved in the care of these patients need to be comfortable with the evaluation and management of thyroid nodules, to include developing experience in reviewing thyroid US images in order to optimize selection of patients for FNA, and to ensure that complete preoperative assessment for regional lymph node disease occurs before surgery.

Significance of the Clinical Problem

Approximately 1% to 2% of pediatric-aged patients have a thyroid nodule(s) noted by physical examination and up to 18% have a thyroid abnormality (cyst or nodule) on US.[1] For the majority of patients, there is no identifiable etiology. However, multiple factors are associated with an increased risk for developing a nodule and/or thyroid cancer, the most common being a history of exposure to radiation for treatment of a nonthyroid malignancy, a history of autoimmune thyroid disease, and a family history of predisposition to thyroid nodules and/or thyroid cancer.

Over the last decade, the annual incidence of pediatric thyroid carcinoma has steadily increased. The increase in the number of adolescent patients diagnosed with thyroid cancer has followed similarly reported data in adults.[2,3] Approximately 40% of pediatric patients are found to have a nodule on palpation by a clinician, 20% are found incidentally on unrelated imaging studies, and 40% are discovered by patients' families or by patients themselves, with the latter group having the largest nodules and highest rates of thyroid cancer metastasis.[4] While the greatest increase has been for tumors between 0.5 and 1 cm, there has been an increase in the diagnosis of tumors across all sizes, suggesting that more frequent use of imaging is not solely responsible for the upward trend.[3]

In general, pediatric endocrinologists, surgeons, and radiologists receive minimal training and have limited experience in performing and reading thyroid US. Efforts to improve the completeness of the exam and the accuracy of diagnosis for thyroid and neck US in pediatric patients is critical to accurately stratify patients who may benefit from further evaluation and/or surveillance.

Barriers to Optimal Practice

- The lower incidence of thyroid nodular disease in children and adolescents is associated with decreased expertise in performing and reading thyroid and neck US.

- The lack of training and expertise in reading thyroid US increases the reliance of pediatric providers (endocrinologist and surgeons) on radiology reports in selecting patients for FNA and surgery.

- Less training and experience for pediatric US technicians and radiologists increases the risk for incomplete exams and greater intraobserver and interobserver variability in accurate study interpretation.

Strategies for Diagnosis, Therapy, and/or Management
Patients at Increased Risk

The most common risk factors for developing thyroid nodules and thyroid cancer include the following:

1. Previous exposure to ionizing radiation (radiation used to treat a nonthyroid-related malignancy, repeated exposure to diagnostic radiologic imaging, or environmental exposure [nuclear power plant accident or ambient])

2. Patient history of autoimmune thyroid disease

3. Familial predisposition

    a. Nonsyndromic; not associated with a clinical phenotype or an increased risk of developing other tumors

    b. Syndromic; associated with a clinical phenotype and an increased risk of developing other tumors

        i. *PTEN* hamartoma syndrome
        ii. *DICER1*-related syndrome
        iii. Familial adenomatous polyposis
        iv. Multiple endocrine neoplasia type 2

Most patients are diagnosed with differentiated thyroid cancer (DTC) after discovery of an asymptomatic nodule or persistent cervical lymphadenopathy in a patient with no identifiable risk factors. For patients in the high-risk categories, there is disagreement and variation in practice regarding if and when surveillance US should be performed. Those in favor of screening refer to an increased risk of thyroid malignancy within these subpopulations with a goal of identifying the cancer at an earlier state of disease where less aggressive treatment may be needed to achieve remission. Those against surveillance raise concern over the potential increased number of procedures needed for detection of a small number of clinically significant thyroid malignancies, as well as the identification of patients with indolent cancers that may not ever result in clinically significant disease over the patient's lifetime. Incidental, indolent thyroid cancer is found in approximately 10% of the adult population on autopsy.[5]

Survivors of Nonthyroid Childhood Malignancies Exposed to Therapeutic Ionizing Radiation
For survivors of nonthyroid childhood malignancies exposed to therapeutic ionizing radiation, there is a 10- to 18-fold increased incidence of developing thyroid carcinoma, with a latency range of 5 to 35 years. Younger age at the

time of exposure to radiation and female gender are both associated with an increased risk and shorter latency to develop thyroid nodules and thyroid cancer. Within this group of patients, annual physical exam of the thyroid should be instituted with the first 3 years postexposure with consideration for annual thyroid US surveillance starting 3 to 5 years postexposure.

Autoimmune Thyroid Disease (Hashimoto/Lymphocytic Thyroiditis)

Several articles support an increased risk of thyroid nodules in pediatric patients with a history of autoimmune thyroid disease. However, there are mixed reports regarding whether there is an increased risk of thyroid cancer. Interpreting thyroid US in the setting of autoimmune thyroid disease may be challenging, as the tissue typically has a patchy or pseudonodular (cobblestoned) appearance. This may make it difficult to determine if a region is a true nodule or a "germinal center" that is altering the sonographic appearance of the tissue. Viewing the area in video (CINE mode) and with color Doppler may be helpful to determine whether the area is a nodule or a pseudonodule.

Familial Nonmedullary Thyroid Carcinoma

Familial nonmedullary thyroid carcinoma is defined by the presence of 2 or more first-degree relatives with a history of differentiated thyroid carcinoma. Familial thyroid cancer may display genetic anticipation from one generation to the next; that is, the earlier development of thyroid cancer in succeeding generations. Thus, it is reasonable that the first US be performed sometime during early adolescence.

Genetic Syndromes

PTEN hamartoma tumor syndrome, *DICER1* pleuropulmonary blastoma syndrome, and familial adenomatous polyposis are the most frequent syndromes associated with an increased risk of developing thyroid nodules and DTC. Lateral neck and distant metastasis are uncommon in syndromic DTC, with most patients having disease confined to the thyroid or central neck.

Multiple Endocrine Neoplasia Type 2

Multiple endocrine neoplasia type 2 is associated with an increased risk for developing medullary thyroid cancer. In pediatric patients, 75% or more of medullary thyroid cancer cases are associated with germline pathogenic variants in the *RET* proto-oncogene (in adults, 75% or more of medullary thyroid cancer is sporadic). Please refer to the American Thyroid Association guidelines and GeneReviews for individual risk and recommended timing for prophylactic thyroidectomy.

Ultrasonography

Thyroid US is the preferred and most informative method for evaluating and screening for thyroid nodules. US can detect lesions as small as 1 to 2 mm in size and provides information on the multiplicity, laterality, and sonographic characteristics of lesions and background thyroid parenchyma, as well as the status of regional lymph nodes. Characteristics specifically worrisome for malignancy include solitary nodules, larger size, solid parenchyma, presence of punctate echogenic foci, extrathyroidal extension, lobulated or irregular margins, and abnormal lymph nodes.[6,7] Taller-than-wide shape and very hypoechoic echotexture are also high-risk features. Characteristics associated with benign cytology include highly cystic content, spongiform appearance, and echogenic echotexture.[7,8] Blood flow by color Doppler is not a useful differentiating characteristic.[9]

Several systems may be used to stratify nodules for FNA, including the American Thyroid Association thyroid nodule sonographic pattern system and the American College of Radiology Thyroid Imaging Reporting and Data System (TI-RADS – https://www.acr.org/clinical-resources/reporting-and-data-systems/TI-RADS). There are preliminary data on the clinical application for both of these systems in pediatrics, with data suggesting that the systems are useful but not independently sufficient to identify thyroid malignancy. The most recent study examining TI-RADS in the evaluation of nodules in children concluded that the system can identify high-risk nodules accurately and decrease the number of benign nodules undergoing biopsy; however, the management system is not appropriate for pediatric patients in that up to 22% of thyroid cancers would be assigned to follow-up or discharged completely without an FNA.[10] If the TI-RADS system is used in children, a much lower size threshold for biopsy is advised so no cancers are missed. Across all age groups, the presence of cervical lymphadenopathy is important and should overrule the likelihood of thyroid malignancy in nodules that would otherwise be considered benign based on sonographic features or those too small to pursue FNA. Additional important points to remember:

- Within pediatric and young adult patients, a diffusely infiltrative form of papillary thyroid carcinoma (PTC) (diffuse sclerosing variant) presents with a large, heterogeneous gland, scattered microcalcifications ("snow-storm"), hyperemia, and lateral neck lymphadenopathy. This may occupy one-half or the entire gland. There is no distinct nodule on US.

- Cystic composition is the single most reliable feature to predict a lower-risk thyroid nodule (>50%-75% cystic).[11,12] However, larger, solid nodules may undergo cystic degeneration and large cystic nodules should be considered solid in regard to risk assessment.

- US of the lateral neck is a critical, necessary step to help determine the malignant potential of the thyroid lesion and should be included in the initial exam for all patients found to have a thyroid nodule on US (https://www.acr.org/-/media/ACR/Files/Practice-Parameters/ExtracranialHeadandNeck.pdf?la=en).[13] Careful and deliberate US of the neck should also be a routine part of the preoperative evaluation, with the highest incidence of lymph node metastasis found in cervical levels VI (central neck) followed by levels III, IV, and II depending on location of the thyroid nodule (upper vs lower pole of the thyroid lobe).

- Features that are diagnostic and/or concerning for metastatic disease to lymph nodes include the following:[14]

Concerning	Diagnostic
Rounded shape	Peripheral blood flow on Doppler
Increased echogenicity	Microcalcifications (echogenic foci)
Absent fatty hilum	Cystic changes

- For patients with extensive lymphadenopathy, neck CT with contrast or MRI may be considered to more thoroughly evaluate deep regions of the neck, as well as the aerodigestive track.

Sonographic Patterns Associated With Benign Thyroid Disease

The sonographic pattern of Hashimoto thyroiditis may be *diffuse*, with the majority of the gland being hypoechoic with heterogeneous echotexture and having scattered echogenic septations, or *nodular*, with either normal sonographic appearance to the background thyroid parenchyma (called "nodular Hashimoto") or with diffusely heterogenous background parenchyma (cobblestone appearance). These sonographic features reflect variation in the location and degree of lymphocytic infiltration and inflammatory response to the T-cell–mediated destruction of the thyroid with the nodular areas typically representing lymphocytic aggregation into germinal centers. On color Doppler, the blood flow may be slightly or markedly increased (hyperemic) with proposed correlation between hypothyroidism and blood flow mediated through the trophic effects of TSH. In adults, 10% to 20% of patients may have absent to low level alterations in thyroid autoantibody levels with a lower incidence of hypothyroidism in patients with nodular Hashimoto.

In patients with diffuse Hashimoto, benign nodules are more likely to appear hyperechoic compared with the hypoechoic background with smooth margins and no calcifications, while malignant nodules are frequently associated with a very hypoechoic appearance, lobulated margins, and microcalcifications (punctate, macro, and peripheral eggshell). In patients with nodular Hashimoto, there are shared sonographic features between benign nodules (spongiform, cystic/complex, hyperechoic, and anechoic, smooth margin) and malignant nodules (lobulated, irregular margins, increased intramodular blood flow, and echogenic foci), making it difficult at times to distinguish between a benign and malignant nodule without FNA. Perithyroidal (inferior to the thyroid and above the isthmus) reactive lymph nodes are also common and may be distinguished from pathologic lymph nodes by blood flow limited to the hilum on Doppler imaging.[15-17]

Patients with Graves disease may also be at increased risk for developing thyroid nodules. Sonographic assessment of the thyroid before definitive treatment is recommended, as there is an increased risk of malignancy associated with nodular Graves disease.[18]

Intrathyroidal thymic remnant (ITTR) is a variation of normal embryonic development where a piece of thymic tissue is ectopically located within the thyroid gland during organ migration in the first trimester of fetal development. ITTR lesions may mimic thyroid malignancy due to the common sonographic finding of multiple echogenic foci in the setting of a hypoechoic lesion. The distinguishing features of an ITTR from a thyroid nodule include smooth margin, nonshadowing coarse echogenic foci, and an unusual, often angular, shape that may be completely intrathyroidal or extend inferiorly and be associated with a similar appearing lesion in the inferior aspect of the central neck (the caudal aspect of level VI into level VII). Comparing the sonographic appearance of the lesion to the normal thymus is extremely useful. Between 1% and 5% of the pediatric population have an ITTR that follows the same pattern of involution as eutopic thymic tissue, disappearing by the time a patient is in their early 20s. ITTRs may be solitary lesions or there may be multiple unilateral or bilateral lesions; however, as ITTRs represent a variation of normal development, there should

be no evidence of abnormal lymph nodes with features concerning for PTC. If the sonographic features are not distinct for an ITTR, then FNA should be performed to determine the etiology of the lesion. Benign-appearing lymphocytes with a predominance of CD4 and CD8 on flow cytometry are consistent with an ITTR.[19-21]

Clinical Case Vignettes

Case 1

A 14-and-6/12-year-old girl presents with an enlarged thyroid and complaints of dry, brittle hair and fatigue. On physical examination, her vital signs are normal but her thyroid is visible in a neck-neutral position, exaggerated with neck extension. Fullness to the right lobe is reported along with a palpable lymph node in her right lateral neck. Thyroid function tests are ordered and reveal the following:

TSH = 23.8 mIU/L (0.5-4.3 mIU/L)
Free T_4 = 0.9 ng/dL (0.9-1.4 ng/dL) (SI: 11.6 pmol/L [11.6-18.0 pmol/L])
Thyroglobulin antibodies, elevated
TPO antibodies, not detected

Her medical history and family history are notable for autoimmune thyroid disease (her mother and older sister). Thyroid US is ordered, and she is referred to pediatric endocrinology for further evaluation. Imaging reveals diffuse tissue heterogeneity with areas of increased echogenicity but no nodules. There is increased blood flow on Doppler (*see images*).

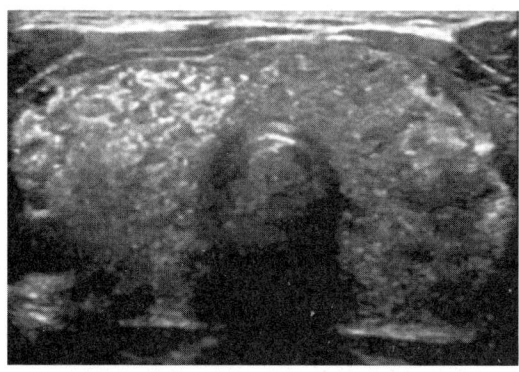

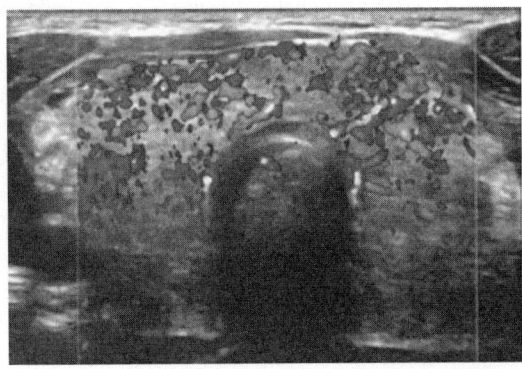

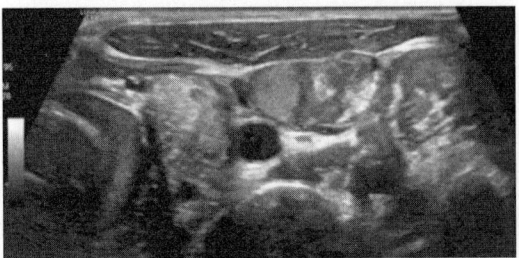

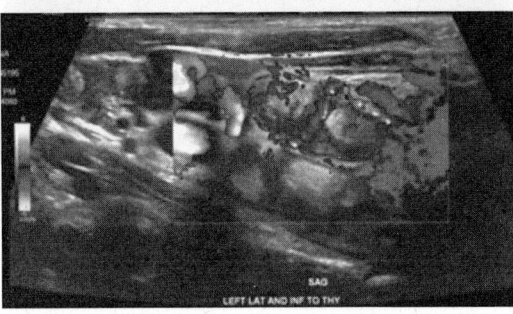

Levothyroxine, 75 mcg daily, is initiated. The radiology report suggests follow-up US in 6 months and based on this, clinical surveillance is continued. Repeated laboratory tests 6 weeks after starting levothyroxine show normalization of TSH and free T_4. Clinically, the patient is doing well, with decreased complaints of dry hair but continued concerns of fatigue, although this may be slightly improved. Repeated examination still shows an enlarged thyroid, firm on palpation. Repeat thyroid US reveals similar images and the radiologist recommends continued surveillance. The lack of decrease in thyroid size and the firmness of the thyroid on the exam are unsettling.

Question 1: Which of the following is the best next step in this patient's evaluation and management?

A. Obtain axial imaging of the neck with CT or MRI

B. Continue surveillance with repeated thyroid US in 6 months

C. Perform FNA biopsy

D. Review thyroid US to determine if the lateral neck was assessed

Answer: D) Review thyroid US to determine if the lateral neck was assessed

On review of the imaging (Answer D), there is no assessment of the central or lateral neck lymph nodes. You order neck US with the following representative images recorded (*see images*).

Axial imaging of the neck with CT or MRI (Answer A) is incorrect, as US provides high-resolution images of the superficial lateral neck lymph nodes and the characteristic sonographic features (listed in the chapter's text) are the standard in assessment for evidence of thyroid cancer metastasis. Continuing surveillance with repeated thyroid US in 6 months (Answer B) is not adequate if there is a concern for malignancy, and performing FNA biopsy (Answer C) is the step that should occur if there is concern for lateral neck lymph node metastasis after US is performed.

Question 2: With US evidence concerning for lateral neck lymph node metastasis, which of the following is the best next step in evaluation and management?

A. Obtain axial imaging of the neck with CT or MRI

B. Continue surveillance with thyroid US in 6 months

C. Perform FNA

D. Perform excisional biopsy of the abnormal lymph node

Answer: C) Perform FNA

This vignette highlights the challenge and potential pitfalls associated with diagnosing diffuse sclerosing variant PTC (dsvPTC). This variant of PTC is more common in pediatric and young adult patients than in older patients. It is commonly associated with elevations in thyroglobulin antibodies and has a diffusely infiltrative behavior that may be associated with increased TSH. The sonographic appearance may mimic autoimmune thyroiditis based on diffuse tissue heterogeneity and increased blood flow on Doppler. However, the presence of too-numerous-to-count echogenic foci (the "snow-storm" appearance) and typical lymph node metastasis should reduce the chances of a missed diagnosis. DsvPTC has a high propensity for both regional (lymph node) and distant (pulmonary) metastasis.

The patient in this vignette underwent FNA (Answer C) after complete, preoperative neck US. FNA confirmed PTC, as well as metastasis to right and left levels III and IV. Total thyroidectomy with bilateral central and bilateral lateral neck dissection was performed with 45/70 lymph nodes positive for metastasis and several lymph nodes having extranodal extension. Oncogene analysis revealed a *RET*-fusion driver pathogenic variant, the most common oncogene associated with dsvPTC.

Axial imaging using CT with contrast or MRI (Answer A) may be performed after cytologic confirmation of lateral neck lymph node metastasis to aid in surgical planning. Thus, this option is not incorrect, but it is not the next best step in the evaluation. Excisional biopsy (Answer D) should be avoided, as it is a more invasive procedure than FNA and does not provide any additional information over cytology. Lastly, continued surveillance (Answer B) should be avoided, as the sonographic images in this case support thyroid cancer with regional metastasis.

Case 2

A 6-year-old child is referred for FNA of a suspicious thyroid nodule. Head and neck CT performed at an outside hospital to investigate chronic neck pain showed a right-sided thyroid nodule and US confirmed the right-sided lesion. The nodule was reported as a solid mass with microcalcifications, suspicious for thyroid cancer. Repeated US shows a well-defined lesion in the

right lobe of the thyroid with nonshadowing bright foci of variable size (*see image*). Imaging inferior to the thyroid gland demonstrates the normal thymus. There are no enlarged or abnormal lymph nodes.

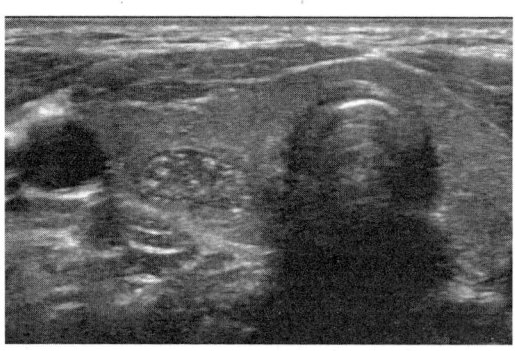

Which of the following is the most appropriate next step?

A. FNA

B. Core-needle biopsy

C. Right lobectomy

D. 6-Month follow-up US to confirm stability of this lesion

Answer: D) 6-Month follow-up US to confirm stability of this lesion

This sonographic finding is an intrathyroidal thymic remnant. The margins of the lesion are sharp, and the echogenic foci are larger and less reflective than the punctate calcifications of PTC. The sonographic characteristics are exactly that of the normal thymus. This remnant can be found in up to 5% of the pediatric population. Follow-up to confirm lack of growth (Answer D) can be useful to confirm the diagnosis. An experienced imager who recognizes this finding can make a confident diagnosis and discharge the patient without follow-up.

This finding should be recognized as a benign lesion and does not require FNA (Answer A), core-needle biopsy (Answer B), or surgical resection (Answer C).

Case 3

A 15-year-old boy reports feeling a lump in his throat and some difficulty swallowing. On palpation, the thyroid feels enlarged with nodular contours. US (*see image*) demonstrates an enlarged heterogeneous gland with linear echogenic strands. No discrete nodule is seen. Several enlarged benign-appearing nodes are noted in levels III and IV.

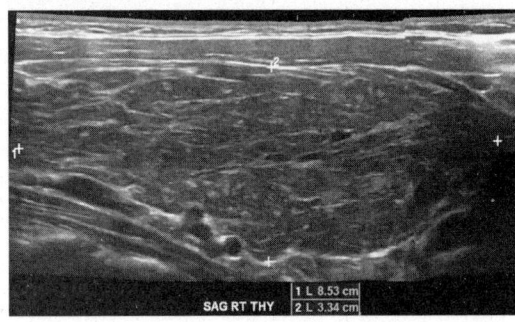

Which of the following is the most appropriate next step?

A. FNA

B. Thyroid function tests and measurement of TPO antibodies

C. Consultation with a pediatric surgeon

D. Core-needle biopsy

Answer: B) Thyroid function tests and measurement of TPO antibodies

The sonographic findings are highly suggestive of Hashimoto (lymphocytic) thyroiditis. Enlarged benign lymph nodes on US are typical of this disease. The presence of TPO antibodies will confirm the diagnosis, and thyroid function tests determine whether thyroid hormone replacement is indicated (Answer B). Tissue sampling with either FNA (Answer A) or core-needle biopsy (Answer D) is not necessary in patients with Hashimoto thyroiditis, and there is no role for surgery (Answer C).

Case 4

A 14-year-old girl undergoes head CT for neck pain following a motor vehicle accident. The CT report describes abnormalities in the thyroid gland bilaterally, which cannot be categorized. US is performed (*see image*).

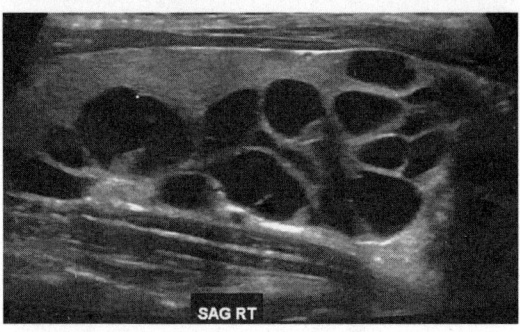

Which of the following is the most appropriate next step?

A. FNA

B. MRI of the neck

C. Complete thyroid function testing

D. No immediate treatment; follow-up US in 6 to 12 months to assess for change

Answer: D) No immediate treatment, follow-up US in 6 to 12 months to assess for change

US shows multiple simple cysts. The risk of malignancy is zero. Follow-up US to determine if the cysts continue to increase in size and number (Answer D) would be appropriate. Tissue sampling with FNA (Answer A) is not necessary in patients with simple cysts. There is never a role for MRI (Answer B) in evaluation of the thyroid gland; US is the best imaging modality for the thyroid. If the thyroid gland becomes completely replaced with cysts, thyroid function might be impacted and should be evaluated at that point (Answer C), but it is highly unlikely to be abnormal at this time, as there is normal thyroid tissue well visualized at the upper anterior aspect of the lobe.

References

1. Avula S, Daneman A, Navarro OM, Moineddin R, Urbach S, Daneman D. Incidental thyroid abnormalities identified on neck US for non-thyroid disorders. *Pediatr Radiol.* 2010;40(11):1774-1780. PMID: 20490485

2. Burkhamer J, Kriebel D, Clapp R. The increasing toll of adolescent cancer incidence in the US. *PLoS One.* 2017;12(2):e0172986. PMID: 28235028

3. Qian ZJ, Jin MC, Meister KD, Megwalu UC. Pediatric thyroid cancer incidence and mortality trends in the United States, 1973-2013. *JAMA Otolaryngol Head Neck Surg.* 2019;145(7):617-623. PMID: 31120475

4. Gupta A, Ly S, Castroneves LA, et al. How are childhood thyroid nodules discovered: opportunities for improving early detection. *J Pediatr.* 2014;164(3):658-660. PMID: 24345455

5. Furuya-Kanamori L, Bell KJL, Clark J, Glasziou P, Doi SAR. Prevalence of differentiated thyroid cancer in autopsy studies over six decades: a meta-analysis. *J Clin Oncol.* 2016;34(30):3672-3679. PMID: 27601555

6. Richman DM, Benson CB, Doubilet PM, et al. Thyroid nodules in pediatric patients: sonographic characteristics and likelihood of cancer. *Radiology.* 2018;288(2):591-599. PMID: 29714678

7. Tessler FN, Middleton WD, Grant EG. Thyroid imaging reporting and data system (TI-RADS): a user's guide. *Radiology.* 2018;287(1):29-36. PMID: 29558300

8. Haugen BR, Alexander EK, Bible KC, et al. 2015 American Thyroid Association management guidelines for adult patients with thyroid nodules and differentiated thyroid cancer: the American Thyroid Association Guidelines Task Force on Thyroid Nodules and Differentiated Thyroid Cancer. *Thyroid.* 2016;26(1):1-133. PMID: 26462967

9. Frates MC, Benson CB, Doubilet PM, Cibas ES, Marqusee E. Can color Doppler sonography aid in the prediction of malignancy of thyroid nodules? *J Ultrasound Med.* 2003;22(2):127-131. PMID: 12562117

10. Richman DM, Benson CB, Doubilet PM, et al. Assessment of American College of Radiology Thyroid Imaging Reporting and Data System (TI-RADS) for pediatric thyroid nodules. *Radiology.* 2019;191326. PMID: 31821121

11. Gannon AW, Langer JE, Bellah R, et al. Diagnostic accuracy of ultrasound with color flow Doppler in children with thyroid nodules. *J Clin Endocrinol Metab.* 2018;103(5):1958-1965. PMID: 29546281

12. Gupta A, Ly S, Castroneves LA, et al. A standardized assessment of thyroid nodules in children confirms higher cancer prevalence than in adults. *J Clin Endocrinol Metab.* 2013;98(8):3238-3245. PMID: 23737541

13. AIUM-ACR-SPR-SRU practice parameter for the performance and interpretation of a diagnostic ultrasound examination of the extracranial head and neck. *J Ultrasound Med.* 2018;37(11):E6-E12. PMID: 30308087

14. Leboulleux S, Girard E, Rose M, et al. Ultrasound criteria of malignancy for cervical lymph nodes in patients followed up for differentiated thyroid cancer. *J Clin Endocrinol Metab.* 2007;92(9):3590-3594. PMID: 17609301

15. Anderson L, Middleton WD, Teefey SA, et al. Hashimoto thyroiditis: part 2, sonographic analysis of benign and malignant nodules in patients with diffuse Hashimoto thyroiditis. *AJR Am J Roentgenol.* 2010;195(1):216-222. PMID: 20566819

16. Anderson L, Middleton WD, Teefey SA, et al. Hashimoto thyroiditis: part 1, sonographic analysis of the nodular form of Hashimoto thyroiditis. *AJR Am J Roentgenol.* 2010;195(1):208-215. PMID: 20566818

17. Janus D, Wojcik M, Drabik G, Wyrobek L, Starzyk JB. Ultrasound variants of autoimmune thyroiditis in children and adolescents and their clinical implication in relation to papillary thyroid carcinoma development. *J Endocrinol Invest.* 2018;41(3):371-380. PMID: 28866751

18. MacFarland SP, Bauer AJ, Adzick NS, et al. Disease burden and outcome in pediatric and young adults with concurrent Graves disease and differentiated thyroid carcinoma. *J Clin Endocrinol Metab.* 2018;103(8):2918-2925. PMID: 29788090

19. Frates MC, Benson CB, Dorfman DM, Cibas ES, Huang SA. Ectopic intrathyroidal thymic tissue mimicking thyroid nodules in children. *J Ultrasound Med.* 2018;37(3):783-791. PMID: 28850707

20. Monaco SE, Escobar F, Simons JP. Hassall's corpuscles in the fine-needle aspiration cytology of pediatric ectopic thymic tissue. *Diagn Cytopathol.* 2017;45(8):735-737. PMID: 28556508

21. Segni M, di Nardo R, Pucarelli I, Biffoni M. Ectopic intrathyroidal thymus in children: a long-term follow-up study. *Horm Res Paediatr.* 2010;75(4):258-263. PMID: 21196700

Pediatric Bone Fragility: When to Worry and What to Do?

Laura K. Bachrach, MD. Division of Endocrinology, Stanford University School of Medicine, Stanford, CA; E-mail: lkbach@stanford.edu

Learning Objectives

As a result of participating in this session, learners should be able to:

- Identify the risk factors for pediatric bone fragility.

- Order appropriate laboratory and radiographic studies to assess fracture risk.

- Discuss the indications for bisphosphonate or sex steroid therapy in pediatric patients.

Main Conclusions

The foundation for lifetime bone strength is established in the first 2 decades. Bone size, geometry, microarchitecture, and material properties each contribute to resistance of bone to fracture.[1] The expected gains in bone strength can be compromised during this critical developmental period by genetic and acquired disorders. Early identification and treatment of younger patients at risk for bone fragility is key to avoiding fractures in not only in childhood but throughout later life. Each 10% (1 SD) gain in peak bone strength has been estimated to reduce an individual's lifetime fracture risk by 50%.[2]

There have been several advances in the assessment and treatment of pediatric bone fragility in the past 30 years. Despite improvements in DXA, peripheral quantitative CT, and high-resolution peripheral quantitative CT, these have proven to be imperfect surrogate predictors of fracture risk. For this reason, a panel of pediatric bone experts recommended that the diagnosis of pediatric osteoporosis be restricted to those with a significant fracture history.[3] The armamentarium to treat pediatric osteoporosis is still limited.[4,5] Bisphosphonates have proved helpful in reducing fractures in both primary (genetic) and most forms of secondary osteoporosis. Low-dosage estrogen has been shown to increase bone mineral density (BMD) in hypothalamic amenorrhea (eating disorders, exercise-associated amenorrhea), but the impact on fractures remains uncertain. In the absence of randomized controlled trials, the choice of drug, dosage, and duration of treatment for younger patients remain based on expert opinion.

Significance of the Clinical Problem

Pediatric providers are increasingly asked to address bone fragility in younger patients. Referrals are made for children who already have had fractures and those considered "at risk" because of conditions associated with osteoporosis (*Box*). Although attention to early skeletal health is encouraging, the provider faces persistent dilemmas related both to the evaluation and treatment of bone fragility. There is no established pediatric bone "fracture threshold" based on DXA or peripheral quantitative CT. Additionally, there is no tool comparable to FRAX used in adults to weight the clinical factors that aid in calculating fracture risk. For these reasons, pediatric patients who have not yet sustained a fracture are usually managed with general bone health measures only. These include optimizing nutrition, calcium and vitamin D intake, physical activity, and treatment of the underlying chronic diseases, while minimizing exposure to osteotoxic drugs.

For patients meeting the criteria for pediatric osteoporosis (based on fractures), there are still controversies regarding the choice of optimal drug, dosage, and duration of treatment. Data on the safety and efficacy of bisphosphonates are inadequate to recommend these agents for routine use; offering these drugs on a compassionate use basis to treat fractures and bone pain is accepted as standard of care. Intravenous zoledronic acid has replaced pamidronate in many centers because of the shorter infusion time and longer duration of action of this newer drug. Pediatric dosing of zoledronic acid ranges from 0.05 to 0.10 mg/kg per year delivered every 6 months; pamidronate dosing ranges from 4 to 9 mg/kg per year divided every 2 to 4 months depending on age. The maximal gains from bisphosphonate therapy are achieved by 2 to 4 years. However, it appears risky to institute a "drug holiday" for growing patients who face ongoing threats from chronic conditions such as osteogenesis imperfecta or Duchenne muscular dystrophy. Fractures can occur at the interface between older "treated" bone and the weaker, newly acquired distal bone. To avoid over-suppression of bone turnover, the dosage of bisphosphonates used for the initial treatment is typically halved during the maintenance phase. Data on safety and efficacy of newer agents, including denosumab and sclerostin antibody, remain quite limited. Anabolic agents, including teriparatide, have a black box warning prohibiting use in patients with open epiphyses.

Barriers to Optimal Practice

- Challenges to deciding when to use a pharmacologic agent to treat bone fragility in young patients.

- Bone densitometry alone cannot be used to diagnose pediatric osteoporosis.

- Uncertainty about choice of osteoporosis drugs because of randomized controlled trials with

functional endpoints (bone pain, fractures) are lacking.

- Randomized controlled trials of sex steroids for hypothalamic amenorrhea have been short term with biochemical bone markers and BMD as outcome measures.

Strategies for Diagnosis, Therapy, and/or Management
Defining Pediatric Osteoporosis

According to the International Society of Clinical Densitometry (ISCD) guidelines, the diagnosis of osteoporosis is reserved for patients with the following:

- One or more vertebral compression fractures occurring without local disease or major trauma (with or without densitometry measures)

  OR

- Low bone mineral content or density for age (a standard deviation for age or Z-score less than −2) plus 2 or more long bone fractures by age 10 years or 3 or more by age 19 years

These criteria reflect the fact that BMD Z-scores vary depending on the normative reference database used. They also account for the observation that fragility fractures can occur at a relatively "better" bone mineral content or BMD, particularly in patients treated with glucocorticoids. The guidelines emphasize the differing clinical significance of fractures at various skeletal sites. Fractures of long bones but not fingers and toes are important in decision making about treatment.

Evaluation
For Whom?
A bone health assessment is appropriate for patients with a diagnosis of the genetic disorders or acquired diseases associated with bone fragility, several of which are listed in the *Box*. Other

Box. Causes of Osteoporosis

Causes of Primary Osteoporosis

- Osteogenesis imperfecta
- Syndromes:
  - Bruck syndrome
  - Marfan syndrome
  - Ehlers-Danlos syndrome
  - Osteoporosis-pseudoglioma syndrome
- Paget disease
- Metabolic syndromes:
  - Wilson disease
  - Homocystinuria
  - Menkes kinky hair syndrome
  - Galactosemia
- Idiopathic juvenile osteoporosis

Causes of Secondary Osteoporosis

- Chronic inflammatory disorders
  - Inflammatory bowel disease
  - Juvenile idiopathic arthritis
  - Celiac disease
  - Cystic fibrosis
- Immobilization
  - Cerebral palsy
  - Myopathic disease (eg, Duchenne muscular dystrophy)
  - Epidermolysis bullosa
- Endocrine disturbance
  - Turner syndrome
  - Anorexia nervosa
  - Type 1 diabetes mellitus
- Cancer and therapies with adverse effects on bone health
  - Acute lymphoblastic leukemia
  - Post chemotherapy for childhood cancer
  - Post transplant (non-renal)
- Hematologic disorders
  - Thalassemia
  - Sickle-cell disease
- Drug-induced
  - Glucocorticoids
  - Immunosuppressants
  - Anticonvulsant agents
  - Medroxyprogesterone

candidates include seemingly healthy children with recurrent fractures. Deciding how much evaluation is needed in the latter situation is challenging since fractures are a common injury in children.[6] Features of a concerning fracture history include low-trauma injuries (from standing height or less) or vertebral or femur fractures since injuries at these skeletal sites are rare in healthy youth.

How?

A detailed clinical history should be obtained about prior bone pain or fractures and how the injuries occurred. The family history should explore if relatives have had recurrent fractures or hip fractures. Baseline laboratory studies include measurement of serum 25-hydroxyvitamin D, calcium, phosphate, creatinine, PTH, antibodies for celiac disease, and urinary calcium excretion. Testing for thyroid, growth, sex hormone abnormalities, or underlying pathogenic genetic variants may be appropriate depending on the clinical history and physical exam. Urine and blood biochemical markers of bone turnover have proven less useful surrogate measures of bone health because of their greater interindividual and intraindividual variability in childhood and adolescence. These tests are not recommended for diagnosis or decision making for treatment, but they may be useful to monitor for over-suppression of bone turnover during pharmacologic therapy. The most commonly measured parameters are procollagen type I N-terminal propeptide (PINP; a marker of bone formation) and serum collagen type I cross-linked C-telopeptide (CTx; a marker of bone resorption).

Bone densitometry may be included as part of the evaluation; in clinical practice this is typically done using DXA. The ISCD guidelines recommend performing an initial DXA when the patient might benefit from intervention and when the densitometry results would influence management.[3] There are now robust pediatric reference data to allow calculation of standard deviation Z-scores for age, sex, ethnicity, and height.[7] As discussed above, however, the diagnosis of pediatric osteoporosis can be made only in the presence of a significant fracture history. For this reason, determining whether a vertebral fracture has occurred is often an important part of the evaluation. Since 40% of vertebral fractures are asymptomatic, the absence of back pain does not rule out this injury. Expertise is required to differentiate vertebral fractures from normal variants of pediatric vertebral development. Lateral thoracolumbar spine radiographs using the Genant semiquantitative scoring method to calculate the spinal deformity index are considered the "gold standard" to identify vertebral fractures.[8] Vertebral fractures can also be detected using vertebral fracture assessment software available on newer DXA equipment.

Management

General Measures

A key first step is to address all risk factors for poor bone health. Although this seems obvious, attention to these general measures can be overlooked in the care of these complex disorders. Nutritional goals include achieving a healthy BMI since both overweight and underweight have been linked to pediatric fractures. Counseling should focus on intake of calories, protein, calcium, and vitamin D. Although the definition of vitamin D "sufficiency" is debated, supplementation is appropriate for all. If the serum 25-hydroxyvitamin D concentration is less than 20 ng/mL (<50 nmol/L), a 6- to 12-week course of high-dosage vitamin D supplementation (50,000 IU weekly or 4000 IU daily) is recommended. The 25-hydroxyvitamin D measurement should be repeated at the end of therapy since higher dosages may be needed in patients with obesity, cystic fibrosis, or other malabsorption disorders. Activity should be encouraged as tolerated but may be limited in those with immobilization disorders. Control of the underlying chronic disease is key to improving bone health. The use of biologics instead of glucocorticoids to reduce inflammatory cytokines has proven effective in enhancing BMD.[9] Sex steroid replacement is appropriate for patients with gonadal failure from chemotherapy, Turner syndrome, or other causes and appears to enhance BMD. Less is known about the impact of hormone replacement on fracture risk.

Drug Therapy

Osteoporosis in pediatric patients often results from a *failure to gain* bone strength rather than from the *accelerated bone loss* experienced by elderly and postmenopausal patients. For this reason, it would be ideal to treat with an anabolic agent to build bone. The most commonly prescribed of these, synthetic parathyroid hormone (teriparatide), carries a black box warning against its use in growing patients.

Bisphosphonates are the most commonly prescribed pharmacologic agents for both primary and secondary osteoporosis.[4,5] None are FDA-approved for use in pediatric patients because of a lack of adequate randomized controlled trials in younger patients. The outcome measures in most studies have been surrogates (such as BMD) rather than the functional variables (bone fracture or pain). Bisphosphonates appear to be effective in most causes of primary and secondary osteoporosis with the exception of anorexia nervosa.

The benefits of sex steroid therapy to increase BMD or reduce fractures to treat "hypothalamic amenorrhea" (anorexia nervosa, exercise associated amenorrhea) remain controversial. Bone fragility in these disorders reflects nutritional (energy) deficits, as well as deficits in both estrogen and the insulinlike growth factors (IGFs). Nutritional therapy is recommended as first-line treatment with reduction in excessive activity if present.[10] Supplementation with both sex steroids and IGF-1 or use of low-dosage sex steroids have shown positive effects on BMD.[11] These may be reasonable to initiate if nutritional rehabilitation has been unsuccessful. More research is needed to clarify the benefits of sex hormone therapy to reduce fracture risk for these patients.

Clinical Case Vignettes

Case 1

A 14-year-old girl with primary amenorrhea comes with her parents to discuss bone health after sustaining a stress fracture of her right foot. She is a ballet dancer hoping to be accepted into an elite dance troupe. Her days are filled with school and dance practice, leaving little time for socializing with peers. The foot fracture occurred after 6 months of beginning toe dance maneuvers and appears to be healing slowly.

On physical examination, she has Tanner stage 4 breast and pubic hair development but has not had menarche. Her height plots at the 40th percentile and her BMI at the 10th percentile.

Her parents request further evaluation and treatment, so she can safely continue to return to her training.

Which of the following is the best next step in her evaluation?

A. DXA of spine and hip

B. DXA of whole body and spine

C. Prolactin, LH, FSH, estradiol, and 25-hydroxyvitamin D measurements and celiac screen

D. Lateral spine x-ray

E. Serum pregnancy test

Answer: C) Prolactin, LH, FSH, estradiol, 25-hydroxyvitamin D measurements and celiac screen

This patient's stress fracture represents an overuse injury in the setting of intensive training, chronic energy deficits, and hypogonadism. This clinical scenario is often referred to as "the athletic triad." The diagnosis is one of exclusion, and it is important to exclude other causes of amenorrhea, including primary ovarian insufficiency or hyperprolactinemia (Answer C). Ruling out vitamin D insufficiency is reasonable, although these athletes are often taking vitamins in an effort to maintain a healthy body. Screening for celiac disease is always reasonable in the setting of fractures. Performing a pregnancy test

(Answer E) is appropriate in any adolescent girl with amenorrhea, but it might not be done as a first-line evaluation given the history that her hours in school and dance practice leave her no time for socializing.

Perhaps the most controversial question is the role for bone densitometry in the evaluation of this patient. If DXA were to be performed, the preferred regions of interest would be whole body and spine (Answer B) and not spine and hip (Answer A). Whether DXA findings would change management is not clear. If results were normal, would they provide false reassurance about the risks for future fractures? If abnormal, would this increase adherence to recommendations for skeletal health?

In this case, the parents insisted upon DXA, which showed whole-body and spine BMD values of –0.8 and –0.7, respectively. Laboratory test results were normal, including a 25-hydroxyvitamin D value of 32 ng/mL (79.9 nmol/L) and negative celiac antibodies. She had a spontaneous period during the 4-month hiatus from dancing while her stress fracture healed. She is being allowed to return to dance with a graded exercise program closely supervised by the sports medicine team.

Case 2

You are asked to see a 14-year-old boy with a history of 7 long bone fractures. At age 3 years, he sustained a spiral femur fracture when an older child landed on him at play. Six weeks later, he fell backwards with his heavy leg cast and suffered a left arm greenstick fracture. At age 5 years, he fractured both radius and ulna while sliding; at age 7 years, he fractured his collarbone playing football; at age 10 years, he broke his humerus rollerblading; at age 12 years, he fractured his wrist rollerblading, and at 14 years, he had a radial fracture playing basketball. All injuries healed normally and left no skeletal deformities. He has no back pain, hearing deficits, or dental caries. He consumes a normal diet, has no gastrointestinal complaints, and takes no medications.

On physical examination, he has normal height at the 95th percentile, BMI at the 70th percentile, and Tanner stage 4 genitalia. His sclerae are white and teeth are noncarious. There is no tenderness and no deformities on skeletal exam, including the spine.

His 8-year-old brother has had 3 fractures, but there is otherwise no family history of recurrent fractures or osteoporosis in his other 3 siblings, parents, or extended family. Prior laboratory tests show normal levels of calcium, phosphate, PTH, 25-hydroxyvitamin D, complete blood cell count, and erythrocyte sedimentation rate. Celiac antibodies are negative.

Which of the following evaluations (if any) should be performed now?

A. Reassurance only; fractures very common in boys and all of his fractures occurred with trauma

B. DXA of whole body and spine

C. Bone biopsy

D. LH, FSH, prolactin, and testosterone measurements

E. Genetic studies for osteogenesis imperfecta

Answer: E) Genetic studies for osteogenesis imperfecta

Fractures in otherwise healthy youth are a common injury. By 16 years of age, up to 40% of otherwise healthy girls and 64% of boys will have experienced at least 1 broken bone, with a peak incidence in the peripubertal years.[6] Epidemiological studies have shown that these injuries are not distributed evenly; some children fracture more than once, while others escape injury. The risk of a second fracture has been estimated to double for a child who has already had 1 fracture. This increase in fracture rates persists after controlling for risk-taking behavior, suggesting there may be underlying differences in bone strength among those with fractures.

The concerning features in this teen's history are the large number of fractures beginning before age 5 years, the occurrence of a femur facture, and the low-trauma nature of the first arm fracture (fall from standing height). Two-thirds of the fractures in healthy youth involve the distal radius and hand. By contrast, femur, hip, and spine fractures occurring without major trauma suggest abnormal bone fragility. There are enough concerning features in this patient's history to argue against reassurance alone (Answer A). DXA of the whole body and spine (Answer B), even if abnormal, does not establish a diagnosis of osteoporosis. DXA was indeed performed in this patient and showed spine and whole-body BMD Z-scores of –1.7 and –1.1, respectively. These were not corrected for height and may have overestimated his actual areal BMD. A bone biopsy (Answer C) would be indicated only if noninvasive testing were nondiagnostic. His growth, BMI, and Tanner staging are normal, making assessment of sex steroids (Answer D) less helpful. Genetic testing (Answer E) was performed in this patient, which confirmed a pathogenic variant in the *COL1A1* gene. He was treated with bisphosphonates for 3 years, stopped playing contact sports, and remained fracture-free during the subsequent 4 years.

Case 3

A 9-year-old boy with Duchenne muscular dystrophy (DMD) is referred for discussion of bisphosphonate therapy to prevent fractures. DMD was diagnosed at age 5 years, and deflazacort, 0.8 mg/kg, was started at that time. He remains ambulatory at home but uses a wheelchair at school and participates in adaptive physical education. He has never had a long bone fracture and does not complain of back pain. Serial DXAs at another facility show a decline in spine BMD Z-scores from –1.7 to –2.1 over the past 2 years. His parents are concerned about his fracture risk after reading posts on a DMD parents' website, and they want to start medication now to prevent their son from having a broken bone.

Which of the following do you advise at this visit?

A. Start once-weekly oral alendronate

B. Start intravenous zoledronic acid

C. Start intravenous pamidronate

D. Obtain lateral spine x-ray

E. Repeat DXA in 6 months and treat if Z-score is less than −2.5

Answer: D) Obtain lateral spine x-ray

It is well established that the reduced mobility, chronic inflammation, delayed growth and puberty, and exposure to long-term, high-dosage glucocorticoids in patients with DMD create a clinical "perfect storm" for bone fragility. Low-impact fractures both in long bones and in the vertebrae (once glucocorticoids are initiated) are common. The lack of skeletal loading contributes to narrower bones with thinner cortices. Glucocorticoids appear to have a greater impact on trabecular bone in the spine. Similar risk factors for osteoporosis complicate other chronic disorders characterized by inflammation, growth delay, reduced activity, and pharmacologic dosages of glucocorticoids. The decline in BMD Z-score in this patient is not unexpected and reflects the slower rate of growth and bone mineral accrual in DMD, perhaps compounded by accelerated bone loss from the glucocorticoids. However, the change in BMD Z-score alone is not a sufficient indication for drug therapy (thus, Answer E is incorrect). The best next step is a lateral spine radiograph (Answer D) or vertebral fracture assessment by DXA. Finding a vertebral fracture would establish the diagnosis of osteoporosis and would be an indication to offer bisphosphonates.

The question raised by this case is the indication for bisphosphonates as primary prevention for patients at high risk such as this one. Are there sufficient data to guide who should be treated and when? At present, the standard of care has been to initiate pharmacologic therapy only *after* a first fracture has occurred in the hopes of preventing more. Bisphosphonates (Answers A, B, and C) would not be recommended based on changes in BMD alone. Furthermore, oral bisphosphonates such as alendronate have not been shown to be as effective as intravenous agents in preventing vertebral fractures in children.[4] Given the increased incidence of vertebral fracture in patients receiving glucocorticoids, alendronate would not be a preferred drug.

Primary prevention drug trials are worthy of future investigation if the population of children to be targeted can be determined. Valuable insights into predicting fractures have come from longitudinal observational studies conducted by the Steroid-Associated Osteoporosis in the Pediatric Population (STOPP) network, a consortium of pediatric bone centers across Canada. This research has identified several clinical and laboratory correlates of fragility fractures in patients with acute lymphoblastic leukemia, nephrotic syndrome, and rheumatologic disorders. At the time of diagnosis, 16% of children with acute lymphoblastic leukemia had at least 1 fracture. The cumulative risk of incident vertebral fracture and nonvertebral fracture was 32.5% and 23%, respectively, over the next 6 years; 71% occurred in the first 2 years of treatment.[12] The presence of even 1 mild grade 1 vertebral fracture predicted future fractures, a phenomenon called the "vertebral fracture cascade." Cumulative, average daily dose, and short bursts of high-dose "pulse therapy" of glucocorticoids were strong correlates of fracture. Other factors associated with vertebral fracture include younger age, lower BMD, cranial and spinal radiation, endocrine deficits, decreased physical activity, and vitamin D deficiency. Randomized controlled trials could be designed to target those at highest risk for incident fracture and those least likely to exhibit healing (reshaping) of the vertebral deformities.

References

1. Gordon CM, Zemel BS, Wren TA, et al. The determinants of peak bone mass. *J Pediatr.* 2016;180:261-269. PMID: 27816219

2. Rizzoli R, Bianchi ML, Garabedian M, McKay HA, Moreno LA. Maximizing bone mineral mass gain during growth for the prevention of fractures in the adolescent and the elderly. *Bone.* 2010;46(2):294-305. PMID: 19840876

3. Gordon CM, Leonard MB, Zemel BS; International Society for Clinical Densitometry. 2013 Pediatric Position Development Conference: executive summary and reflections [published correction appears in *J Clin Densitom.* 2014;17(4):517]. *J Clin Densitom.* 2014;17(2):219-224. PMID: 24657108

4. Ward LM, Konji VN, Ma J. The management of osteoporosis in children. *Osteoporosis Int.* 2016;27(7):2147-2179. PMID: 27125514

5. Grover M, Bachrach LK. Osteoporosis in children with chronic illnesses: diagnosis, monitoring, and treatment. *Curr Osteoporos Rep.* 2017;15(4):271-282. PMID: 28620868

6. Clark EM. The epidemiology of fractures in otherwise healthy children. *Curr Osteoporos Rep.* 2014;12(3):272-278. PMID: 24973964

7. Zemel BS, Leonard MB, Kelly A, et al. Height adjustment in assessing dual energy x-ray absorptiometry measurements of bone mass and density in children. *J Clin Endocrinol Metab.* 2010;95(3):1265-1273. PMID: 20103654

8. Genant HK, Wu CY, van Kuijk C, Nevitt MC. Vertebral fracture assessment using a semiquantitative technique. *J Bone Miner Res.* 1993;8(9):1137-1148. PMID: 8237484

9. Griffin LM, Thayu M, Baldassano RN, et al. Improvements in bone density and structure during anti-TNF-α therapy in pediatric crohn's disease. *J Clin Endocrinol Metab.* 2015;100(7):2630-2639. PMID: 25919459

10. Southmayd EA, Hellmers AC, De Souza MJ. Food versus pharmacy: assessment of nutritional and pharmacological strategies to improve bone health in energy-deficient exercising women. *Curr Osteoporos Rep.* 2017;15(5):459-472. PMID: 28831686

11. Ackerman KE, Singhal V, Baskaran C, et al. Oestrogen replacement improves bone mineral density in oligo-amenorrhoeic athletes: a randomised clinical trial. *Br J Sports Med.* 2019;53(4):229-236. PMID: 30301734

12. Ward LM, Ma J, Lang B, Ho J, et al; Steroid-Associated Osteoporosis in the Pediatric Population (STOPP) Consortium. Bone morbidity and recovery in children with acute lymphoblastic leukemia: Results of a six-year prospective study. *J Bone Miner Res.* 2018;33(8):1435-1443. PMID: 29786884

Diabetes Insipidus in Children

Craig A. Alter, MD. Division of Endocrinology and Diabetes, Children's Hospital of Philadelphia, Pearlman School of Medicine at the University of Pennsylvania, Philadelphia, PA; E-mail: alterc@email.chop.edu

Learning Objectives

As a result of participating in this session, learners should be able to:

- Determine when and when not to perform a water-deprivation study.

- Formulate a plan to determine the cause of central diabetes insipidus (DI).

- Describe the pros and cons of various therapies for DI.

Main Conclusions

Although DI is considered as a possible diagnosis when children have polyuria, other diagnoses should be considered. In addition to hyperglycemia, other conditions such as thyrotoxicosis, hypercalcemia, and hypokalemia can lead to polyuria. Protein malnutrition can produce dilute urine. Some medications such as lithium can lead to poor renal water reabsorption. Psychogenic polydipsia is the most common state that must be distinguished from central DI. In children with polyuria and polydipsia, a serum osmolality exceeding 300 mOsm/kg with a simultaneous urine osmolality less than 300 mOsm/kg confirms the diagnosis of DI. The threshold of urine osmolality used to exclude DI ranges from 600 to 750 mOsm/kg. In clinical practice, it has been observed that some patients whose initial urine osmolality is between these values are subsequently diagnosed with partial DI. Thus, it is advised to use a urine osmolality threshold of at least 750 mOsm/kg to assess the possibility of DI when there is clinical suspicion for disease.

Once the diagnosis of central DI is established, an organized approach to diagnosing the cause is crucial. The most common causes are idiopathic (likely hypophysitis), tumor, histiocytosis, germ-cell tumors, structural defects, and congenital (genetic) defects.

Treatment may involve ensuring specific water intake, desmopressin (oral, intranasal, or subcutaneous formulations), and occasionally diuretics.

Significance of the Clinical Problem

After establishing a diagnosis of central DI, MRI of the pituitary is mandatory if the etiology is not known. The pediatric endocrinologist is often faced with various findings on MRI and must decide when repeat scanning is needed or whether a central nervous system biopsy is mandated. This chapter will outline an organized approach to using MRI to formulate a plan. Correlations of MRI findings to clinical parameters will be reviewed. In addition, the pros and cons of choosing different formulations of desmopressin will be discussed.

Barriers to Optimal Practice

- One of the challenges in establishing the etiology of central DI is that the diagnosis is usually not known after the initial MRI.

- The most important decision is how often to repeat MRI and when to obtain a central nervous system biopsy.

Strategies for Diagnosis, Therapy, and/or Management

Introduction

Arginine vasopressin (AVP) is crucial to maintaining water and osmolar homeostasis. The condition of DI may be due to inability of the kidneys to respond to AVP or to a disordered release or deficiency of AVP (central DI).

AVP is released in response to dehydration, along with activation of the renin-angiotensin system and thirst. The neurons that synthesize AVP are hypothalamic in origin, but they convene at the posterior pituitary. AVP is stored in granules in the posterior pituitary and are seen as the posterior pituitary "bright spot" on T1-weighted MRI imaging (a bright area in the posterior pituitary on a noncontrast film). AVP binds to the AVP V2 receptors in the collecting ducts of the renal tubules. Through a cyclic AMP signal transduction mechanism, this results in activation, transport, and insertion of aquaporin-2 water channels into the membranes of the collecting duct. As a result, there is increased permeability of the collecting duct to water and reabsorption of water back into the circulation. AVP also stimulates V1 α receptors on blood vessels, causing vasoconstriction. AVP is involved in von Willebrand factor production, as well as factor VIII synthesis.[1]

Blood pressure and plasma osmolality are maintained by a combined effort of thirst, AVP, the adrenal glands, and the kidneys. AVP increases in a linear fashion in response to even a 1% increase in osmolality or a 10% or more decrease in intravascular volume. For more details, please see *Pituitary Disorders of Childhood* (Humana Press, 2019).

Given the short half-life of AVP, it is difficult to use it in the clinical workup of a child with symptoms of DI. However, copeptin, a 39-amino acid glycosylated peptide that is synthesized along with AVP and neurophysin II in the hypothalamus, may prove to be useful clinically given its longer half-life. Copeptin measurement after infusion of hypertonic saline may be an alternative approach to water-deprivation testing in diagnosing DI, but this has not been studied in pediatric patients.[2]

The Child With Polydipsia and Polyuria

When a child presents with increased thirst or urination, there are important clues to pursue not only by history, but also on physical examination. New-onset or worsening enuresis should be questioned. Drinking from unusual sources such as puddles, bathtub faucets, the toilet, or other people's drinks suggests abnormal thirst. Trying to quantify the liquids can be useful. Fatigue is common and may be due to poor sleep, dehydration, potentially concomitant central hypothyroidism, or another systemic process. Occasionally, the degree of polydipsia decreases without therapy, but this should not be interpreted as reassurance that the underlying process has resolved. Primary polydipsia can be just as potent as the polydipsia from central DI. Growth chart analysis is crucial to the evaluation. Unusual rashes or bone abnormalities may support a diagnosis of Langerhans cell histiocytosis. Weight loss can signify a systemic process such as a germ-cell tumor or can result from the marked polyuria. While type 1 diabetes mellitus is at the top of the differential diagnosis list in patients with polyuria, it has usually been ruled out by the time central DI is considered. Asking questions about vision change is important, as it is common for a child and their family to be unaware of vision changes. For example, it would be important to know that a child recently diagnosed with central DI had been moved to the front row in the classroom due to concerns of mild blurriness.

Polyuria: Differential Diagnosis

Although central DI is considered a possible diagnosis when children have polyuria, other diagnoses should be considered before evaluating for central DI. These etiologies include endocrine and metabolic disorders, as well as medications that can lead to increased urine output. Hyperglycemia is a prime example. Hyperglycemia with a blood glucose concentration well above the renal threshold (145-160 mg/dL [8.0-8.9 mmol/L]) leads to an osmotic diuresis that resolves with initiation of diabetes therapy. Other endocrine disorders are associated with polyuria. Thyrotoxicosis can produce polyuria due to decreased expression of aquaporin water channel expression, despite adequate amounts of AVP, along with increased solute excretion. Hypercalcemia, regardless of etiology, can produce deficits in renal concentrating capacity. Hypokalemia can lead to defects in renal concentrating capacity via mechanisms that are not completely understood but may be related to accelerated autophagy-mediated degradation of aquaporin-2. Protein malnutrition can also produce increased output of dilute urine.

Diuretics can make the assessment of polydipsia and polyuria difficult. Lithium is unique because it reduces the renal responsiveness to AVP, leading to defects in urinary concentrating capacity.

Hypernatremia (Hyperosmolality)

Hypernatremia in the absence of polyuria most often reflects hypernatremic dehydration, as may occur in the setting of febrile illness, excessive losses of body free water (eg, diarrhea, burns), or impaired fluid intake. Hypernatremia can occur when thirst is impaired or there is inability to request increased fluids, which may be seen in those with neurological conditions, including brain trauma. Polydipsia in the absence of hypernatremia is less often related to a central lesion and may rather indicate a psychiatric disorder. In these cases, persistently low or low-normal serum sodium should raise suspicion for a psychiatric diagnosis. Psychogenic polydipsia is often mild, but in severe cases it may result in hyponatremic seizures.

Central DI

DI is diagnosed when the serum sodium concentration exceeds 145 mEq/L (>145 mmol/L), urine osmolality is less than 300 mOsm/kg, urine output is persistently greater than 4 mL/kg per h, and other causes of polyuria have been excluded.

Making the formal diagnosis of DI can be challenging and involves confirming a dilute urine in the setting of plasma hyperosmolality. Plasma osmolality can be calculated by measuring the concentration of sodium, glucose, and serum urea nitrogen. Sodium is the major effective plasma solute. When serum glucose and serum urea nitrogen are in the normal range, the sodium concentration correlates closely with serum osmolality.

$$pOsm = 2[sodium] + (glucose\ in\ mg/dL/18) + (serum\ urea\ nitrogen\ in\ mg/dL/2.8)$$

If the glucose value is in mmol/L, then there is no need to divide by 18.

In children with polyuria and polydipsia, a plasma osmolality exceeding 300 mOsm/kg, reflecting hyperosmolality, with a simultaneous urine osmolality less than 300 mOsm/kg confirms the diagnosis of DI. Additional testing can determine whether DI is central (responsive to AVP) or nephrogenic (nonresponsive to exogenous forms of AVP). In contrast, if a simultaneous serum osmolality is less than 270 mOsm/kg and the urine osmolality is maximally concentrated, the diagnosis of DI is excluded. The threshold of urine osmolality used to exclude DI ranges from 600 to 750 mOsm/kg. In our clinical practice, we have cared for patients who were subsequently diagnosed with partial DI whose initial urine osmolality was between these values. Thus, it is advised to use a urine osmolality threshold of at least 750 mOsm/kg to assess the possibility of DI when there is strong clinical suspicion for disease.

Water-deprivation testing carries associated risks (most notably dehydration) and should be performed in a carefully monitored setting. Water-deprivation studies in patients with longstanding partial DI may not reveal classic results. In such patients, the urine may only concentrate partially with the addition of pharmacological AVP, even though they have central DI.[3]

Establishing the Etiology of Central DI

Once the diagnosis of central DI is established, it is important, yet challenging, to determine its etiology. Any infiltrative process that involves the hypothalamic-pituitary axis can cause central DI, as well as anterior pituitary hormone deficiencies. Embryologic neurodevelopmental disorders presenting with anterior pituitary hormone deficiencies, such as septo-optic dysplasia, can result in central DI, even if not present clinically at birth. Central DI may occur in conjunction with multiple anterior pituitary hormone deficiencies; hence, anterior pituitary testing and surveillance is warranted. The appearance of anterior pituitary hormone deficits may occur years later, especially if the cause is Langerhans cell histiocytosis. Genetic defects of either AVP production or of its complex with neurophysin II can lead to central DI.

After establishing a diagnosis of central DI, MRI of the pituitary gland and hypothalamus is the first step in identifying the etiology.[4,5] MRI of the whole brain is insufficient to evaluate the pituitary gland. A dedicated MRI of the pituitary should be requested with and without gadolinium contrast to optimally visualize the pituitary gland. MRI of the pituitary without contrast should show a bright appearance of the posterior pituitary, termed the *posterior pituitary "bright spot"* on T1-weighted imaging. This bright spot is often, although not invariably, absent in central DI of any cause. Many clinicians do not advise diagnosing DI based on the presence or absence of the posterior pituitary bright spot alone. However,

in select cases, absence of the posterior pituitary bright spot can be used to provide additional evidence supporting the diagnosis of DI—either central DI or nephrogenic DI.

A child who has an ectopic posterior pituitary gland recognized on T1-weighted images as an ectopic posterior pituitary bright spot does not typically have central DI but is at risk for anterior pituitary hormone deficiencies.[6,7]

When there is a sellar or suprasellar mass on MRI, an important diagnosis to consider is craniopharyngioma. Calcifications strongly suggest craniopharyngioma. CT is more reliable than MRI in detecting calcifications. Other possibilities of masses that can cause central DI include arachnoid cyst, meningioma, teratoma, or lymphoma. Inflammatory and infiltrative disorders including Langerhans cell histiocytosis, germ-cell tumor, hypophysitis, or sarcoidosis can present with pituitary stalk thickening (germ-cell tumors include not only germinomas, but also teratomas, yolk sac tumors, choriocarcinoma, and embryonal carcinoma).

MRI in children with central DI shows a thickened stalk in approximately one-third of cases. Of the children with a thickened stalk, one study showed that 17% were eventually diagnosed with a germ-cell tumor and 17% were diagnosed with Langerhans cell histiocytosis. In the absence of bone lesions and a clear diagnosis of Langerhans cell histiocytosis, serum and cerebrospinal fluid tumor markers for quantitative hCG and α-fetoprotein should be obtained at initial presentation to assess for the possibility of a central nervous system germ-cell tumor.

It is recommended to measure tumor markers and anterior pituitary hormone levels in children presenting with central DI and a thickened infundibulum. Pituitary MRI and measurement of serum tumor markers and anterior pituitary hormones should be performed every 3 months for 1 to 2 years, then yearly for 2 years. Resolution of pituitary stalk thickening is more often associated with lymphocytic hypophysitis and confers a positive prognosis. Sometimes lesions from Langerhans cell histiocytosis can also decrease, or increase, in size. In one study, an infundibular stalk greater than 4.5 mm in thickness was correlated with a greater likelihood of developing multiple anterior pituitary hormone deficiencies.

A normal-appearing stalk and normal anterior pituitary hormone levels at the time central DI is diagnosed is generally reassuring, but these findings do not always exclude an underlying pathology. For example, the stalk was normal in appearance in one child who was subsequently diagnosed with a germ-cell tumor. In children presenting with central DI, a normal pituitary stalk on MRI, and no additional central nervous system risk factors (eg, headaches, seizures, or vision concerns), it is recommended to perform a repeated MRI in 3 to 6 months, then every 6 to 12 months for the next 2 years.[8]

While most cases of central DI are acquired, some may be genetic. Genetic cases of central DI are typically associated with an autosomal dominant inheritance pattern, although rarely an autosomal recessive or X-linked pattern is observed. On MRI, the bright spot is absent and the stalk size is normal. More than 55 pathogenic variants that cause central DI have been described; most are associated with autosomal dominant inheritance. Pathogenic variants have been described in the gene that encodes the AVP peptide, resulting in reduced AVP biological activity.

Other cases of central DI result from congenital or acquired anatomic disruption to the posterior pituitary. In one series of 147 children with central DI, 24% had an associated central nervous system malformation.[5] Congenital malformations include septo-optic dysplasia, holoprosencephaly, vascular malformations, and encephalocele. Central DI can occur following traumatic brain injury or pituitary-hypothalamic surgery. Transient central DI can be seen after transsphenoidal pituitary surgery.

Treatment of the Child With Central DI

The approach to the treatment of children with central DI should be tailored to each family. Desmopressin was introduced in the 1970s and remains the main treatment. Desmopressin is a synthetic analogue of the hormone 8-arginine AVP and has a longer half-life than AVP. The antidiuretic action is more specific than that of AVP, and it has less pressor activity. The duration of action of desmopressin is variable; therefore, the dosage and schedule are titrated to each child. Desmopressin is available for outpatient therapy as a pill, nasal spray, or subcutaneous injection. The adverse effects of desmopressin include fluid retention and hyponatremia.

Central DI Following Neurosurgery: The Triphasic Response

Complete or transient DI can develop in children following neurosurgical procedures involving the pituitary/hypothalamus region. A well-described triphasic response of DI/SIADH/DI is seen in the immediate postoperative period following complete stalk resection, as observed in many children following surgery for craniopharyngioma.

The Infant With Central DI

Management of neonatal DI is particularly difficult, as infants cannot communicate thirst and are dependent on caretakers for providing fluids. Often, fluids alone are used to treat DI, although adding a thiazide class of diuretics with a low solute intake can be effective. If desmopressin is added, typically a low dosage is chosen.[9,10]

Summary

The management of DI in children involves several areas of focus. The first challenge is in establishing the diagnosis, which in itself, has risks. In addition, those with partial or evolving central DI can have reassuringly normal laboratory results and may require prolonged water deprivation to prove there is DI. After the diagnosis of central DI is established, the search for the cause is vital. Germ-cell tumors and Langerhans cell histiocytosis may only be found after a few years of frequent MRI assessments. The treatment of central DI should be tailored to each patient.

Clinical Case Vignettes

Case 1

A 12-year-old boy presents with excessive thirst and urination of 6 months duration. He is otherwise well, with no central nervous system concerns. He has started puberty (Tanner stage 2), and his growth chart is unremarkable other than some weight loss in the past few months. School performance has been fine, but he reports fatigue out of the ordinary. His sodium concentration is 143 mEq/L (143 mmol/L), and his urine is dilute.

Which of the following statements is true?

A. MRI is indicated to look for a pituitary tumor

B. The weight loss and fatigue suggest that tumor markers should be obtained

C. Careful examination is indicated to look for a rash

D. His age rules out familial DI

Answer: C) Careful examination is indicated to look for a rash

About 15% to 20% of children presenting with central DI have Langerhans cell histiocytosis. Langerhans cell histiocytosis can affect the bone and skin and lead to a rash on the arms and groin. Thus, careful examination for a rash (Answer C) is correct. MRI (Answer A) is incorrect because MRI is typically performed after the diagnosis of central DI is established. It is not indicated for nephrogenic DI. The patient's symptoms are typical of polyuria/polydipsia and by themselves do not imply there is a malignancy. Therefore, obtaining tumor markers (Answer B) is not indicated now. Tumor markers are indicated if the diagnosis of central DI is confirmed, even if those

symptoms are not present. Familial DI can present even in older teenagers, so his age does not rule out familial DI (Answer D).

Case 2

A 5-year-old girl with behavioral issues is found to be drinking from unusual sources such as puddles. She has new-onset enuresis.

Laboratory test results:

> Serum sodium = 152 mEq/L (136-142 mEq/L) (SI: 152 mmol/L [136-142 mmol/L])
> Serum urea nitrogen = 8 mg/dL (8-23 mg/dL) (SI: 2.9 mmol/L [2.9-8.2 mmol/L])
> Blood glucose = 80 mg/dL (70-99 mg/dL) (SI: 4.4 mmol/L [3.9-5.5 mmol/L])
> Urine osmolality = 193 mOsm/kg (150-1150 mOsm/kg) (SI: 190 mmol/kg [150-1150 mmol/kg])

Which of the following is true regarding the diagnosis of central DI in this patient?

A. A low copeptin concentration would establish the diagnosis of DI of any cause

B. A water-deprivation study is indicated but should be done on an inpatient basis

C. Therapy with desmopressin can be initiated

D. Serum and urine osmolality should be measured

Answer: C) Therapy with desmopressin can be initiated

This child has a calculated serum osmolality already above 304 mOsm/kg (twice the sodium), plus the additional component from the glucose (5 mOsm/kg). This finding, coupled with the urine, establishes the diagnosis of DI. A low copeptin concentration in the face of hyperosmolality might imply central DI (Answer A); however, this remains to be proven in children. In addition, it would be a test only for central DI, not nephrogenic DI. The main point of this vignette is to show that sometimes a water-deprivation study (Answer B) is not needed, as the diagnosis is already established. The calculated osmolality is well above 305 mOsm/kg. It would have been nice to measure the osmolality (Answer D), but the diagnosis of DI is already established. This patient could have nephrogenic DI, so a trial of desmopressin (Answer C) and MRI (if there is a response to desmopressin) should be the next steps.

References

1. Majzoub JA, Srivatsa A. Diabetes insipidus: clinical and basic aspects. *Pediatr Endocrinol Rev.* 2006;4(Suppl 1):60-65. PMID: 17261971

2. Fenske W, Refardt J, Chifu I, et al. A copeptin-based approach in the diagnosis of diabetes insipidus. *N Engl J Med.* 2018;379(5):428-439. PMID: 30067922

3. Di Iorgi N, Napoli F, Allegri AE, et al. Diabetes insipidus--diagnosis and management. *Horm Res Paediatr.* 2012;77(2):69-84. PMID: 22433947

4. Maghnie M, Cosi G, Genovese E, et al. Central diabetes insipidus in children and young adults. *N Engl J Med.* 2000;343(14):998-1007. PMID: 11018166

5. Werny D, Elfers C, Perez FA, Pihoker C, Roth CL. Pediatric central diabetes insipidus: brain malformations are common and few patients have idiopathic disease. *J Clin Endocrinol Metab.* 2015;100(8):3074-3080. PMID: 26030323

6. Murray PG, Hague C, Fafoula O, et al. Associations with multiple pituitary hormone deficiency in patients with an ectopic posterior pituitary gland. *Clin Endocrinol (Oxf).* 2008;69(4):597-602. PMID: 18331606

7. Chen S, Leger J, Garel C, Hassan M, Czernichow P. Growth hormone deficiency with ectopic neurohypophysis: anatomical variations and relationship between the visibility of the pituitary stalk asserted by magnetic resonance imaging and anterior pituitary function. *J Clin Endocrinol Metab.* 1999;84(7):2408-2413. PMID: 10404812

8. Alter CA, Bilaniuk LT. Utility of magnetic resonance imaging in the evaluation of the child with central diabetes insipidus. *J Pediatr Endocrinol Metab.* 2002;15(Suppl 2):681-687. PMID: 12092681

9. Korkmaz HA, Demir K, Kilic FK, et al. Management of central diabetes insipidus with oral desmopressin lyophilisate in infants. *J Pediatr Endocrinol Metab.* 2014;27(9-10):923-927. PMID: 24854529

10. Rivkees SA, Dunbar N, Wilson TA. The management of central diabetes insipidus in infancy: desmopressin, low renal solute load formula, thiazide diuretics. *J Pediatr Endocrinol Metab.* 2007;20(4):459-469. PMID: 17550208

Screening of the Newborn for Adrenoleukodystrophy

Molly O. Regelmann, MD. Division of Pediatric Endocrinology and Diabetes, Department of Pediatrics, Children's Hospital at Montefiore, Albert Einstein Medical College, Bronx, NY; E-mail: moregelm@montefiore.org

Learning Objectives

As a result of participating in this session, learners should be able to:

- Describe the various presentations and pathophysiology of adrenoleukodystrophy (ALD).

- Explain the newborn screening process and apply adrenal insufficiency surveillance and treatment recommendations to boys identified with ALD.

Main Conclusions

ALD is the most common peroxisomal disorder and presents variably with adrenal insufficiency, neurologic disease, and testicular dysfunction. Recently, ALD was added to state newborn screening panels. Initial newborn screening data suggest that ALD may be more prevalent than previously described and adrenal insufficiency may develop in some affected boys during early infancy. Early monitoring, diagnosis, and treatment of adrenal insufficiency can prevent life-threatening adrenal crisis. The Pediatric Endocrine Society developed an algorithm to guide clinicians caring for boys with ALD identified by newborn screening. The publication suggests a monitoring schedule for adrenal insufficiency, addresses the ambiguities in cortisol and ACTH test results, and guides therapeutic decisions for boys with ALD.[1]

Significance of the Clinical Problem

ALD is a heterogeneous disease that frequently causes primary adrenal insufficiency in affected males.[2,3] Unrecognized and untreated adrenal insufficiency is associated with morbidity and mortality.[1,4] Following the passage of Aidan's Law, New York was the first state to initiate newborn screening for ALD on December 30, 2013. ALD was added to the Recommended Uniform Screening Panel in 2016.[1,5] As of October 2019, newborn screening for ALD has been expanded to 13 states and the District of Columbia with plans to be added to several more states' screening panels in the next 2 years. Adrenal insufficiency develops in most males with ALD, but predicting onset of and diagnosing adrenal insufficiency remain clinical challenges given the limited knowledge of the natural history of adrenal insufficiency in ALD and the subtle and variable clinical presentations.[1-3]

Barriers to Optimal Practice

- Infants do not have established predictable diurnal variation in ACTH and cortisol secretion.

- Normal reference ranges for ACTH and cortisol during infancy are not well established.

- There is no known predictable time course for when adrenal insufficiency will develop in males with ALD.

Strategies for Diagnosis, Therapy, and/or Management

Pathophysiology and Epidemiology

ALD has 6 clinical presentations (*Table*) and is caused by pathogenic variants in the *ABCD1* gene, located on chromosome Xq28. *ABCD1* encodes adrenoleukodystrophy protein, an ATP-binding cassette protein that normally forms a transmembrane channel responsible for the transport of very long-chain fatty acids (VLCFA) into the peroxisome for degradation.[2,3] Pathogenic variants in *ABCD1* (more than 800 described variants - https://adrenoleukodystrophy. info/mutations-and-variants-in-abcd1) lead to elevations in VLCFA. Eighty percent of women heterozygous for and all men hemizygous for pathogenic *ABCD1* variants have elevations in VLCFA.[2] In males, the excess VLCFA accumulate in the adrenal cortex, nervous system, and testicular Leydig cells. There is no correlation between the *ABCD1* variant and the degree of VLCFA elevation. Furthermore, there is no genotype-phenotype correlation, and the degree of VLCFA elevation is not predictive of onset of adrenal insufficiency or neurologic symptoms.[2,6]

In the adrenal cortex, VLCFA preferentially accumulate in the zona fasciculate and zona glomerulosa, leading to glucocorticoid and androgen deficiencies, most commonly. However, mineralocorticoid deficiency is described in some patients with ALD. VLCFA are thought to be directly cytotoxic to adrenocortical cells. In vitro studies also support VLCFA disrupting ACTH receptor function and leading to adrenocortical atrophy.[1]

Before newborn screening, the estimated incidence of ALD in the United States was 1 in 21,000 males and 1 in 14,000 females. The sex discrepancy has been proposed possibly to be secondary to unrecognized adrenal insufficiency.[1] Lower than expected diagnoses rates have also been reported in ethnic minorities.[7] In a prospective study of 49 asymptomatic male patients (mean age 4.5 ± 3.5 years) identified to have ALD based on family history, 80% had abnormal or borderline abnormal adrenal function tests at baseline and 86% did by the end of the study period (mean follow-up 2 ± 1.7 years). None of the 18 patients tested had mineralocorticoid deficiency.[8] In a retrospective review of 159 male

Table. Clinical Presentations of Adrenoleukodystrophy[2,3]

Type of ALD (Frequency)	Description	Age of Onset
Childhood cerebral ALD (~31%-35% of affected males)	Typically presents with symptoms similar to attention-deficit hyperactivity disorder and then rapidly progresses to impaired cognition and motor dysfunction, followed by complete disability (without supportive measures, fatal within 2 to 4 years of symptom onset). Most patients with cerebral ALD have adrenal insufficiency at diagnosis.	First decade (typically not before 2 years)
Adolescent cerebral ALD (~4%-7% of affected males)		Second decade
Adult cerebral ALD (~2%-5% of affected males)		After second decade
Adrenomyeloneuropathy (AMN) (~40%-46% of affected males)	Progressive stiffness/weakness in the legs (spasticity), bowel and bladder incontinence, sexual dysfunction, mood disturbance. Approximately 70% have adrenal insufficiency at diagnosis.	Third to fourth decade
Adrenal insufficiency only (decreases with age)	Primary adrenal insufficiency symptoms (hyperpigmentation, weight loss/growth failure, nausea/anorexia/abdominal pain, fatigue, lack of pubic/axillary hair, and less often salt-wasting if mineralocorticoid deficiency is present).	First decade (peak reported between 3 and 10 years)
Asymptomatic	No symptoms of ALD but at high risk for both adrenal insufficiency and neurologic disease.	Newborn

patients with ALD in 2 large neurology clinics, there was an estimated 80% lifetime prevalence of adrenal insufficiency, with most developing adrenal insufficiency during childhood and adolescence (median age of diagnosis, 14 years). There was an average delay in diagnosis of adrenal insufficiency of 3.5 years (range, 0.25-21 years) based on reported symptoms, and more than two-thirds had endocrine symptoms at the time of ALD diagnosis. A significant number of patients were treated with mineralocorticoid, but the median time to therapy initiation was significantly older at 56 years.[6]

Newborn Screening

ALD is considered an ideal condition for screening, as there is a presymptomatic phase and life-saving interventions are available to treat both the primary adrenal insufficiency and cerebral ALD. State programs have varying protocols, but all measure VLCFA from filter paper specimens. In some states, after confirmation of elevated VLCFA, *ABCD1* gene sequencing is available. The sensitivity and specificity of the filter paper VLCFA measurements are reported to be excellent for males hemizygous for pathogenic *ABCD1* variants. As 20% of females heterozygous for *ABCD1* pathogenic variants do not have VLCFA elevations, they are not expected to be identified by newborn screening. VLCFA are also elevated in other, rarer peroxisomal disorders, including but not limited to Zellweger syndrome, acyl CoA oxidase deficiency, and D-bifunctional protein deficiency, which do not have good therapeutic interventions for neurologic disease at this time. Once a patient is identified to have elevated VLCFA on newborn screening, most state protocols refer infants and families to a metabolic center for confirmatory testing and genetic counseling. Because ALD is X-linked, it is common to identify additional family members at risk for ALD, some of whom may require urgent evaluations for adrenal insufficiency or cerebral ALD.[5]

Surveillance for Adrenal Insufficiency

Initial recommendations for adrenal insufficiency surveillance did not address the unpredictable secretory pattern or lack of robust reference data for ACTH and cortisol during the first few years of life.[5] The Pediatric Endocrine Society Drug and Therapeutics/Rare Diseases Committee recognized the gap in knowledge and the need for clinical guidance when caring for boys with ALD.[1] Other than case reports and the referenced studies above,[6,8] there is little published about the natural history of adrenal insufficiency associated with ALD. The youngest patients reported to have biochemical evidence of adrenal dysfunction were 5 months old,[8] 7 months old,[6] and, in a recent case series, 5 weeks and 4.5 months old.[9] Given the limited experience with male infants known to have ALD and case reports found in the literature, as well as clinician experience, the recommendation was made to start screening shortly after ALD diagnosis. Follow-up surveillance for adrenal insufficiency was recommended every 3 to 4 months for children younger than 2 years and every 4 to 6 months for children older than age 2 years (more frequent screening was recommended in the younger age group due to the challenge of identifying symptoms of adrenal insufficiency in patients younger than 2 years). The algorithm developed for adrenal insufficiency surveillance in males with ALD was not only designed to address the unpredictable nature of adrenal insufficiency associated with ALD, but also to consider the potential pitfalls of ACTH and cortisol interpretation during the first few years of life (*Figure*).[1]

Figure. Suggested Algorithm for Surveillance of Adrenal Function[1]

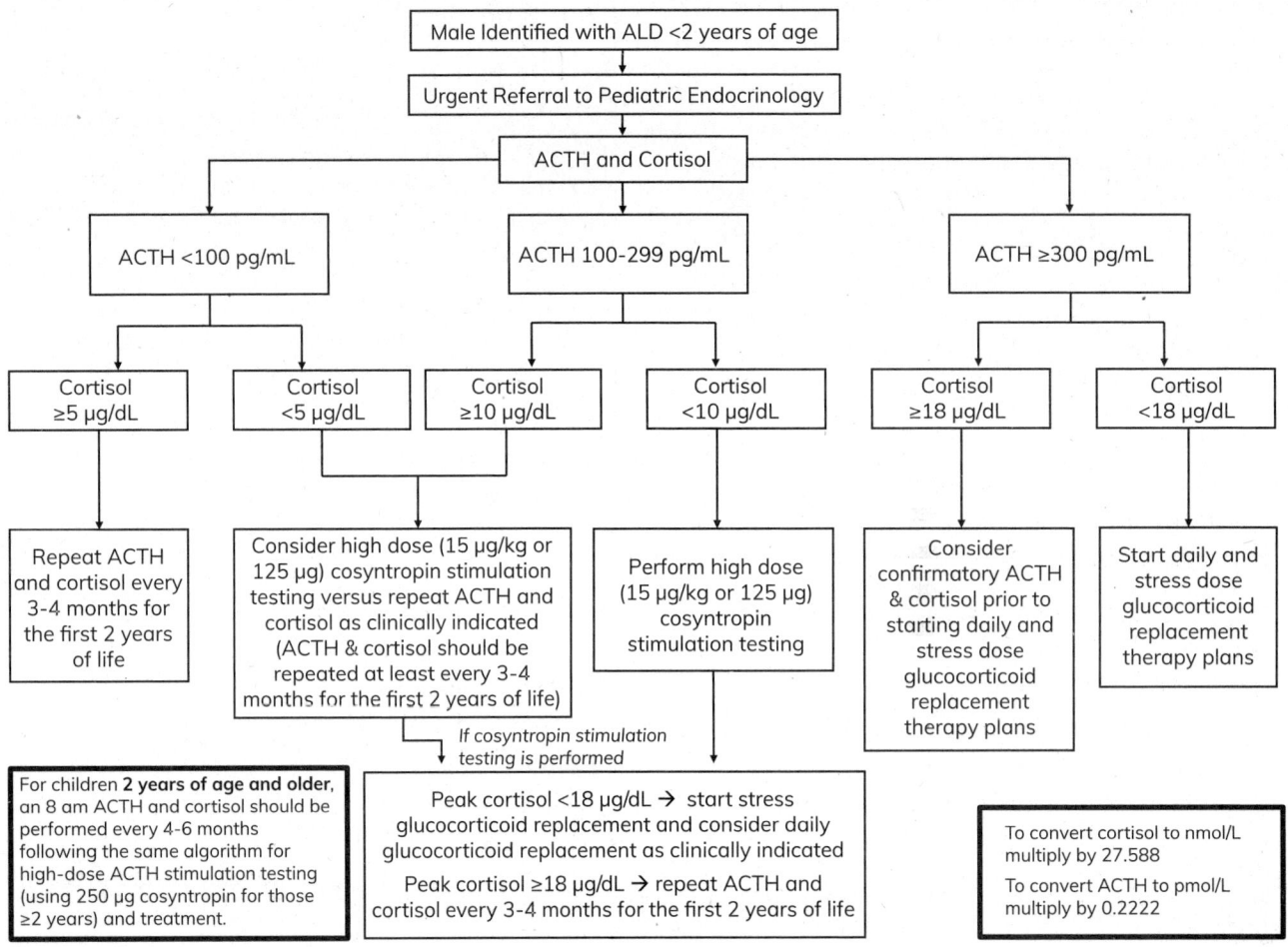

For children **2 years of age and older**, an 8 am ACTH and cortisol should be performed every 4-6 months following the same algorithm for high-dose ACTH stimulation testing (using 250 µg cosyntropin for those ≥2 years) and treatment.

To convert cortisol to nmol/L multiply by 27.588
To convert ACTH to pmol/L multiply by 0.2222

Management of Adrenal Insufficiency

Treatment of adrenal insufficiency associated with ALD is the same as treatment for most other causes of primary adrenal insufficiency.[10] Hydrocortisone is the preferred glucocorticoid and, for ALD, the starting dosage is 8 to 12 mg/m² daily divided into 3 doses. Doses should be increased with stress, and a standardized "Adrenal Insufficiency Action Plan" has recently been published to provide guidance for safe outpatient and emergency department management of adrenal insufficiency. It is recommended that all patients receive an individualized treatment plan, including instructions to increase oral hydrocortisone (2 to 3 times physiologic doses administered every 6 to 8 hours in times of stress) and to administer injectable hydrocortisone when unable to take oral stress doses. All caregivers should be provided training for administration of injectable hydrocortisone. Patients with adrenal insufficiency should be instructed to wear medical identification alerting emergency medical care providers to the need for steroid therapy.[4]

Neurologic Disease: Cerebral ALD and Adrenomyeloneuropathy

An extensive review of the pathophysiology, surveillance, and treatment of neurologic disease is beyond the scope of this chapter. Surveillance MRI protocols for cerebral ALD vary, but generally, MRI of the brain is initiated around 12 months of age and performed annually until age 3 years, when the risk for cerebral ALD increases. Surveillance MRI of the brain is then repeated every 6 months until age 10 years. After 10 years of age, brain MRI is performed annually, as risk for cerebral ALD decreases. Brain MRI is performed more frequently when concerning lesions are noted. Cerebral ALD, when detected in its earliest stages, can be treated with hematopoietic stem-cell therapy. Gene therapy has also been reported to halt cerebral ALD, although this therapy is still considered investigational. At present, only supportive therapies are available to manage adrenomyeloneuropathy.[2,3]

Additional Resources for Providers, Patients, and Families

- ALD Info – https://adrenoleukodystrophy.info
- ALD Connect – https://aldconnect.org
- Aidan Jack Seeger Foundation – https://aidanhasaposse.org
- Leukodystrophy Network (Hunter's Hope) – https://www.huntershope.org/family-care/leukodystrophies/adrenoleukodystrophy/

Clinical Case Vignettes

Case 1

A 3-month-old male infant is identified on New York State newborn screening as having elevations in VLCFA and a de novo variant of uncertain clinical significance in the *ABCD1* gene. The variant is predicted to be pathogenic based on models. His parents receive genetic counseling at an outside institution, and the baby's initial screening cortisol and ACTH are reported to be "normal." His mother is of Western European descent and his father is of African descent. He now presents for a pediatric endocrine consultation visit at 1 PM. He is exclusively breastfed and typically gets up at night to feed every 4 hours. Stool and urine patterns are reported as typical for age, without concerns for constipation.

On physical examination, his length and weight are at the 50th percentile and consistent with the pediatrician's parameters from the 3-month-old well-child visit. He seems to have a skin tone that is between his mother's and father's (both present for the visit), but it is possible that the scrotum and areolae are slightly hyperpigmented. His tone is normal, and findings on neurologic examination are normal.

Which of the following is the best next step in this patient's evaluation?

A. Draw sample for ACTH measurement today

B. Draw sample for cortisol measurement today

C. Draw sample for both ACTH and cortisol measurement today

D. Have the baby return for an 8-AM draw for ACTH and cortisol measurement

E. Perform a high-dose cosyntropin-stimulation test today

Answer: C) Draw sample for both ACTH and cortisol measurement today

This baby is at high risk for adrenal insufficiency due to ALD. After taking a detailed history and performing the exam, the clinician should counsel the parents about signs and symptoms of adrenal insufficiency. Signs and symptoms can often be subtle, and there are reports of male infants with ALD as young as 5 weeks with test results consistent with adrenal insufficiency. The parents should be given an explanation of options for evaluation. The baby is unlikely to have predictable diurnal secretion of ACTH and cortisol, as he is not sleeping through the night and is younger than 6 months. Therefore, ACTH and cortisol can be drawn in the clinic in the early afternoon (thus, Answer C is correct and Answer D is incorrect). One may be able to measure ACTH alone (Answer A), but if the level is borderline elevated, cortisol measurement is needed to interpret whether the level is appropriate. Evolving primary adrenal insufficiency may be missed by measuring cortisol without ACTH (Answer B), as ACTH will rise before the cortisol is frankly low. If travel to the clinic is a significant burden for a family, a cosyntropin-stimulation test (Answer E) can be discussed. It is not unusual to obtain ambiguous test results at baseline and need to recall for a cosyntropin-stimulation test. Parents should be counseled about the ambiguity of test results and be included in decisions regarding additional testing and treatment.[1]

Case 2

A 16-month-old boy presents to the pediatric endocrinology clinic for routine adrenal insufficiency surveillance. He was identified on Connecticut newborn screening to have elevated VLCFA and was subsequently diagnosed with ALD based on confirmatory testing with a peroxisomal screen (confirmed elevated VLCFA) and *ABCD1* gene sequencing, which identified a known pathogenic variant. He has had routine adrenal insufficiency surveillance since diagnosis was confirmed at 6 weeks of age. He had an 8-AM blood draw a few days ago in anticipation of today's visit.

Laboratory test results are shown in the table.

On physical examination, his weight is at the 25th percentile (previously was at the 35th percentile) and length is at the 25th percentile (previously at the 23rd percentile). He seems developmentally appropriate and is climbing on the chairs in the exam room. He is of Hispanic descent and appears to have more pigmentation on his scrotum and in the axillary creases than you recall from the previous visit.

Question 1: At what age would you have started stress doses of hydrocortisone?

A. 6 weeks

B. 4 months

C. 7 months

D. 13 months

E. 16 months

Answer: A) 6 weeks

On the basis of the algorithm (*Figure*), stress doses of hydrocortisone should have been started at 6 weeks of age (Answer A), when the peak cortisol concentration was 17.1 µg/dL (471.8 nmol/L). It is notable that the cutoff of 18 µg/dL (496.6 nmol/L) is based on older polyclonal assays and it is possible that newer monoclonal assays may have lower normal cutoffs.[1]

Question 2: At what age would you have started daily doses of hydrocortisone?

A. 6 weeks

B. 4 months

C. 7 months

D. 13 months

E. 16 months

Answer: D) 13 months

Age	ACTH	Cortisol	Stimulated Cortisol
6 weeks	92 pg/mL (SI: 20.2 pmol/L)	1.2 µg/dL (SI: 33.1 nmol/L)	...
6 weeks	...	4.3 µg/dL (SI: 118.6 nmol/L)	17.1 µg/dL (SI: 471.8 nmol/L)
4 months	176 pg/mL (SI: 38.7 pmol/L)	8.0 µg/dL (SI: 220.7 nmol/L)	16.9 µg/dL (SI: 466.2 nmol/L)
7 months	212 pg/mL (SI: 46.6 pmol/L)	9.0 µg/dL (SI: 248.3 nmol/L)	...
10 months	120 pg/mL (SI: 26.4 pmol/L)	13.0 µg/dL (SI: 358.6 nmol/L)	...
13 months	314 pg/mL (SI: 69.1 pmol/L)	12.1 µg/dL (SI: 333.8 nmol/L)	...
16 months	429 pg/mL (SI: 94.4 pmol/L)	10.2 µg/dL (SI: 281.4 nmol/L)	...

Based on the algorithm, daily hydrocortisone doses should have been started at age 13 months (Answer D). The ACTH cutoff of 300 pg/mL or higher (≥66 pmol/L) was chosen, as it is reported that the adrenal cortex is maximally stimulated with an ACTH concentration of 300 pg/mL (66 pmol/L). However, it is important to emphasize that the algorithm is intended to be a guide and is not meant to replace good clinical judgment. In an otherwise asymptomatic child who is being monitored closely and is receiving stress doses of hydrocortisone, the decision to continue stress doses of hydrocortisone as clinically indicated and to monitor for another short interval before starting daily doses may be a viable option at 13 months (as it appears was done in this patient's case). It is not unusual for ACTH and cortisol levels to fluctuate, and if the ACTH concentration were in the 200s pg/mL (44 pmol/L) with a cortisol concentration greater than 10 µg/dL (>275.9 nmol/L), the algorithm suggests holding off on daily doses. Conversely, if at 7 months, the baby were not gaining weight well and had evidence of hyperpigmentation, even with the ACTH concentration being less than 300 pg/mL (<66 pmol/L), it may have been reasonable to consider starting daily hydrocortisone therapy. The decisions regarding hydrocortisone therapy should be based on a combination of clinical signs and symptoms, as well as laboratory testing.[1]

References

1. Regelmann MO, Kamboj MK, Miller BS, et al; Pediatric Endocrine Society Drug and Therapeutics/Rare Diseases Committee. Adrenoleukodystrophy: guidance for adrenal surveillance in males identified by newborn screen. *J Clin Endocrinol Metab.* 2018;103(11):4324-4331. PMID: 30289543

2. Raymond GV, Moser AB, Fatemi A. X-linked adrenoleukodystrophy. GeneReviews. February 15, 2018. Available at: from https://www.ncbi.nlm.nih.gov/books/NBK1315/. Accessed for verification December 2019.

3. Engelen M, Kemp S, de Visser M, et al. X-linked adrenoleukodystrophy (X-ALD): clinical presentation and guidelines for diagnosis, follow-up and management. *Orphanet J Rare Dis.* 2012;7:51. PMID: 22889154

4. Miller BS, Spencer SP, Geffner ME, et al. Emergency management of adrenal insufficiency in children: advocating for treatment options in outpatient and field settings. *J Investig Med.* 2019 [Epub ahead of print]. PMID: 30819831

5. Vogel BH, Bradley SE, Adams DJ, et al. Newborn screening for X-linked adrenoleukodystrophy in New York State: diagnostic protocol, surveillance protocol and treatment guidelines. *Mol Genet Metab.* 2015;114(4):599-603. PMID: 25724074

6. Huffnagel IC, Laheji FK, Aziz-Bose R, et al. The natural history of adrenal insufficiency in X-linked adrenoleukodystrophy: an international collaboration. *J Clin Endocrinol Metab.* 2019;104(1):118-126. PMID: 30252065

7. Bonkowsky JL, Wilkes J, Bardsley T, Urbik VM, Stoddard G. Association of diagnosis of leukodystrophy with race and ethnicity among pediatric and adolescent patients. *JAMA Netw Open.* 2018;1(7):e185031. PMID: 30646379.

8. Dubey P, Raymond GV, Moser AB, Kharkar S, Bezman L, Moser HW. Adrenal insufficiency in asymptomatic adrenoleukodystrophy patients identified by very long-chain fatty acid screening. *J Pediatr.* 2005(4);146(4):528-532. PMID: 15812458

9. Eng L, Regelmann MO. Early onset primary adrenal insufficiency in males with adrenoleukodystrophy: case series and literature review. *J Pediatr.* 2019;211:211-214. PMID: 31101408

10. Bornstein SR, Allolio B, Arlt W, et al. Diagnosis and treatment of primary adrenal insufficiency: an Endocrine Society clinical practice guideline. *J Clin Endocrinol Metab.* 2016;101(2):364-389. PMID: 26760044

Diagnosis and Management of Congenital Adrenal Hyperplasia in Children

Phyllis W. Speiser, MD. Department of Pediatrics, Zucker School of Medicine at Hofstra, Cohen Children's Medical Center of New York, Northwell Health, Lake Success, NY; E-mail: pspeiser@northwell.edu

Learning Objectives

As a result of participating in this session, learners should be able to:

- Describe the clinical presentation of various types of congenital adrenal hyperplasia (CAH) in the pediatric age group.
- Recall the latest Endocrine Society Clinical Practice Guidelines for managing CAH.

Main Conclusions

Timely diagnosis, treatment, and monitoring of CAH in infants, children, and adolescents can optimize outcomes in terms of growth, puberty, reproductive potential, and emotional health throughout the lifespan. Persons with classic CAH are most often diagnosed by mandatory newborn screening. Such individuals require lifelong steroid replacement treatment with periodic evaluation of adrenocortical hormone levels. In children, ancillary biomarkers of adrenal control include steady growth, normal body weight, normally timed puberty, and epiphyseal maturation as seen on serial bone age x-rays. Persons with nonclassic CAH (NCAH) most often present after infancy and are usually not at risk for clinically significant adrenal insufficiency. Glucocorticoid treatment may be selectively considered in patients manifesting adrenal hormone excess, such as precocious puberty, hirsutism, oligomenorrhea, acne, or infertility. Multidisciplinary specialty care is desirable to address comorbidities.

Significance of the Clinical Problem

CAH is a disease due to one of several enzyme defects in steroidogenesis that leads to decreased cortisol feedback and excess ACTH (*Table*). The most common defect is in the activity of steroid 21-hydroxylase (encoded by *CYP21A2*), found in 1:14,000 to 1:18,000 live births worldwide.[1] Consequences of severe forms of this enzyme deficiency include insufficient production of cortisol and, in about 75% of patients, insufficient aldosterone to maintain sodium homeostasis, resulting in potentially lethal salt-wasting. These perturbations simultaneously cause the overproduction of adrenal sex hormone precursors, with genital atypia or ambiguity in newborn females. Most classic or severe cases of CAH are detected by newborn screening programs via filter paper assay with typical marked elevations of blood 17-hydroxyprogesterone. Affected females have genital differences as a flag for the diagnosis, whereas newborn males show no physical signs of the disease until adrenal salt-wasting crisis occurs.[2] Surprisingly, up to 20% of affected females may be missed based on clinical criteria alone, demonstrating the value of screening to begin treatment to prevent morbidity and mortality.[3] Glucocorticoid replacement, preferably as hydrocortisone, is usually lifelong. Mineralocorticoid replacement as fludrocortisone and sodium chloride supplements is required in infancy but may eventually be tapered as dietary salt consumption increases.

Nonclassic milder forms of CAH, with a prevalence of approximately 1 in 1000 persons in the general population, are not usually detected by newborn screening programs, nor is this the target of screening, as NCAH is not a fatal disease. NCAH presents in childhood, or even adult life. Typically, females with NCAH do not have genital ambiguity; however, there is a wide phenotypic spectrum.[1] As a consequence of the variable adrenal androgen excess seen in NCAH, some affected children grow rapidly, undergo premature pubarche, and have advanced epiphyseal maturation detected on bone age x-ray. Nonetheless, average adult height is well within the normal range.[4] Affected adolescents may have hirsutism (approximately 60% of affected females), oligomenorrhea or amenorrhea (54%), and acne vulgaris (33%).[5] It should be noted that signs of androgen excess are also associated with the even more prevalent polycystic ovary syndrome.[6] Thus, thorough evaluation should be performed and treatment targeted to the cause of hyperandrogenism, as not all individuals with androgen excess symptoms have adrenal pathology. Precise diagnostic markers for polycystic ovary syndrome are lacking, and the diagnosis in adolescence is still debated.[7]

Barriers to Optimal Practice

Barriers to optimal practice include lack of familiarity with these conditions among health care providers and the absence of newborn screening for CAH in some areas. Additionally, it is frequently challenging to balance steroid replacement so as to avoid undertreatment or overtreatment.

Strategies for Diagnosis, Therapy, and/or Management

Newborn screening is universal in the United States and many developed countries, although protocols differ in terms of heel-stick filter paper sample timing, type of assay, secondary screening tests, cut-points for each test, and how abnormal results are triaged. The gold standard diagnostic test for CAH is a cosyntropin (ACTH 1-24)-stimulation test. Although *CYP21A2* genotyping is feasible, it is not commonly used as the test of first choice. This is because of the complexity of the gene locus, comparatively high cost of genetic testing, and lag time to getting results. After infancy, screening for NCAH may be accomplished by measuring early morning serum 17-hydroxyprogesterone (17-OHP) by specific assay methods (eg, tandem mass spectrometry, LC-MS/MS). In postpubertal female patients, blood sampling should be done in the early follicular phase of the menstrual cycle, if possible.

Serum 17-OHP should be less than 200 ng/dL (<6.1 nmol/L) when measured in the early morning for screening purposes by LC-MS/MS. Radioimmunoassay results are less reliable. If one cannot use the preferred assay method, then a cosyntropin-stimulation test should be done with measurement of baseline and 1-hour serum values of adrenal steroids to establish the hormonal diagnosis. Genotyping is useful if hormonal diagnosis is equivocal and for the purposes of genetic counseling.

Medical treatment for classic CAH consists of hormone replacement with glucocorticoid and mineralocorticoid. Hydrocortisone (10 to 15 mg/m² per day in children) is the preferred glucocorticoid for maintenance therapy because of its shorter duration of action and fewer adverse effects, especially growth suppression, compared with more potent medications (eg, prednisolone and dexamethasone). The dosage is titrated to maintain serum 17-OHP and androstenedione in the high-normal range for age and gender. Serum testosterone may also be measured in prepubertal males and in females at all ages. Mineralocorticoid is given as oral fludrocortisone (0.05-0.2 mg daily).

Table. Features of Various Types of CAH

Feature/Adrenal Deficiency	21-Hydroxylase	11β-Hydroxylase	17α-Hydroxylase	3β-Hydroxysteroid Dehydrogenase	Lipoid Hyperplasia	P450 Oxidoreductase
Defective Gene	CYP21A2	CYP11B1	CYP17A1	HSD3B2	STAR or 20,22 Lyase	POR
Genital Atypia	+ XX	+ XX	+ XY	+ XY, mild XX	+ XY	Variable
Puberty	Early if untreated	Early if untreated	Absent in XX	Early if untreated	Absent	Variable
Acute Adrenal Insufficiency	+	Rare	None	+	+	Variable
Incidence	1:15000	1:100,000	Rare	Rare	Rare	Rare
Cortisol	Low	Low	Compensated by high corticosterone	Low	Low	+/- Low
Mineralocorticoids	Low	High	High	Low	Low	Variable
Androgens	High	High	Low	Low XY; high XX	Low	Variable
Marker Metabolites	17-hydroxy-progesterone	DOC, 11-deoxycortisol	DOC; corticosterone	DHEA; 17-hydroxy-pregnenolone	None, all low	Steroid profiling
Blood Pressure and Sodium Balance	Low	High	High	Low	Low	Variable

Meta-analysis has shown that mineralocorticoid treatment is associated with improved height.[4] Sodium chloride supplements are prescribed for infants, typically at a dosage of 1 g in divided doses in feedings; these supplements may continue in later life, as needed. Mineralocorticoid and sodium dosing should be titrated to serum electrolytes and plasma renin activity.[1]

Ancillary parameters that should be monitored in children with CAH are growth charts showing height, weight, and BMI over time, bone age x-rays, and blood pressure. Testicular adrenal rests, benign tumors detected on ultrasonography, are common among boys and men with classic forms,[8] but relatively rare in boys and men with NCAH.

Clinical Case Vignettes
Case 1

On third-trimester fetal ultrasonography in a G1P0 mother, a potential fetal genital anomaly is observed. The baby girl is born at term with a birth weight of 3130 g in a small community hospital. Genital ambiguity is observed, and the baby is transferred to a university medical center for endocrine consultation. The endocrinologist's examination findings are notable for external genital virilization, Prader stage 3, consisting of a 1 × 1-cm clitoro-phallic structure, nonrugated labial folds, and a single perineal urethral-vaginal opening. After obtaining blood for diagnostic studies, the baby is started on oral hydrocortisone, 2.5 mg every 8 hours; oral fludrocortisone, 0.05 mg daily; and sodium chloride, 1 g daily as oral 7% NaCl solution with feeds every 3 hours.

Pelvic ultrasonography shows a normal uterus. No gonads are identified. Renal ultrasonography is negative for hydronephrosis or renal anomalies.

On day 3 of life, the newborn screen for 17-hydroxyprogesterone is markedly elevated at 576 ng/mL (<35 ng/mL), indicative of classic CAH. Her pretreatment serum 17-OHP concentration returns as 25,700 ng/dL (779 nmol/L), confirming classic salt-wasting CAH. Karyotype is 46,XX. Genotype analysis shows homozygous deletions in *CYP21A2* consistent with severe, classic, salt-wasting 21-hydroxylase deficiency CAH.

After hospital discharge, her medication dosages are adjusted, with the hydrocortisone dosage reduced to 1.25 mg 3 times daily (as crushed, weighed tablets), and fludrocortisone increased to 0.1 mg daily due to a low serum sodium concentration of 130 mEq/L (130 mmol/L) and elevated plasma renin activity of 155 ng/mL per h.

Her adrenal profile at 6 months of age reveals an acceptable serum 17-OHP concentration of 648 ng/dL (19.6 nmol/L). Androstenedione and testosterone are suppressed (13 ng/dL [0.45 nmol/L] and <3 ng/dL [<0.10 nmol/L], respectively). Plasma renin activity is low-normal at 2.2 ng/mL h, and serum sodium and potassium are also normal. She has had no interval illnesses or salt-wasting crises and is growing well, between the 25th and 50th percentile for height and weight.

There is no family history of infertility, infant demise, or adrenal disease.

Does this infant need a cosyntropin-stimulation test for diagnosis?

Answer: No. With a baseline 17-OHP concentration greater than 20,000 ng/dL (>606 nmol/L), cosyntropin stimulation is not needed if the phenotype is consistent with classic 21-hydroxylase deficiency CAH.

Does the genotype alter clinical management in this case?

Answer: No. There is already ample evidence that this child is affected with classic salt-wasting CAH, and her phenotype is typical for this condition. Knowing the *CYP21A2* pathogenic variants is helpful for genetic counseling should the parents wish to have more children.

How long should one keep her on the high hydrocortisone dosage (ie, 25-30 mg/m² per day) before reducing the dosage?

Answer: Repeated adrenal hormone profiling should be done in 2 to 3 weeks, and the hydrocortisone dosage should be reduced if the hormone levels are suppressed.

What is the maximum hydrocortisone dosage one should give infants?

Answer: No more than 15 to 17 mg/m² per day is advised to avoid adverse effects.

When should one reduce fludrocortisone and/or sodium supplements?

Answer: Once plasma renin activity is within the normal range, fludrocortisone may be reduced. Similarly, once serum sodium is normal on at least 2 measurements, one may begin tapering the sodium chloride supplements.

How often should one measure electrolytes?

Answer: This depends on the baby's clinical status, but at least twice within the first 4 to 6 weeks. If the infant is clinically and biochemically stable, one may rely on plasma renin activity for monitoring thereafter.

How should one counsel these parents regarding surgical intervention?

Answer: Parents should have an opportunity to discuss medical and surgical treatment plans with a multidisciplinary team. Parental preferences and values should be considered, and they should be informed of all options, including avoiding surgery or deferring surgery to age 6 to 12 months or even older to allow the mature adolescent to make this decision. There is no strong evidence to support either early or late surgery for CAH at this time.

How would you counsel the parents about future pregnancies?

Answer: Prenatal diagnosis is feasible. However, the Endocrine Society clinical practice guidelines do not support prenatal dexamethasone treatment because of the long-term safety concerns set forth in detail in that document. Preimplantation genetic diagnosis and embryo selection is an alternative to this quandary.

Case 2

A 16-year-old girl presents to her physician for excess weight gain and irregular menses. Menarche was at age 13 years, and thereafter she began to gain a great deal of weight. Menses are unpredictable and sometimes heavy, lasting from just 2 days to more than 1 week with irregular intervals, occurring up to 4 months apart. At age 16 years, she developed worsening acne and hirsutism on her face and lower abdomen requiring monthly waxing. There is no family history of polycystic ovary syndrome or adrenal disease.

On physical examination, she is an overweight adolescent girl with chin stubble. Her height is 60 in (152.5 cm) (5th percentile), and weight is 145 lb (65.8 kg) (81th percentile) (BMI = 28 kg/m^2 [93rd percentile]). Her blood pressure is 112/61 mm Hg. Ferriman-Gallwey score is 15 (normal <8) with grade 3 hirsutism on the chin, sideburns, chest, lower abdomen, and legs, following waxing 2 weeks earlier. She has moderate facial acne. Pubertal status is Tanner stage 5. Genital examination reveals no clitoromegaly or labial fusion.

A cosyntropin-stimulation test confirms the diagnosis of NCAH due to 21-hydroxylase deficiency. Genotyping reveals compound heterozygosity for the most common classic *CYP21A2* pathogenic variant (the intron 2 splice mutation), in combination with the typical nonclassic *CYP21A2* pathogenic variant, Val281Leu. This compound heterozygote genotype is associated with NCAH. Her parents and siblings are tested and determined to be heterozygous carriers. Pelvic ultrasonography shows a normal uterus with multifollicular ovaries that are not enlarged.

A lipid profile, thyroid function profile, and measurements of fasting glucose and insulin, gonadotropins, prolactin, and SHBG are normal.

The patient is initially treated with hydrocortisone, beginning at a dosage of 10 mg daily, then 20 mg daily, then 10 mg 3 times daily. Despite increasing the hydrocortisone dosage, she does not achieve satisfactory suppression of adrenal hormones, with persistently high early-morning predose serum 17-OHP, androstenedione, and testosterone. She gains another 10 lb (4.5 kg) within the year on a hydrocortisone dosage of 30 mg daily, even though

she has been following a diet and exercising regularly. However, she has noticed a decrease in body hair and more regular menses.

How might the treatment regimen be altered to improve adrenal cortical hormone levels?

Answer: The patient is now 16 years old and has likely attained her full height. Thus, there should no longer be a concern about potential growth suppression with long-acting glucocorticoids such as prednisolone.

What criteria should be used to assess adrenal control?

Answer: Since growth is complete, the important parameters to follow in this patient include weight, blood pressure, and principally, her adrenal steroid profile. The latter may include serum 17-OHP, androstenedione, and testosterone measured by LC-MS/MS. Before dosage changes are considered, there should be a consistent pattern observed in all of these analytes on at least 2 measurements.

When should blood samples be obtained?

Answer: Ideally, blood samples should be obtained at a consistent time in relation to medication dosing. There have been research attempts to measure blood or urine steroid profiles or obtain frequent 17-OHP levels by either saliva or fingerstick sampling, but these methods are not standard.

Does this patient have polycystic ovary syndrome?

Answer: The symptoms of polycystic ovary syndrome and NCAH often overlap and the two conditions may coexist. There is no single accepted diagnostic test specific for polycystic ovary syndrome. In the United States, the diagnosis of polycystic ovary syndrome is made by clinical and/or biochemical signs of hyperandrogenism and irregular menses. One must exclude known disorders causing hyperandrogenism, such as NCAH. In Europe, the demonstration of polycystic ovarian morphology is a requisite for diagnosis.[7] The young woman in this vignette is unlikely to have polycystic ovary syndrome if glucocorticoid treatment has resulted in hyperandrogenic symptom improvement.

Does this patient require additional medication such as contraceptives or insulin-sensitizing drugs?

Answer: If menses are regular and androgens remain suppressed with glucocorticoids, no other medications are needed. She should be encouraged to lose weight by diet and exercise. Adjunctive dermatologic treatments for hirsutism can be considered.[6]

What is this patient's prognosis for fertility?

Answer: Women with NCAH are most often fertile even without hormone treatments. There may be a mildly prolonged time lag to conception and slightly higher rate of miscarriage in the absence of treatment.[9]

Does she need to remain on long-term glucocorticoid treatment?

Answer: Not necessarily. If symptoms abate and there are no fertility issues, glucocorticoids may eventually be tapered and discontinued in patients with NCAH. This is not true for classic forms of CAH.

References

1. Speiser PW, Arlt W, Auchus RJ, et al. Congenital adrenal hyperplasia due to steroid 21-hydroxylase deficiency: an Endocrine Society clinical practice guideline. *J Clin Endocrinol Metab.* 2018;103(11):4043-4088. PMID: 30272171

2. White PC. Optimizing newborn screening for congenital adrenal hyperplasia. *J Pediatr.* 2013;163(1):10-12. PMID: 23522380

3. Heather NL, Seneviratne SN, Webster D, et al. Newborn screening for congenital adrenal hyperplasia in New Zealand, 1994-2013. *J Clin Endocrinol Metab.* 2015;100(3):1002-1008. PMID: 25494862

4. Muthusamy K, Elamin MB, Smushkin G, et al. Clinical review: adult height in patients with congenital adrenal hyperplasia: a systematic review and metaanalysis. *J Clin Endocrinol Metab.* 2010;95(9):4161-4172. PMID: 20823467

5. Moran C, Azziz R, Carmina E, et al. 21-Hydroxylase-deficient nonclassic adrenal hyperplasia is a progressive disorder: a multicenter study. *Am J Obstet Gynecol.* 2000;183(6):1468-1474. PMID: 11120512

6. Martin KA, Anderson RR, Chang RJ, et al. Evaluation and treatment of hirsutism in premenopausal women: an Endocrine Society clinical practice guideline. *J Clin Endocrinol Metab.* 2018;103(4):1233-1257. PMID: 29522147

7. Ibáñez L, Oberfield SE, Witchel S, et al. An International Consortium update: pathophysiology, diagnosis, and treatment of polycystic ovarian syndrome in adolescence. *Horm Res Paediatr.* 2017;88(6):371-395. PMID: 29156452

8. Claahsen-van der Grinten HL, Sweep FC, Blickman JG, Hermus AR, Otten BJ. Prevalence of testicular adrenal rest tumours in male children with congenital adrenal hyperplasia due to 21-hydroxylase deficiency. *Eur J Endocrinol.* 2007;157(3):339-344. PMID: 17766717

9. Eyal O, Ayalon-Dangur I, Segev-Becker A, Schachter-Davidov A, Israel S, Weintrob N. Pregnancy in women with nonclassic congenital adrenal hyperplasia: time to conceive and outcome. *Clin Endocrinol (Oxf).* 2017;87(5):552-556. PMID: 28731586

Youth-Onset Type 2 Diabetes Mellitus

Philip Zeitler, MD, PhD. Section of Endocrinology, Department of Pediatrics, University of Colorado School of Medicine, Aurora, CO; E-mail: philip.zeitler@childrenscolorado.org

Petter Bjornstad, MD. Section of Endocrinology, Department of Pediatrics, University of Colorado School of Medicine, Aurora, CO; E-mail: petter.bjornstad@childrenscolorado.org

Learning Objectives

As a result of participating in this session, learners should be able to:

- Describe the initial approach to evaluation and management of new-onset diabetes mellitus in the obese adolescent.

- Select and modify pharmacologic agents for treatment of youth with type 2 diabetes (T2DM).

- Develop an approach to the management of complications and cardiovascular risk in youth with T2DM.

Main Conclusions

Youth-onset T2DM is a complex metabolic disorder characterized by progressive β-cell injury and insulin resistance. With the rapidly rising number of obese adolescents with T2DM, it is critical to check pancreatic autoantibodies in the workup of youth-onset T2DM. Compared with T1DM, youth-onset T2DM also carries higher risk and earlier onset of severe complications, such as heart disease, diabetic kidney disease, and fatty liver disease. Options for management are limited and have been largely understudied in youth-onset T2DM. Currently FDA-approved medications include insulin, metformin, and liraglutide.

Significance of the Clinical Problem

Youth-onset T2DM is an emerging disorder in children, adolescents, and young adults, and it has unique clinical challenges. The incidence of T2DM in youth has increased dramatically over the last 20 years, although it remains a rare disorder. In the United States, the best estimates are that the incidence is as high as 5000 new cases per year, with a total prevalence of less than 50,000.[1,2] The pathophysiology of T2DM in youth resembles that in adults: insulin resistance and nonautoimmune β-cell injury. However, studies indicate that youth-onset T2DM has a number of unique aspects. For example, there is an important association of T2DM with pubertal development—the median age of onset of T2DM in youth is approximately 14 years. This observation is most likely related to the transient reduction in insulin sensitivity that occurs in children as they enter puberty[3] and the need for compensation in insulin secretion, which may lead to hyperglycemia in youth with limited β-cell capacity. Furthermore, diabetes onset during puberty may be reversible in some youth due to the dynamic nature of the underlying insulin resistance. And, while rates in adult men and women are similar, adolescent girls have a 60% higher prevalence rate than that of adolescent boys.[2] In addition, while decline in β-cell function also occurs in adults with T2DM, β-cell failure appears to be more rapid in youth than in adults, leading to loss of glycemic control on oral therapy that is more rapid.[4-11] Finally, there is evidence of microvascular complications and risk markers for macrovascular complications at the time of diagnosis, along with rapid progression of these complications.[12-15]

T2DM has a disproportionate impact on youth from ethnic/racial minorities and disadvantaged backgrounds and occurs in complex psychosocial and cultural environments that make durable lifestyle change elusive and adherence to medical recommendations a struggle. Furthermore, these complexities hinder successful recruitment into and completion of research programs, leaving large gaps in knowledge regarding pathophysiology and treatment optimization.[2,16-18]

Barriers to Optimal Practice

- Complex social milieu.
- Knowledge gaps in understanding underlying pathophysiology.
- Rapidly progressive course with frequent oral treatment failure.
- High risk of vascular complications.
- Limited clinical experience.
- Restricted access to diabetes medications.
- No evidence-based treatment guidelines.

Strategies for Diagnosis, Therapy, and/or Management
Diagnosis

The diagnosis of T2DM in youth requires 2 steps: confirmation of the presence of diabetes mellitus followed by determination of diabetes type. The criteria and classification of diabetes mellitus are provided in the American Diabetes Association annual guidelines and the International Society for Pediatric and Adolescent Diabetes Clinical Practice Consensus Guidelines.[19,20] However, there are several important points. First, while the American Diabetes Association has added hemoglobin A_{1c} as a diagnostic criterion, this assumes measurement in a laboratory with a

DCCT-aligned assay, not point-of-care testing, and it has not been specifically validated in youth. Second, in the absence of symptoms, hyperglycemia detected incidentally or under conditions of acute physiologic stress may be transitory and should not be regarded as diagnostic of diabetes. Accordingly, a second test on a different day is required.

After the diagnosis of diabetes is established, consideration should be given to determining diabetes type. There are features of presentation and phenotype that may be useful in developing a presumption of T2DM, although there is substantial overlap between characteristics of T2DM and T1DM in the obese adolescent, making these features of limited value. The degree of pubertal development may be the most useful, although in a negative fashion; youth with T2DM are almost always in puberty, with a mean age of diagnosis of 13 to 14 years and Tanner stage 4 to 5 and are rarely prepubertal.[21,22] Most importantly, diabetes autoantibody testing (glutamic acid decarboxylase antibodies [GAD], microinsulin autoantibodies [mIAA], zinc transporter 8 antibodies [ZnT8], tyrosine phosphatase-based islet antigen 2 antibody [IA2]) should be done in all youth with the clinical diagnosis of T2DM because of the high frequency of islet-cell autoimmunity in patients with otherwise "typical" T2DM.[21] The presence of antibodies predicts rapid development of insulin requirement, as well as risk for development of other autoimmune disorders. Diabetes autoantibody testing also should also be considered in overweight/obese pubertal children with a clinical picture of T1DM (weight loss, ketosis/ketoacidosis), some of whom may have T2DM and be able to be weaned off of insulin for extended periods of time.[23-25] Finally, single-gene forms of diabetes, such as maturity-onset diabetes of the young should be considered in individuals who have a presentation and course that is not characteristic of either T1DM or T2DM.

Management

Initial treatment of the obese adolescent with diabetes must take into account that diabetes type is often not certain in the first few weeks of treatment, that 10% to 15% of obese adolescents have T1DM, and that a substantial percentage of adolescents with T2DM present with clinically significant ketoacidosis.[21,26] Therefore, initial treatment should be based on the clinical presentation, while maintaining an open mind regarding both the diabetes type and eventual therapy.[19]

Obese adolescents presenting with acidosis require initiation of intravenous insulin. However, once acidosis is resolved, subsequent therapy depends on the provisional clinical diagnosis. When the clinical impression is T2DM, basal insulin at a dosage of 0.2 to 0.4 units/kg once daily is started and titrated based on fingerstick glucose measurements. Insulin is administered at whatever time of day is the most likely to promote good adherence. At the same time, metformin is initiated at 500 mg once daily and titrated weekly to a maximally tolerated dosage, with a target of 2000 mg daily. Insulin can generally be discontinued within a few weeks once antibody negativity has been confirmed.

Asymptomatic patients with an initial hemoglobin A_{1c} level greater than 9% or 10% (>75 or 86 mmol/mol) may also require initiation of once-daily basal insulin therapy to allow sufficient recovery of β-cell function for successful monotherapy with an oral medication. However, results from the TODAY study suggest that initiation of metformin and basic dietary intervention will result in a hemoglobin A_{1c} level in the nondiabetes range, with or without insulin.[25] Obese, asymptomatic adolescents presenting with a lesser degree of decompensation can be started on metformin alone, with a high likelihood of initial success. Patients not on insulin are asked to check their fingerstick glucose twice daily a few days each week and whenever they feel ill. This frequency of blood glucose monitoring represents a sustainable balance between providing adequate safety to identify gradual deterioration, while avoiding excessive burden on this generally poorly adherent population, particularly as adolescents quickly recognize that daily glucose readings are not used for medication adjustment.

Lifestyle change is critical to treatment of T2DM, and clinicians should initiate a lifestyle modification program, including nutrition and physical activity, for children and adolescents at the time of diagnosis.[27] The interventions include promoting a healthy lifestyle through behavior change, including nutrition, exercise training, weight management, and smoking cessation. However, the challenges in implementing lifestyle modifications in adolescents are greater than in adult patients, since many adolescent patients with T2DM come from families where overeating and a sedentary lifestyle are considered the norm. Thus, many adolescents with T2DM will not maintain the recommended lifestyle changes and will remain overweight with poor diabetes control.[28]

The target of therapy is to attain and maintain hemoglobin A_{1c} below 6.5% (<48 mmol/mol). In most cases, this target can be successfully achieved and maintained for extended periods with metformin monotherapy, combined with focused lifestyle counseling and support. The approach to the adolescent with T2DM who does not attain and/or maintain target hemoglobin A_{1c} has not been studied systematically. In most cases, pediatric endocrinologists will add basal insulin as a second agent and titrate to achieve target hemoglobin A_{1c}.[19] This combination of basal insulin and metformin is often effective and may provide reliable glycemic control for extended periods. Failure to achieve target at an insulin dose of 1 unit/kg or evidence for poor control of postprandial glycemia may prompt consideration of the addition of rapid-acting insulin, but the known challenges with adherence in this population should be kept in mind. Premixed insulins may offer some benefits over rapid-acting insulin regarding ease of administration, but they require a degree of attention to mealtimes and snacks that is not always achievable.

Although major therapeutic advances have been made in diabetes care for adults with T2DM, the only FDA-approved medications as of June

2019 for youth with T2DM were metformin and insulin, although liraglutide, a GLP-1 receptor agonist, has recently been approved for youth based on data from the ELLIPSE trial.[29] Further compounding the issue, pharmacotherapy may have different effects in youth-onset T2DM vs adult-onset T2DM as illustrated in the recently completed Restoring Insulin Secretion (RISE) trial.[10,11]

Clinical Case Vignettes

Case 1

A 16-year-old Latina girl was diagnosed with diabetes mellitus 3 years ago by her primary care physician. At that time, diabetes type was determined based on clinical presentation and family history of T2DM. Metformin, 2000 mg daily, was prescribed, but she reports that she took this for only a few months. Since that time, she has taken no medications and reports no symptoms of diabetes, including polyuria, polydipsia, or weight loss. One month ago, she was admitted to the hospital following a suicide attempt. During that admission, she was noted to have a glucose value of 550 mg/dL (30.5 mmol/L) and glucosuria, with small ketonuria and normal venous pH. Her hemoglobin A_{1c} level was 12.5% (113 mmol/mol). She was treated by the inpatient team with subcutaneous basal and bolus insulin and restarted on metformin. She was referred to the diabetes center for further evaluation. At that visit, her BMI was 28 kg/m² and blood pressure was 125/72 mm Hg.

Given the length of time since original diagnosis, which of the following investigations is the most important next step in this patient's evaluation?

A. Fasting lipid panel

B. Fasting and stimulated C-peptide measurements

C. Home glucose measurements

D. Liver enzyme measurements

E. Pancreatic autoantibody measurements

Answer: E) Pancreatic autoantibody measurements

Even though this patient has had diabetes for 3 years without severe metabolic decompensation off treatment, there is no clinical characteristic with 100% sensitivity in excluding T1DM. Since T1DM remains more common than T2DM at all ages and in most ethnicities, the a priori risk for T1DM is higher than T2DM, despite "typical" characteristics. Furthermore, even among those race/ethnicity groups (African American, American Indian) in which T2DM is more common in adolescents, T1DM still occurs. A substantial percentage of adolescents with T1DM in the United States are obese, and obesity does not protect from autoimmunity.[30]

Therefore, even in this setting, the most important step in the evaluation of an adolescent with diabetes is rigorous determination of diabetes type. The presence of positive antibodies (Answer E), no matter what the phenotype, is associated with more rapid progression to insulin requirement, and patients with positive antibodies should be treated with insulin regardless of how they are doing on oral therapy.

Measurement of fasting C-peptide may be helpful in determining degree of insulin resistance and stimulated C-peptide (Answer B) may be a reasonable measure of insulin secretory capacity, potentially contributing to the distinction of T2DM from T1DM. However, this is only true in the setting of stable metabolic status. During acute decompensation, insulin and C-peptide secretion are transiently decreased. Measurement of C-peptide may be more useful in asymptomatic patients, patients who have recovered from decompensation, or in patients with presumed T2DM who have a persistent insulin requirement.

Fasting lipid panel (Answer A), home glucose measurements (Answer C), and liver enzyme measurement (Answer D) would be important to obtain at diagnosis in an obese individual with diabetes, regardless of diabetes type, but would be unlikely to make an immediate difference in therapeutic decisions. However, the specific screening done would depend on whether the individual has positive antibodies (TSH, celiac antibodies, lipids) or negative antibodies (lipids, AST/ALT, urine albumin, creatinine clearance).

Case 2

A 15-year-old Latino boy with long history of being overweight was recently found to have a fasting glucose concentration of 289 mg/dL (16.0 mmol/L) during a yearly exam for school. He has no complaints initially, but on questioning, he recalls some polyuria, polydipsia, and fatigue for the last few months. His mother has noted increased thirst, but thought it was due to the hot summer. The patient has been healthy and takes no medications.

On physical examination, his BMI is 32 kg/m² and blood pressure is 120/58 mm Hg. Pubertal development is Tanner stage 5, and the rest of the exam findings are unremarkable.

His hemoglobin A_{1c} level is 8.7% (72 mmol/mol) and antibodies (GAD, IA2, ZnT8, mIAA) are negative.

You prescribe metformin and titrate to 2000 mg daily. He returns in 3 months and reports that he has been taking his metformin every day and his mother confirms that she has been watching him. His hemoglobin A_{1c} level is now 7.1% (54 mmol/mol).

Which of the following is the best next step in this patient's management?

A. Measure fasting C-peptide

B. Measure stimulated C-peptide

C. Start liraglutide, 1.8 mg daily

D. Start basal insulin once daily

E. Start multiple daily injections with glargine and glulisine

Answer: D) Start basal insulin once daily

The patient is nearly at the American Diabetes Association and International Society for Pediatric and Adolescent Diabetes targets for glycemia,[17,18] and a common response would be that no changes are needed. However, recently published results from the TODAY study[9]

indicate that a hemoglobin A_{1c} level greater than 6.3% (>45 mmol/mol) after a few months of metformin monotherapy is associated with a 4- to 10-fold increased risk for loss of glycemic control, depending on sex and race/ethnicity, with a median time to loss of control of approximately 11 months. While it may be premature to start basal insulin at this initial visit, failure to achieve a hemoglobin A_{1c} level in the nondiabetes range on metformin monotherapy suggests that the provider taking care of this patient should initiate discussion with the family (the response to metformin has not been sufficient to date and add-on therapy may be necessary soon). Initiation of basal insulin (Answer D) is the standard approach to add-on therapy in the absence of evidence for oral or injected agents other than metformin and insulin.[19,28] Starting multiple daily injections (Answer E) would help with glycemia, but adherence among youth with T2DM is generally poor and it is preferable to use the simplest regimen possible.

Measurement of fasting C-peptide (Answer A) will provide information on insulin sensitivity, and measurement of stimulated C-peptide (Answer B) will provide information on β-cell reserve, but these factors are already incorporated into the hemoglobin A_{1c} measurement and will not affect management. Liraglutide (Answer C), a GLP-1 receptor agonist, was FDA approved in June 2019[29] and is a reasonable alternative for this patient. However, the starting dosage of liraglutide is 0.6 mg daily for 1 week, increasing to 1.2 mg injections thereafter. Starting liraglutide at the maximum dosage of 1.8 mg daily is not recommended due to a higher likelihood of adverse reactions (nausea, vomiting, diarrhea, anorexia, dyspepsia, and constipation). Additional agents, including SGLT-2 inhibitors, DPP-4 inhibitors, and dual gastric inhibitor polypeptide and GLP-1 receptor agonist are likely also useful, but not yet FDA approved in pediatrics and can therefore not be formally recommended.

Case 3

A 15-year-old Latina girl was recently diagnosed with T2DM during a routine physical examination. Her primary care physician prescribed metformin and referred her to the diabetes center. She has been healthy and takes no medications other than metformin. Her review of systems is negative. On physical examination, her BMI is 35 kg/m^2. Her hemoglobin A$_{1c}$ level is 7.8% (62 mmol/mol).

Which of the following should be prescribed as the most important next step in this patient's management?

A. Atorvastatin, 10 mg daily, for an LDL-cholesterol level of 160 mg/dL (4.14 mmol/L)

B. Fenofibrate, 67 mg daily, for a triglyceride level of 745 mg/dL (8.42 mmol/L)

C. Lisinopril, 10 mg daily, for a blood pressure of 145/82 mm Hg

D. Lisinopril, 20 mg daily, for a urinary albumin-to-creatinine ratio of 48 mg/g

E. Vitamin E, 600 IU daily, for an ALT level of 87 U/L (1.45 μkat/L)

Answer: B) Fenofibrate, 67 mg daily, for a triglyceride level of 745 mg/dL (8.42 mmol/L)

T2DM generally occurs in the setting of other insulin-resistant abnormalities, including lipid abnormalities, endothelial and cardiac dysfunction, increased procoagulant and inflammatory markers, increased hepatic and muscle lipid deposition, mitochondrial dysfunction, increased plasma uric acid, ovarian hyperandrogenism, and sleep disorders, all of which increase cardiovascular risk. Given the prevalence of comorbidities at the time of diagnosis,[31,32] evaluation should occur either at the time of initial diagnosis or upon reestablishment of metabolic stability.[19,27]

Blood pressure should be measured at every clinic visit and normalized for sex, height, and age. Initial treatment of blood pressure above the 95th percentile consists of weight loss, limitation of dietary salt, and increased physical activity. Thus, prescribing lisinopril now (Answer C) is incorrect.

After 6 months, if blood pressure is still above the 95th percentile, an ACE inhibitor could be started to achieve blood pressure values that are less than the 90th percentile. If the ACE inhibitor is not tolerated because of adverse effects (mainly cough), an angiotensin-receptor blocker may be used. Combination therapy may be required if hypertension does not normalize on single-agent therapy. Workup of hypertension not responsive to initial medication should also include renal ultrasonography and echocardiography.

Urinary albumin excretion should be assessed at diagnosis and annually. Microalbuminuria is defined as an albumin-to-creatinine ratio of 30 to 299 mg/g in a spot urine sample. Because an elevated value can be secondary to exercise, cigarette smoking, menstruation, and orthostasis, the diagnosis of persistent abnormal microalbuminuria requires documentation of 2 of 3 consecutive abnormal values obtained on different days, preferably on rising, as benign orthostatic proteinuria is common in adolescents. Thus, starting lisinopril now (Answer D) is incorrect. ACE inhibitors are the agents of choice due to proven renal protection, even if blood pressure is normal. Measurement of albumin excretion should be repeated at 3- to 6-month intervals, and therapy should be titrated to achieve a normal albumin-to-creatinine ratio. Non-diabetes–related causes of renal disease should be excluded, and consultation should be obtained if the albumin-to-creatinine ratio is greater than 300 mg/g.

Testing for dyslipidemia should be performed soon after diagnosis when blood glucose control has been achieved and annually thereafter. Goals for lipids are an LDL-cholesterol concentration less than 100 mg/dL (<2.59 mmol/L), triglyceride concentration less than 150 mg/dL (<1.70 mmol/L), and HDL-cholesterol concentration greater than 40 mg/dL (>1.04 mmol/L). If LDL cholesterol is above goal, blood glucose control should be maximized and dietary counseling provided (dietary cholesterol <200 mg daily, saturated fat <7% of total calories, and <30% calories from fat). If LDL cholesterol remains greater than 130 mg/dL (>1.04 mmol/L) after 6 months, statin therapy should be started with a target of less than 100 mg/dL (<2.59 mmol/L) (thus, Answer A is incorrect). The use of statins in sexually active adolescent females must be carefully considered and the risks explicitly discussed. Elevated triglycerides are not treated for cardiovascular disease prevention. However, if fasting triglycerides are greater than 500 mg/dL (>5.65 mmol/L), a fibric acid is started (Answer B) due to significantly increased risk for acute pancreatitis, with a treatment goal of less than 150 mg/dL (<1.70 mmol/L).

Hepatic steatosis is present in 25% to 50% of adolescents with T2DM, and more advanced forms of fatty liver disease are increasingly common and associated with progression to cirrhosis, portal hypertension, and liver failure.

Fatty liver is now the most frequent cause of chronic liver disorders among obese youth and is the most common reason for liver transplant in adults in the United States. T2DM therapies that improve insulin resistance appear to improve fatty liver. Vitamin E therapy (Answer E) may improve fatty liver, but it has also been linked with elevated all-cause mortality. Vitamin E is currently not recommended to treat hepatic steatosis in adolescents. Due to the potential for progression to steatohepatitis, fibrosis, and cirrhosis, ongoing monitoring of liver enzymes is recommended in youth with T2DM, with referral for biopsy if enzymes remain markedly elevated.

In addition, the clinician should explore the presence of polycystic ovary syndrome, depression, eating disorders, and sleep disturbance and address these as appropriate.

References

1. Lawrence JM, Imperatore G, Dabelea D, et al; SEARCH for Diabetes in Youth Study Group. Trends in incidence of type 1 diabetes among non-Hispanic white youth in the U.S., 2002-2009. *Diabetes.* 2014;63(11):3938-3945. PMID: 24898146

2. Dabelea D, Mayer-Davis EJ, Saydah S, et al; SEARCH for Diabetes in Youth Study. Prevalence of type 1 and type 2 diabetes among children and adolescents from 2001 to 2009. *JAMA.* 2014;311(17):1778-1786. PMID: 24794371

3. Hannon TS, Janosky J, Arslanian SA. Longitudinal study of physiologic insulin resistance and metabolic changes of puberty. *Pediatr Res.* 2006;60(6):759-763. PMID: 17065576

4. TODAY Study Group, Zeitler P, Hirst K, et al. A clinical trial to maintain glycemic control in youth with type 2 diabetes. *N Engl J Med.* 2012;366(24):2247-2456. PMID: 22540912

5. Rascati K, Richards K, Lopez D, Cheng LI, Wilson J. Progression to insulin for patients with diabetes mellitus on dual oral antidiabetic therapy using the US Department of Defense Database. *Diabetes Obes Metab.* 2013;15(10):901-905. PMID: 23531154

6. Kahn SE. Clinical review 135: the importance of beta-cell failure in the development and progression of type 2 diabetes. *J Clin Endocrinol Metab.* 2001;86(9):4047-4058. PMID: 11549624

7. Kahn SE, Lachin JM, Zinman B, et al; ADOPT Study Group. Effects of rosiglitazone, glyburide, and metformin on β-cell function and insulin sensitivity in ADOPT. *Diabetes.* 2011;60(5):1552-1560. PMID: 21415383

8. TODAY Study Group. Effects of metformin, metformin plus rosiglitazone, and metformin plus lifestyle on insulin sensitivity and β-cell function in TODAY. *Diabetes Care.* 2013;36(6):1749-1757. PMID: 23704674

9. Zeitler P, Hirst K, Copeland KC, et al; TODAY Study Group. HbA1c after a short period of monotherapy with metformin identifies durable glycemic control among adolescents with type 2 diabetes. *Diabetes Care.* 2015;38(12):2285-2292. PMID: 26537182

10. RISE Consortium; RISE Consortium Investigators. Effects of treatment of impaired glucose tolerance or recently diagnosed type 2 diabetes with metformin alone or in combination with insulin glargine on beta-cell function: comparison of responses in youth and adults. *Diabetes.* 201968(8):1670-1680. PMID: 31178433

11. RISE Consortium. Impact of insulin and metformin versus metformin alone on beta-cell function in youth with impaired glucose tolerance or recently diagnosed type 2 diabetes. *Diabetes Care.* 2018;41(8):1717-1725. PMID: 29941500

12. Copeland KC, Zeitler P, Geffner M, et al; TODAY Study Group. Characteristics of adolescents and youth with recent-onset type 2 diabetes: the TODAY cohort at baseline. *J Clin Endocrinol Metab.* 2011;96(1):159-167. PMID: 20962021

13. Sellers EA, Yung G, Dean HJ. Dyslipidemia and other cardiovascular risk factors in a Canadian First Nation pediatric population with type 2 diabetes mellitus. *Pediatr Diabetes.* 2007;8(6):384-390. PMID: 18036065

14. Hannon TS, Arslanian SA. The changing face of diabetes in youth: lessons learned from studies of type 2 diabetes. *Ann N Y Acad Sci.* 2015;1353:113-137. PMID: 26448515

15. Dart AB, Martens PJ, Rigatto C, Brownell MD, Dean JH, Sellers EA. Earlier onset of complications in youth with type 2 diabetes. *Diabetes Care.* 2014;37(2):436-443. PMID: 24130346

16. Zeitler P, Chou HS, Copeland KC, Geffner M. Clinical trials in youth-onset type 2 diabetes: needs, barriers, and options. *Curr Diab Rep.* 2015;15(5):28. PMID: 25777998

17. Fazeli Farsani S, van der Aa MP, van der Vorst mmJ, Knibbe CA, de Boer A. Global trends in the incidence and prevalence of type 2 diabetes in children and adolescents: a systematic review and evaluation of methodological approaches. *Diabetologia.* 2013;56(7):1471-1488. PMID: 23677041

18. Petitti DB, Klingensmith GJ, Bell RA, et al; SEARCH for Diabetes in Youth Study Group. Glycemic control in youth with diabetes: the SEARCH for Diabetes in Youth Study. *J Pediatr.* 2009;155(5):668-672. PMID: 19643434

19. Zeitler P, Arslanian S, Fu J, et al. ISPAD clinical practice consensus guidelines 2018: type 2 diabetes mellitus in youth. *Pediatr Diabetes.* 2018;19(Suppl 27):28-46. PMID: 29999228

20. American Diabetes Association. 13. Children and adolescents: standards of medical care in diabetes-2019. *Diabetes Care.* 2019;42(Suppl 1):S148-S164. PMID: 30559239

21. Fagot-Campagna A, Pettitt DJ, Engelgau mm, et al. Type 2 diabetes among North American children and adolescents: an epidemiological review and public health perspective. *J Pediatr.* 2000;136(5):664-672. PMID: 10802501

22. Copeland KC, Zeitler P, Geffner M, et al; TODAY Study Group. Characteristics of adolescents and youth with recent-onset type 2 diabetes: the TODAY cohort at baseline. *J Clin Endocrinol Metab.* 2011;96(1):159-167. PMID: 20962021

23. Klingensmith GJ, Pyle L, Arslanian S, et al; TODAY Study Group. The presence of GAD and IA-2 antibodies in youth with a type 2 diabetes phenotype: results from the TODAY study. *Diabetes Care.* 2010;33(9):1970-1975. PMID: 20519658

24. Laffel L, Chang N, Grey M, et al; TODAY Study Group. Metformin monotherapy in youth with recent onset type 2 diabetes: experience from the prerandomization run-in phase of the TODAY study. *Pediatric Diabetes.* 2012;13(5):369-375. PMID: 22369102

25. Kelsey MM, Geffner ME, Guandalini C, et al; Treatment Options for Type 2 Diabetes in Adolescents and Youth Study Group. Presentation and effectiveness of early treatment of type 2 diabetes in youth: lessons from the TODAY study. *Pediatr Diabetes.* 2016;17(3):212-221. PMID: 25690268

26. Pinhas-Hamiel O, Dolan LM, Zeitler P. Diabetic ketoacidosis among obese African-American adolescents with NIDDM. *Diabetes Care.* 1997;20(4):484-486. PMID: 9096965

27. Copeland KC, Silverstein J, Moore KR, et al; American Academy of Pediatrics. Management of newly diagnosed type 2 diabetes mellitus (T2DM) in children and adolescents [published correction appears in *Pediatrics.* 2013;131(5):1014]. *Pediatrics.* 2013;131(2):e648-e664. PMID: 23359574

28. Nadeau KJ, Anderson BJ, Berg EG, et al. Youth-Onset Type 2 Diabetes Consensus Report: Current Status, Challenges, and Priorities. *Diabetes Care.* 2016;39(9):1635-1642. PMID: 27486237

29. Tamborlane WV, Barrientos-Perez M, et al; Ellipse Trial Investigators. Liraglutide in children and adolescents with type 2 diabetes. *N Engl J Med.* 2019;381(7):637-646. PMID: 31034184

30. Foster NC, Beck RW, Miller KM, et al. State of type 1 diabetes management and outcomes from the T1D exchange in 2016-2018. *Diabetes Technol Ther.* 2019;21(2):66-72. PMID: 30657336

31. West NA, Hamman RF, Mayer-Davis EJ, et al. Cardiovascular risk factors among youth with and without type 2 diabetes: differences and possible mechanisms. *Diabetes Care.* 2009;32(1):175-180. PMID: 18945923

32. Pinhas-Hamiel O, Zeitler P. Acute and chronic complications of type 2 diabetes mellitus in children and adolescents. *Lancet.* 2007;369(9575):1823-1831. PMID: 17531891

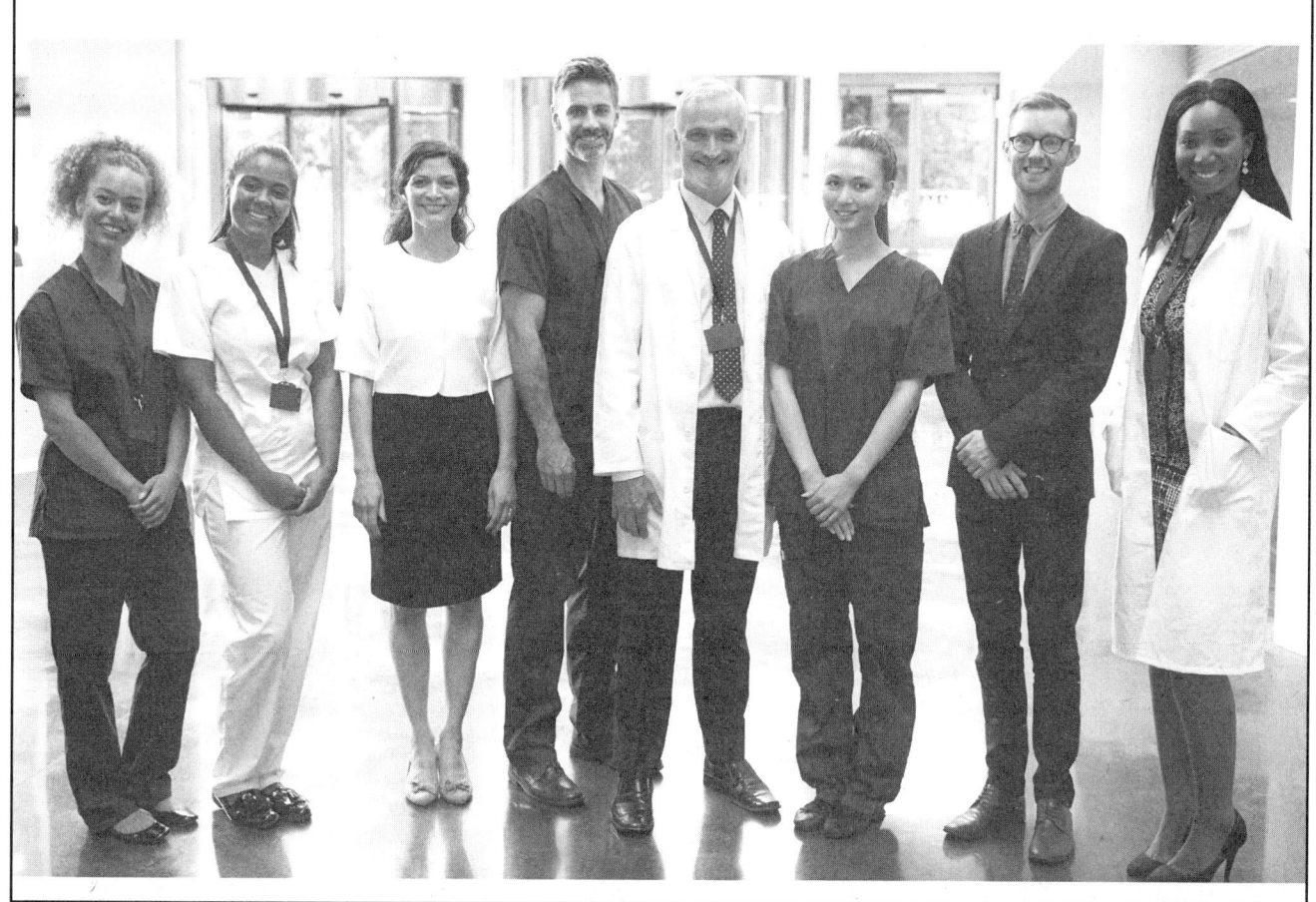

REPRODUCTIVE
ENDOCRINOLOGY

Diagnosis and Management of Functional Hypogonadism in the Male Patient

Mathis Grossmann, MD, PhD, FRACP. University of Melbourne Austin Health, Heidelberg, Victoria, Australia; E-mail: mathisg@unimelb.edu.au

Learning Objectives

As a result of participating in this session, learners should be able to:

- Assess and evaluate men for clinically significant androgen deficiency in the setting of confounding comorbidities.

- Manage men presenting with functional hypogonadism using an evidence-based approach for nontestosterone- and testosterone-based treatment.

Main Conclusions

Functional suppression of the male hypothalamic-pituitary-testicular (HPT) axis due to acute or chronic health conditions is a common clinical problem in older men, but it can also occur in young men. Functional hypogonadism is a diagnosis of exclusion and requires careful, individualized assessment to exclude organic hypogonadism due to anatomic pathology of the HPT axis.

While definitive randomized controlled trials are lacking, the available evidence suggests that measures to optimize ill health (eg, achieving a healthy body weight, optimizing comorbidities, stopping offending medications) can improve androgen deficiency-like symptoms and lead to a modest increase in circulating testosterone. Moreover, such men can respond to targeted treatments addressing relevant symptoms (eg, phosphodiesterase-5 inhibitors for sexual dysfunction) or end-organ deficits (eg, antiresorptive therapy for osteoporosis).

Not uncommonly, measures to reverse suppression of the functional HPT axis are difficult to implement successfully and, even if successful, may not be sufficient. In this situation, the question arises as to whether testosterone treatment is appropriate. While recent randomized controlled trials in carefully selected middle-aged and older men have reported short-term effects of testosterone treatment, effects of testosterone treatment on important long-term health outcomes remain unknown. If testosterone treatment is considered, it should be directed towards men with significant clinical features and persistently low circulating testosterone after exclusion of contraindications and appropriate counseling, with guideline-conforming monitoring for efficacy and adverse effects.

Significance of the Clinical Problem

Older men, especially if overweight or obese and experiencing comorbidities, often present with nonspecific androgen deficiency-like symptoms, such as low energy and sexual dysfunction, and modestly lowered serum testosterone relative to reference ranges based on healthy young men. Most such men do not have organic hypogonadism due to classic pituitary or testicular disease, but instead have functional hypogonadism.

Hence, they have potentially reversible HPT axis suppression due to acute and chronic health conditions external to the HPT axis, such as medication use and/or lifestyle behaviors. Notably, ill health can also cause functional hypogonadism in young men in the context of energy deficit (eg, the reversible energy deficit of sport syndrome, eating disorders, and body dysmorphic disorders) or during recovery from anabolic steroid use.

In the clinical approach to such men, making the distinction between organic and functional hypogonadism is important. This is because organic hypogonadism can be due to potentially serious pathology, such as a pituitary lesion. Moreover, the treatment approach differs. While organic hypogonadism is generally treated with testosterone replacement, in men with functional hypogonadism, lifestyle measures—especially achieving a healthy body weight, optimizing comorbidities, and stopping offending medications—may improve symptoms and increase serum testosterone.

Barriers to Optimal Practice

In some men, clinical and biochemical features consistent with androgen deficiency may persist despite optimization of body weight and comorbidities. In such men, reevaluation for organic HPT axis pathology should be considered, as this can be missed.

Measures to reverse functional hypogonadism may be unsuccessful in some patients (eg, weight loss is not achieved or sustained) or are not feasible (eg, cessation of opioids for chronic pain). Therefore, the clinician is commonly faced with the question as to whether testosterone therapy should be considered, and there is vigorous debate about this issue. Although recent randomized controlled trials have provided data on the short-term benefits and risks of testosterone treatment in older men, definitive studies assessing the long-term effects of testosterone treatment on important health outcomes are currently not available.

Strategies for Diagnosis, Therapy, and/or Management

Background: Organic vs Functional Hypogonadism

In the clinical approach to men with suspected androgen deficiency, distinguishing organic from functional hypogonadism is important (*Table 1*), because organic hypogonadism can be due to potentially serious pathology (eg, a pituitary tumor). Moreover, this distinction influences the treatment approach.

Organic Hypogonadism
Organic hypogonadism due to medical disease of the HPT axis, such as a pituitary tumor or Klinefelter syndrome, is an important diagnosis not to be missed. Organic hypogonadism should be considered in a man of any age who presents with clinical and biochemical features suggestive of androgen deficiency, including unexplained psychosexual complaints, osteoporosis, anemia, or sarcopenia.[2]

While randomized controlled trials are lacking, clinical experience and uncontrolled studies of testosterone replacement in men with organic hypogonadism demonstrate marked benefits on sexual function, energy, hemoglobin, bone density, and body composition.[3] Testosterone replacement should be considered irrespective of age, noting that testosterone does not improve fertility but instead can suppress spermatogenesis.

Functional Hypogonadism
Many older men, especially when overweight or obese and living with chronic disease (such as diabetes, depression, liver, or renal disease), present with nonspecific, androgen deficiency-like symptoms such as fatigue, low energy, and sexual dysfunction (low libido and/or erectile dysfunction). They may also have clinical features overlapping with those of organic hypogonadism such as central adiposity, sarcopenia, and reduced bone mineral density. Such men commonly have modest reductions in their circulating testosterone concentrations, fluctuating in the lower range

Table 1. Organic Hypogonadism vs Functional Hypogonadism in Middle-Aged and Older Men

Clinical Aspects	Organic Hypogonadism	Functional Hypogonadism
Condition	Proven HPT axis pathology (structural, destructive, or congenital disease)	No recognizable structural intrinsic HPT axis pathology No specific pathologic etiologies of functional hypogonadism (diagnosis of exclusion)
Reversibility	Established disease state, organic, and generally irreversible HPT axis pathology	HPT axis suppression is functional and may be reversible
Symptoms/signs	Specific: eunuchoidism More specific/objective: low libido, small testes, loss of male hair, gynecomastia	Less specific: erectile dysfunction, low energy and mood
Testosterone levels	Unequivocally, consistently, and severely low	Borderline low, fluctuating around the lower limit of assay range, occasionally severely low
Gonadotropin levels	Elevated (primary hypogonadism) or low/inappropriately normal (secondary hypogonadism)	Usually in the normal range, occasionally low (secondary hypogonadism)
Association of low testosterone with symptoms	Causal	Uncertain, symptoms may be predominantly or partially due to comorbid illness
Testosterone therapy	Replacement	Replacement?
Benefits of therapy	Marked symptomatic and somatic response (except fertility)	Symptomatic and somatic response less well established
Risks of therapy	Considered low relative to benefits	Unknown

Abbreviation: HPT, hypothalamic-pituitary-testicular. Adapted in part from *Endocr Pract.* 2013;19(5):853-863.[1]

relative to reference ranges based on healthy young men (typically ranging from 173-288 ng/dL (6.0-10.0 nmol/L).[4]

The estimated prevalence of functional hypogonadism (in older men also referred to as late-onset hypogonadism), defined as the coexistence of androgen deficiency-like features and lowered circulating testosterone in the absence of organic HPT axis pathology, is estimated to be 2% to 5% in community-dwelling older men.[5] However, the extent to which lowered testosterone concentrations contribute to the aging male phenotype is not known. It is also possible that lowered testosterone is primarily a consequence of functional hypothalamic-pituitary suppression due to ill health. Low testosterone, at the very least, is a sensitive marker of poor health.

Of note, functional hypogonadism due to acute or chronic ill health can also occur in young men. Both under- and overnutrition can suppress the male HPT axis. Functional hypogonadism in young men in the context of energy deficit (overtraining, eating and body dysmorphic disorders) or during recovery from anabolic steroid use is increasingly recognized.[6,7]

Workup of Older Men Presenting With Features Suggestive of Androgen Deficiency

The clinical workup is primarily geared towards excluding a diagnosis of organic hypogonadism. Given that hypogonadism is a clinical diagnosis supported by consistent biochemical findings, men who present with features suggestive of androgen deficiency should have a thorough history and physical examination to determine the degree of clinically significant androgen deficiency.[2] Clinical assessment should be focused on eliciting the more specific features of androgen deficiency, such as gynecomastia, recent loss of body hair, and decreasing testicular volume. Many features such as fatigue, low libido, and reduced muscle bulk are nonspecific and can be caused by almost any chronic disease.[4] Initial assessment should include the identification of comorbidities that may confound the clinical picture or represent potentially reversible causes such as obesity, depression, uncontrolled sleep apnea, or medications (eg, opioids or glucocorticoids). Clues to underlying organic etiology, such as signs of pituitary dysfunction or mass effect, should not be missed. Surreptitious anabolic steroid use should be considered.

The clinical impression of androgen deficiency should be confirmed by documenting at least 2 low serum total testosterone concentrations by an accurate and reliable assay, with the sample drawn in the morning in the fasted state.[2] Testosterone should not be measured during an intercurrent illness, as this can lead to temporary HPT axis suppression. Measurement of SHBG and determination of free testosterone (usually calculated) may provide additional information in men with borderline total testosterone and/or conditions in which abnormalities in SHBG are suspected.

Most men with functional hypogonadism have low-normal gonadotropin concentrations due to nondestructive hypothalamic-pituitary inhibition from chronic disease, including being obese or underweight.[4] Especially in older men, evaluation for underlying organic HPT axis pathology is commonly of low yield and should be individualized. In men with nonelevated gonadotropins, the probability of organic hypothalamic-pituitary pathology is inversely related to BMI, age, number of comorbidities, and testosterone concentrations. In the absence of clinical suspicion of pituitary disease, biochemical workup can be limited to measuring prolactin, and in men younger than 65 years, iron studies to exclude hemochromatosis. The testosterone cutoff below which pituitary imaging is necessary is not well defined, but imaging should be considered in men with a total testosterone concentration less than 150 ng/dL (<5.2 nmol/L) and low to normal gonadotropins, even in the absence of clinical suspicion of hypothalamic pituitary disease.[2]

Management of Functional Hypogonadism

Lifestyle and Optimization of Comorbidities

Priority should lie in the management of reversible causes, most importantly the implementation of lifestyle measures to optimize body weight and comorbidities (eg, depression, sleep apnea, or glycemic control in diabetes) and, if possible, removal of offending medications (eg, opioids, glucocorticoids) (Figure). This strategy can improve nonspecific symptoms, lead to modest increases in testosterone, and have general health benefits. In some observational studies, implementation of continuous positive airway pressure for sleep apnea, improvement of glycemic control in men with diabetes, and opioid or glucocorticoid cessation, have been associated with increases in testosterone concentrations of around 58 to 144 ng/dL (2.0-5.0 nmol/L).[4] Explaining this to affected men can increase their motivation to engage with these measures.

Obesity is the strongest risk factor for low testosterone, even overriding the effects of age, in part because obesity blunts the age-related rise in LH that can compensate for testicular dysfunction occurring in some older men.[8] Consistent with this, successful weight loss, whether by diet or surgery, can lead to substantial increases in testosterone in obese men. The increase in testosterone is proportional to the amount of weight lost: 10% weight loss increases testosterone by 58 to 86 ng/dL (2.0-3.0 nmol/L), whereas profound weight loss after bariatric surgery in morbidly obese men can raise testosterone by more than 288 ng/dL (>10 nmol/L).[4]

In addition to general measures, predominant clinical features can be addressed with targeted therapy (Table 2).

Testosterone Therapy

In some men, measures to reverse functional hypogonadism may be unsuccessful, either because implementation is not feasible (eg, cessation of opioids) or they are not achieved or maintained (eg, weight loss). In others, symptoms may persist even despite successful implementation of these

Figure. Approach to Possible Hypogonadism

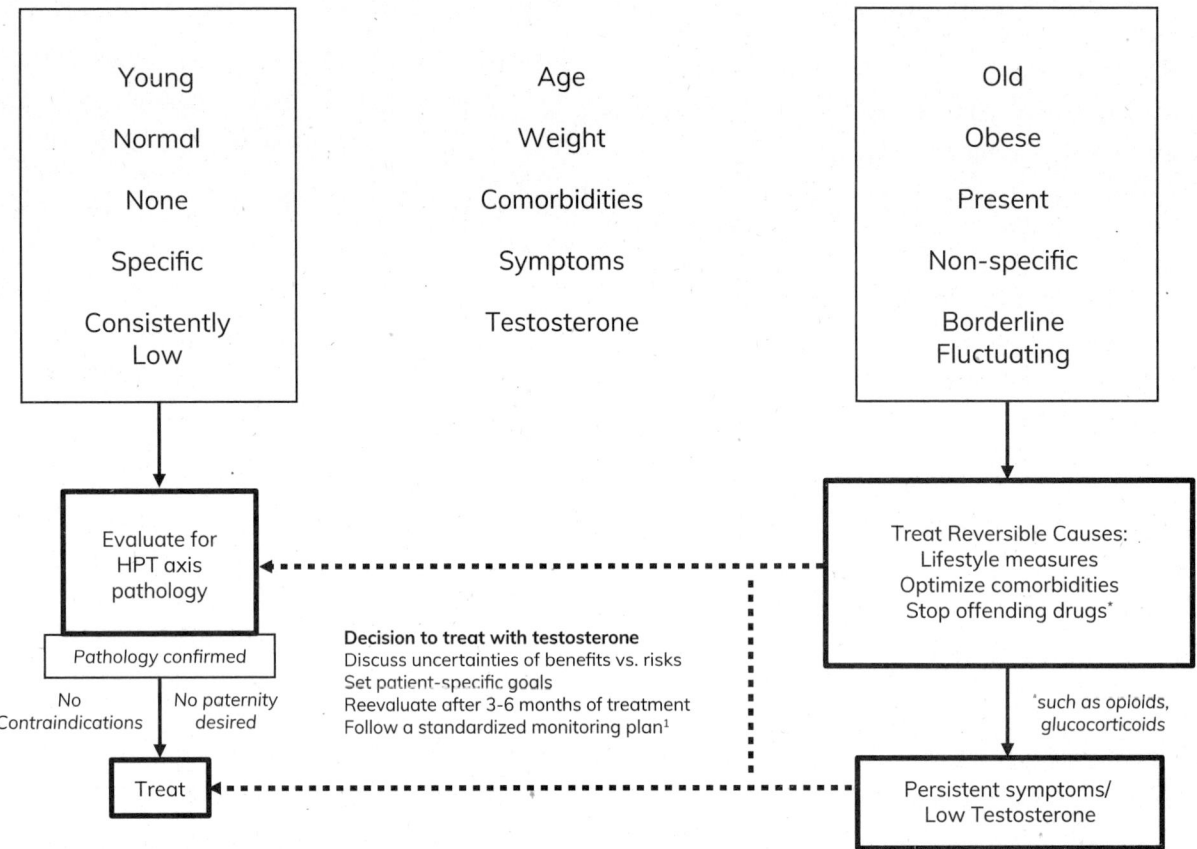

measures. In some men, the low testosterone may contribute to fatigue or poor motivation that reduces their ability to initiate healthy lifestyle measures. This raises the question as to whether testosterone therapy should be considered in selected circumstances, and what the benefits and risks of testosterone treatment are. Of note, in such men, reevaluation for organic HPT axis pathology should be considered, as this can be missed.

Possible Benefits of Testosterone Therapy
The Testosterone Trials (T-Trials), the largest randomized controlled clinical trials of testosterone treatment in older men, have provided new data on organ-specific outcomes for testosterone treatment in older men. The T-Trials were a coordinated set of trials (a main trial and several substudies) conducted in the United States, which included 790 men aged 65 years or older who were randomly assigned to receive transdermal testosterone (dosed to maintain

serum testosterone within the normal range for healthy young men) or placebo for 12 months. Eligible participants had a baseline testosterone concentration less than 275 ng/dL (<9.54 nmol/L) (averaged from 2 measures) and at least 1 symptom or sign consistent with hypogonadism (eg, decreased libido, difficulty walking, or low vitality). Men with organic hypogonadism were excluded from the study.[9] Testosterone treatment resulted in modest benefits in sexual function and slightly improved mood and depressive symptoms, but it did not improve cognitive function. Concomitant substudies demonstrated improvements in volumetric bone mineral density and anemia.[10] Other smaller randomized controlled trials of testosterone treatment have reported a 4.4-lb (2-kg) gain in muscle mass (with associated increases in muscle strength) and 4.4-lb (2-kg) loss of fat mass, as well as modest improvements in insulin resistance. However, in men with generally well-controlled diabetes,

Table 2. Effects of Testosterone Treatment in Randomized Controlled Trials of Middle-Aged and Older Men: Evidence to Date[a]

Concern	Testosterone Treatment Effect	Targeted Treatment
Sexual	Modest improvement in most domains of sexual function (if testosterone <275-346 ng/dL [<9.5-12.0 nmol/L]) In most randomized controlled trials, effect on libido more marked than on erectile function	Phosphodiesterase 5 inhibitor (for erectile dysfunction)
Muscle	3.5-5.9 lb (1.6-2.7 kg) increase in mass, and, in some studies, increased muscle strength; modest improvements in some measures of muscle performance (eg, small increase in walking distance)	Exercise
Fat	3.5-4.4 lb (1.6-2.0 kg) decrease	Weight loss
Glucose metabolism	Modest improvement in insulin resistance in some randomized controlled trials[b]; no effect on hemoglobin A_{1c}	Lifestyle, antidiabetes medications
Bone	2%-7% increase in lumbar spine bone mineral density, with generally smaller increases in femoral bone mineral density; randomized controlled trials have not been large enough to assess effects on fractures	Osteoporotic drug therapy
Mood	Slight improvement in mood/depressive symptoms	eg, Counseling, antidepressants
Cognition	No effect on cognition, memory	eg, Cholinesterase inhibitors

[a] In these randomized controlled trials, men with organic hypogonadism were excluded.

[b] In these randomized controlled trials, men had relatively well-controlled diabetes at baseline.

no improvements in glycemic control have been observed (*Table 2*).[11]

Whether testosterone treatment reduces important clinical endpoints such as fractures, disability, or mortality in older men is not known. This is because existing randomized controlled trials of testosterone therapy in older men have been relatively small and of short duration. Some randomized controlled trials have included men who either had no clinical evidence of androgen deficiency or did not have confirmed low testosterone.[2]

Possible Risks of Testosterone Therapy

Trials to date have been underpowered to provide definitive outcome data regarding prostate and cardiovascular events, and long-term risks are unknown. It has been estimated that a randomized controlled trial enrolling several thousand men over 3 to 5 years would be needed to define true long-term risks. The largest randomized controlled trial to date enrolled 790 men over 12 months.[9]

Regarding prostate events, the data have been reassuring. Despite the fact that androgen deprivation therapy is an effective treatment for established prostate cancer, clinical studies to date have not demonstrated that testosterone treatment increases the risk of developing prostate cancer. Prostate monitoring during testosterone therapy may, however, lead to overdiagnosis of preexisting, clinically insignificant prostate cancer. Guidance to minimize this risk is available.[2]

The current evidence regarding testosterone treatment and cardiovascular outcomes is contradictory and inconclusive, with some studies suggesting increased risks, whereas most studies do not.

If treatment is considered, men with functional hypogonadism should be informed about the absence of high-level evidence regarding long-term benefits and risks. Clear patient-specific goals should be identified, and treatment should be stopped if these goals are not achieved. Monitoring for adverse events should follow consensus recommendations.[2]

Conclusions

Men with organic hypogonadism should be identified and considered for testosterone replacement. More research is needed to clarify the role for testosterone therapy in other settings. In most older men, low testosterone is a marker of poor health and should prompt a holistic approach with focus on lifestyle measures and optimization of comorbidities. Successful weight loss combined with optimization of comorbidities can be sufficient to improve symptoms and increase testosterone concentrations and will lead to other important health benefits in such men.

Clinical Case Vignettes

Case 1

A 51-year-old man consults you for a second opinion. He previously saw a medical practitioner for androgen deficiency-like symptoms and a low testosterone measurement, which the practitioner attributed to his comorbid metabolic syndrome and being overweight. He was advised to engage in healthy lifestyle measures. With dietary changes, he lost 8.8 lb (4 kg) without any symptomatic improvement. He has been unable to exercise, which he attributes to ongoing lethargy, muscle weakness, and low mood. He reports poor libido. Work has been stressful, and he is concerned about losing his job.

On physical examination, his BMI is 29.0 kg/m^2, waist circumference is 41 in (104 cm), and blood pressure is 152/90 mm Hg. He has mild gynecomastia and 15-mL testes bilaterally. Visual fields are normal to confrontation.

Laboratory test results (sample drawn at 8 AM while fasting):

> Total testosterone = 133 ng/dL (300-900 ng/dL) (SI: 4.6 nmol/L [10.4-31.2 nmol/L]) (repeated measurement = 144 ng/dL [SI: 5.0 nmol/L])
> Hemoglobin = 12.7 g/dL (13.8-17.2 g/dL) (SI: 127 g/L [138-172 g/L])
> Glucose = 125 mg/dL (70-99 mg/dL) (SI: 6.9 mmol/L [3.9-5.5 mmol/L])
> Hemoglobin A$_{1c}$ = 6.6% (4.0%-5.6%) (49 mmol/mol [20-38 mmol/mol])

Liver function, normal
Renal function, normal
Iron studies, normal

Which of the following is the best next step in this patient's management?

A. Evaluate for sleep obstructive sleep apnea

B. Refer to a dietician to achieve a healthy body weight

C. Evaluate for organic HPT axis pathology

D. Refer to a psychologist for counseling

Answer: C) Evaluate for organic HPT axis pathology

This middle-aged man presents with clinical findings suggestive of organic pathology (gynecomastia, borderline testicular size). His serum testosterone is frankly and repeatedly low. There is no intercurrent illness suggesting temporary HPT axis suppression. He has mild unexplained anemia, which is compatible with androgen deficiency. His clinical presentation should not be attributed to functional hypogonadism, a diagnosis of exclusion. Further evaluation of his HPT axis is indicated (Answer C). Upon further investigation, his LH concentration was 2.4 mIU/L (2.4 IU/L), inappropriately low in the face of his repeatedly and frankly low serum testosterone. His prolactin concentration was mildly elevated at 31 ng/mL (1.3 nmol/L), suggestive of pituitary stalk effect rather than a prolactin-secreting pituitary. Pituitary imaging demonstrated a 2-cm macroadenoma well away from the optic chiasm, consistent with a nonfunctioning adenoma on further workup.

Obstructive sleep apnea (Answer A) is not uncommon in older, obese men with functional hypogonadism and it may contribute to fatigue. However, this is not the foremost consideration in this middle-aged, overweight man with mild anemia (untreated obstructive sleep apnea may increase hemoglobin due to hypoxemia). Likewise, a weight-loss program (Answer B) or counseling (Answer D) might be appropriate flanking measures, but they are not the best next step. This man, following review by a neurosurgeon, opted for expectant management of his pituitary adenoma. Testosterone replacement was subsequently initiated after noting that he had no desire for paternity. He reported marked improvement of energy levels and sexual function. His motivation to engage in healthy lifestyle measures increased, and, over the next 12 months, he successfully lost 13.2 lb (6 kg).

Case 2

A 67-year-old man presents with low energy, low libido, and erectile dysfunction. He has well-controlled hypertension treated with an ACE inhibitor. He has no history of cardiovascular disease or diabetes mellitus. He is a former cigarette smoker (40 pack-year history). He reports poor dietary habits and does not exercise. He has no symptoms of sleep apnea.

On physical examination, his BMI is 34.6 kg/m^2 and blood pressure is 132/84 mm Hg. He has normal male-pattern body hair, and testes are 20 mL bilaterally. There is no gynecomastia or visual field defect.

Laboratory test results (sample drawn at 8 AM while fasting):

> Total testosterone = 202 ng/dL (300-900 ng/dL) (SI: 7.0 nmol/L [10.4-31.2 nmol/L]) (repeated measurement = 210 ng/dL [SI: 7.3 nmol/L])
> SHBG = 2.7 µg/mL (1.1-6.7 µg/mL) (SI: 24 nmol/L [10-60 nmol/L])
> Calculated free testosterone = 5.0 ng/dL (9.0-30.0 ng/dL) (SI: 0.17 nmol/L [0.31-1.04 nmol/L])
> LH = 4.3 mIU/mL (1.0-9.0 mIU/mL) (SI: 4.3 IU/L [1.0-9.0 IU/L])
> FSH = 3.7 mIU/mL (1.0-13.0 mIU/mL) (SI: 3.7 IU/L [1.0-13.0 IU/L])
> Prolactin, normal
> Thyroid function, normal
> Iron studies, normal

Which of the following is the best next step in this patient's management?

A. Perform pituitary-directed MRI

B. Initiate lifestyle measures to achieve weight loss and prescribe a phosphodiesterase 5 inhibitor

C. Prescribe an aromatase inhibitor

D. Prescribe a selective estrogen-receptor modulator

Answer: B) Initiate lifestyle measures to achieve weight loss and prescribe a phosphodiesterase 5 inhibitor

In this man, the clinical suspicion of organic hypogonadotropic hypogonadism is low, and pituitary-directed MRI (Answer A) is not necessary. His obesity is most likely the major contributor to his lowered testosterone, and successful weight loss may improve his energy levels and increase circulating testosterone. His erectile function should improve with the use of a phosphodiesterase 5 inhibitor. Therefore, among the options given, initiating lifestyle measures to achieve weight loss and prescribing a phosphodiesterase 5 inhibitor (Answer B) is the best next step.

Selective estrogen-receptor modulators (Answer D) or aromatase inhibitors (Answer C) such as anastrozole are sometimes prescribed off-label by practitioners for the treatment of functional hypogonadism, with the expectation that by decreasing the estradiol-mediated central negative feedback on the hypothalamic pituitary unit, LH increases and subsequently serum testosterone increases. These agents are not approved for male hypogonadism, and there is no convincing evidence for clinical benefit. Moreover, by decreasing estradiol production, aromatase inhibitors have been reported to reduce bone density in men.

Case 2 (Continued)

Over the next 9 months, with diligent implementation of dietary measures and increased physical activity, the patient manages to lose 24 lb (11 kg). He reports a modest improvement in sexual function with the use of a phosphodiesterase 5 inhibitor, but still rates his libido and energy levels as "lower than they should be." His morning fasting total testosterone is now 256 ng/dL (8.9 nmol/L) and 245 ng/dL (8.5 nmol/L) on repeated measurement. Recent bone mineral density measurements by DXA demonstrated T-scores of +0.5 at the lumbar spine, –0.3 at the total hip, and –0.1 at the femoral neck. He now seeks your advice regarding testosterone therapy.

On the basis of current evidence from randomized controlled trials, which of the following is the least likely effect of starting testosterone in this patient?

A. Increased hemoglobin

B. Increased PSA

C. Reduced coronary artery plaque volume

D. Increased bone mineral density

Answer: C) Reduced coronary artery plaque volume

The clinical characteristics of the patient in this vignette are similar to those of eligible T-Trial participants. Most men enrolled in the T-Trials had cardiovascular risk factors such as obesity (63%) and hypertension (72%), and men participating in the bone trial had normal bone mineral density as quantified by DXA, with T-scores ranging from –0.3 to +1.3 at baseline.

In the main trial, testosterone treatment improved all aspects of sexual function (libido and sexual activity more so than erectile function) and improved mood and depressive symptoms to a small degree.

The cardiovascular trial reported a greater increase in coronary plaque volume in testosterone-treated men than in placebo-treated men, raising a possible concern over adverse cardiovascular effects of testosterone. While there was no difference in cardiovascular events between groups, the trial was not large enough or long enough to assess cardiovascular outcomes. Overall, considering the literature as a whole, the evidence regarding cardiovascular effects of testosterone in older men remains inconclusive.

In the anemia trial, testosterone increased hemoglobin and corrected mild to moderate anemia. In the bone trial, testosterone treatment substantially improved volumetric bone mineral density in the spine, increasing 6.8% more in testosterone-treated patients than in placebo-treated patients. Testosterone also improved estimated bone strength. The study was not powered for fracture outcomes. While more testosterone treated men experienced an increase in PSA of 1.0 ng/mL or greater (≥1.0 µg/L) (23 men compared with 8 men receiving placebo), only 1 man (assigned to testosterone) was diagnosed with prostate cancer during the 12-month randomized controlled trial.

References

1. Basaria S. Testosterone therapy in older men with late-onset hypogonadism: a counter-rationale. *Endocr Pract.* 2013;19(5):853-863. PMID: 24014017

2. Bhasin S, Brito JP, Cunningham GR, et al. Testosterone therapy in men with hypogonadism: an Endocrine Society clinical practice guideline. *J Clin Endocrinol Metab.* 2018;103(5):1715-1744. PMID: 29562364

3. Snyder PJ, Peachey H, Berlin JA, et al. Effects of testosterone replacement in hypogonadal men. *J Clin Endocrinol Metab.* 2000;85(8):2670-2677. PMID: 10946864

4. Grossmann M, Matsumoto AM. A perspective on middle-aged and older men with functional hypogonadism: focus on holistic management. *J Clin Endocrinol Metab.* 2017;102(3):1067-1075. PMID: 28359097

5. Wu FC, Tajar A, Beynon JM, et al; EMAS Group. Identification of late-onset hypogonadism in middle-aged and elderly men. *N Engl J Med.* 2010;363(2):123-135. PMID: 20554979

6. Wong HK, Hoermann R, Grossmann M. Reversible male hypogonadotropic hypogonadism due to energy deficit. *Clin Endocrinol (Oxf).* 2019;91(1):3-9. PMID: 30903626

7. Goldman AL, Pope HG, Bhasin S. The health threat posed by the hidden epidemic of anabolic steroid use and body image disorders among young men. *J Clin Endocrinol Metab.* 2019;104(4):1069-1074. PMID: 30239802

8. Tajar A, Forti G, O'Neill TW, et al; EMAS Group. Characteristics of secondary, primary, and compensated hypogonadism in aging men: evidence from the European Male Ageing Study. *J Clin Endocrinol Metab.* 2010;95(4):1810-1818. PMID: 20173018

9. Snyder PJ, Bhasin S, Cunningham GR, et al; Testosterone Trials Investigators. Effects of testosterone treatment in older men. *N Engl J Med.* 2016;374(7):611-624. PMID: 26886521

10. Snyder PJ, Bhasin S, Cunningham GR, et al. Lessons from the testosterone trials. *Endocrine Rev.* 2018;39(3):369-386. PMID: 29522088

11. Kaufman JM, Lapauw B, Mahmoud A, T'Sjoen G, Huhtaniemi IT. Aging and the male reproductive system. *Endocrine Rev.* 2019;40(4):906-972. PMID: 30888401

Evaluation of Female Fertility: Antimullerian Hormone and Ovarian Reserve Testing

Marcelle I. Cedars, MD. University of California, San Francisco, San Francisco, CA; E-mail: marcelle.cedars@ucsf.edu

Learning Objectives

As a result of participating in this session, learners should be able to:

- Evaluate the infertile woman.

  - Describe an approach to assessing reproductive aging.

  - Describe available tests and their implications.

- Select treatments that optimize patient physiology and reduce risk.

- Summarize the likelihood of livebirths after treatment of infertility.

Main Conclusions

The elements of the management of the infertile couple are the following:

- Importance of evaluation of the couple.

- Primacy of the evaluation and management of the woman.

  - Young women who are ovulating will generally conceive with a subfertile male—restoration of ovulation in young women who are infertile will often result in conception for a couple.

  - Decreased ovarian reserve in young women is not implicated in infertility and/or lowered fecundity.

  - Older women, especially those with diminished ovarian reserve, may have a shortened timeline for conception and should be managed more aggressively. They often require assisted reproductive technology to conceive after a short course of medical therapy and/or intrauterine insemination.

- Women with polycystic ovary syndrome (PCOS) are best treated with weight reduction; if this fails to induce ovulation and/or the women is older, ovulation induction with letrozole is indicated.

- Women with hypogonadotropic hypogonadism should have the underlying cause corrected (hypothyroidism, hyperprolactinemia, weight gain). For women with functional hypothalamic amenorrhea, ovulation induction with pulsatile GnRH is the most effective and physiological.

Significance of the Clinical Problem

Approximately 1 in 8 couples have trouble conceiving or sustaining a pregnancy according to the Centers for Disease Control 2006-2010 National Survey of Family Growth. In the United

States, infertility is typically defined as the inability to conceive after 1 year, at which time an evaluation should begin. For women older than 35 years, evaluation is advised after 6 months. While the percentage of women with infertility and no living children has increased largely due to the increasing age at the time of first pregnancy, the overall percentage of women with infertility has been relatively stable over several decades. Although infertility is frequently considered a "women's disease," about 35% of couples have both a male and female etiology of their infertility with another 10% to 20% having a sole male factor as the identifiable cause.

Normal fertility requires a competent oocyte (requiring normal ovulatory function in the female); a functional sperm (requiring normal endocrinological function and spermatogenic capacity in the male); an anatomic capacity for sperm/egg interaction (functional cervix, uterus and fallopian tubes in female and functional vasa, epididymis, and penis in the man); and the capacity for implantation (endocrinological and anatomic uterine environment). Infertility or reduced fecundity (ability to produce a live born) can result from abnormalities in any of these areas. We are aware that today, there are many ways to build a family and many types of families. This session will focus on the role of ovarian reserve in chances for conception.

Barriers to Optimal Practice

- Delay in attempts at pregnancy (increasing age of the female partner).

- Incomplete understanding of physiology of normal female and male reproductive function.

- Cost and lack of access to fertility care, particularly due to lack of insurance or underinsurance.

- Perception that infertility is caused by the patient or couple (eg, lifestyle choices such as delay in decision to conceive or exposure to sexually transmitted infections).

- Press/public focus on high-tech treatments such as in vitro fertilization (suggesting these expensive treatments are the only appropriate care and/or are so powerful they can overcome all factors, including age).

Strategies for Diagnosis, Therapy, and/or Management
Initial Evaluation of the Infertile Couple

Couples should begin an evaluation if they have not conceived after 1 year of active attempts. This assumes that the woman is having regular cycles and that there have been 12 "ovulatory, exposed" cycles. A woman who has had irregular cycles with long episodes of amenorrhea should present earlier for evaluation because she is likely anovulatory. Women older than 35 years should be evaluated for infertility after 6 months of unsuccessful active attempts.

Both members of an infertile couple should be evaluated, and the couple should be queried as to whether they are having frequent (2-3 times weekly) vaginal intercourse ("exposure"). A careful history should be taken for each member of the couple for causes of infertility such as anovulation in the woman or hypogonadism in the man.

Approach to the Subfertile/ Infertile Woman

The evaluation always begins with the woman, as women with normal fecundity usually conceive even with men who have subnormal reproductive function. The first approach to an infertile woman is to characterize the menstrual pattern. A history of regular, cyclic, predictable periods is associated with ovulation in greater than 98% of cases. However, it is also important to further characterize even "regular" cycles. Important questions include changes in cycle interval (a shortening of the intermenstrual interval may suggest a decline in ovarian reserve). New-onset spotting prior to menstrual flow may suggest a reduction in luteal phase progesterone, also a symptom of ovarian aging. For women whose cycles are irregular, and specifically for those women with oligomenorrhea and amenorrhea, a careful history is important. This should begin with the onset of menses and the transition (if any) to irregularity. Additional questions should ascertain the presence or absence of symptoms of hypothyroidism, hyperprolactinemia, hypoestrogenism, and hyperandrogenism. These questions can guide the examination and laboratory investigation. Additionally, the history should focus on factors that would interfere with normal tubal function such as a history of sexually transmitted infections, pelvic surgery, dysmenorrhea, or dyspareunia.

Physical examination of the woman should include assessment of vital signs (may point to thyroid or adrenal dysfunction), presence or absence of hyperandrogenism (hair growth, acne, androgenic alopecia), thyromegaly, galactorrhea, and evidence of past and current estrogen (breast development, vaginal and cervical lubrication). A pelvic examination to feel the size and mobility of the uterus and any adnexal pain/tenderness should be performed. For those with unexplained infertility (no risk factors) or symptoms of endometriosis, a recto-vaginal examination can reveal uterosacral nodularity or tenderness that might further suggest this diagnosis. Laboratory testing for the anovulatory woman should include measurement of TSH, prolactin, FSH, and estradiol. Additional testing of DHEA-S, testosterone, and LH may be warranted in certain instances. All women should have an evaluation of ovarian reserve by measurement of serum antimullerian hormone (AMH) and/or ultrasound-guided antral follicle count.

If AMH is low, decreased ovarian reserve is suspected. AMH is a glycoprotein in the TGF-β family. It is produced by the granulosa cells of preantral and small antral follicles. As such, it correlates with the residual ovarian pool of primordial follicles. AMH was heralded as a better marker of ovarian reserve, compared with FSH and estradiol, as it was thought to not vary across (or between) menstrual cycles and not to be affected by contraception or anovulation. Early studies suggested a correlation with natural fecundability. However, 2 large studies have not shown a correlation between AMH and fecundability.[1,2] Thus, it is clear that AMH is not a "fertility marker."

AMH is a predictor of response to stimulation (in vitro fertilization cycle), but it does not correlate with pregnancy.[3] This suggests AMH is a marker of "quantity" but not "quality" of the oocytes. It is a marker of the residual oocyte pool. Additionally, there is intracycle variability of AMH. And perhaps most important for assessment of "ovarian reserve" in a general population, AMH is lowered with the use of oral contraceptive pills, by as much as 50%, and thus may not be reflective of true ovarian reserve.[4,5]

The 2 most common causes of anovulation include PCOS, which is characterized by 2 of the following 3 findings: irregular cycles, hyperandrogenism and polycystic-appearing ovaries, and hypogonadotropic hypogonadism (which can be genetic, functional, or due to hypothyroidism or hyperprolactinemia). For women with PCOS, screening should exclude dyslipidemia, fatty liver, and/or impaired glucose tolerance/diabetes that may require further assessment, treatment, and/or weight loss before conception.[6,7] For patients who are metabolically normal, ovulation induction is the first treatment approach. Agents that can be used include clomiphene citrate, metformin, and letrozole. Randomized controlled trials have identified letrozole as most effective first-line treatment.[8,9] Given intact feedback mechanisms in women with PCOS, only a short course of the antiestrogen letrozole is enough to "jump start" the cycle by increasing FSH and allowing physiological response of the ovaries for development of the dominant follicle. Due to intact feedback from the hypothalamic-pituitary axis, most cycles are followed by ovulation of a single follicle, but a small risk (about 5%-8%) of multiple pregnancy is possible. About 85% of women with PCOS conceive with these drugs.

Interestingly, while preantral development has been thought to be unaffected by FSH, women with hypogonadotropic hypogonadism may have significantly suppressed antral follicle count and AMH.[10] For women with hypogonadotropic hypogonadism, the etiology of the low gonadotropins should be identified.[11] Then, the primary source should be treated, including thyroid replacement or reduction in prolactin with dopamine agonists as appropriate. For women with Kallmann syndrome or functional hypothalamic amenorrhea, the ideal treatment is pulsatile administration of GnRH.[12,13] This agent is not available in the United States, but it is under FDA review. Unless pulsatile GnRH becomes available, the standard treatment is the use of exogenous gonadotropins. Gonadotropin therapy is effective, but it is much more likely than GnRH therapy to be complicated by a high risk of multiple pregnancy and ovarian hyperstimulation due to its direct action on the ovaries. Women with hypogonadotropic hypogonadism seem to have a very narrow window between under-response and over-response, making dosing quite difficult. Additionally, they typically have a high number of responsive follicles and are at high risk for multiple pregnancy.

Clinical Case Vignettes

Case 1

A 28-year-old woman is seen for management of Hashimoto disease. She is concerned about future fertility and asks about egg freezing. She has taken continuous oral contraceptive pills for the last 5 years.

Which of the following is the best course of action?

A. Suggest she stop oral contraceptive pill and attempt conception
B. Measure serum AMH
C. Refer to reproductive endocrinology for egg freezing
D. Reassure her that given her young age, future fertility will not be a problem

Answer: B) Measure serum AMH

While this patient is still young, the fact she is asking the question and that she has Hashimoto disease with risk for other autoimmune disorders (including premature ovarian insufficiency) warrants testing (Answer B). Conception should never be suggested (Answer A) until a patient is ready for family building. Egg freezing (Answer C) may or may not be advised based on the patient's ovarian reserve. Lastly, while age is a strong predictor of successful conception, age alone is more relevant as a poor prognosticator in a woman older than 40 years than as a good prognosticator for a young woman (Answer E).

Case 1 (Continued)

Her AMH concentration is 0.5 ng/mL (3.6 pmol/L).

Which of the following is the best next step?

A. Suggest she stop oral contraceptive pills and repeat the testing
B. Refer to reproductive endocrinology for egg freezing
C. Counsel her regarding risk for early menopause
D. Advise her of low chances for conception

Answer: A) Suggest she stop oral contraceptive pills and repeat the testing

Oral contraceptive pills, especially when given in a continuous fashion, can suppress antral follicle growth and AMH levels. Most recovery is seen in the first 2 months, but levels can continue to rise for 6 months. The next step would be to stop the oral contraceptive pills and repeat testing in 2 to 3 months.

Again, egg freezing (Answer B) may or may not be indicated based on the patient's ovarian reserve and her social situation. While there is an association between AMH and menopausal onset, this cannot currently be prospectively predicted and this AMH level may be falsely suppressed by the oral contraceptive pills. Thus, counseling her regarding risk for early menopause (Answer C) would be inappropriate. AMH levels do not correlate with chances for spontaneous conception when she starts trying to conceive (Answer D).

Case 2

A couple presents for evaluation. The 28-year-old woman stopped oral contraceptive pills 6 months prior to consultation. Her cycle interval seems shorter than she recalls before starting oral contraceptive pills 10 years ago. Her cycles are currently every 25 to 26 days. Additionally, she has noticed 3 days of precycle spotting.

On physical examination of the woman, her BMI is 24 kg/m². She has no thyromegaly. Skin is normal. Pelvic examination documents estrogenized mucus and no masses or tenderness.

Laboratory testing documents normal levels of TSH and prolactin.

Which of the following is the best course of management for this couple?

A. Advise them to keep trying to conceive and increase intercourse frequency to 4 times weekly

B. Measure serum AMH in the woman

C. Measure serum AMH in the woman and perform semen analysis in her husband

D. Start a trial of letrozole for the woman

Answer: B) Measure serum AMH in the woman

Although this couple does not meet the United States definition of infertility (no conception after 1 year of trying), the woman may have diminished ovarian reserve given the shortened intermenstrual interval and precycle spotting. Assessing ovarian reserve may indicate a shortened reproductive window while not impacting the chance for spontaneous conception at the current time. Based on family planning goals, a shortened reproductive window may be relevant to the couple.

Some experts would evaluate this man with a semen analysis, but healthy young men are more than 90% likely to have a sperm in the ejaculate. Thus, the focus should be evaluation and treatment of menstrual changes and not assessment of the man. All men with a risk factor for infertility, symptoms or signs of hypogonadism, or small testes should be assessed with measurement of serum testosterone and gonadotropins and semen analysis.

Case 2 (Continued)

Her AMH concentration is 0.5 ng/mL (3.6 pmol/L). Her antral follicle count is 5.

Which of the following is the best course of action for this couple?

A. Advise them to keep trying

B. Recommend controlled ovarian stimulation

C. Recommend in vitro fertilization

D. Advise to freeze eggs

Answer: B) Recommend controlled ovarian stimulation

While any of these options may be reasonable based on the couple's desire for family building (number and spacing of pregnancies), starting controlled ovarian stimulation (Answer B) (typically with clomiphene citrate) and intrauterine insemination, to shorten time to pregnancy, may be warranted. Given her young age and the apparent slower decline in oocyte loss with lower egg numbers, her management may not need to change. She likely would be able to conceive both now and with a subsequent pregnancy. She may want to freeze eggs (embryo) (Answer D) for a subsequent pregnancy, but the greatest likelihood is that this would not be necessary. As AMH does not predict fecundability, it is not clear that in vitro fertilization (Answer C) as a treatment (vs for protection of future pregnancy) would be warranted. An advisement to continue trying (Answer A) may be reasonable, but most likely some low-dosage medication (eg, clomiphene citrate) is indicated to stop the precycle spotting and likely lowered progesterone production.

Case 3

A couple presents for evaluation. The 32-year-old woman has had oligomenorrhea (fewer than 6 episodes of menstrual bleeding per year) since puberty. She has mild hirsutism and no history of conception. Her 34-year-old husband has no medical illnesses and no history of fathering a child. They have not been able to conceive after 9 months of trying to conceive (vaginal intercourse twice weekly without contraception).

On physical examination of the woman, her BMI is 28 kg/m². She has no thyromegaly. She has mild hirsutism on the chin and chest and acne on her face, chest, and back. Her waist circumference is 39 in (99 cm) and she has hair up to the umbilicus. Pelvic examination documents estrogenized mucus and no masses or tenderness.

Laboratory testing documents normal levels of TSH and prolactin.

Which of the following is the best course of management for this couple?

A. Advise them to keep trying to conceive and increase intercourse frequency to 4 times weekly

B. Measure serum AMH in the woman

C. Measure serum AMH in the woman and perform semen analysis in her husband

D. Start a trial of letrozole for the woman

Answer: D) Start a trial of letrozole for the woman

Although this couple does not meet the United States definition of infertility (no conception after 1 year of trying), the woman is very likely anovulatory. Her history and examination findings indicate that she has PCOS, and a history of fewer than 6 menstrual cycles per year suggests that most, if not all, of her periods are anovulatory. Given the chronic oligoanovulation, additional attempts at "trying" (Answer A) will have a very low likelihood of success. Measuring AMH (Answers B and C) will not add to the likely diagnosis of PCOS with anovulation and hyperandrogenism. Ovulation induction with the oral agent letrozole (Answer D) is most effective and the correct answer.

However, measurement of AMH has been suggested as helpful in assessing response to ovulation induction, so some would suggest measurement. In this patient, as in most, if not all, women with PCOS, AMH would be elevated (most likely above 5 ng/mL [>35.7 pmol/L]). This value would also suggest which women would be at highest risk for multifollicular development and risk for multiple pregnancy, suggesting the need for ultrasonography monitoring of ovulation induction.

Healthy young men are more than 90% likely to have a sperm in the ejaculate. Thus, the focus should be treatment of her chronic anovulation and not assessment of the man. All men with a risk factor for infertility, symptoms or signs of hypogonadism, or small testes should be assessed with measurement of serum testosterone and gonadotropins and semen analysis.

Case 4

A couple presents for evaluation after 5 months of infertility. The 35-year-old woman has not had a menstrual cycle since she stopped oral contraceptive pills 5 months ago. Her 31-year-old partner is healthy and has no significant medical history and no risk factors for infertility. The woman has always been thin and was a competitive athlete in her teens and twenties. She had regular menstrual cycles after puberty but became amenorrheic in high school. She has been on oral contraceptive pills since that time.

On physical examination of the woman, her pulse rate is 54 beats/min and BMI is 18 kg/m². She has a normal thyroid gland. She has no hirsutism or acne. On pelvic examination, she has pale, atrophic vaginal mucosa and no cervical mucus. Bimanual examination does not detect any pelvic masses or tenderness. The uterus is small.

Laboratory test results:

Prolactin, normal
TSH, normal
FSH = 1.5 mIU/mL (SI: 1.5 IU/L)

Estradiol (ultrasensitive assay) = 10 pg/mL
  (SI: 36.7 pmol/L)
AMH = 0.01 ng/mL (SI: 0.07 pmol/L)

Which of the following is the most likely diagnosis?

A. Primary ovarian insufficiency

B. PCOS

C. Hypogonadotropic hypogonadism

D. Postpill amenorrhea

Answer: C) Hypogonadotropic hypogonadism

While this patient's AMH level is quite low, perhaps suggesting primary ovarian insufficiency (Answer A), the FSH level is also low in the face of a low estradiol. This combination of findings suggests a central cause of amenorrhea (Answer C). While oral contraceptive pills (Answer D) may suppress endogenous FSH and hence ovarian estradiol, this suppression would not persist for 5 months after stopping the pills and to this extent. Additionally, after 5 months off the oral contraceptive pills, recovery of ovarian suppression (low AMH) would be expected. Patients with PCOS (Answer B) are not hypoestrogenic, and AMH would be expected to be high due to increased ovarian reserve.

Case 4 (Continued)

For this woman, which of the following would be the best treatment to improve her fertility?

A. Pulsatile GnRH therapy

B. Letrozole

C. Recombinant FSH and hCG

D. Referral to an assisted reproductive technology expert for assessment through an ovarian biopsy and in vitro fertilization

Answer: A) Pulsatile GnRH therapy

Based on her history and laboratory results, this patient has hypogonadotropic hypogonadism. This is most likely functional in nature. She should be queried about her diet and exercise patterns, and she should be counseled that a slightly higher body weight might be useful for ovulation. However, the appropriate medical treatment is to replace the missing hormone: GnRH (Answer A). The patient would not be expected to respond to aromatase inhibitors (Answer B) or clomiphene since her serum estradiol is already low. FSH and hCG can be given (Answer C), but the risk for ovarian hyperstimulation and multiple pregnancy is high in a young, likely otherwise fertile woman, so careful management is required by an experienced provider. Ovarian biopsy would not be indicated, and in vitro fertilization (Answer D) is reserved for circumstances when single follicular development is not achieved with exogenous gonadotropin and pulsatile GnRH therapy is not available.

References

1. Steiner AZ, Pritchard D, Stanczyk FZ, et al. Association between biomarkers of ovarian reserve and infertility among older women of reproductive age. *JAMA.* 2017;318(14):1367-1376. PMID: 29049585

2. Zarek SM, Mitchell EM, Sjaarda LA, et al. Is anti-müllerian hormone associated with fecundability? Findings from the EAGeR trial. *J Clin Endocrinol Metab.* 2015;100(11):4215-4521. PMID: 26406293

3. Depmann M, Broer SL, Eijkemans MJC, et al. Anti-Müllerian hormone does not predict time to pregnancy: results of a prospective cohort study. *Gynecol Endocrinol.* 2017;33(8):644-648. PMID: 28393651

4. Birch Petersen K, Hvidman HW, Forman JL, et al. Ovarian reserve assessment in users of oral contraception seeking fertility advise on their reproductive lifespan. *Hum Reprod.* 2015;30(10):2364-2375. PMID: 26311148

5. Letourneau JM, Cakmak H, Quinn M, et al. Long-term hormonal contraceptive use is associated with a reversible suppression of antral follicle count and a break from hormonal contraception may improve oocyte yield. *J Assist Reprod Genet.* 2017;34(9):1137-1144. PMID: 28669055

6. Goodman NF, Cobin RH, Futterweit W, et al; American Association of Clinical Endocrinologists (AACE); American College of Endocrinology (ACE); Androgen Excess and PCOS Society (AES). American Association of Clinical Endocrinologists, American College of Endocrinology, and Androgen

Excess and PCOS Society disease state clinical review: guide to best practices in the evaluation and treatment of polycystic ovary syndrome--Part 1. *Endocr Pract.* 2015;21(11):1291-1300. PMID: 26509855

7. Goodman NF, Cobin RH, Futterweit W, et al; American Association of Clinical Endocrinologists (AACE); American College of Endocrinology (ACE); Androgen Excess and PCOS Society. American Association of Clinical Endocrinologists, American College of Endocrinology, and Androgen Excess and PCOS Society Disease State Clinical Review: guide to the best practices in the evaluation and treatment of polycystic ovary syndrome - Part 2. *Endocr Pract.* 2015;21(12):1415-1426. PMID: 26642102

8. Legro RS, Barnhart HX, Schlaff WD, et al; Cooperative Multicenter Reproductive Medicine Network. Clomiphene, metformin, or both for infertility in the polycystic ovary syndrome. *N Engl J Med.* 2007;356(6):551-566. PMID: 17287476

9. Legro RS, Brzyski RG, Diamond MP, et al; NICHD Reproductive Medicine Network. Letrozole versus clomiphene for infertility in the polycystic ovary syndrome [published correction appears in *N Engl J Med.* 2014;317(15):1465]. *N Engl J Med.* 2014;371(2):119-129. PMDI: 25006718

10. Tran ND, Cedars MI, Rosen MP. The role of anti-müllerian hormone (AMH) in assessing ovarian reserve. *J Clin Endocrinol Metab.* 2011;96(12):3609-3614. PMID: 21937624

11. Gordon CM, Ackerman KE, Berga SL, et al. Functional Hypothalamic Amenorrhea: An Endocrine Society Clinical Practice Guideline. *J Clin Endocrinol Metab.* 2017;102(5):1413-1439. PMID: 28368518

12. Dumont A, Dewailly D, Plouvier P, Catteau-Jonard S, Robin G. Comparison between pulsatile GnRH therapy and gonadotropins for ovulation induction in women with both functional hypothalamic amenorrhea and polycystic ovarian morphology. *Gynecol Endocrinol.* 2016;32(12):999-1004. PMID: 27258574

13. Tranoulis A, Laios A, Pampanos A, Yannoukakos D, Loutradis D, Michala L. Efficacy and safety of pulsatile gonadotropin-releasing hormone therapy among patients with idiopathic and functional hypothalamic amenorrhea: a systematic review of the literature and a meta-analysis. *Fertil Steril.* 2018;109(4):708-719.e8. PMID: 29605411

Health Care of the Transgender Woman Across the Lifespan

Vin Tangpricha, MD, PhD. Professor of Medicine, Division of Endocrinology, Metabolism, and Lipids, Department of Medicine, Emory University School of Medicine, Atlanta, GA; E-mail: vin.tangpricha@emory.edu

Learning Objectives

As a result of participating in this session, learners should be able to:

- Initiate and monitor hormone therapy in transgender women.

- Counsel transgender women on health concerns from young, middle, and senior ages.

- Screen for conditions in transgender women that may arise from gender-affirming hormone therapy.

Main Conclusions

Transgender women are women who were recorded with a male gender at birth but have a female gender identity. Transgender women have unique health care needs starting from early adulthood to their senior years. Endocrinologists should be able to manage the initiation and monitoring of hormone therapy and be aware of potential health conditions unique among transgender women. Topics important for transgender women include fertility preservation, cancer screening, osteoporosis screening, HIV disease prevention, and cardiovascular/cerebrovascular disease prevention. Larger and longer-term studies of high quality are needed to guide future recommendations specific to transgender women.

Significance of the Clinical Problem

Transgender people represent a growing segment of the US and world population. The current estimated population of adults who identify as transgender is 0.6% in the United States.[1] Guidelines for transgender and gender nonconforming individuals have been developed by the Endocrine Society and other associations to address the health needs of this population.[2] Although high-quality evidence is lacking to inform current recommendations, endocrinologists and other health care practitioners should be able to counsel transgender women at all stages of the lifespan—young, middle, and senior ages. Current guidelines suggest screening for chronic diseases per recommendations for the cisgender population. Since the release of the guidelines, more evidence has emerged regarding the risks of gender-affirming hormone therapy in transgender women. Endocrinologists should counsel young transgender women on reproductive options, HIV prevention, and safe hormone level targets. Middle-aged and senior-aged transgender women need counseling on screening for hormone-sensitive cancers, osteoporosis, and cardiovascular/cerebrovascular disease. This chapter focuses on unique health care needs of transgender women across the lifespan.

Barriers to Optimal Practice

- Most endocrinologists have not had formal fellowship training on transgender medicine, as this is an emerging field in endocrinology.

- Guidelines for the care of transgender people have largely been extrapolated from other populations, but new data are emerging for conditions that may be associated with gender-affirming hormone therapy.

- Management of transgender women requires an individualized approach and understanding of potential adverse events associated with gender-affirming hormone therapy.

Strategies for Diagnosis, Therapy, and/or Management

Transgender women have a female gender identity and seek medical assistance in aligning their physical appearance with their gender identity by a combination of gender-affirming hormones, typically estrogen and testosterone-lowering medications, and/or gender-affirming surgeries, which include genital and nongenital surgeries. Most transgender women have gender dysphoria, which describes the uneasiness expressed when an individual's gender identity does not match the physical and behavioral social norms associated with one's gender recorded at birth. The diagnosis of a transgender identity is made primarily by a detailed history and use of the diagnostic criteria for gender dysphoria in the *Diagnostic and Statistical Manual of Mental Disorders, Fifth Edition (DSM-5)*.[3] There are plans to move these criteria to a separate chapter focused on sexual health in future editions of the DSM, as having a transgender identity is not a disorder.

Most experienced clinicians can diagnose transgender identity in adults and youth older than age 16 years presenting for gender-affirming medical care. However, in cases where the diagnosis is not clear or the presentation could be confounded by mental health conditions, clinicians should refer these individuals to a mental health specialist for management of the potentially confounding mental health conditions and for confirmation of the transgender identity. For transgender youth younger than age 16 years, the diagnosis of a transgender identity should be made in consultation with a multidisciplinary team with medical and mental health specialists who have expertise in gender dysphoria in transgender and gender-diverse youth.

Before the initiation of gender-affirming hormone therapy, clinicians should evaluate for medical conditions that can be exacerbated by hormone therapy. This includes health conditions that can be exacerbated by estrogen such as hormone-sensitive cancers, thromboembolic disorders, and potentially cardiovascular and cerebrovascular diseases. Gender-affirming hormone therapy for transgender women consists of estrogen (oral estradiol, 2-6 mg daily; transdermal patch, 0.025-0.2 mg daily; or parenteral estradiol valerate, 5-20 mg intramuscularly every 2 weeks) in combination with a testosterone-lowering medication (oral spironolactone, 100-300 mg daily; GnRH agonist monthly or quarterly subcutaneously; or cyproterone acetate, 50-100 mg daily). The Endocrine Society recommends monitoring hormone levels every 3 months in the first year and 1 to 2 times yearly to ensure values are in the suggested target ranges (estradiol, 100-200 pg/mL, and testosterone, <50 ng/dL).

Most importantly, before starting hormone therapy, clinicians should discuss future fertility plans since hormone therapy will decrease fertility potential. In a survey of transgender women in Belgium, 51% of participants stated that they wished to store sperm for future fertility if they had been provided with that option.[4] The most widely available option available for fertility preservation for transgender women is sperm cryopreservation.[5] Other options that are currently under investigation include spermatogonium stem cell and testicular tissue cryopreservation.[5] Reproductive services for transgender women already taking hormone therapy are very limited.[6] One study of 135 transgender women undergoing orchiectomy as part of gender-affirmation surgery found that 79% of the patients had no evidence of spermatogenesis on microscopic examination.[7] A similar study of 86 transgender women undergoing orchiectomy found 80% maturation arrest of the spermatogonia.[8] The time course of recovery of normal spermatogenesis following cessation of gender-affirming hormones is not known and is most likely dependent on the dose, duration, and regimens used. For those transgender women who have already started hormone therapy, there are no published guidelines to assist in the recovery of spermatogenesis. One published case report of a 26-year-old transgender woman taking parental estradiol and oral spironolactone for 16 months discontinued her hormone regimen for 2 months and started therapy with follitropin alfa (FSH), 3 times weekly, and clomiphene citrate, 25 mg daily. At 6 weeks, there was recovery of spermatogenesis, and levels of sex steroid hormones reached the male reference range.[9] While there is hope for further refinement in recovery of fertility potential in transgender women, clinicians should first discuss whether the patient is willing and able to discontinue gender-affirming hormone therapies to allow for recovery of spermatogenesis.

Cancer screening for transgender women should follow guidelines currently put forth for cisgender women. Two large cohort studies have investigated the risk of breast cancer in transgender women. A study from the Netherlands reported the incidence of breast cancer among 2260 transgender women who were a mean of 51 years of age and on hormone therapy for approximately 20 years. There were only 18 cases of breast cancer found in this cohort (15 invasive and 3 noninvasive cancers). The standardized incidence ratio of breast cancer was 0.3 (95% confidence interval (CI), 0.2-0.4) compared with cisgender women and 46.7 (95% CI, 27.2-75.4) compared with cisgender men. In a cohort of 2791 transgender women in the United States, there were 3 cases of breast cancer (1 incident and 2 prevalent).[10]

Long-term health concerns for transgender women include cardiovascular, cerebrovascular, and thromboembolic disease. A Dutch cohort of 6793 transgender women seen in the gender clinic in Amsterdam from 1972 to 2015 found significant increases in events of stroke, myocardial infarction, and venous thromboembolism as compared to a female reference range.[11] A US cohort of 2842 transgender women found higher incidence of venous thromboembolism at 2 and 8 years of follow-up compared with reference groups of cisgender males or females.[12] Also, there was higher incidence of ischemic stroke and venous thromboembolism following initiation of gender-affirming hormone therapy relative to the incidence in cisgender males and females. The rate of myocardial infarction was similar between transgender women and reference cisgender males and females. Given the mixed findings for the rate of myocardial infarction, transgender women should have calculation of their 10-year risk of cardiovascular disease using the Atherosclerotic Cardiovascular Disease Risk Algorithm by the American Heart Association/American College of Cardiology to determine whether statin therapy is required. However, the current challenge is determining which gender to use for the risk calculator. A conservative approach would be to use the gender recorded at birth to provide the highest risk category. Individuals with greater than a 10% risk of cardiovascular disease may also consider the addition of aspirin to prevent cardiovascular disease according to the US Preventive Services Task Force guidelines.[13]

Compared with cisgender women, transgender women have higher rates of HIV infection.[14] The increased risk of HIV infection in transgender women is due to many factors, including inequalities in accessing health care and psychosocial, behavioral, and biologic factors.[14] The Centers for Disease Control recommend that individuals between the ages of 13 and 64 years get tested at least once and that individuals with risk factors undergo annual testing.[15] Clinicians should consider annual HIV testing in transgender women and counsel on safer sex practices.

Clinicians should also discuss preexposure prophylaxis with transgender women who are HIV negative.

Transgender women have increased risk for venous thromboembolism, which due to the known biologic effects of estrogen on blood-clotting proteins. The transdermal route of administration seems to be associated with lowered risk of venous thromboembolism. Certain estrogen preparations such as ethinyl estradiol and conjugated estrogens are associated with increased risk of venous thromboembolism. It is currently unknown if there is a threshold serum estradiol concentration whereby risks of venous thromboembolism are increased or if the risks of estrogen hormone are dose and duration dependent in transgender women. In the absence of such data, the Endocrine Society recommendations state that estradiol concentrations should be targeted at a range of 100 to 200 pg/mL and should be used in combination with an androgen-lowering medication in order for the estrogen to have its best desired effect. Counseling on signs and symptoms of venous thromboembolism should be provided to transgender women. Furthermore, transgender women should have a preoperative and postoperative venous thromboembolism plan when undergoing major surgery. Transgender women at highest risk of venous thromboembolism, such as those with preexisting or history of unprovoked venous thromboembolism, may need lifelong anticoagulation therapy to remain on estrogen therapy.

For older transgender women, osteoporosis screening should also follow guidelines for cisgender women. A meta-analysis of 9 studies representing 392 transgender women found significant increases in bone density at the spine 12 and 24 months following hormone therapy but no significant changes at the total hip and femoral neck. Fractures were only evaluated in a small study of 53 transgender women where no fractures were reported. Similar to the recommendations by the Endocrine Society, the International Society for Clinical Densitometry released a position statement in 2019 that bone density testing be performed according to guidelines recommended for cisgender women and earlier screening be performed in transgender women who may have experienced interruptions in their gender-affirming hormone therapy or have traditional risk factors for bone loss.[16] The International Society for Clinical Densitometry also stated that Z-scores and T-scores should be calculated from the reference population that conforms with an individual's gender identity and that there are no data to suggest that bone mineral density predicts fracture risk differently in the transgender population than in the cisgender population. Therefore, in the absence of data, treatment decisions should be made based on the combination of bone density results and FRAX risk score.

Clinical Case Vignettes
Case 1

A 24-year-old transgender woman presents to your office to discuss potential fertility options. She was recently married and would like to explore potential options for having children using her own genetic material. For the past 2 years, she has been on estradiol, 2 mg orally twice daily, and spironolactone, 100 mg twice daily. Her partner is a cisgender woman who has not had children in the past. The patient's laboratory tests include an estradiol concentration of 150 pg/mL (550.7 pmol/L) and a total testosterone concentration of 10 ng/dL (0.3 nmol/L). Her electrolytes are normal.

Which of the following is the best next step given this patient's concern?

A. Start clomiphene, 50 mg orally 3 times weekly

B. Discontinue estradiol and spironolactone and check semen analysis in 3 months

C. Inform her that adoption is the only option since she has already started hormone therapy

D. Refer her for microsurgical epididymal sperm aspiration

E. Discuss whether discontinuation of hormone therapy would be an option for her

Answer: E) Discuss whether discontinuation of hormone therapy would be an option for her

This transgender woman wishes to discuss fertility options. She has already started gender-affirming hormone therapy. Initiating clomiphene (Answer A) is incorrect because starting clomiphene without discontinuing estradiol and spironolactone will not likely result in successful sperm recovery. Discontinuing estradiol and spironolactone and checking semen analysis in 3 months (Answer B) is incorrect because the clinician should first discuss how she would respond to discontinuation of hormone therapy. Stating that adoption is the only option (Answer C) is incorrect as there are several options for infertility for transgender women. Referring her for microsurgical epididymal sperm extraction (Answer D) is incorrect since at the present time there is unlikely to be sufficient sperm for aspiration. The first step is to determine whether the patient could tolerate discontinuation of hormone therapy (Answer E) and to discuss the potential time course off therapy. It is unknown how much time is required for sperm to recover spontaneously. She will most likely need additional therapies such as clomiphene and/or FSH treatment.

Case 2

A 55-year-old transgender woman comes to your office for her annual physical examination and refills of her gender-affirming hormone therapy. She has been on gender-affirming hormone therapy for 10 years. She is currently on an estradiol patch, 0.1 mg daily changed weekly. She completed gender-affirmation surgery with penile inversion technique and orchiectomy 6 years ago. She is monogamous and happily married to a cisgender male. She does not have children. Her only other medical problem is hypertension for which she takes hydrochlorothiazide, 25 mg daily.

On physical examination, her BMI is 28.2 kg/m², and blood pressure is 128/76 mm Hg. The rest of the examination findings are normal.

She wants to know which tests she requires for health screening this year.

Which of the following tests is NOT currently indicated in her case?

A. Serum estradiol measurement

B. Breast mammography

C. Fasting lipid profile

D. Bone mineral density by DXA

E. Carotid ultrasonography

Answer: E) Carotid ultrasonography

This middle-aged transgender woman presents for her routine annual physical examination. Annual serum estradiol measurement (Answer A) is recommended by the Endocrine Society. She is older than 50 years, and she should have screening mammography (Answer B) as recommended for the cisgender population. She has hypertension and elevated BMI, and she should have a fasting lipid profile (Answer C) to calculate her 10-year risk of cardiovascular disease to determine whether she should start statin therapy. She should have annual bone density screening (Answer D). Carotid ultrasonography (Answer E) is not a recommended test for screening for cardiovascular disease in transgender women.

Case 3

A 75-year-old transgender woman presents to your clinic to discuss osteoporosis. She recently underwent bone mineral density testing by DXA and was told that she had osteoporosis. She has lost about 3 cm from her maximum reported height. She consumes 3 servings of dairy daily. She smoked cigarettes for 10 years and quit when she was 40 years old. She has not had any fractures. She does not drink alcohol. She has been taking estradiol, 2 mg daily. She had gender-affirmation surgery, which included orchiectomy, when she was 55 years old. Her current estradiol concentration is 120 pg/mL (440.5 pmol/L), and her total testosterone concentration is less than 5 ng/dL (<0.2 nmol/L). Her DXA report documents the following:

> Spine (L1-L4) T-score = –2.9
> Left femoral neck T-score = –2.3
> Left total hip T-score = –1.7

The T-scores were calculated using the female reference range.

Which of the following is the best next treatment step?

A. Start raloxifene, 60 mg daily

B. Start vitamin D, 2000 IU daily, and calcium, 2500 mg daily

C. Increase the estradiol dosage to 6 mg daily

D. Start oral alendronate, 70 mg once weekly

E. Start low-dose transdermal testosterone daily

F. Start oral DHEA, 50 mg daily

Answer: D) Start oral alendronate

This transgender woman has osteoporosis. Starting oral alendronate (Answer D) is the best option since she meets the criteria for treatment based on her spine T-score of –2.9. Starting raloxifene (Answer A) would not be correct because a selective estrogen-receptor modulator plus estradiol would increase the risk of venous thromboembolism. Starting vitamin D and calcium (Answer B) is incorrect because vitamin D and calcium are insufficient to treat osteoporosis in this patient. Increasing the estradiol dosage (Answer C) is incorrect since her serum estradiol levels are in the correct range. Starting low-dosage transdermal testosterone (Answer E) and starting oral DHEA (Answer F) are incorrect because there are no data to support adding these therapies to the regimen of transgender women.

References

1. Flores AR, Herman JL, Gates GJ, Brown TN. How many adults identify as transgender in the United States? Los Angeles: The Williams Institute; 2016. Available at: https://williamsinstitute.law.ucla.edu/wp-content/uploads/How-Many-Adults-Identify-as-Transgender-in-the-United-States.pdf. Accessed for verification December 2019.

2. Hembree WC, Cohen-Kettenis PT, Gooren L, et al. Endocrine treatment of gender-dysphoric/gender-incongruent persons: an Endocrine Society clinical practice guideline. *J Clin Endocrinol Metab.* 2017;102(11):3869-3903. PMID: 28945902

3. American Psychiatric Association. *Diagnostic and Statistical Manual of Mental Disorders, 5th ed.* Arlington, VA: American Psychiatric Publishing. 2013.

4. De Sutter P, Kira K, Verschoor A, Hotimsky A. The desire to have children and the preservation of fertility in transsexual women: a survey. *Int J Transgend.* 2002;6(3).

5. Mattawanon N, Spencer JB, Schirmer DA 3rd, Tangpricha V. Fertility preservation options in transgender people: a review. *Rev Endocr Metab Disord.* 2018;19(3):231-242. PMID: 30219984

6. James-Abra S, Tarasoff LA, Green D, et al. Trans people's experiences with assisted reproduction services: a qualitative study. *Hum Reprod.* 2015;30(6):1365-1374. PMID: 25908658

7. Kent MA, Winoker JS, Grotas AB. Effects of feminizing hormones on sperm production and malignant changes: microscopic examination of post orchiectomy specimens in transwomen. *Urology.* 2018;121:93-96. PMID: 30092303

8. Matoso A, Khandakar B, Yuan S, et al. Spectrum of findings in orchiectomy specimens of persons undergoing gender confirmation surgery. *Hum Pathol.* 2018;76:91-99. PMID: 29555572

9. Alford AV, Theisen KM, Kim N, Bodie JA, Pariser JJ. Successful ejaculatory sperm cryopreservation after cessation of long-term estrogen therapy in a transgender female. *Urology.* 2019;pii:S0090-4295(19)30739-3. PMID: 31465795

10. Silverberg MJ, Nash R, Becerra-Culqui TA, et al. Cohort study of cancer risk among insured transgender people. *Ann Epidemiol.* 2017;27(8):499-501. PMID: 28780974

11. Nota NM, Wiepjes CM, de Blok CJM, Gooren LJG, Kreukels BPC, den Heijer M. Occurrence of acute cardiovascular events in transgender individuals receiving hormone therapy. *Circulation.* 2019;139(11):1461-1462. PMID: 30776252

12. Getahun D, Nash R, Flanders WD, et al. Cross-sex hormones and acute cardiovascular events in transgender persons: a cohort study. *Ann Intern Med.* 2018;169(4):205-213. PMID: 29987313

13. US Preventive Services Task Force. Final recommendation statement: aspirin use to prevent cardiovascular disease and colorectal cancer: preventive medication. Available at: https://www.uspreventiveservicestaskforce.org/Page/Document/RecommendationStatementFinal/aspirin-to-prevent-cardiovascular-disease-and-cancer. Accessed for verification December 2019.

14. Ackerley CG, Poteat T, Kelley CF. Human immunodeficiency virus in transgender persons. *Endocrinol Metab Clin North Am.* 2019;48(2):453-464. PMID: 31027552

15. Centers for Disease Control and Prevention. Screening in Clinical Settings. Available at: https://www.cdc.gov/hiv/clinicians/screening/clinical-settings.html. Accessed for verification December 2019.

16. Rosen HN, Hamnvik OR, Jaisamrarn U, et al. Bone densitometry in transgender and gender nonconforming (TGNC) individuals: the 2019 ISCD Official Positions. *J Clin Densitom.* 2019;pii:S1094-6950(19)30150-7. PMID: 31327665

Management of Hormone Replacement Therapy in Post–Reproductive-Aged Women

Genevieve Neal-Perry, MD, PhD. Reproductive Endocrinology, Department of Obstetrics and Gynecology, University of Washington School of Medicine, Seattle, WA; E-mail: nealperr@uw.edu

Learning Objectives

As a result of participating in this session, learners should be able to:

- Explain the basic physiology of menopause and modifiers of symptomology.

- Manage common symptoms of the menopausal transition and describe the risks associated with treatment.

Main Conclusions

Female reproductive senescence reflects the gradual loss of oocytes as the reproductive axis matures in a continuous, natural process from menarche to menopause. It reflects the loss of the finite numbers of oocytes produced during fetal development. *Menopause* is defined as the permanent cessation of menses; by convention, the diagnosis of menopause is not made until the individual has had 12 months of amenorrhea. Menopause is thus characterized by the loss of menses. However, hormonal changes, rather than the cessation of menstruation itself, often give rise to bothersome vasomotor symptoms that disrupt the quality of life of affected women. When used in the appropriate patient population, hormone replacement therapy (HT) is highly effective and safe.

Significance of the Clinical Problem

Reduced and variable circulating levels of estradiol during the menopausal transition and early menopause are associated with vasomotor symptoms, disrupted sleep patterns, and increased morbidity. The population at risk for menopausal symptoms numbers in the hundreds of millions and varies by race, ethnicity, and socioeconomics. HT is currently the most effective treatment for these life-disrupting symptoms. However, study outcomes from the Women's Health Initiative have affected appropriate use of HT.

Barriers to Optimal Practice

- Fears of patients regarding the appropriate use of HT.

- Misinterpretation of clinical studies regarding HT.

Strategies for Diagnosis, Therapy, and/or Management

Menopause is characterized by the permanent cessation of menses and follicular depletion of the ovaries and defined retrospectively by the absence of menses for a minimum of 12 months. Menopause typically occurs in the fifth to sixth decades of life, with a median age of 52.5 years. However, this definition relies upon a woman having menstrual cycles of some degree of regularity. Menopause and the final menstrual period are preceded by the menopausal transition, a window of time that is characterized by several years of menstrual cycle instability and erratic hormone secretion. The average woman takes about 4 years to make the transition into menopause. However, there is a wide variation about this median.[1] Women who enter the transition at a younger age tend to have more symptoms and a longer duration, whereas those who enter it later in life are more likely to have a more rapid transit to the final menstrual period. There are racial and ethnic differences in menopausal symptoms and multiple other factors that may influence the timing of the final menstrual period for any given woman (see Table).

The menopausal transition is heralded by ovarian follicular pool depletion (ovarian reserve), menstrual cycle length changes, reduced luteal phase progesterone synthesis, variable estradiol levels, and elevated FSH.[2] The associated hormonal fluctuations may trigger debilitating symptoms in the early menopausal transition, symptoms that may worsen and persist throughout the early postmenopausal period.

Table. Factors That Influence the Age at Menopause

Factor	Direction	Degree
Genetic/familial		
MSH6	Earlier menopause	NA
MCM8	Earlier menopause	NA
Pvull estrogen receptor (ER) polymorphism	Earlier menopause, hysterectomy	6 months
Turner syndrome mosaic	Earlier menopause	Variable
Fragile X	Earlier menopause	Variable
Environmental		
Endocrine-disrupting chemicals	Earlier menopause	1.8-3.8 years
High altitude	Earlier menopause	1-1.5 years
Lifestyle		
Cigarette smoking	Earlier menopause	1-2 years
Low socioeconomic status	Earlier menopause	1-2 years
Oral contraceptive use	Later menopause	6 months
Race/ethnicity		
African American	Earlier menopause[*]	2 years
Hispanic	Earlier menopause	2 years
Asian	Later menopause	1-2 years
Menstrual characteristics		
Shorter cycles (<26 days)	Earlier menopause	1.4 years

[*] Relative to Caucasian women.

Diagnosis of Menopause

Laboratory tests are typically not indicated if history and physical examination rule out other potential causes of amenorrhea and bothersome symptoms.

Measurement of FSH and estradiol or antimullerian hormone may be indicated for women who:

- have had a hysterectomy without oophorectomy

- are younger than 40 years

- are using estrogen-containing contraceptives (suppress FSH and elevate estradiol)

- continue to have menses after age 55 years (may be postmenopausal but with bleeding endometrial neoplasm or other uterine pathology)

Menopausal Symptoms

Menopausal symptoms are often composed of 4 cardinal symptoms that directly relate to menopause. These include vasomotor symptoms/hot flashes, vaginal dryness, sleep, and mood/cognition.

Vasomotor symptoms affect up to 80% of women. Thermoregulatory dysfunction begins in hypothalamus in response to hormonal fluctuations. The threshold in core temperature for cooling (flushes, sweats) is lowered, and the threshold for warming (shivering) is raised. KNDy neurons (kisspeptin/neurokinin B/dynorphin), located adjacent to the thermoregulatory center, are hypothesized to be the primary driver of vasomotor symptoms.[3] Vasomotor symptoms have a median duration of 7.4 years, with a mean post-final menstrual period persistence of 4.5 years.[4] However, further clinical history can help predict the duration of vasomotor symptoms with more precision. Shared decision making about treatment type and duration can be facilitated by taking these additional factors into account.

Vaginal dryness, dyspareunia, and urogenital symptoms are less common than vasomotor symptoms, but are highly prevalent and disruptive of the quality of life. Affected women often report vaginal dryness, chronic irritation, or burning of both the vagina and vulva; decreased lubrication; pain during sex; or bleeding after sex. Urinary frequency, urethritis, and frequent urinary tract infections may also occur. Symptoms that women experience are believed to reflect hypogonadism. Genitourinary syndrome of menopause rather than atrophic vaginitis is a term used to describe vaginal dryness apart from intercourse, dyspareunia, and associated urinary symptoms.[5] Unlike vasomotor symptoms, symptoms of genitourinary syndrome of menopause do not spontaneously resolve over time. Therefore, long-term treatment may be required to preserve quality of life. Ospemifene, a selective estrogen receptor modulator with estrogen receptor β-agonist properties, is available; however, it is administered systemically. To treat dyspareunia, the FDA recently approved vaginal dehydroepiandrosterone. Additionally, several studies have raised the possibility that laser treatment of the vagina may provide relief from genitourinary syndrome of menopause symptoms, although there is insufficient information to recommend this approach at this time. Adverse mood is associated with traversal of menopause in a complex manner.

Depressive symptoms are associated with night-time hot flashes and sleep disruption, suggesting an intimate relationship between sleep and mood. Cohort studies have identified the late transition as a period of vulnerability for depression in midlife women. Women are 2- to 4-fold more likely to experience new-onset major depression during the menopausal transition than premenopausal women or after their final menstrual period.[6] Neither major depression nor depressive symptoms are associated with absolute levels of hormones. However, concomitant anxiety and hot flashes predict the risk for major depression during this time of life. Heavier flow (menorrhagia), irregular cycle length (metrorrhagia), and intermenstrual bleeding can reflect high estrogen relative to low progesterone associated with anovulation. This hormonal imbalance can cause endometrial overgrowth, precancer (endometrial hyperplasia), or cancer. Postmenopausal bleeding or perimenopausal bleeding at intervals less than 21 days warrants evaluation.

Sleep disturbances are common in women, but also worsen with age. Thus, it may be challenging to distinguish between age-related sleep changes and poor sleep due to menopause. While some epidemiologic studies suggest the menopausal transition contributes to sleep dysfunction in advanced reproductive-aged women, others do not, except for a small, vulnerable subset of women with relatively poor sleep at baseline. Vasomotor symptoms can mediate sleep disruption in perimenopausal and recently menopausal women, in part by prompting night-time awakenings. HT may help sleep dysfunction exacerbated by vasomotor symptoms.

Treatment of Bothersome Menopausal Symptoms

Hormonal management includes estradiol, estrogens, and progestin when a uterus is present. When selecting a menopausal HT regimen, the following should be considered: (1) the presence of a uterus, (2) the type of menopausal symptoms for which treatment is desired, and (3) comorbid medical conditions that might influence management options.

Estrogen therapy given to women younger than 60 years without a uterus carries minimal risk. Estrogen and progestogen therapy should be given to women with a uterus, but it carries an increased breast cancer risk for women of all ages. Estrogen and progestogen risks may be dose dependent and may vary by progestogen type. Progestin intrauterine devices may also be used; however, their impact on breast cancer risk has not been determined. Progesterone alone can decrease hot flashes, but it is rarely used due to breast cancer concerns.

The FDA recommends that HT be used in women with bothersome symptoms, at the lowest possible dosage, and for the shortest duration required to ease symptoms. Tissue-targeted therapies should be used whenever possible to decrease overall systemic dose (eg, vaginal estrogen for vaginal symptoms). Transdermal preparations may carry lower risk of thromboembolic events while providing the same efficacy for treatment management. Progestogen is indicated for women with a uterus, but the dosage should be carefully considered. All women taking HT should be evaluated annually.

Risks and Adverse Effects of HT

Risks and adverse effects of HT are modulated by the route of administration, hormonal formulation, patient age, time since the final menstrual period, the presence or absence of a uterus, and coexisting morbidities such as cardiovascular disease, dementia, and diabetes.[7]

Uterine Neoplasia

The incidence of uterine neoplasia is increased under conditions of chronic unopposed estrogen exposure in a woman with an intact uterus. Thus, the primary indication of progestin therapy during menopause is to prevent estradiol-induced endometrial hyperplasia and cancer. Commonly used progestins include medroxyprogesterone acetate, norethindrone acetate, and micronized progestin (native progesterone). Progestin administered continuously or sequentially provides adequate endometrial protection. However, controversy exits as to whether micronized progestin protects the uterus as effectively as synthetic progestin.

Breast Cancer

Breast cancer risk and menopausal HT are reported in randomized controlled trials and observational studies. Different types of menopausal HT formulations, the duration of therapy, and the time at which menopausal HT is initiated may modify the risk for breast cancer.[8]

Venous Thromboembolism

Venous thromboembolism and stroke risk increases with advancing age and a diagnosis of thrombophilia. The risk is related to oral administration and estradiol dosage.[9,10] Venous thromboembolism events are more likely to occur within the first year of HT, and the risk is magnified with coexisting risk factors such as obesity or thrombophilia. Venous thromboembolism risk is not significantly affected by micronized progesterone, medroxyprogesterone acetate, or norethindrone but may be increased by norpregnane derivatives.

Cognitive Function

The effects of HT on cognitive function are variable. Observational studies suggested cognitive function may improve with HT. Results from the Kronos Early Estrogen Prevention Study and Early vs Late Intervention Trial with Estradiol suggest that HT does not affect cognitive function when it is taken by younger women and in early menopause. In contrast, the Women's Health Initiative Memory Study found an increased incidence of dementia in women older than 65 years initiating HT. These studies suggest that cognitive health may be adversely affected by an interaction between age and HT.

Discontinuing Menopausal HT

Many women choose to discontinue hormones after the worst of their menopausal symptoms have subsided. For women planning to stop HT, they should stop taking HT 1 week before an annual visit to allow assessment of symptom severity. Most women prefer to slowly wean, while others just stop. However, a small proportion of women (3% to 15%) have persistence of severe symptoms and will require continued hormones or nonhormonal alternatives.

Summary

The hypogonadism of menopause can adversely affect multiple organ systems and increase the risk for morbidities such as osteoporosis, dementia, and heart disease. Observational studies and randomized controlled trials suggest the risk for morbidity is increased with advanced age and time since the onset of menopause. Additionally, the risk and benefit of HT vary by organ system, HT formulation, and the time since the final menstrual period. Observational studies, as well as randomized controlled trials, also suggest that HT, when administered within the first 5 years of the final menopause attenuates some but not all adverse effects of menopause that are related to hypogonadism.

Symptoms commonly associated with menopause (hot flashes, sleep dysfunction, mood, and genitourinary syndrome of menopause) are readily improved with HT. Nonetheless, fear of hormones has led to widespread undertreatment of symptoms and a proliferation of nonrigorously tested but popular treatments such as custom compounded hormones, pellets, and a large variety of herbal preparations. Clinicians should assess a patient's symptoms and offer evidence-based treatment, with periodic reevaluation of the necessity of treatment.

Clinical Case Vignettes
Case 1

A 48-year-old, G2P2, African American woman presents with complaints of hot flashes that are disruptive to her sleep and daily activity. She wakes up 6 to 8 times each night and reports feeling uncomfortable multiple times during the day.

Which of the following factors is likely to affect the duration of this patient's hot flashes?

A. Race

B. Age

C. Depression

D. Socioeconomic status

Answer: A) Race

There are racial and ethnic differences in the duration and persistence of hot flashes (Answer

A). For this patient, black race is a modifier. When compared with other races and ethnic groups, African American women are more likely to have a longer duration and persistence of hot flashes. Other modifiers of the severity of hot flashes include a high BMI, lower socioeconomic status, and depression.

See references 4 and 11.

Case 2

A 48-year-old, G0, sexually active woman presents with extremely heavy bleeding after amenorrhea for 6 months. Prior to that, menses were every 18 to 90 days. Her BMI is 62 kg/m^2, and she has a diagnosis of polycystic ovary syndrome, but she is otherwise healthy. She has no allergies. She is married and has an unremarkable family history. She would like help with her heavy periods and a contraceptive method.

Which of the following would be the best treatment for her heavy bleeding?

A. Combined oral contraception

B. Copper intrauterine device

C. Progestin intrauterine device

D. Vaginal contraceptive ring

E. Barrier contraception

Answer: C) Progestin intrauterine device

In women older than 45 years, combined oral contraceptives and vaginal contraceptive rings impose an increased risk for venous thromboembolism,[12] myocardial infarction,[13] and breast neoplasia.[14] A copper intrauterine device and a barrier would provide contraception, but they would not reduce the bleeding related to ovulatory dysfunction observed during perimenopause. A progestin intrauterine device would provide contraception and reduce the risk for endometrial neoplasia.[15]

References

1. Gold EB, Crawford SL, Avis NE, et al. Factors related to age at natural menopause: longitudinal analyses from SWAN. *Am J Epidemiol.* 2013;178(1):70-83. PMID: 23788671

2. Santoro N, Crawford SL, El Khoudary SR, et al. Menstrual cycle hormone changes in women traversing the menopause: study of women's health across the nation. *J Clin Endocrinol Metab.* 2017;102(7):2218-2229. PMID: 28368525

3. Prague JK, Roberts RE, Comninos AN, et al. Neurokinin 3 receptor antagonism as a novel treatment for menopausal hot flushes: a phase 2, randomised, double-blind, placebo-controlled trial. *Lancet.* 2017;389(10081):1809-1820. PMID: 28385352

4. Avis NE, Crawford SL, Greendale G. Duration of menopausal vasomotor symptoms over the menopause transition. *JAMA Intern Med.* 2015;175(4):531-539. PMID: 25686030

5. Portman DJ, Gass ML; Vulvovaginal Atrophy Terminology Consensus Conference Panel. Genitourinary syndrome of menopause: new terminology for vulvovaginal atrophy from the International Society for the Study of Women's Sexual Health and the North American Menopause Society. *Menopause.* 2014;21(10):1063-1068. PMID: 25160739

6. Bromberger JT, Kravitz HM, Chang YF, Cyranowski JM, Brown C, Matthews KA. Major depression during and after the menopausal transition: study of Women's Health Across the Nation (SWAN) [published correction appears in *Psychol Med.* 2011;41(9):1879-1888]. *Psychol Med.* 2011;41(9):1879-1888. PMID: 21306662

7. The NAMS 2017 Hormone Therapy Position Statement Advisory Panel. The 2017 hormone therapy position statement of The North American Menopause Society. *Menopause.* 2017;24(7):728-753. PMID: 28650869

8. Breast cancer and hormone replacement therapy: collaborative reanalysis of data from 51 epidemiological studies of 52,705 women with breast cancer and 108,411 women without breast cancer. Collaborative Group on Hormonal Factors in Breast Cancer [published correction appears in *Lancet.* 1997;350(9089):1484]. *Lancet.* 1997;350(9084):1047-1059. PMID: 10213546

9. Chlebowski RT, Rohan TE, Manson JE, et al. Breast cancer after use of estrogen plus progestin and estrogen alone: analyses of data from 2 Women's Health Initiative Randomized Clinical Trials. *JAMA Oncol.* 2015;1(3):296-305. PMID: 26181174

10. Canonico M, Plu-Bureau G, Lowe GD, Scarabin PY. Hormone replacement therapy and risk of venous thromboembolism in postmenopausal women: systematic review and meta-analysis. *BMJ.* 2008;336(7655):1227-1231. PMID: 18495631

11. Gold EB, Sternfeld B, Kelsey JL, et al. Relation of demographic and lifestyle factors to symptoms in a multi-racial/ethnic population of women 40-55 years of age. *Am J Epidemiol.* 2000;152(5):463-473. PMID: 10981461

12. Burkman RT, Collins JA, Shulman LP, Williams JK. Current perspectives on oral contraceptive use. *Am J Obstet Gynecol.* 2001;185(Suppl 2):S4-S12. PMID: 11521117

13. Carr BR, Ory H. Estrogen and progestin components of oral contraceptives: relationship to vascular disease. *Contraception.* 1997;55(5):267-272. PMID: 9220222

14. Marchbanks PA, McDonald JA, Wilson HG, et al. Oral contraceptives and the risk of breast cancer. *N Engl J Med.* 2002;346(26):2025-2032. PMID: 12087137

15. Bitzer J. Overview of perimenopausal contraception. *Climacteric.* 2019;22(1):44-50. PMID: 30562124

Detection and Management of Abuse of Androgenic Performance-Enhancing Drugs

Bradley D. Anawalt, MD. University of Washington School of Medicine, Seattle, WA;
E-mail: banawalt@medicine.washington.edu

Learning Objectives

As a result of participating in this session, learners should be able to:

- Recognize the clinical presentation of androgenic performing-enhancing drug (PED) abuse (including infertility).

- Identify the laboratory studies that are useful for identifying androgenic PED abuse.

- Recognize the pattern of serum hormone results that are consistent with specific forms of androgenic PED abuse.

- Develop a rational approach to the use of psychotherapy and hormone therapy in the management of patients who wish to discontinue androgenic PED abuse.

Main Conclusions

Androgens and drugs that raise endogenous androgen production are the most commonly abused PEDs. In clinical practice, androgenic PEDs are used almost exclusively by men. The proven health consequences include infertility, acne, and erythrocytosis in men. The other potential adverse effects include increased cardiovascular disease, hepatopathy (with oral alkylated androgens), neuropsychopathology, and ruptured upper-extremity tendons. The common clinical presentations of androgenic PED abuse are male infertility and requests for testosterone prescriptions to treat low serum testosterone. Serum gonadotropins are suppressed, and seminal fluid analyses show azoospermia or very low sperm concentrations. Recovery of gonadal axis function occurs spontaneously after discontinuation of androgenic PEDs. Treatment consists of encouraging cessation by respectful and nonjudgmental education about the health consequences of androgenic PEDs and management of underlying anxiety and depressive disorders. For some men who have abused high dosages of PEDs for years, there might be a role for adjunctive hormone therapy with a short course of testosterone or clomiphene to treat anabolic androgenic steroid withdrawal syndrome or a short course of gonadotropin or clomiphene therapy to hasten spermatogenic recovery and improve fertility.

Significance of the Clinical Problem

Many drugs are used to enhance athletic performance and appearance, including androgens and drugs that increase serum androgen concentrations, insulin, and growth hormone. Androgens administered at pharmacological dosages are the most commonly used PEDs, and they are the only class of drugs with definitive evidence that they enhance strength and athletic performance. Members of the general public are much less likely to use growth hormone, insulin, and other nonandrogens as potential PEDs.

For the purposes of this review and session, the focus will be androgenic PED abuse, and the use of pharmacological dosages of androgens or drugs that increase endogenous androgens will be defined as androgenic PED use. Individuals who are eugonadal and take androgenic PEDs are abusing them; prescription of androgen and gonadotropin replacement to hypogonadal patients is not PED abuse.

It has been difficult to assess the prevalence of androgenic PED abuse, but the lifetime prevalence of ever using these PEDs is probably 1% to 5% in men worldwide.[1] There is a trend toward decreased incidence in teenagers and young adults, but there might be increased incidence in middle-aged and older men. The chronic abuse of androgenic PEDs is much lower. The prevalence of androgenic PED abuse is much higher in men than in women (>50:1), and long-term abusers are almost exclusively male. Most chronic androgenic PED abusers begin in their twenties and are former elite or near-elite athletes or weightlifters with a fixation on being more muscular (often referred to as muscle dysmorphia or bigorexia).

It has been difficult to assess the short-term and long-term adverse effects of androgenic PEDs. There are well-described adverse effects of androgen therapy, including acne (more common in younger patients), erythrocytosis (more common in older patients), and infertility.[1,2] Chronic androgenic PED use accelerates male-pattern alopecia and causes hirsutism, alopecia, and defeminization and virilization in women. Hepatopathy occurs with use of oral alkylated androgens only, and there appears to be increased risk of tendinous ruptures, particularly in muscles of the arms and chest.[3,4] There is increasing evidence that there is an androgenic PED withdrawal syndrome of depressed mood, anxiety, and low self-esteem after acute cessation.[5,6]

Other potential adverse effects of high dosages of androgenic PEDs include increased risk of cardiovascular events, hypertension, and psychiatric disorders,[3,7] but the causal relationship is unclear because chronic androgenic PED abusers are also more likely to have baseline depression and anxiety and to use tobacco and marijuana products, alcohol, illicit drugs, and high dosages of dietary supplements and nutraceuticals that have not been studied rigorously for safety. In addition, androgenic PEDs are often purchased on the open market or through the Internet, and these drugs might contain or be contaminated with unsafe substances.

Barriers to Optimal Practice

- Social stigma and laws against androgenic PED abuse are barriers to disclosure of abuse.

- Many clinicians do not recognize the clues of possible androgenic PED abuse.

- Except for disclosure of androgenic abuse by the patient, there are no methods of making a definitive diagnosis of androgenic PED abuse in members of the general public.

- There are very limited data on the best therapeutic approach for individuals who abuse androgenic PEDs and want to discontinue.

- The data about the short-term and long-term effects of androgenic PED abuse are based on epidemiological studies with numerous confounders.

Strategies for Diagnosis, Therapy, and/or Management
Clinical Presentation of Androgenic PED Abuse

Men who chronically abuse androgenic PEDs typically present with infertility or with requests for evaluation for testosterone therapy. Men who are chronic androgenic PED abusers may present with androgenic PED withdrawal syndrome, with symptoms and signs of hypogonadism, or infertility. The use of aromatizable, androgenic PEDs may cause gynecomastia, and the use of nonaromatizable androgenic PEDs may be associated with sexual dysfunction.

Women who are chronic androgenic abusers are almost exclusively elite athletes and are rarely seen by most endocrinologists; they may present with amenorrhea, infertility, and variable degrees of defeminization and virilization. This session will not address this rare endocrine disorder.

Diagnosis of Androgenic PED Abuse

The diagnosis of androgenic PED abuse should be suspected in muscular men who present with infertility or an evaluation for testosterone therapy. Most men who abuse androgenic PEDs exercise frequently and many lift weights regularly. These men usually have bigorexia or muscular dysmorphia, a distorted body image that they are not muscular enough.[1] They will often spontaneously report that their strength and muscle bulk benefit has plateaued in the weight room. Another clue that may suggest chronic androgenic PED abuse is a history of use of nutraceuticals and supplements to build muscles (eg, creatine powder).

In addition to increased musculature, the physical examination may demonstrate gynecomastia and small testes, but these findings are not sensitive or specific. Chronic androgenic PED abuse is associated with variably decreased testicular volumes (typically ~25%-35%), and men with baseline testicular volumes of 25 mL or more may not have small testes after chronic androgenic PED abuse. Testicular texture (eg, softness or firmness) is not a specific or sensitive physical examination finding of androgenic PED abuse.

The biochemical evaluation for suspected androgenic PED abuse begins with measurement of serum testosterone and gonadotropins on a blood sample obtained between 7 and 10 AM. Serum testosterone and gonadotropin concentrations differ depending on the type of androgenic PED use (*Table*). The use of nontestosterone androgenic anabolic steroids (eg, nandrolone, oxandrolone, danazol, stanozolol, or tetrahydrogestrinone) is associated with low testosterone and gonadotropin concentrations. The standard evaluation for secondary

Table. Serum Hormone Concentrations During Androgenic PED Use

Androgenic PED	Serum Testosterone	Serum FSH	Serum LH
Testosterone	↑	↓	↓
Testosterone precursors[a]	↑	↓	↓
Nontestosterone AAS	↓	↓	↓
hCG	↑	↓	↓
Aromatase inhibitor alone	↑	↑	↑
Clomiphene	↑	↑	↑

Abbreviation: AAS, anabolic androgenic steroid.

[a] Very high dosages are required.

hypogonadism, including sellar imaging and measurement of serum prolactin, should be done in patients with this biochemical profile who do not report the use of androgenic PEDs. If androgenic PED use is suspected in a patient with laboratory evidence of secondary hypogonadism, it is worthwhile to repeat a respectful and nonjudgmental enquiry about androgenic PED use. Sometimes, patients will report androgenic PED use if they understand that further evaluation for other secondary causes of hypogonadism will cost them time and money.

Androgens raise serum hematocrit and decrease serum HDL cholesterol, SHBG, and thyroxine-binding globulin. In patients with suspected androgenic PED use, it is useful to measure hematocrit and often helpful to measure HDL cholesterol, SHBG, and/or thyroxine-binding globulin. Seminal fluid analyses generally show azoospermia or very low sperm concentrations.

There are methods for detecting androgenic PEDs and their metabolites in urine samples of elite athletes, but these methods are not available in commercial laboratories.[8] In addition, there are many ways to create spurious results, including dilution, substitution of someone else's sample, and submitting a sample at a time when the patient is not using androgenic PEDs. For elite athletes, urine samples are obtained under very strict circumstances, including random times and observed micturition into a sample container. Thus, methods to accurately measure androgenic PEDs and their metabolites in urine are not relevant diagnostic studies in clinical practice.

Treatment of Androgenic PED Abuse and Withdrawal Syndrome

There are no clinical trials or guidelines on the management of patients who abuse androgenic PEDs or the management of cessation of androgenic PEDs and androgenic PED withdrawal syndrome. Therefore, care of patients who abuse androgenic PEDs is based on the following: (1) readiness to cease androgenic PEDs; (2) duration and intensity of androgenic PED abuse; (3) near-team goals for fertility; and (4) a risk-benefit analysis of the treatment options compared with continuation or resumption of use of androgenic PEDs.[1]

A key principle for the care of androgenic PED users is the establishment a relationship of trust based on respectful and nonjudgmental behavior. While this principle guides all patient-clinician relationships, it is particularly important for this group of patients. They are often distrustful of traditional health care providers and scientists. After all, scientists disputed the benefits of androgenic PEDs decades after athletes empirically proved the performance-enhancing effects; why should androgenic PED abusers believe scientists and clinicians about potential adverse effects? All androgenic PED users must be queried about anxiety and depression and abuse of alcohol or illicit drugs and offered a referral for treatment if appropriate.

Some men are not prepared to stop using androgenic PEDs. The endocrinologist should counsel patients about the known adverse effects (including reduced fertility that might take 1 to 2 years to normalize after discontinuation of androgenic PEDs, erythrocytosis, and dyslipidemia) and potential adverse effects with a focus on the cardiovascular system. Some men who are not willing to discontinue androgenic PEDs are willing to "convert" to prescription testosterone. Conversion to intramuscular testosterone formulations at up to 2 to 3 times the usual replacement dosage with a tapering of the dosage over several months is likely to be safer than very high dosages of androgenic PEDs of unknown safety and purity purchased from unregulated sources. High dosages of testosterone are initially required because androgenic PED users generally use high dosages of various androgens simultaneously ("stacking"), and they will experience symptoms of withdrawal if immediately converted directly to typical testosterone replacement dosages used for treatment of male hypogonadism. This approach permits the establishment of a relationship between the patient and clinician over time; this might facilitate eventual discontinuation of androgenic PED use.

For men who are ready to quit androgenic PED use, there are the following options: (1) immediate discontinuation without medical therapy; (2) conversion to testosterone therapy with a tapering dosage over many months (see above); (3) discontinuation with initiation of a limited course of subcutaneous hCG therapy, or (4) discontinuation with initiation of a limited course of oral clomiphene therapy.

Immediate discontinuation of androgenic PEDs without additional medical therapy is the best choice for men who have used these drugs for 1 year or less. Based on limited, low-quality data, it appears that after androgenic PED discontinuation, serum gonadotropin concentrations spontaneously normalize within 3 to 6 months, followed by recovery of serum testosterone to normal serum concentrations within 6 months in most men who report a year or less of androgenic PED use. Spermatogenesis typically returns to normal 3 to 6 months after serum testosterone normalizes.[1,9]

For men who report chronic androgenic PED use longer than 1 year, there is a higher risk of withdrawal syndrome, and the gonadal axis may take years to recover.[1,10,11] Intramuscular testosterone that is tapered over many months might be a good option for many of these men, but this approach is not an option for men who are interested in conceiving. Exogenous testosterone therapy will continue to suppress spermatogenesis and fertility. For men who are infertile because of androgenic PED use for more than 1 year and who want to have a child within the next 2 years, the best options may be hCG therapy or clomiphene therapy. There is much more clinical experience and safety data for hCG therapy than for clomiphene, but there are scanty data on the effectiveness for improving spermatogenesis and fertility in this setting for either drug.

Clinical Case Vignettes

Case

A 32-year-old man requests evaluation for testosterone or clomiphene therapy. He reports decreased libido and decreased sexual pleasure. He also reports that he is experiencing less benefit (muscle mass and strength) with his weightlifting workouts at the local gym. He reports no easy bruisability, purple striae, hand arthralgias, or use of corticosteroids or androgens. He went through puberty at age 13 or 14 years. He reports no history of medical illness, and his only surgery was an appendectomy at age 9 years. He takes no medications. He states that he does not take anabolic androgenic steroids ("steroids"). He reports taking no opioids or other illicit drugs. He drinks 2 to 3 cocktails weekly.

On physical examination, his blood pressure is 135/85 mm Hg, pulse rate is 80 beats/min, respiratory rate is 12 breaths/min, and BMI is 21 kg/m². He is muscular. There is no gynecomastia, and testes are 15 mL bilaterally. No acne is observed.

Laboratory test results:

> Hematocrit = 46% (38%-48%)
> Serum total testosterone = 110 ng/dL (264-915 ng/dL)
> (SI: 3.8 nmol/L [9.2-31.8 nmol/L])
> Serum FSH = 0.2 mIU/mL (1.0-7.0 mIU/mL)
> (SI: 0.2 IU/L [1.0-7.0 IU/L])
> Serum LH = 0.1 mIU/mL (1.0-9.0 mIU/mL)
> (SI: 0.1 IU/L [1.0-9.0 IU/L])

What additional evaluation would you order now to help confirm your suspicion that he is using androgenic PEDs?

A. Serum lipid panel and cortisol-binding globulin measurement

B. Serum lipid panel and SHBG measurement

C. Serum thyroxine-binding globulin and cortisol-binding globulin measurement

D. Screen of urinary metabolites of testosterone and testosterone precursors and known androgenic steroids by mass spectrometry

Answer: B) Serum lipid panel and SHBG measurement

This man has a discordance between his physical appearance (muscularity) and his serum testosterone concentration (very low), and he is a member of a social group at higher risk for use of androgenic PEDs (weightlifter at a gym). His hematocrit is higher than would be expected for his serum testosterone concentration, too. Androgens suppress serum HDL cholesterol, SHBG, and thyroxine-binding globulin concentrations. Low concentrations of HDL cholesterol, SHBG, and thyroxine-binding globulin concentrations would support the clinical suspicion of androgenic PED abuse (Answer B).

Androgens do not affect serum cortisol-binding globulin concentrations (thus, Answers A and C are incorrect). Sophisticated methods for detection of androgen abuse are used by the World Anti-Doping Agency to screen for androgenic PED use by elite athletes. These methods are not widely available in commercial laboratories (thus, Answer D is incorrect). Furthermore, unlike athletes who must provide urine samples under observation at random times, a patient has many methods of creating false results (eg, dilution, providing a urine sample from another individual, or providing a urine sample when not taking androgenic PEDs).

Case (Continued)

The patient's serum HDL-cholesterol, SHBG, and thyroxine-binding globulin concentrations are very low. His serum prolactin and ferritin concentrations are normal. Sellar MRI demonstrates a normal pituitary gland.

Which of the following is the most likely diagnosis?

A. Androstenedione abuse

B. Clomiphene abuse

C. Tetrahydrogestrinone ("Clear") abuse

D. Androgen-producing adrenal tumor

Answer: C) Tetrahydrogestrinone ("Clear") abuse

This patient has low serum testosterone and gonadotropin concentrations. A nontestosterone androgenic PED such as tetrahydrogestrinone (Answer C) would produce these results by suppressing gonadotropin secretion and reducing endogenous androgen production.

Androstenedione (Answer A) is a precursor in the pathway of testosterone synthesis. Consumption of very large dosages of androstenedione can raise serum testosterone concentration (by mass action) and act indirectly as a PED. In that setting, the serum testosterone concentration would be high-normal or elevated. Clomiphene (Answer B) is a selective estrogen-receptor modulator that increases gonadotropin secretion and circulating gonadotropin and testosterone concentrations in men with intact gonadotrope and Leydig-cell function. Adrenal tumors (Answer D) do not commonly produce enough testosterone to affect serum testosterone concentrations in men. When these tumors produce significant amounts of testosterone, serum gonadotropins may be suppressed, but the serum testosterone concentration is not low.

Case (Continued)

When the patient returns to your clinic in 2 weeks to review the results of his evaluation, he confides that he has been taking anabolic androgenic steroids for the past year. He reports that he takes a combination of several at once ("stacking") and rotates the combination ("cycling"). His wife has been urging him to stop taking them because she is concerned about his health. He is under the care of a mental health professional for treatment of anxiety and depression. He is very concerned about losing muscle mass, and he would like to know if there is any medical therapy that he can take after stopping androgenic PEDs.

In addition to advising immediate cessation of androgenic PEDs, which of the following would you recommend?

A. No additional therapy

B. Testosterone gel taper over 6 months

C. Clomiphene taper over 12 months

D. hCG taper over 6 months

Answer: A) No additional therapy

In patients who have been taking androgenic PEDs for 1 year or less, the best management of cessation of androgens is supportive care (eg, treatment of depression and anxiety) with no additional medical therapy (Answer A). These patients generally recover normal function of the gonadal axis within 6 to 12 months.

Additional medical therapy is unnecessary, and the cost or potential risks are not justified. Exogenous testosterone and hCG (Answers B and D) may delay gonadal axis recovery. Based on inferential data from women, clomiphene (Answer C), a selective estrogen-receptor modulator, may increase the risk of thromboembolic events, and that potential risk is not justified in this setting.

Case (Continued)

He returns 2 months later with his wife. He reports that he has felt tired and despondent since stopping the androgenic PEDs. He has low libido and low sexual satisfaction. He now reports that he has been taking androgenic PEDs for many years. His wife confirms his symptoms and reports that they have been trying to conceive during the past 6 months. She is 33 years old, healthy, takes no medications, and has regular menses every 28 to 32 days.

Laboratory test results at this clinic visit:

Hematocrit = 41% (38%-48%)
Serum total testosterone = 80 ng/dL (264-915 ng/dL)
 (SI: 2.8 nmol/L [9.2-31.8 nmol/L])
Serum FSH = 0.3 mIU/mL (1.0-7.0 mIU/mL)
 (SI: 0.3 IU/L [1.0-7.0 IU/L])
Serum LH = 0.2 mIU/mL (1.0-9.0 mIU/mL)
 (SI: 0.2 IU/L [1.0-9.0 IU/L])
Seminal fluid analysis, no sperm

Which of the following would you recommend?

A. Reassurance

B. Intramuscular testosterone taper

C. hCG therapy

D. Anastrozole therapy

Answer: C) hCG therapy

This man continues to be significantly hypogonadal after 2 to 3 months of cessation of androgenic PED abuse. His decline in hematocrit supports that he has discontinued. It is unclear how quickly his gonadal axis will recover, but his additional history that he took androgenic PEDs for many years suggests that it might be more than 1 to 2 years before he recovers spermatogenesis. His wife will be 35 in 2 years, an age when female fertility begins to decline (on average). Gonadotropin therapy is very effective in most men (~90%) with postpubertal hypogonadotropic hypogonadism. His testicular volumes indicate that he completed normal puberty. Treatment with hCG therapy (Answer C) (that has LH) is likely to be effective in restoring his normal endogenous testosterone concentrations and may restore spermatogenesis within 6 to 12 months. FSH therapy (usually as recombinant human FSH) may be added if conception has not occurred and spermatogenesis remains low after serum testosterone concentrations have been normalized with hCG therapy. Treatment with hCG to normalize his serum testosterone concentration would also help alleviate his withdrawal symptoms.

This patient is likely to have prolonged absence or markedly decreased spermatogenesis; reassurance (Answer A) is incorrect. An intramuscular testosterone taper (Answer B) would lessen his withdrawal symptoms, but exogenous testosterone would continue to suppress serum gonadotropin concentrations and spermatogenesis. Aromatase inhibitors suppress serum estradiol concentrations, thereby increasing gonadotropin secretion; there is anecdotal evidence for using this class of drugs in selected men with hypospermatogenesis and infertility (eg, men with infertility due to morbid obesity). Anastrozole (Answer D) might increase spermatogenesis in this man, but there is much stronger evidence for effectiveness with gonadotropin replacement therapy. Furthermore, aromatase inhibitor therapy may cause loss of bone mineral density, increase body fat, and decrease sexual function in men.

References

1. Anawalt BD. Diagnosis and management of anabolic androgenic steroid use. *J Clin Endocrinol Metab.* 2019;104(7):2490-2500. PMID: 30753550

2. Christou MA, Christou PA, Markozannes G, Tsatsoulis A, Mastorakos G, Tigas S. Effects of anabolic androgenic steroids on the reproductive system of athletes and recreational users: a systematic review and meta-analysis. *Sports Med.* 2017;47(9):1869-1883. PMID: 28258581

3. Pope HG Jr, Wood RI, Rogol A, Nyberg F, Bowers L, Bhasin S. Adverse health consequences of performance-enhancing drugs: an Endocrine Society scientific statement. *Endocr Rev.* 2014;35(3):341-375. PMID: 24423981

4. Kanayama G, DeLuca J, Meehan WP 3rd, et al. Ruptured tendons in anabolic-androgenic steroid users: a cross-sectional cohort study. *Am J Sports Med.* 2015;43(11):2638-2644. PMID: 26362436

5. Onakomaiya MM, Henderson LP. Mad men, women and steroid cocktails: a review of the impact of sex and other factors on anabolic androgenic steroids effects on affective behaviors. *Psychopharmacology (Berl).* 2016;233(4):549-569. PMID: 26758282

6. Piacentino D, Kotzalidis GD, Del Casale A, et al. Anabolic-androgenic steroid use and psychopathology in athletes. A systematic review. *Curr Neuropharmacol.* 2015;13(1):101-121. PMID: 26074746

7. Baggish AL, Weiner RB, Kanayama G, et al. Cardiovascular toxicity of illicit anabolic-androgenic steroid use. *Circulation.* 2017;135(21):1991-2002. PMID: 28533317

8. Anawalt BD. Detection of anabolic androgenic steroid use by elite athletes and by members of the general public. *Mol Cell Endocrinol.* 2018;464:21-27. PMID: 28943276

9. Liu PY, Swerdloff RS, Christenson PD, Handelsman DJ, Wang C; Hormonal Male Contraception Summit Group. Rate, extent, and modifiers of

spermatogenic recovery after hormonal male contraception: an integrated analysis. *Lancet.* 2006;367(9520):1412-1420. PMID: 16650651

10. Kanayama G, Hudson JI, DeLuca J, et al. Prolonged hypogonadism in males following withdrawal from anabolic-androgenic steroids: an under-recognized problem. *Addiction.* 2015;110(5):823-831. PMID: 25598171

11. Rasmussen JJ, Selmer C, Østergren PB, et al. Former abusers of anabolic androgenic steroids exhibit decreased testosterone levels and hypogonadal symptoms years after cessation: a case-control study. *PLoS One.* 2016;11:e0161208. PMID: 275532478

Evaluation of Male Infertility

Channa Jayasena, MD, PhD. Division of Diabetes and Endocrinology, Imperial College London, London, United Kingdom; E-mail: c.jayasena@imperial.ac.uk

Learning Objectives

As a result of participating in this session, learners should be able to:

- Investigate the diagnostic pathway for male infertility.

- Explain classic and contemporary management options for treating men with infertility.

Main Conclusions

Male infertility may be classified into secondary hypogonadism, testicular failure, and obstruction. Secondary hypogonadism (hypogonadotropic hypogonadism) is congenital or acquired and is most familiar to endocrinologists. Several genetic pathogenic variants have been identified that cause congenital hypogonadotropic hypogonadism. Gonadotropin injections are highly effective at inducing spermatogenesis in men with secondary hypogonadism. GnRH pulsatile therapy is usually restricted to research settings when inducing spermatogenesis in men with secondary hypogonadism. Most cases of male infertility are due to testicular failure (ie, hypergonadotropic hypogonadism). The most severe form of testicular failure is called nonobstructive azoospermia (NOA). The last decade has seen notable developments in the diagnostic evaluation and management of NOA. Microsurgical testicular sperm extraction (mTESE) is used to successfully retrieve sperm in 20% to 40% of men with NOA, including men with Klinefelter syndrome. Hormonal stimulation with gonadotropins or selective estrogen modulators are used routinely before mTESE in men with NOA, but there are insufficient data to support their widespread use. Obstructive azoospermia (OA) is a common and underrecognized form of male infertility, most often caused by genitourinary tract infection. However, it may also be associated with cystic fibrosis carrier status (pathogenic variants in the *CFTR* gene). There is no role for endocrine therapy in the management of OA, but endocrinologists should be aware of the diagnostic features of OA to ensure appropriate urological referral. This session will provide endocrinologists with a state-of-the art overview of the evaluation and management of men with any form of male infertility in a multidisciplinary clinic setting.

Significance of the Clinical Problem

Infertility is the inability to achieve pregnancy after 12 months of regular unprotected intercourse. Up to half of cases of infertility are attributed to a problem in the male partner ("male-factor infertility"). Recent reports suggest that sperm counts in North America and Europe have halved since the 1970s. Combined with increasing maternal age at first pregnancy worldwide, the management of male infertility is likely to become even more important in the future.

Barriers to Optimal Practice

- Endocrine therapies are being increasing used empirically (by urologists) for men with testicular failure, but most endocrinologists are unaware of this practice.

- Successful treatment of male fertility increasingly requires coordinated management with other specialties (eg, obstetrics/gynecology, reproductive endocrinology, and urology).

Strategies for Diagnosis, Therapy, and/or Management

Physiology of Male Fertility

Male fertility requires activity of the hypothalamic-pituitary-gonadal axis. GnRH is released to the portal circulation in a pulsatile manner, stimulating the anterior pituitary to secrete pulses of the gonadotropin hormones, LH and FSH. LH stimulates the testicular Leydig cells to synthesize testosterone, and FSH stimulates Sertoli cells in the seminiferous tubules to support spermatogenesis. LH and FSH secretion are negatively regulated by testosterone and inhibin, respectively. A cycle of spermatogenesis is 60 to 80 days in duration.

Etiology

See *Table 1* for a summary of etiologies of male infertility.[1]

Secondary Hypogonadism

Secondary hypogonadism is caused by hypothalamic or pituitary disease resulting in low testosterone with low LH and FSH secretion (hypogonadotropic hypogonadism). Secondary hypogonadism may arise from congenital or acquired GnRH deficiency. Congenital GnRH deficiency or congenital hypogonadotropic hypogonadism is a rare disorder characterized by the deficient production, secretion, or action of GnRH resulting in low FSH, LH, and testosterone with otherwise normal pituitary function.[2]

Table 1. Causes of Male Infertility

Etiology	Examples	Diagnostic Features
Hormonal (hypogonadotropic hypogonadism)	<ul><li>Pituitary tumor</li><li>Anabolic steroids</li><li>Androgens (prescribed and illicit)</li><li>Strong opioids (eg, morphine)</li><li>Congenital hypogonadotropic hypogonadism</li><li>Diabetes mellitus</li></ul>	<ul><li>Azoospermia or oligospermia</li><li>FSH: low</li><li>LH: low</li><li>Testosterone: low</li><li>Testicular volume: low</li><li>Low libido, sparse body hair, erectile dysfunction</li></ul>
Testicular	<ul><li>Primary testicular failure</li><li>Previous cancer therapy</li><li>Undescended testes (cryptorchidism)</li><li>Varicocele</li><li>Lifestyle factors (obesity, tobacco smoking, cannabis)</li><li>Infections (eg, mumps)</li><li>Drugs (eg, sulfasalazine, methotrexate, calcium-channel blockers, nitrofurantoin, erythromycin, tetracycline, spironolactone)</li><li>Genetic disorders (eg, Klinefelter syndrome, Y-chromosome microdeletions, primary ciliary dyskinesia)</li></ul>	<ul><li>Azoospermia or oligospermia</li><li>FSH: high</li><li>LH: high or normal</li><li>Testosterone: low or normal</li><li>Testicular volume: often low</li></ul>
Obstruction	<ul><li>Genitourinary infection (chlamydia, ureaplasma, mycoplasma)</li><li>Previous surgery (eg, hernia repair, orchidopexy)</li><li>Vasectomy</li><li>Cystic fibrosis (associated with congenital bilateral absence of vas deferens)</li></ul>	<ul><li>Usually azoospermia</li><li>FSH: normal</li><li>Testosterone: normal</li><li>Testicular volume: normal</li><li>Elevated semen leukocytes or round cells indicate possible infection</li></ul>
Others	<ul><li>Retrograde ejaculation (eg, α-adrenergic blockers, diabetes, pelvic surgery)</li><li>Sexual dysfunction</li></ul>	<ul><li>Low volume or no ejaculate</li></ul>

Clinical features of congenital GnRH deficiency are incomplete or absent puberty and infertility, which may or may not occur in association with other developmental abnormalities (eg, cleft lip or palate, hearing impairment). Congenital GnRH deficiency in association with anosmia or hyposmia is termed Kallmann syndrome, which results from incomplete migration in utero of GnRH neurons from the olfactory placode to the hypothalamus. Alternatively, GnRH neuronal function may be deficient, but smell can be intact (ie, normosmic congenital GnRH deficiency). Pathogenic variants in several genes have been identified that cause either normosmic congenital GnRH deficiency, Kallmann syndrome, or both.[2] Hypothalamic GnRH deficiency may also be acquired due to obesity, chronic disease, opioid use, or severe weight loss or exercise.

Testicular Failure

Testicular failure classically results in low testosterone, high LH and FSH secretion, and either impaired or absent spermatogenesis. Azoospermia may arise from complete testicular failure associated with genetic factors, cryptorchidism, mumps orchitis, testicular cancer, radiotherapy, and cytotoxic agents such as cyclophosphamide.

Klinefelter Syndrome

Approximately 10% of men with NOA have Klinefelter syndrome caused by a 47,XXY karyotype. Klinefelter syndrome causes primary testicular failure during early adulthood, with increased gonadotropins and low testosterone. It had previously been assumed that these patients had complete azoospermia, but it has now been reported that 25% may have evidence of spermatozoa on semen analysis, although spontaneous conception is rare. mTESE followed by intracytoplasmic sperm injection can be used to successfully achieve conception in patients with Klinefelter syndrome,3 but there is a lack of data regarding the live birth rate following this methodology for such couples. Men with NOA may rarely have a 46,XX karyotype; a fragment of

the Y chromosome containing the *SRY* gene causes male sexual differentiation, but the absence of other genes on the Y chromosome is incompatible with spermatogenesis and is untreatable.

Y-Chromosome Microdeletions

The Y chromosome contains genes crucial for spermatogenesis.[4] Microdeletions in the Yq11 region on the long arm of the Y chromosome (also called the azoospermic factor, AZF region) may involve several genes, and these microdeletions are present in 5% to 10% of men with NOA (or severe oligoasthenospermia [<5 million sperm/mL]). Deletions of the AZFa and AZFb regions are largely incompatible with spermatogenesis, and mTESE is not advised. However, deletions of the AZFc region may be compatible with a degree of spermatogenesis in some patients, so mTESE may be considered with subsequent intracytoplasmic sperm injection if surgical sperm retrieval is successful.

Monogenic Causes

Pathogenic variants in *INSL3*, *TEX11*, and the gene encoding the androgen receptor (*AR*) have been found in men with NOA, but screening is currently not performed routinely. Discovery of more single genes associated with male infertility is anticipated in the future.

Acquired Causes of Testicular Failure

Obesity, type 1 or type 2 diabetes mellitus, trauma, cancer treatment, and several drugs may impair spermatogenesis.

Obstructive Azoospermia

Obstructive azoospermia can be caused by genitourinary tract infections such as chlamydia, ureaplasma, and mycoplasma, which lead to scarring and blockage of the epididymis. Epididymal obstruction is a recognized complication of any testicular surgery. OA may also be associated with *CFTR* gene carrier status.[4]

Assessment

When evaluating a male patient with infertility, the clinician should ask questions about loss of libido, early morning erections, anosmia, and onset of puberty. Aspects of the history suggesting a specific etiology include mumps, sexually transmitted infections, previous malignancy, any systemic or chronic disease, and undescended testes. Cigarette smoking, alcohol, cannabis, opioids, and anabolic steroids can all contribute to infertility.

Clinical examination should look for facial, axillary, and pubic hair and gynecomastia. Both testes should be palpated to exclude undescended testes. Testicular volume should be assessed using a Prader orchidometer or ultrasonography. Semen analysis should be performed in all patients following abstinence of a minimum of 2 days and maximum of 7 days (*Table 2*).[5] Hormonal analysis should include early morning fasted serum testosterone, SHBG, estradiol, LH, FSH, and prolactin. Free testosterone may be calculated or measured using equilibrium dialysis. Genetic testing should be performed for all patients with azoospermia; these tests should include karyotype analysis and assessment for Y-chromosome microdeletions and *CFTR* pathogenic variants. OA should be suspected if men have azoospermia despite having normal testicular volume and no features of hypogonadism.

Table 2. World Health Organization Minimum Thresholds of Semen Parameters in Men Fathering Children Without Fertility Problems[2]

Parameter	Lower Reference Limit (95% confidence interval)
Semen volume	1.5 mL
Sperm concentration	15×10^6 per mL
Total motility	40%
Progressive motility	32%
Sperm morphology (normal forms)	4%

Management

Induction of Spermatogenesis With Gonadotropin Injections

Gonadotropin therapy is the most common form of sperm induction for men with secondary hypogonadism desiring fertility with their partner.[2] Pulsatile GnRH is an alternative treatment for secondary hypogonadism due to hypothalamic dysfunction, but it is unavailable in most countries. A typical gonadotropin therapy protocol includes the initiation of hCG to mimic the biological activity of LH and induce the testes to produce testosterone. This may be sufficient to induce sperm in some patients, so semen analysis should be performed after 6 months of hCG therapy. The dose of hCG should be titrated to maintain a normal serum testosterone level. FSH-containing injections (such as menotropin) should be added to hCG therapy in patients who remaining azoospermic following 6 months of hCG treatment. A small randomized controlled trial has reported that patients with a testicular volume less than 4 mL may have better outcomes from an alternative treatment regimen commencing with FSH therapy for 6 months (to aid testicular maturation) before starting hCG therapy.[6]

Selective Estrogen Receptor Modulators and Aromatase Inhibitors

Both selective estrogen receptor modulators and aromatase inhibitors indirectly stimulate gonadotropin secretion by reducing estrogenic pituitary feedback in men, so therefore elevate levels of serum testosterone in men with hypogonadism while preserving spermatogenesis.[7] Clomiphene citrate, anastrozole, and letrozole have therefore been proposed as alternatives to testosterone therapy in hypogonadal men of reproductive age who wish to actively conceive. However, little safety data exist for use of selective estrogen receptor modulators and aromatase inhibitors in male hypogonadism, and neither drug class is licensed for the treatment of male hypogonadism or male infertility.[8] Selective estrogen receptor modulators and aromatase inhibitors work by reducing negative pituitary feedback, so they are ineffective in men with panhypopituitarism and extremely low testosterone levels.

Surgical Management of Male Infertility

Surgical techniques have a vital role in the management of obstructive infertility and an emerging role in the management of testicular failure. Percutaneous epididymal sperm aspiration or microsurgical epididymal sperm aspiration are highly effective techniques for collecting sperm in men with OA, since spermatogenesis is often intact in affected patients. Surgical sperm retrieval may also be used to obtain sperm from men with NOA or severe oligoasthenospermia, which is otherwise insufficient for assisted reproductive technologies (such as intracytoplasmic sperm injection. The technique of TESE may have high associated rates of hematoma and testicular devascularization. Therefore, mTESE was introduced in 1999 and is now considered the gold standard surgical procedure for surgical sperm retrieval. mTESE allows for the microdissection and identification of individual tubules appearing to be engorged with spermatogenesis in situ. During mTESE, tubules are dissected and examined microscopically for sperm during surgery. Testicular samples are homogenized with storage medium, and either cryopreserved for future use or used fresh for fertilization of eggs collected during a synchronized cycle of assisted reproductive technology. Hormonal stimulation with gonadotropins or selective estrogen receptor modulators are often used before mTESE to maintain serum testosterone secretion in hypogonadal men with NOA without suppressing spermatogenesis; however, there are insufficient interventional data to support their safety or efficacy in treating men with NOA.

Clinical Case Vignettes

Case 1

A 38-year-old man has been on testosterone replacement since he had delayed puberty as a teenager. He is taking intramuscular testosterone enanthate every 4 weeks. He now has a long-term partner and they would like to start a family. On physical examination, testicular volume is 3 mL bilaterally.

Laboratory test results after 3 months off testosterone therapy:

LH = 0.2 mIU/mL (1.0-9.0 mIU/mL) (SI: 0.2 IU/L [1.0-9.0 IU/L])
FSH = 1.5 mIU/mL (1.0-13.0 mIU/mL) (SI: 1.5 IU/L [1.0-13.0 IU/L])
Serum testosterone (8 AM in fasted state) = 58 ng/dL (300-900 ng/dL) (SI: 2.0 nmol/L [10.4-31.2 nmol/L])

Semen analysis shows azoospermia.

Which of the following statements is correct?

A. Prior testosterone therapy impairs chance of successful sperm induction in men with hypogonadism

B. The goal should be a sperm count in the World Health Organization reference range (15 million/mL) to achieve spontaneous pregnancy

C. Pretreatment with 6 months of FSH will increase sperm count more when compared with starting treatment with hCG or GnRH

D. He should be counseled about the risk of gynecomastia when starting hCG therapy

Answer: D) He should be counseled about the risk of gynecomastia when starting hCG therapy

Recent meta-analyses suggest that testosterone therapy does not significantly reduce the effectiveness of sperm induction for hypogonadotropic hypogonadism (thus, Answer A is incorrect).[9] Couples can become pregnant with sperm counts much lower than the World Health Organization reference range (thus, Answer B is incorrect). A recent article suggested that recombinant FSH pretreatment may aid seminiferous tubule development.[5] However, no significant increase in sperm count or testicular volume was observed in this small study (thus, Answer C is incorrect). hCG may cause gynecomastia in a minority of cases, which can occasionally be irreversible and disfiguring (Answer D).

Case 2

A 32-year-old man has a 3-year history of infertility with his 34-year-old partner. Investigations reveal azoospermia on 3 occasions, and his karyotype is documented to be 47,XXY (nonmosaic). He feels otherwise well and has normal libido and erectile function.

On physical examination, his height is 70.1 in (178 cm), he has slightly reduced male-pattern hair growth, and testicular volume is 10 mL bilaterally.

Laboratory test results:

Serum LH = 10.3 mIU/mL (1.0-9.0 mIU/mL) (SI: 10.3 IU/L [1.0-9.0 IU/L])
Serum FSH = 20.1 mIU/mL (1.0-13.0 mIU/mL) (SI: 20.1 IU/L [1.0-13.0 IU/L])
Serum testosterone (8 AM in fasted state) = 251 ng/dL (300-900 ng/dL) (SI: 8.7 nmol/L [10.4-31.2 nmol/L])

He is interested in learning more about surgical sperm retrieval.

Which of the following statements is correct?

A. Testosterone therapy should be started without delay to prevent osteoporosis
B. It is highly unlikely that sperm can be retrieved with mTESE since he has nonmosaic Klinefelter syndrome
C. Men with Klinefelter syndrome have increased surgical risk due to thrombophilia
D. Men have a 5% chance of developing new symptomatic hypogonadism following mTESE

Answer: C) Men with Klinefelter syndrome have increased surgical risk due to thrombophilia

The patient is not symptomatic and may undergo mTESE soon. Testosterone therapy should not be started, otherwise any residual spermatogenesis is likely to be suppressed (thus, Answer A is incorrect). It remains controversial whether hCG or selective estrogen receptor modulators increase chances of sperm retrieval before mTESE in men with Klinefelter syndrome. Sperm retrieval following mTESE is reported widely in men with nonmosaic Klinefelter syndrome (thus, Answer B is incorrect). Men with Klinefelter syndrome should be counseled about their increased risk of thromboembolic disease (Answer C). New hypogonadism has been reported in 20% of men with NOA following mTESE (thus, Answer D is incorrect), but the incidence has not been studied previously in men with Klinefelter syndrome.

References

1. Wall J, Jayasena CN. Diagnosing male infertility. *BMJ*. 2018;363:k3202. PMID: 30287677
2. Boehm U, Bouloux PM, Dattani MT, et al. Expert consensus document: European consensus statement on congenital hypogonadotropic hypogonadism--pathogenesis, diagnosis and treatment. *Nat Rev Endocrinol*. 2015;11(9):547-564. PMID: 26194704
3. Schlegel PN. Testicular sperm extraction: microdissection improves sperm yield with minimal tissue excision. *Hum Reprod*. 1999;14(1):131-135. PMID: 10374109
4. Wosnitzer MS. Genetic evaluation of male infertility. *Transl Androl Urol*. 2014;3(1):17-26. PMID: 26813518
5. World Health Organization. WHO laboratory manual for the examination and processing of human semen. World Health Organization. Available at: http://www.who.int/reproductivehealth/publications/infertility/9789241547789/en/. Accessed for verification January 2020.
6. Dwyer AA, Sykiotis GP, Hayes FJ, et al. Trial of recombinant follicle-stimulating hormone pretreatment for GnRH-induced fertility in patients with congenital hypogonadotropic hypogonadism. *J Clin Endocrinol Metab*. 2013;98(11):E1790-E1795. PMID: 24037890
7. Scovell JM, Khera M. Testosterone replacement therapy versus clomiphene citrate in the young hypogonadal male. *Eur Urol Focus*. 2018;4(3):321-323. PMID: 30131284
8. Bhasin S, Brito JP, Cunningham GR, et al. Testosterone therapy in men with hypogonadism: an Endocrine Society clinical practice guideline. *J Clin Endocrinol Metab*. 2018;103(5):1715-1744. PMID: 29562364
9. Rastrelli G, Corona G, Mannucci E, Maggi M. Factors affecting spermatogenesis upon gonadotropin-replacement therapy: a meta-analytic study. *Andrology*. 2014;2(6):794-808. PMID: 25271205

Approach to Reproductive Strategies in the Young Patient With Cancer

Lillian Meacham, MD. Emory University School of Medicine, Atlanta, GA; E-mail: lmeacha@emory.edu

Learning Objectives

As a result of participating in this session, learners should be able to:

- Describe cancer therapies that place pediatric patients with cancer at risk for future infertility.

- Identify barriers to fertility preservation in pediatric patients with cancer.

- Identify which pediatric patients with cancer are eligible for standard of care fertility preservation options.

- Discuss emerging experimental modalities of fertility preservation in pediatric patients with cancer.

Main Conclusions

Infertility can be a late occurring adverse effect of pediatric and adolescent cancer treatment. Traditional alkylating agent and heavy metal chemotherapy; ovarian, testicular, or hypothalamic exposure to radiation; surgery on reproductive organs; and hematopoietic stem-cell transplant (HSCT) that includes alkylating agents or total-body irradiation place patients at risk for future infertility. Fertility preservation should be done before beginning cancer treatment. Standard of care fertility preservation includes sperm, oocyte, and embryo cryopreservation. These standard of care interventions can only be offered to pubertal male patients (typically ≥13 years and ≥Tanner stage 3) and postmenarchal female patients. Additional interventions that may offer some protection to the ovaries/testes include gonadal transposition (moving the ovary or the testes out of the radiation field), gonadal shielding from radiation, and gonadotropin agonist therapy in female patients. Experimental fertility preservation for prepubertal patients and pubertal patients not able to undergo standard of care interventions include ovarian tissue cryopreservation and testicular tissue cryopreservation. Experimental fertility preservation should be offered through institutional review board protocols. Lastly, for female patients, fertility preservation can be considered after the completion of cancer therapy and before the onset of premature ovarian insufficiency. Barriers to fertility preservation include the awkwardness of the discussion about fertility preservation at the time of diagnosis, inadequate time for the intervention before beginning cancer therapy, the lack of standard of care options for prepubertal patients, the high financial burden of fertility preservation procedures, and poor health literacy around the complex issues of fertility preservation.

Significance of the Clinical Problem

With advances in pediatric oncology, more than 80% of patients diagnosed with cancer before age 21 years will experience long-term survival.[1] However, 73% to 95% of patients will live with long-term health consequences often referred to as late effects of cancer treatment.[2,3] One such late effect is gonadal dysfunction, which can include infertility. Patients treated with traditional alkylating agent or heavy metal chemotherapy; radiation therapy fields that include the ovaries, testes, or hypothalamus; surgery on the reproductive organs; or HSCT are at risk for future infertility.[4-6] Rates of infertility in childhood cancer survivors and the level of risk for future infertility associated with different cancer treatment modalities are hard to ascertain because infertility as an outcome is very difficult to measure. Infertility, the inability to achieve pregnancy after 1 year of trying, requires self-report, which is difficult to capture, and the infertile state is not typically recognized until young adulthood when many patients are no longer followed in pediatric centers. The studies that have measured self-reported infertility in childhood cancer survivors describe rates of 46% in male patients and 13% in female patients.[7,8] Most studies of reproductive potential in survivors of childhood cancer use surrogate measures for infertility such as lack of pregnancy, acute ovarian failure, premature ovarian insufficiency, diminished ovarian reserve, elevated FSH levels, oligomenorrhea/amenorrhea, or oligospermia/azoospermia.[9-16] Regardless of the challenges in capturing infertility data in childhood cancer survivors, the potential for future infertility remains one of the top concerns of adolescent young adult cancer survivors, and many report lack of clarity regarding their personal risk for infertility and their fertility status.[17-20] Most pediatric oncology programs offer standard of care fertility preservation interventions: sperm, oocyte, or embryo cryopreservation. Other services offered may include ovarian or testicular transposition (surgically moving the gonad out of the radiation field), shielding from radiation, or the use of GnRH agonists in female patients. Some programs offer eligible patients experimental ovarian or testicular tissue cryopreservation.[21,22]

Barriers to Optimal Practice

Although potential infertility is identified as a prominent health concern in adolescent young adult cancer survivors, few patients or their families have this on their mind at the time of diagnosis. The *first barrier* to fertility preservation is beginning an emotionally laden conversation during an overwhelming time for newly diagnosed patients and their families. Therefore, initiating the discussion of risk for future infertility and fertility preservation options requires a sensitive discussion led by providers—preferably by a member of a fertility preservation team or someone trained in fertility preservation.

The *second barrier* to fertility preservation is lack of time. For many pediatric patients with cancer, treatment must start very quickly within days of diagnosis. Many female patients cannot delay cancer treatment the 2 weeks required for ovarian stimulation and oocyte harvest. For male patients, if there is a delay in requesting the fertility consult, the patient may have only hours, not days, to produce a specimen for sperm banking.

The *third barrier* to fertility preservation is the lack of standard of care options for a large proportion of pediatric patients with cancer because of their prepubertal status at diagnosis.

The *fourth barrier* to fertility preservation is the financial burden of fertility preservation procedures that is typically borne by the patient and/or family. Fertility preservation services are often not covered by insurance and the cost to cryopreserve reproductive material can range from a couple hundred dollars for sperm banking to more than 10,000 dollars to harvest and cryopreserve oocytes. In addition, the family has to be prepared to pay annual cost to maintain the cryopreserved materials, potentially for decades.

The *fifth barrier* to fertility preservation is the lack of health literacy. Health literacy is more than education; it requires ensuring that patients understand the information provided and can use it to make decisions.[23] Teach-back is a patient-centered technique that can be used to ensure that patients understand key concepts communicated during a fertility preservation consult.[24] Patients and families may need repeated conversations and/or access to handouts or websites they can use to review their specific options for fertility preservation in order to make an actionable decision.

Strategies for Diagnosis, Therapy, and/or Management

Having a fertility preservation team facilitates prompt, sensitive, and informative consults for patients facing gonadotoxic treatments. A dedicated provider or team for fertility consults also ensures consistent messaging, facilitates capturing all eligible patients and provides fertility navigation to ensure successful fertility preservation interventions. Once a new patient has been identified, it is important to ascertain their level of risk for future infertility. The Children's Oncology Group Long-Term Follow-Up Guidelines for Survivors of Childhood, Adolescent, and Young Adult Cancers have identified cancer therapeutic exposures that place patients at risk for gonadal damage and infertility.[4] Traditional alkylating agent and heavy metal chemotherapy; ovarian, testicular, or hypothalamic exposure to radiation; surgery on reproductive organs; and HSCT that includes alkylating agents or total-body irradiation place patients at risk for future infertility. There is a differential effect by sex, as male patients are more sensitive than female patients to damage, and in female patients, being prepubertal may afford some protection against gonadal damage. Collaborators in the Pediatric Initiative Network of the Oncofertility Consortium are working to establish a risk stratification grid that is based on literature review and expert opinion that can be used to counsel patients regarding their specific level of risk for future infertility. Although there is some variation in practice regarding what constitutes minimally increased risk and a moderate level of risk, most oncology centers agree on the therapies that place patients at a high level of increased risk for infertility (*Table 1*).

The fertility preservation options that can be offered to a patient vary by sex and age (*Table 2*). When referring to sex of the patient, we are referring to the type of gonad present: for females, ovaries, and for males, testes. Widely accepted standard of care fertility preservation options are sperm cryopreservation in male patients and ovarian stimulation with oocyte harvest for oocyte or embryo cryopreservation in female patients.

Table 1. Cancer Therapies That Place Patients at a High Level of Increased Risk for Future Infertility

Cancer Therapies	Female Patients	Male Patients
Alkylating agent chemotherapy as cyclophosphamide equivalent dose[a,b,c]	Prepubertal >12 g/m^2	Cyclophosphamide equivalent dose ≥4 g/m^2
	Pubertal >8 g/m^2	
Gonadal exposure to radiation[d,e]	Prepubertal ≥15 Gy	≥4 Gy
	Pubertal ≥10 Gy	
Hypothalamic exposure to radiation	≥40 Gy	
Bone marrow transplant	Alkylator-based and/or total-body irradiation	
	Myeloablative and reduced intensity	

[a] Most traditional alkylating agents can be converted to cyclophosphamide equivalents, allowing for the calculation of a cumulative alkylating agent exposure.[25]

[b] Criteria for high-risk cyclophosphamide equivalent dose for female patients.[9,10]

[c] Criteria for high-risk cyclophosphamide equivalent dose for male patients.[12,26]

[d] Criteria for high-risk ovarian radiation exposure.[9,16]

[e] Criteria for high-risk testicular radiation exposure.[12]

Table 2. Fertility Preservation Options for Pediatric and Adolescent Patients With Cancer

	Targeted Patients[a]	Barriers
Standard of Care Fertility Preservation Interventions		
Sperm cryopreservation[b]	Pubertal male patients Tanner stage 3 pubertal development Typically ≥13 years History of ejacularche	Awkward conversation around masturbation for semen specimen Collection can be challenging in the inpatient setting
Oocyte cryopreservation[b]	Pubertal female patients Postmenarchal	2 weeks needed for ovarian stimulation Vaginal ultrasonography, home injections, and frequent visits to the fertility clinic Patient cost (typically $10,000)
Embryo cryopreservation[b]	Typically partnered patients	Similar to barriers for oocyte cryopreservation and, in addition, a partner must be identified
Other Interventions to Protect Fertility		
Gonadal shielding	Male and female patients	Only protects from radiation, not gonadotoxic chemotherapy
Gonadal transposition	Male and female patients	Only protects from radiation, not chemotherapy Possible infertility related to manipulation of the adnexa
GnRH agonist	Pubertal female patients	Symptoms of hypogonadism Equivocal efficacy
Experimental/Investigational (Should Be Done Under Institutional Review Board/Study Protocol)		
Ovarian tissue cryopreservation	Prepubertal patients Pubertal patients who cannot freeze oocytes	Open institutional review board protocol Patient cost (typically $5000-$7000) Coordination with other procedure (eg, line placement)
Testicular tissue cryopreservation	Prepubertal patients Pubertal patients who are unable produce sperm for cryopreservation	Open institutional review board protocol Patient cost (typically $5000-$7000) Coordination with other procedure (eg, line placement)

[a] Sex refers to the presence of ovaries in female patients and testes in male patients.

[b] Standard of care endorsed by the American Society for Reproductive Medicine and American Society of Clinical Oncology.

The American Society of Reproductive Medicine and the American Society for Clinical Oncology endorse these options as standard practice before starting cancer therapy.[27-29] In general, these standard of care options are commonly available but often not used, especially in female patients, because of lack of time to undergo these procedures before the start of cancer treatments. Pediatric cancers are often aggressive and thus therapy cannot be delayed. In addition, the need for several vaginal ultrasonography and frequent lab samples can be a barrier for oocyte harvest in adolescent female patients. For male patients who are unable to ejaculate a specimen, epidydimal aspiration, testicular biopsy, or the use of electroejaculation may yield sperm that can be cryopreserved. Even marginal samples should be cryopreserved because in vitro fertilization with intracytoplasmic sperm injection can be used in the future.

Other options for protecting fertility include shielding or moving the gonads out of the radiation field. However, radiation scatter or concomitant gonadotoxic chemotherapy may still place the patient at risk for infertility. The use of GnRH agonists has been proposed as an ovarian protectant. However, the data are equivocal, and most studies are of young adult women, not pediatric or adolescent patients.[28] Suppression of the testicular hormonal axis is not beneficial and should not be recommended.

Lastly, experimental forms of fertility preservation for patients who are at high risk for infertility include ovarian tissue cryopreservation and testicular tissue cryopreservation. These procedures should be offered under institutional review board protocols. Ovarian tissue cryopreservation and testicular tissue cryopreservation are the only options for fertility preservation in prepubertal patients whose gonads have not matured to the point to be able to collect mature sperm or oocytes for cryopreservation. Many pediatric oncofertility centers around the world are harvesting ovarian tissue (1 ovary or cortical strips from 1 ovary) and testicular tissue (wedge resection up to 25% of 1 testis—typically <500 mg tissue) for cryopreservation. Research is ongoing as to the best way to freeze and use ovarian and testicular tissue. Use of ovarian tissue cryopreservation and testicular tissue cryopreservation usually involves transplant back to the patient when pregnancy is desired. In some pediatric patients with cancer, especially those with leukemia or lymphoma, this is problematic given the tendency for the gonad to harbor malignant cells. Various techniques have been used to ensure cancer is not being reintroduced to the patient.[30] There have been more than 130 live births from ovarian tissue harvested from pubertal female patients, 1 live birth from tissue harvested from a prepubertal girl, and 1 live birth in a primate after reintroduction of testicular tissue harvested prepubertally.[31-33]

After cancer treatment, fertility preservation can still be considered in female survivors. Gonadal function and ovarian reserve are typically monitored in survivor care. Female patients who have normal FSH levels but diminished ovarian reserve as measured by low antimullerian hormone or low antral follicle count can be referred to a reproductive endocrinologist for consideration of posttreatment ovarian stimulation and oocyte harvest. Male survivors who are able to make sperm after cancer treatment should not experience premature senescence of spermatogenesis.

Clinical Case Vignettes
Case 1

A 16-year-old boy presents with a 1-month history of left leg pain and swelling. Plain films suggest malignancy, and biopsy confirms the diagnosis of Ewing sarcoma of the left distal femur. His oncology team plans to treat him on AEWS0031. Based on this protocol, his treatment will include cyclophosphamide, doxorubicin, etoposide, ifosfamide, and vincristine. His planned cyclophosphamide dose is 8,400 mg/m^2 and planned ifosfamide dose is 63,000 mg/m^2. This will result in a cumulative cyclophosphamide equivalent dose of 23,772 mg/m^2. No radiation is planned.

During the fertility consultation, which of the following should be discussed?

A. He has minimally increased risk for future infertility, and no fertility preservation intervention is recommended

B. He has significantly increased risk for infertility, and sperm banking is recommended prior to the start of chemotherapy

C. He has significantly increased risk for infertility, and sperm banking is recommended at any time that is convenient for him and his family

D. He has significantly increased risk for infertility and should be offered sperm banking; if he is unable to ejaculate a specimen, epidydimal aspiration or testicular sperm extraction by a urologist may be of benefit

E. GnRH therapy may provide some protection to the testes

F. Both B and D

G. Both C and E

Answer: F) Both B and D

Alkylator chemotherapy resulting in a cyclophosphamide equivalent dose greater than 4 g/m^2 places a male patient at significantly increased risk for infertility (thus, Answer A is incorrect). In pubertal male patients, sperm banking should be offered before the start of chemotherapy (thus, Answers C and G are incorrect). Multiple specimens collected several days apart may provide more options should assisted reproduction be needed in the future. If multiple samples are available, intrauterine insemination can be attempted, which is less expensive than in vitro fertilization that requires oocyte harvest. If very few sperm are present, they should still be cryopreserved, as there is the potential to use intracytoplasmic sperm injections in addition to in vitro fertilization. Epididymal aspiration or testicular sperm extraction may be successful in harvesting sperm for cryopreservation if a specimen cannot be ejaculated. In this patient, sperm banking should be recommended before the start of chemotherapy and epididymal aspiration or testicular sperm extraction (Answer F [both Answers B and D]) could be considered. GnRH agonists (Answers E and G) are not used in male patients to protect the testes.

Case 2

Consider the same scenario as Case 1, but the patient is 9 years old (9-year-old male patient with Ewing sarcoma to be treated on AEWS0031, which will include alkylator exposure for a cumulative cyclophosphamide equivalent dose of 23,772 mg/m^2 and no radiation).

During the fertility consultation, which of the following should be discussed?

A. Because he is prepubertal, he is not at risk for infertility and no fertility preservation intervention is recommended

B. He has significantly increased risk for infertility and should be offered sperm banking to be done before the start of chemotherapy

C. He has significantly increased risk for infertility and could be offered experimental testicular tissue cryopreservation under an institutional review board protocol

Answer: C) He has significantly increased risk for infertility and could be offered experimental testicular tissue cryopreservation under an institutional review board protocol

Prepubertal status does not offer protection in male patients (thus, Answer is incorrect). His planned therapy will place the patient at a high level of risk for future infertility. Because he is prepubertal, he has not started to produce mature sperm and is also hormonally immature and will not be able to ejaculate a specimen for sperm banking (Answer B). If an institutional review board protocol is open for enrollment for testicular tissue cryopreservation (Answer C), this would be the only option for fertility preservation in this patient.

Case 3

A 16-year-old girl presents with left-sided sided neck swelling that has been progressively increasing in size for 3 weeks along with fever and a 30-lb (13.6-kg) weight loss. Stage 4B Hodgkin lymphoma is diagnosed. Her oncology team plans to treat her with the BEACOPP regimen, and she will receive 6 cycles. Her planned treatment will include bleomycin, etoposide, doxorubicin, cyclophosphamide, vincristine, procarbazine, and prednisone. The anticipated cumulative cyclophosphamide dose will be 7200 mg/m^2, and the anticipated cumulative procarbazine dose will be 4200 mg/m^2. The cumulative cyclophosphamide equivalent dose will be 10,800 mg/m^2. Radiation therapy is not planned.

During the fertility consultation, which of the following should be discussed?

A. She has minimally increased risk for future infertility

B. She has significantly increased risk for infertility and should be offered ovarian stimulation and oocyte harvest with cryopreservation

C. She has significantly increased risk for infertility and should primarily be offered unilateral oophorectomy for ovarian tissue cryopreservation

D. GnRH therapy may provide some protection to the ovaries

E. Amenorrhea may provide some protection to the ovaries

F. Both B and D

G. Both C and E

Answer: F) Both B and D

This patient is pubertal, and based on her cumulative cyclophosphamide equivalent dose of 10,800 mg/m^2 (>8000 mg/m^2), she will have a significantly increased risk for future infertility and should be offered a standard of care fertility preservation intervention (oocyte cryopreservation [Answer B]) (thus, Answer A is incorrect). Two weeks are required for ovarian stimulation. The process includes frequent visits to a reproductive endocrine infertility office for serial blood draws and vaginal ultrasonography to monitor follicular growth. Patients receive daily injections, culminating in a trigger injection to prepare for harvest. Transvaginal aspiration under conscious sedation is used for oocyte harvest. If the patient cannot tolerate these procedures or cancer therapy cannot be delayed 2 to 3 weeks, experimental ovarian tissue cryopreservation (Answer C) under the purview of an institutional review board protocol may be considered. In addition, many oncologists use GnRH agonist (Answer D) to stop menses. It is the suppression of the hypothalamic-ovarian axis, not the absence of menses, that may be protective to the ovary, but the degree of protection if any remains controversial (thus, Answer E is incorrect).

References

1. National Cancer Institute. SEER Cancer Statistics Review (CSR), 1975-2015. Bethesda, MD: National Cancer Institute; 2019. Available at: https://seer.cancer.gov/csr/1975_2015/. Accessed for verification December 2019.

2. Oeffinger KC, Mertens AC, Sklar CA, et al; Childhood Cancer Survivor Study. Chronic health conditions in adult survivors of childhood cancer. *N Engl J Med.* 2006;355(15):1572-1582. PMID: 17035650

3. Hudson MM, Ness KK, Gurney et al. Clinical ascertainment of health outcomes among adults treated for childhood cancer [published correction appears in *JAMA.* 2013;310(1):99]. *JAMA.* 2013;309(22):2371-2381. PMID: 23757085

4. Children's Oncology Group. Long-Term Follow-Up Guidelines for Survivors of Childhood, Adolescent, and Young Adult Cancers. Children's Oncology Group; 2018. Available at: www.survivorshipguidelines.org. Accessed for verification December 2019.

5. van Dorp W, Mulder RL, Kremer LC, et al. Recommendations for premature ovarian insufficiency surveillance for female survivors of childhood, adolescent, and young adult cancer: a report from the International Late Effects of Childhood Cancer Guideline Harmonization Group in collaboration with the PanCareSurFup Consortium. *J Clin Oncol.* 2016;34(28):3440-3450. PMID: 27458300

6. Skinner R, Mulder RL, Kremer LC, et al. Recommendations for gonadotoxicity surveillance in male childhood, adolescent, and young adult cancer survivors: a report from the International Late Effects of Childhood Cancer Guideline Harmonization Group in collaboration with the PanCareSurFup Consortium. *Lancet Oncol.* 2017;18(2):e75-e90. PMID: 28214419

7. Wasilewski-Masker K, Seidel KD, Leisenring W, et al. Male infertility in long-term survivors of pediatric cancer: a report from the childhood cancer survivor study. *J Cancer Surviv.* 2014;8(3):437-447. PMID: 24711092

8. Barton SE, Najita JS, Ginsburg ES, et al. Infertility, infertility treatment, and achievement of pregnancy in female survivors of childhood cancer: a report from the Childhood Cancer Survivor Study cohort. *Lancet Oncol.* 2013;14(9):873-881. PMID: 23856401

9. Levine JM, Whitton JA, Ginsberg JP, et al. Nonsurgical premature menopause and reproductive implications in survivors of childhood cancer: a report from the Childhood Cancer Survivor Study. *Cancer.* 2018;124(5):1044-1052. PMID: 29338081

10. Chemaitilly W, Li Z, Krasin MJ, et al. Premature ovarian insufficiency in childhood cancer survivors: a report From the St. Jude Lifetime Cohort. *J Clin Endocrinol Metab.* 2017;102(7):2242-2250. PMID: 28368472

11. Chow EJ, Stratton KL, Leisenring WM, et al. Pregnancy after chemotherapy in male and female survivors of childhood cancer treated between 1970 and 1999: a report from the Childhood Cancer Survivor Study cohort. *Lancet Oncol.* 2016;17(5):567-576. PMID: 27020005

12. Green DM, Liu W, Kutteh WH, et al. Cumulative alkylating agent exposure and semen parameters in adult survivors of childhood cancer: a report from the St Jude Lifetime Cohort Study. *Lancet Oncol.* 2014;15(11):1215-1223. PMID: 25239573

13. Romerius P, Stahl O, Moell C, et al. High risk of azoospermia in men treated for childhood cancer. *Int J Androl.* 2011;34(1):69-76. PMID: 20345878

14. Green DM, Kawashima T, Stovall M, et al. Fertility of male survivors of childhood cancer: a report from the Childhood Cancer Survivor Study. *J Clin Oncol.* 2010;28(2):332-339. PMID: 19949008

15. Sklar CA, Mertens AC, Mitby P, et al. Premature menopause in survivors of childhood cancer: a report from the childhood cancer survivor study. *J Natl Cancer Inst.* 2006;98(13):890-896. PMID: 16818852

16. Chemaitilly W, Mertens AC, Mitby P, et al. Acute ovarian failure in the childhood cancer survivor study. *J Clin Endocrinol Metab.* 2006;91(5):1723-1728. PMID: 16492690

17. Stein DM, Victorson DE, Choy JT, et al. Fertility preservation preferences and perspectives among adult male survivors of pediatric cancer and their parents. *J Adolesc Young Adult Oncol.* 2014;3(2):75-82. PMID: 24940531

18. Gilleland Marchak J, Seidel KD, Mertens AC, et al. Perceptions of risk of infertility among male survivors of childhood cancer: a report from the Childhood Cancer Survivor Study. *Cancer*. 2018;124(11):2447-2455. PMID: 29663341

19. Gilleland Marchak J, Elchuri SV, Vangile K, Wasilewski-Masker K, Mertens AC, Meacham LR. Perceptions of infertility risks among female pediatric cancer survivors following gonadotoxic therapy. *J Pediatr Hematol Oncol*. 2015;37(5):368-372. PMID: 25985237

20. Lehmann V, Flynn JS, Foster RH, Russell KM, Klosky JL. Accurate understanding of infertility risk among families of adolescent males newly diagnosed with cancer. *Psychooncology*. 2018;27(4):1193-1199. PMID: 29351367

21. Lee SJ, Schover LR, Partridge AH, et al; American Society of Clinical Oncology. American Society of Clinical Oncology recommendations on fertility preservation in cancer patients [published correction appears in *J Clin Oncol*. 2006;24(36):5790]. *J Clin Oncol*. 2006;24(18):2917-2931. PMID: 16651642

22. Smith BM, Duncan FE, Ataman L, et al. The National Physicians Cooperative: transforming fertility management in the cancer setting and beyond. *Future Oncol*. 2018;14(29):3059-3072. PMID: 30474429

23. Office of Disease Prevention and Health Promotion. National Action Plan to Improve Health Literacy. 2010. Available at: https://health.gov/communication/initiatives/health-literacy-action-plan.asp. Accessed for verification December 2019.

24. Bodenheimer T. Teach-back: a simple technique to enhance patients' understanding. *Fam Pract Manag*. 2018;25(4):20-22. PMID: 29989780

25. Green DM, Nolan VG, Goodman PJ, et al. The cyclophosphamide equivalent dose as an approach for quantifying alkylating agent exposure: a report from the Childhood Cancer Survivor Study. *Pediatr Blood Cancer*. 2014;61(1):53-67. PMID: 23940101

26. Green DM, Zhu L, Wang M, et al. Effect of cranial irradiation on sperm concentration of adult survivors of childhood acute lymphoblastic leukemia: a report from the St. Jude Lifetime Cohort Study†. *Hum Reprod*. 2017;32(6):1192-1201. PMID: 28444255

27. Ethics Committee of the American Society for Reproductive Medicine. Fertility preservation and reproduction in patients facing gonadotoxic therapies: an ethics committee opinion. *Fertil Steril*. 2018;110(3):380-386. PMID: 30098684

28. Oktay K, Harvey BE, Partridge AH, et al. Fertility preservation in patients with cancer: ASCO clinical practice guideline update. *J Clin Oncol*. 2018;36(19):1994-2001. PMID: 29620997

29. Loren AW, Mangu PB, Beck LN, et al; American Society of Clinical Oncology. Fertility preservation for patients with cancer: American Society of Clinical Oncology clinical practice guideline update. *J Clin Oncol*. 2013;31(19):2500-2510. PMID: 23715580

30. Shapira M, Raanani H, Derech Chaim S, Meirow D. Challenges of fertility preservation in leukemia patients. *Minerva Ginecol*. 2018;70(4):456-464. PMID: 29696942

31. Donnez J, Dolmans MM. Fertility preservation in women. *N Engl J Med*. 2017;377(17):1657-1665. PMID: 29069558

32. Matthews SJ, Picton H, Ernst E, Andersen CY. Successful pregnancy in a woman previously suffering from β-thalassemia following transplantation of ovarian tissue cryopreserved before puberty. *Minerva Ginecol*. 2018;70(4):432-435. PMID: 29696941

33. Fayomi AP, Peters K, Sukhwani M, et al. Autologous grafting of cryopreserved prepubertal rhesus testis produces sperm and offspring. *Science*. 2019;363(6433):1314-1319. PMID: 30898927

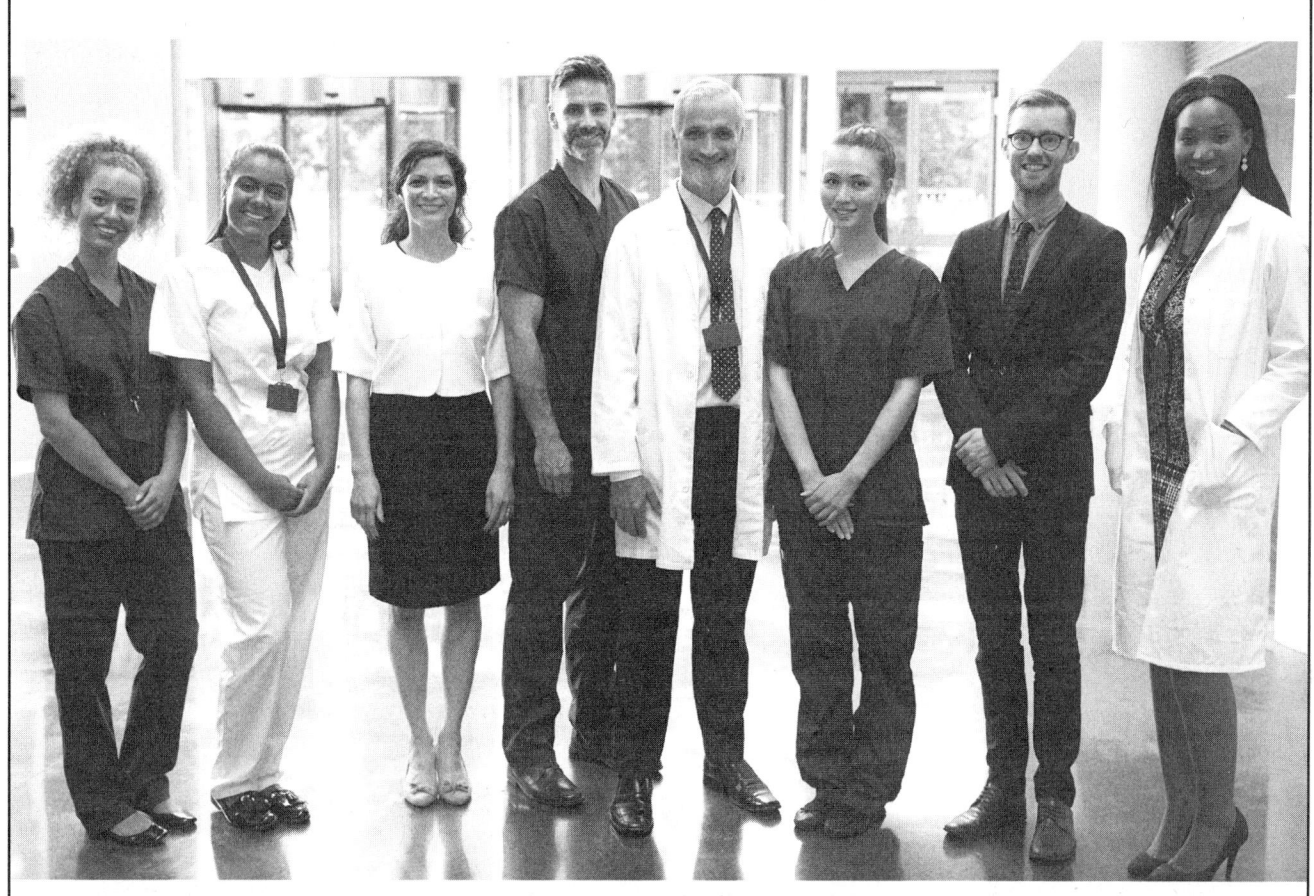

THYROID

Management of Patients With Medullary Thyroid Cancer

Rossella Elisei, MD. Department of Clinical and Experimental Medicine, Unit of Endocrinology, University of Pisa, Pisa, Italy; E-mail: rossella.elisei@med.unipi.it

Learning Objectives

As a result of participating in this session, learners should be able to:

- Increase their ability to recognize and diagnose medullary thyroid carcinoma (MTC).

- Explain the relevance of genetic screening in patients with MTC.

- Improve their knowledge of prognostic factors for survival in patients with MTC.

- Increase their ability to treat and follow-up patients with MTC.

- Describe the clinical impact of the approved receptor tyrosine kinase–targeted therapies in advanced MTC.

- Discuss the clinical trials of new *RET* target therapies.

Main Conclusions

MTC is a rare cancer whose cytologic diagnosis represents a challenge for pathologists. However, serum calcitonin, when elevated, can be helpful in making a correct diagnosis. Early diagnosis, when MTC is still intrathyroidal, is fundamental to definitively cure the patient. Because 6% to 10% of MTC cases that present as sporadic are indeed hereditary, all patients with MTC should undergo *RET* genetic screening. All first-degree relatives of patients with an identified pathogenic variant should undergo genetic testing. Family members who test positive will either immediately be treated or be kept under surveillance with the aim of performing an early thyroidectomy. Despite a rather bad prognosis for patients with advanced stage cancer (M1) at diagnosis, not all patients with MTC have a poor prognosis and several factors can be helpful in providing good information about the prognosis. Among others, a serum calcitonin level before surgery (<500 pg/mL [<146 pmol/L]) and after surgery (<20 pg/mL [<5.8 pmol/L]) portends a good prognosis, as does the absence of laterocervical lymph node metastases at diagnosis. This information is important to better manage patients with MTC, and, in particular, to identify those whose disease will likely progress and require systemic therapies. Two multitarget tyrosine kinase inhibitors, vandetanib and cabozantinib, are available to treat advanced and progressive MTC or patients with symptomatic MTC. Phase 3 clinical trials with these 2 drugs, the ZETA and EXAM trials, demonstrated significant prolongation of progression-free survival in patients treated with the drug compared with survival in those treated with placebo. Despite these good results, patients with MTC can experience progression while being treated with these drugs and they need other therapeutic options. New monotarget *RET* inhibitors, LOXO 292 and BLUE 667, are being evaluated in very promising clinical trials.

Significance of the Clinical Problem

MTC is a rare cancer deriving from neuroendocrine C cells. It can be sporadic or hereditary, and in both cases early diagnosis followed by early treatment is the only way to guarantee definitive cure. Knowledge about this malignancy among endocrinologists must be increased to improve early identification of affected patients and refer them to specialized centers.

Patients who are diagnosed later in the disease course will never be cured and must be followed with periodic examinations and measurement of serum markers (ie, calcitonin and CEA), and treating clinicians must interpret the clinical meaning of their values and, in particular, of observed changes. Targeted therapies have a significant impact on progression-free survival in patients with MTC, but the administration of these medications requires that the prescribing endocrinologist have specific knowledge and competencies in the management of their adverse events.

Barriers to Optimal Practice

- Difficulty in making a cytologic diagnosis due to the nonspecific cytologic features.

- Incurable disease when the diagnosis is delayed, particularly when the tumor is already extrathyroidal.

- Rarity of the disease requires treatment in referral centers.

- Few therapeutic options for advanced, progressive, or symptomatic disease.

Strategies for Diagnosis, Therapy, and/or Management
Epidemiology and Pathogenesis

MTC is a neuroendocrine tumor originating from the parafollicular C cells, which are localized in the thyroid and secrete calcitonin and other peptides such as chromogranin, serotonin, somatostatin, carcinoembryonic antigen (CEA), or calcitonin-gene related peptide.[1] The parafollicular C cells represent only 0.1% of all thyroid cells and, normally, they are not visible on standard hematoxylin-eosin tissue staining, but become detectable if immunohistochemistry with a calcitonin antibodies is performed. Because of its origin, MTC is considered a separate entity from other differentiated thyroid carcinomas.

The incidence of MTC is unknown. It accounts for 5% to 10% of all thyroid malignancies,[2] is present in 0.4% to 1.4% of all thyroid nodules, and is present in less than 1% of thyroid glands of individuals at autopsy. The National Institutes of Health recognizes MTC as a rare disease. The median age at diagnosis is 45 to 55 years, but there is a wide range in terms of age of onset. No difference in sex distribution has been reported. No specific risk factors for the development of MTC have been discovered.

One peculiarity of MTC is that it can be sporadic or arise in the context of familial syndromes (75% and 25% of cases, respectively). When sporadic, it affects 1 single person in the kindred, while in familial cases, a dominant mendelian autosomal transmission of the disease is observed, often associated with other endocrine neoplasias such as pheochromocytoma and/ or hyperparathyroidism due to parathyroid hyperplasia or multiple adenomatosis. These syndromes are known as multiple endocrine neoplasia and are classified into 3 phenotypes according to the combination of endocrine neoplasia and other nonendocrine findings. Only the hereditary form of MTC affects children. Generally, multiple endocrine neoplasia type 2B is the most aggressive form with the earliest presentation.[3]

The pathogenesis of MTC has been extensively studied in the last 25 years after the recognition that activation of the *RET* proto-oncogene was strongly correlated with the development of the hereditary form of MTC.[4] More recently, a very important role of *RET* pathogenic variants has been demonstrated in the sporadic form of the disease as well, since about 50% of cases are positive for a somatic *RET* pathogenic variant that is related to greater aggressiveness and poor outcome.[5] No data are available regarding the possible causes of induction of *RET* pathogenic variants.

Prognostic Factors

The clinical behavior of MTC is much less favorable than that of other well-differentiated thyroid carcinomas, although it is not as unfavorable as that of anaplastic carcinoma. A 10-year survival for about 50% of patients with MTC is reported in several series. Disease stage at diagnosis is the most important prognostic factor for both cure and survival, as demonstrated by the evidence that if an early diagnosis is made, possibly when the neoplastic disease is still intrathyroidal, 90% of patients survive up to 35 years. Also, serum calcitonin can have a prognostic role. If the calcitonin value is less than 500 pg/mL (<146 pmol/L) before surgery, there is a good probability of survival. Clinical remission is almost 100% when calcitonin decreases to less than 20 pg/mL (<5.8 pmol/L) after surgery. Also, the presence of lymph node metastases in the laterocervical neck region, but not those in the central compartment, is considered a bad prognostic factor for both persistence of disease and survival.[6]

Diagnosis

The most common clinical presentation of sporadic MTC is a thyroid nodule, either single or belonging to a multinodular goiter. With the exception of the simultaneous presence of diarrhea and/or flushing syndrome, which is rare and usually related to advanced metastatic disease, there are no symptoms or signs that prompt suspicion for MTC.

When a family history of MTC is present or the patient has already had a pheochromocytoma or hyperparathyroidism, the suspicion for hereditary MTC is more likely. Mucosal neuromas on the tongue and/or in the conjunctiva, marfanoid habitus, and/or skeletal alterations suggest the diagnosis of multiple endocrine neoplasia type 2B and should prompt evaluation for MTC. Similarly, the presence of an interscapular cutaneous itchy lesion (ie, cutaneous lichen amyloidosis) is also highly suggestive of multiple endocrine neoplasia type 2A because this lesion, although rare (affects 10% of patients with multiple endocrine neoplasia type 2A), is almost exclusively found in individuals with this syndrome.

As above mentioned, sporadic MTC appears as a thyroid nodule, single or in the context of a multinodular goiter. Physical examination of the neck does not offer any significant diagnostic elements, especially now that most nodules are not palpable and are incidentally discovered by neck ultrasonography often performed for other purposes. Once the nodule has been discovered, a classic workup for thyroid nodular disease is then performed. Neck ultrasonography usually shows a nodule with an intermediate- or high-suspicion pattern of malignancy but without any specific or peculiar feature to prompt specific suspicion of MTC. FNA cytology with standard staining does not always show the typical MTC "salt and pepper" and "plasmacytoid" appearance of cells. Cell shape varies from oval to round, and they can be large polygonal or spindled and are usually isolated. Although the cytologic pattern of MTC is generally typical, several series show a high percentage of failure in making a presurgical diagnosis by FNA cytology. Calcitonin is the most specific and sensitive MTC marker, both before and after thyroidectomy. It is a small polypeptide hormone of 32 amino acids normally produced almost exclusively by C cells. Several studies have demonstrated that routine measurement of serum calcitonin is the most accurate diagnostic tool for the detection of MTC in patients with thyroid nodules. In all series, the sensitivity of serum calcitonin was more accurate than that of cytology.[7,8] Nevertheless, there are still controversial opinions on the role of routine measurement of basal serum calcitonin in the workup of thyroid nodules. If the routine measurement of serum calcitonin is not adopted in the clinical workup of thyroid nodules, it could be helpful at least when surgical treatment is planned for a nodule with indeterminate cytology. An elevated level is also helpful with malignant cytology to better guide surgical decision making of whether to perform total thyroidectomy and dissection of the central neck node compartment.

Diagnostic Tools When Serum Calcitonin Is In the "Grey Zone"

Elevated basal serum calcitonin, especially a medium-low level (ie, <100 pg/mL [<29.2 pmol/L]), should not be immediately considered to be diagnostic of MTC. These medium-low levels can be further investigated by performing a stimulation test with the intravenous administration of calcium to confirm that the calcitonin is really secreted by MTC: a significant increase in serum calcitonin (usually 3 to 4 times the basal level) is observed in patients with MTC, but not in those with elevated basal serum calcitonin derived from other sources or artifacts. If the cytologic diagnosis is not definitive for MTC and the serum calcitonin value is in the grey zone of the assay (ie, >20 pg/mL [>5.8 pmol/L] but <100 pg/mL [<29.2 pmol/L]), the calcitonin measurement in the washout of the needle used for the FNA cytology of the suspected thyroid nodule may be crucial. This approach is of particular diagnostic utility to ascertain the nature of neck lymph nodes, especially before thyroidectomy, to plan the surgical approach or the most appropriate therapeutic strategies.[9]

Genetic Screening

After 20 years since the discovery that germline *RET* oncogene pathogenic variants are responsible for hereditary cases of MTC, it is now recognized that *RET* genetic screening must be performed in all patients with MTC, even in the absence of a family history of thyroid cancer.[10] The rationale for this screening is that 5% to 10% of patients with apparently sporadic MTC harbor a germline *RET* pathogenic variant—either de novo or misdiagnosed familial cases.[11] This finding is of great relevance for the early identification of carriers in the family who are unaware of their condition and are sometimes already affected. Although not yet introduced as a standard of care, *RET* gene analysis would also be useful if performed in the tumoral tissue, either in fresh or paraffin-embedded tumoral tissue, of ascertained sporadic cases. There are at least 3 main reasons to perform this procedure: (1) the discovery of a somatic pathogenic variant (usually in 45% of cases) confirms the sporadic nature of the tumor; (2) the prognostic value of the presence/absence of the somatic pathogenic variant; (3) the future possibility for patients with *RET* pathogenic variants to be treated with drugs specifically aimed at inhibiting the altered *RET* gene.

Once an index case has been confirmed to be hereditary, all first-degree relatives should be tested for the presence of the same pathogenic variant. Relatives who do not carry the pathogenic variant can avoid being monitored over the years, as they are not at increased risk to develop MTC. However, relatives who carry the pathogenic variant should undergo clinical, biochemical (ie, basal calcitonin measurement), and imaging assessments (neck ultrasonography) for early discovery of the disease. If both basal calcitonin and neck ultrasonography are negative, a calcium-stimulation test for calcitonin is usually recommended.[12] The therapeutic strategies and follow-up protocols for family members carrying pathogenic variants have been changed over the years. Immediately after the discovery that *RET* pathogenic variants were responsible for the hereditary forms, the surgical practice of prophylactic thyroidectomy in all children with pathogenic *RET* variants was strongly recommended. It is clear that *RET* pathogenic variants vary in terms of penetrance and the age of MTC development. The M918T mutation and the noncysteine mutations (ie, V804M, S891A, L790F, etc) are the most and the least transforming and aggressive, respectively.[13] For these reasons, the American Thyroid Association guidelines classify pathogenic variants into different classes of risk, and the timing of thyroidectomy in carriers should be based on several factors, including the level of risk of the pathogenic variant and the basal and stimulated value of serum calcitonin. Periodic evaluation of serum calcitonin, both basal and stimulated, may be very useful in identifying the right time to perform an early and safe thyroidectomy.[2]

Follow-Up and Therapies for Advanced Disease

Independent from the sporadic or hereditary nature of MTC in a given patient, 3 months after surgery, every patient should be evaluated with physical examination, neck ultrasonography, and measurement of serum free T_3, free T_4, TSH, calcitonin, and CEA. Serum calcitonin is the specific marker to be used for the follow-up of patients with MTC. CEA measurement is relevant because it provides a better idea about the tumoral burden and the degree of differentiation of the tumor since, when dedifferentiated, serum calcitonin can be relatively low and CEA rather elevated.

When patients are not cured by the primary surgical treatment, which should include total thyroidectomy and central neck lymph node dissection, other therapeutic procedures are indicated depending on the localization and the number of lesions. In planning a therapeutic strategy, clinicians should take into account that most distant metastases found during follow-up are small at the time of their recognition and that their growth is usually rather slow. These lesions are compatible with a long period of good quality of life. In these cases, an aggressive therapeutic approach may not be indicated, unless an evident rapidly progressive disease is demonstrated. New drugs, tyrosine kinase inhibitors, have been approved for the treatment of advanced and progressive MTC. Nevertheless, before starting these systemic therapies, some considerations must given to the number, size, and growth rate of the lesions. Whenever possible, local treatment is preferred and systemic therapy should be postponed depending on the evidence for multimetastatic progressive disease.[14]

Current systemic therapeutic options for advanced and progressive MTC are represented by targeted tyrosine kinase inhibitor therapies specifically directed against signal transduction pathways and or genetic alteration of MTC. Although several tyrosine kinase inhibitors have been tested in advanced and progressive MTC, only 2 drugs, vandetanib and cabozantinib, have been approved by both the FDA and European Medicines Agency for treatment of these patients after the phase 3 clinical trials, ZETA and EXAM.[15,16] Although they have different patterns, both vandetanib and cabozantinib are small molecules able to block multiple tyrosine kinases with different activities. These medications should be started if the progression of the disease, as assessed according to Response Evaluation Criteria in Solid Tumors (RECIST), has been documented in the last 12 months or according to clinical judgment in very advanced cases. The choice of one or the other drug is very much dependent on the availability of the drug, since not all countries have both drugs approved and reimbursed. However, in those countries where either can be prescribed, the choice must take into consideration the patient's clinical features and each drug's characteristics. According to the results of the phase 3 studies, the effect of cabozantinib seems to be more rapid but with a safety profile more demanding in its management. Cabozantinib has also been tested in patients who had been previously treated with another tyrosine kinase inhibitor, and the results showed that it works in terms of prolongation of progression-free survival, thus suggesting that it can be used as second-line therapy. This information is unavailable for vandetanib, which is apparently more manageable but slower in determining disease control. Vandetanib, but not cabozantinib, has also been tested in children with a dedicated scheme of administration, and the results show that it is safe and effective in childhood MTC.[17] Moreover, there are several reported cases whereby the ectopic ACTH secretion and the consequent paraneoplastic Cushing syndrome, which is frequently present when the disease is multimetastatic and advanced, is reverted and cured by the administration of vandetanib. Vandetanib cannot be used in patients who have a prolonged QTc interval (>450 ms in men and >470 ms in women), while cabozantinib does not have this limitation. Adverse effects are similar, but the prevalence of each one of them is different according to the drug that is used.

Despite the fact that a significant advantage in prolonging the progression-free survival time has been demonstrated by both drugs, so far neither has shown an increase in overall survival.

Both drugs, as are all tyrosine kinase inhibitors, are cytostatic and not cytotoxic; thus, they can stop cell growth, but they do not kill cells. For this reason, they must be continued until there is evidence of clinical benefit. However, from the results of the 2 studies, it is clearly evident that sooner or later a sort of resistance develops and the clinician must decide to continue or stop the drug. Further studies to analyze the possibility of using the 2 drugs in an alternating modality, combining them, or using them with other drugs, either working via the same mechanism or by modulating the immune system, will be the next challenge of the future. There are already 2 new *RET*-specific inhibitors, LOXO 292[18] and BLUE 667, that are characterized by good efficacy similar to that of the tyrosine kinase inhibitors, with a much smaller impact on quality of life.

Conclusions

Early diagnosis of MTC, when the tumor is still intrathyroidal, is the only way to guarantee that surgery can cure the patient. Measurement of serum calcitonin can be helpful in making an early diagnosis. However, not all cases of MTC are aggressive and lethal. There are several markers of a bad prognosis: (1) advanced stage at diagnosis; (2) preoperative serum calcitonin values greater than 500 pg/mL and/or greater than 20 pg/mL after surgery; (3) the presence of laterocervical metastatic lymph nodes; and (4) *RET* somatic pathogenic variants.

Considering the rarity of the disease, the difficulty of making an early diagnosis, the possibility that MTC can be familial, and the fact that management of persistent disease can be challenging, it is recommended that patients with MTC be followed by a multidisciplinary team in a specialized center.

Clinical Case Vignettes
Case 1

A 43-year-old woman notes a right neck lump. Neck ultrasonography reveals a suspicious right 2.4-cm thyroid nodule. She has no local symptoms. Neck ultrasonography does not show any abnormal lymph nodes. The left lobe had a subcentimeter nonsuspicious nodule. FNA cytology is THY III (atypia of undetermined significance or follicular lesion of undetermined significance [AUS/FLUS]). Thyroid function is normal without evidence of thyroid antibodies, and the serum calcitonin concentration is 45 pg/mL (13.1 pmol/L).

Which of the following is the best next step?

A. Wait and see; perform clinical and biochemical examination every 6 months

B. Total thyroidectomy with central neck dissection

C. Lobectomy for diagnostic purpose

D. Repeated FNA for immunocytochemistry for calcitonin and measurement of calcitonin in the needle washout

Answer: D) Repeated FNA for immunocytochemistry for calcitonin and measurement of calcitonin in the needle washout

When the serum calcitonin concentration is greater than 20 pg/mL but less than 100 pg/mL (5.8-29.2 pmol/L), it is not immediately diagnostic of MTC, but it should serve as an alert that MTC might be present and should prompt other diagnostic procedures. Other than these 2 above-mentioned tools, a calcium-stimulation test can be performed since "true" calcitonin secreted by MTC shows a very high increase after stimulation, while calcitonin from other origins (ie, other neuroendocrine tumors, ectopic production, interference from heterophilic antibodies, etc) does not respond to the stimulus.

Case 2

A 56-year-old man undergoes workup for a multinodular goiter with 2 major thyroid nodules of 1.8 and 2.9 cm. The cytology of the 2.9-cm nodule shows the presence of MTC, and the serum calcitonin value is 420 pg/mL (122.6 pmol/L). Neck ultrasonography does not show any lymph node metastases. The patient undergoes total thyroidectomy and central neck dissection. Histology confirms MTC in the 2.9-cm nodule associated with widespread C-cell hyperplasia with no lymph node metastases. The patient asks about his prognosis and, being aware (from Dr Google) that MTC can be hereditary, he wonders whether his relatives should have testing.

Which of the following statements is correct?

A. His prognosis is good with a high probability for long survival: *RET* genetic screening should be first performed in the patient himself

B. The prognosis of MTC is always severe and his relatives should be immediately screened for serum calcitonin

C. His prognosis is good and since there is no history of other familial cases, there is no need to screen his relatives

D. His prognosis depends on the sporadic or hereditary nature of the disease, and his relatives should be screened only if the hereditary nature is confirmed

Answer: A) His prognosis is good with a high probability for long survival: RET *genetic screening should be first performed in the patient himself*

The prognosis of MTC can widely vary according to the extension of the disease at the time of the diagnosis. Usually cases that are still intrathyroidal have a good prognosis and a preoperative serum calcitonin value less than 500 pg/mL (<146 pmol/L) is consistent with a good prognosis, at least in terms of long survival. The prognosis is not influenced by the sporadic or hereditary nature of MTC, but all patients with MTC, regardless of the familial or personal medical history, must be screened for the presence of a germline *RET*

pathogenic variant since there are patients who are positive despite their apparently sporadic nature. Once the case has been ascertained to be hereditary and a *RET* pathogenic variant is identified, his relatives can undergo testing for the same pathogenic variant to identify those at risk to develop MTC (Answer A).

Case 3

A 63-year-old man with a long history of MTC has undergone surveillance for many years. He has several mediastinal metastatic lymph nodes, the largest of which is 23 mm in diameter, and several nodules in the lungs are very suspicious for metastases. For several years, CT showed stable disease. His serum calcitonin concentration varied from 300 to 400 pg/mL (87.6-116.8 pmol/L), and his CEA concentration varied from 40 to 60 ng/mL. The last 2 serum calcitonin measurements were 630 pg/mL and 780 pg/mL (184.0 and 228.0 pmol/L), and the CEA values were 68 ng/mL and 85 ng/mL. Current CT reveals increased size of all already known metastatic lesions (both lymph nodes and lung lesions) and a 50% increase of liver lesions that were previously described as subcentimetric angiomas.

The patient has been in good general health except for the recent development of diarrhea.

Which of the following is the best next step in this patient's management?

A. Start intravenous chemotherapy

B. Start a tyrosine kinase inhibitor

C. Wait and see

D. Start external radiotherapy targeting the mediastinal lymph nodes

Answer: B) Start a tyrosine kinase inhibitor

Although advanced MTC is often rather indolent, having a very long progression time, a short doubling time of serum calcitonin and CEA suggests that the disease is rapidly growing. Moreover, the evidence, according to RECIST (Response Evaluation Criteria in Solid Tumors), of progressive disease involving all the lesions is sufficient to indicate that it is now time to start a systemic therapy. Currently, this would be a new target therapy, such as vandetanib and cabozantinib, able to simultaneously inhibit several tyrosine kinase receptors (Answer B). Both drugs have been demonstrated to significantly prolong the time of progression-free survival. Since the patient is also symptomatic, vandetanib should be the first choice because the ZETA trial demonstrated its ability to work in symptomatic patients.

References

1. Williams ED: Histogenesis of medullary carcinoma of the thyroid. *J Clin Pathol*. 1966;19(2):114-118. PMID: 5948665
2. Wells SA Jr, Asa SL, Dralle H, et al; American Thyroid Association Guidelines Task Force on Medullary Thyroid Carcinoma. Revised American Thyroid Association guidelines for the management of medullary thyroid carcinoma. *Thyroid*. 2015;25(6):567-610. PMID: 25810047
3. Raue F, Frank-Raue K. Epidemiology and clinical presentation of medullary thyroid carcinoma. *Recent Results Cancer Res*. 2015;204:61-90. PMID: 26494384
4. Eng C, Mulligan LM. Mutations of the RET proto-oncogene in the multiple endocrine neoplasia type 2 syndromes, related sporadic tumours, and hirschsprung disease. *Hum Mutat*. 1997;9(2):97-109. PMID: 9067749
5. Elisei R, Cosci B, Romei C, et al. Prognostic significance of somatic RET oncogene mutations in sporadic medullary thyroid cancer: a 10-year follow-up study. *J Clin Endocrinol Metab*. 2008;93(3):682-687. PMID: 18073307
6. Raue F, Kotzerke J, Reinwein D, et al. Clin Investig. Prognostic factors in medullary thyroid carcinoma: evaluation of 741 patients from the German Medullary Thyroid Carcinoma Register. 1993;71(1):7-12. PMID: 8095831
7. Hahm JR, Lee MS, Min YK, et al. Routine measurement of serum calcitonin is useful for early detection of medullary thyroid carcinoma in patients with nodular thyroid diseases. *Thyroid*. 2001;11(1):73-80. PMID: 11272100
8. Essig GF Jr, Porter K, Schneider D, et al. Fine needle aspiration and medullary thyroid carcinoma: the risk of inadequate preoperative evaluation and initial surgery when relying upon FNAB cytology alone. *Endocr Pract*. 2013;19(6):920-927. PMID: 23757627
9. Elisei R. Routine serum calcitonin measurement in the evaluation of thyroid nodules. *Best Pract Res Clin Endocrinol Metab*. 2008;22(6):941-953. PMID: 19041824
10. Romei C, Tacito A, Molinaro E, et al. Twenty years of lesson learning: how does the RET genetic screening test impact the clinical management of medullary thyroid cancer? *Clin Endocrinol (Oxf)*. 2015;82(6):892-899. PMID: 25440022
11. Wiench, M, Wygoda Z, Gubala E, et al. Estimation of risk of inherited medullary thyroid carcinoma in apparent sporadicpatients. J Clin Oncol. 2001;19(5):1374-1380. PMID: 11230481
12. Elisei R, Alevizaki M, Conte-Devolx B et al. 2012 European Thyroid Association guidelines for genetic testing and its clinical consequences in medullary thyroid cancer. *Eur Thyroid J*. 2013;1(4):216-231. PMID: 24783025
13. Romei C, Ciampi R, Elisei R. A comprehensive overview of the role of the RET proto-oncogene in thyroid carcinoma. *Nat Rev Endocrinol*. 2016;12(4):192-202. PMID: 26868437
14. Schlumberger M, Brose M, Elisei R et al. Definition and management of radioactive iodine-refractory differentiated thyroid cancer. *Lancet Diabetes Endocrinol*. 2014;2(5):356-358. PMID: 24795243
15. Elisei R, Schlumberger MJ, Müller SP, et al. Cabozantinib in progressive medullary thyroid cancer [published correction appears in *J Clin Oncol*. 2014;32(17):1864]. *J Clin Oncol*. 2013;31(29):3639-3646. PMID: 24002501
16. Wells SA Jr, Robinson BG, Gagel RF, et al. Vandetanib in patients with locally advanced or metastatic medullary thyroid cancer: a randomized, double-blind phase III trial. *J Clin Oncol*. 2012;30(2):134-141. PMID: 22025146
17. Fox E, Widemann BC, Chuk MK, et al. Vandetanib in children and adolescents with multiple endocrine neoplasia type 2B associated medullary thyroid carcinoma. *Clin Cancer Res*. 2013;19(15):4239-4248. PMID: 23766359
18. Subbiah V, Velcheti V, Tuch BB, et al. Selective RET kinase inhibition for patients with RET-altered cancers. *Ann Oncol*. 2018;29(8):1869-1876. PMID: 29912274

When Thyroid Function Test Results Don't Make Sense

Mark Gurnell, MD, PhD. Wellcome Trust-MRC Institute of Metabolic Science, University of Cambridge and Addenbrooke's Hospital, Cambridge, United Kingdom; E-mail: mg299@medschl.cam.ac.uk

Learning Objectives

As a result of participating in this session, learners should be able to:

- Recognize the potential causes of discordant or anomalous thyroid function test (TFT) results.

- Explain the basis of commonly used laboratory assays for measuring thyroid hormones and TSH and how assay interference can arise.

- Adopt a systematic approach to the patient with discordant or anomalous TFT results to allow accurate diagnosis in a timely manner and avoid inappropriate investigation and treatment.

Main Conclusions

Discordant or anomalous TFT results may arise in the context of:

- Confounding intercurrent illness and/or medication use.

- Erratic or poor adherence to levothyroxine therapy.

- Interference in commonly used laboratory assays for thyroid hormone or TSH measurement.

- Rare genetic or acquired disorders of the hypothalamic-pituitary-thyroid (HPT) axis.

Successful resolution of discordant or anomalous TFT results is dependent on a sound understanding of:

- HPT axis physiology and the mechanisms governing thyroid hormone action at a cellular level.

- Key principles and methodologies underpinning commonly used thyroid hormone and TSH assays.

- Patterns of abnormal TFT results.

- Roles of dynamic tests, radiologic investigation, and genetic testing in the diagnosis of rare genetic and acquired disorders of the HPT axis.

Significance of the Clinical Problem

TFTs are among the most commonly requested laboratory investigations (~10 million TFTs are ordered each year in the United Kingdom to detect thyroid dysfunction in ~4% of adults). While many of these tests yield results that are straightforward to interpret, an important subgroup returns apparently discordant or anomalous results that at first glance "don't make sense." When this occurs, the endocrinologist is required to disentangle abnormal results that are a consequence of confounding intercurrent illness or medications from those due to laboratory artefacts, while bearing in mind the possibility of rarer but important genetic or acquired disorders of the HPT axis.

Raised thyroid hormones (T_4, T_3) with nonsuppressed TSH levels are an important, and relatively commonly encountered, pattern of discordant TFTs; many cases can be explained by confounding intercurrent illness, concomitant medication use, or analytic interference in thyroid hormone or TSH assays, but differentiating between these and other rarer causes (eg, resistance to thyroid hormone, TSH-secreting pituitary tumor) can be difficult.

Misdirected investigation of these entities results in wastage of resources and/or incorrect therapeutic intervention.

Barriers to Optimal Practice

- Limited awareness and knowledge of the diverse array of conditions that can give rise to discordant or anomalous TFT results.

- Failure to recognize the inherent susceptibility of commonly used laboratory assays (for T_4, T_3, and TSH measurement) to analytical interference.

- Relative rarity of genetic and acquired disorders of the HPT axis such as resistance to thyroid hormone and TSH-secreting pituitary tumors—distinguishing between these conditions is often challenging, and typically requires a combination of investigations, several of which are only rarely performed in routine clinical endocrine practice.

Strategies for Diagnosis, Therapy, and/or Management

Review the Causes of Different TFT Patterns[1,2]

Recognition of the myriad causes of different patterns of TFT results is an essential first step in the investigation and management of TFT results that "don't make sense." The most important conditions to consider are shown in *Figure 1*, along with those that account for most cases of classic primary hypothyroidism and thyrotoxicosis.

Consider Potential Confounding Factors[1,2]

It is important to pay attention to the clinical context, as several factors may have particular relevance for the interpretation of TFTs, including:

- *Age*: Many laboratories do not report age-specific reference ranges, with potential implications for interpreting TFT results at the extremes of age.

- *Pregnancy*: Thyroid hormone and TSH levels vary during normal pregnancy, and trimester-specific reference ranges should be used wherever possible.

- *Levothyroxine therapy*: Levothyroxine replacement in a physiological dosage to optimize TSH may be associated with mildly elevated free T_4 (but normal free T_3) levels in some patients. Owing to their differing half-lives, intermittent hormone ingestion may result in normal or even elevated thyroid hormone levels but fails to normalize TSH.

- *Confounding medications/supplements*: Medications and supplements have the potential to alter thyroid physiology (eg, amiodarone) or cause artifactual laboratory results (eg, heparin or biotin—see below).

- *Nonthyroidal illness*: Several different TFT patterns may be seen during nonthyroidal illness depending on the stage of the illness and laboratory assays used (*Figure 1*).

Exclude Laboratory Assay Interference[3-5]

TSH Measurement

Most TSH assays use a "sandwich" format with 2 antibodies—capture and (labeled) detection—directed against different epitopes on TSH, with the TSH moiety acting as a bridge between the them. The presence of human anti-animal antibodies in a patient's serum can interfere with TSH measurement if directed against the same

Figure 1. Different Patterns of Thyroid Function Tests and Their Causes

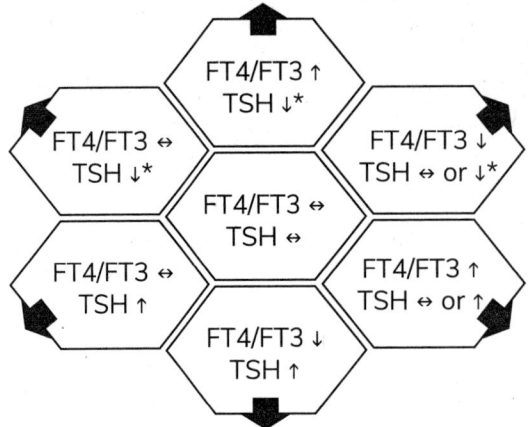

- Graves disease
- Toxic multinodular goiter
- Toxic adenoma
- Thyroiditis (post-viral, post-partum)
- Drugs (amiodarone); excess iodine intake
- Excess thyroxine ingestion
- Pregnancy-related (hyperemesis gravidarum; hydatidiform mole)
- Congenital hyperthyroidism

- Subclinical hyperthyroidism
- Recent treatment for hyperthyroidism
- Drugs (eg, steroids, dopamine)
- Assay interference
- NTI

FT4/FT3 ↑
TSH ↓*

FT4/FT3 ↔
TSH ↓*

FT4/FT3 ↓
TSH ↔ or ↓*

FT4/FT3 ↔
TSH ↔

FT4/FT3 ↔
TSH ↑

FT4/FT3 ↑
TSH ↔ or ↑

FT4/FT3 ↓
TSH ↑

- NTI
- Central hypothyroidism
- Isolated TSH deficiency
- Assay interference

- Subclinical hypothyroidism
- Poor adherence to levothyroxine
- Malabsorption of levothyroxine
- Drugs (eg, amiodarone)
- Assay interference
- NTI recovery phase
- TSH resistance

- Assay interference; FDH
- Levothyroxine replacement therapy (including poor adherence)
- Drugs (eg, amiodarone, heparin)
- NTI (including acute psychiatric disorders)
- Neonatal period
- TSH-secreting pituitary adenoma
- Resistance to thyroid hormone
- Disorders of thyroid hormone transport or metabolism

- Autoimmune thyroiditis (Hashimoto, atrophic)
- Post-radioiodine therapy/thyroidectomy
- Hypothyoid phase of thyroiditis
- Drugs (amiodarone, lithium, TKIs, ATDs)
- Iodine deficiency or excess
- Neck irradiation
- Riedel thyroiditis
- Thyroid infiltration (tumor, amyloid)
- Congenital hypothyroidism

Abbreviations: ATDs, antithyroid drugs; FDH, familial dysalbuminemic hyperthyroxinemia; FT3, free triiodothyronine; FT4, free thyroxine; NTI, nonthyroidal illness; TKI, tyrosine kinase inhibitors.

species as the assay antibodies. Thus, a human anti-animal antibody that blocks TSH binding to either capture or detection antibodies will result in "negative interference," causing a falsely low TSH value. Conversely, a human anti-animal antibody that is capable of cross-linking the capture and detection antibodies may cause "positive interference," leading to a falsely high TSH value. Heterophile (weak, polyspecific) antibodies may cause similar interference. Laboratory strategies for confirming interference include the demonstration of:

- Discordant TSH results in different assays that use different antibody pairs/methodology.

- Nonlinear TSH measurement following sample dilution.

- Altered TSH result following immunosubtraction (using PEG or protein G/A).

Free T$_4$ and Free T$_3$ Measurement

The relatively small size of T$_4$ (and T$_3$) precludes use of a "sandwich" assay format, so competition assays are commonly used. Here, labeled T$_4$ (the tracer) competes with serum T$_4$ for a fixed number of T$_4$ antibody-binding sites. Free hormone assays are designed such that the equilibrium between T$_4$ and its binding proteins is conserved during measurement, so the amount of tracer displaced reflects the "free" rather than "total" hormone concentration. The presence of factors in serum that affect this equilibrium will confound hormone measurement. Examples include:

- Fractionated and unfractionated heparin: both can cause an artifactual elevation in measured concentrations of free T_4 and free T_3 by displacement of T_4 and T_3 from their carrier proteins; the mechanism is poorly understood, but it is likely to involve generation of free fatty acids via heparin-mediated activation of endothelial lipoprotein lipase, with free fatty acids displacing thyroid hormones from albumin.

- Iodothyronine antibodies that bind the tracer.

- Human anti-animal antibodies or heterophilic antibodies that block the assay antibody.

- Variant thyroid hormone–binding proteins: dominantly-inherited genetic variants of albumin (familial dysalbuminemic hyperthyroxinemia [FDH] or transthyretin [transthyretin-associated hyperthyroxinemia (TTR-AH)]), may alter affinity for iodothyronines, and can cause free T_4 (and less frequently free T_3) to be overestimated, particularly in "1-step" analogue hormone assays.

The use of a 2-step ("back titration") assay method (which is less susceptible to such interference), equilibrium dialysis, or mass spectrometry can be useful in confirming or excluding this possibility.

Biotin (Vitamin B$_7$)
Biotin used either as a medication or dietary supplement presents a specific challenge for laboratory platforms that use biotin as part of the core assay configuration (eg, streptavidin-biotin complex). This issue can affect a multitude of assays, not simply thyroid hormone or TSH measurements.

Consider Specific Conditions

Once potential confounding factors and artifactual results have been excluded, then consideration can be given to the investigations required to diagnose rarer genetic and acquired disorders, such as resistance to thyroid hormone and TSH-secreting pituitary tumors, which often present a specific challenge.

Resistance to Thyroid Hormone vs TSH-Secreting Pituitary Tumor[6-10]
Resistance to thyroid hormone (estimated incidence 1 in 40,000 to 50,000 live births) and TSH-secreting pituitary tumors (estimated prevalence 1 to 3 per million) occur in patients of a similar age range and either gender. A subset of patients with predominant central/pituitary resistance also exhibit thyrotoxic symptoms and signs, such that these features are not discriminatory. An algorithm for distinguishing resistance to thyroid hormone and TSH-secreting pituitary tumors is shown in *Figure 2*.

However, several potential pitfalls should be kept in mind, including:

- *Serum α-subunit*: Elevated serum α-subunit levels are also found in nonfunctioning and GH-secreting pituitary tumors, while normal levels are a recognized finding in TSH-secreting microadenomas.

- *SHBG*: falsely low levels can occur in mixed GH/TSH-secreting tumors due to inhibition of SHBG synthesis by GH; conversely, synthetic estrogen therapy in resistance to thyroid hormone can falsely elevate SHBG.

- *Pituitary imaging*: TSH-secreting microadenomas may be difficult to visualize, while patients with resistance to thyroid hormone do harbor "incidental" abnormalities on imaging. In addition, persistently elevated TSH levels following thyroid ablation in resistance to thyroid hormone results in thyrotroph hyperplasia and pituitary enlargement.

Figure 2. Algorithm to Aid in Distinction Between Resistance to Thyroid Hormone and TSH-Secreting Pituitary Tumors

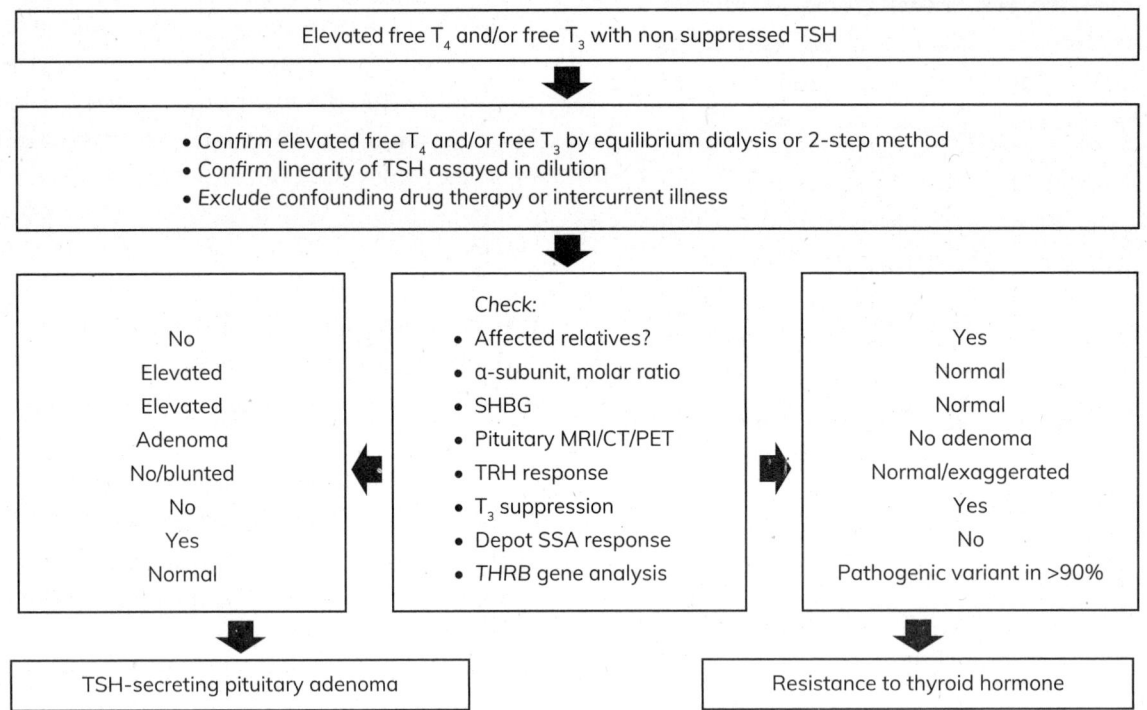

Abbreviation: TRH, thyrotropin-releasing hormone.

- *Thyrotropin-releasing hormone test:* 10% to 20% of patients with TSH-secreting pituitary tumors show an apparent preserved TSH response.

- *THRB gene analysis:* Approximately 15% of cases of resistance to thyroid hormone are not associated with *THRB* pathogenic variants.

Clinical Case Vignettes

Case 1

A 43-year-old woman has regular palpitations and reports a 20-lb (9-kg) weight loss over the past 3 months. On questioning, she also has poor quality sleep and heat intolerance with occasional headaches. Her resting pulse rate is 110 beats/min and regular, and blood pressure is 150/85 mm Hg. She has a fine resting tremor, warm peripheries, and a small symmetric goiter. Visual fields are normal to confrontation testing, and there are no signs of dysthyroid eye disease.

Laboratory test results:

Free T_4 = 3.5 ng/dL (0.8-1.6 ng/dL) (SI: 45 pmol/L [10-20 pmol/L])
Free T_3 =11.7 pg/mL (2.3-4.2 pg/mL) (SI: 18 pmol/L [3.5-6.5 pmol/L])
TSH = 4.8 mIU/L (0.4-4.0 mIU/L)

Which of the following is the most appropriate next step in this patient's management?

A. Perform contrast-enhanced MRI of the pituitary

B. Perform thyrotropin-releasing hormone test

C. Measure serum α-subunit

D. Measure serum SHBG

E. Seek advice on further laboratory analyses

Answer: E) Seek advice on further laboratory analyses

Before embarking on further investigations to distinguish a TSH-secreting pituitary adenoma (thyrotropinoma) from resistance to thyroid hormone, it is first necessary to exclude laboratory assay interference as a cause for the unusual TFT pattern. This patient manifests several features that suggest she has genuine thyrotoxicosis, and therefore suspicion lies more with the TSH result—is this a potentially erroneous/artifactual result and in fact she has primary thyrotoxicosis (with a fully suppressed TSH)? Most endocrine laboratories can readily screen for TSH assay interference. Thus, seeking advice on further laboratory analyses (Answer E) is correct.

Case 2

A 73-year-old woman has fractured her left femoral neck following a fall. She is otherwise fit and healthy, aside from mild hypertension that is well-controlled with amlodipine. She undergoes emergency hip replacement. Twenty-four hours after surgery, she is noted to be in fast atrial fibrillation (120 beats/min) without cardiovascular compromise (her blood pressure is 135/80 mm Hg and the remaining cardiorespiratory examination is unremarkable).

The examining physician notes that she has a small, smooth goiter and queries the possibility of underlying thyroid disease.

Initial laboratory test results:

> Free T_4 = 2.2 ng/dL (0.8-1.6 ng/dL) (SI: 28 pmol/L [10-20 pmol/L])
> TSH = 1.8 mIU/L (0.4-4.0 mIU/L)

Additional investigations (on the same serum sample):

> Total T_4 = 9.2 µg/dL (4.3-10.9 µg/dL) (SI: 118 nmol/L [55-140 nmol/L])

Which of the following is the most likely explanation for the TFT findings?

A. Familial dysalbuminemic hyperthyroxinemia

B. Iodinated contrast-induced thyrotoxicosis

C. Medication-induced artifactual elevation of free T_4

D. Resistance to thyroid hormone due to *THRB* pathogenic variant

E. TSH-secreting pituitary adenoma (thyrotropinoma)

Answer: C) Medication-induced artifactual elevation of free T_4

Although the patient has an apparently raised free T_4 level, the TSH is not suppressed and subsequent investigations on the same serum sample show an entirely normal total T_4 level. Taken together, the normal TSH and total T_4 levels argue against genuine thyrotoxicosis and also exclude familial dysalbuminemic hyperthyroxinemia (due to a pathogenic variant in the albumin gene). Most patients undergoing elective or emergency surgery receive thromboprophylaxis with low-molecular-weight heparin, and this likely explains the apparently raised free T_4 result in this patient. Heparin (both conventional and low-molecular-weight in prophylactic and treatment dosages) is able to activate endothelial lipoprotein lipase. In some patients, the accompanying rise in serum free fatty acid levels is sufficient to cause displacement of T_4 from its binding sites (eg, on thyroxine-binding globulin), thereby raising free, but not total, thyroid hormone levels. This is an in vitro phenomenon, which is exacerbated by delayed processing of the blood sample.

Case 3

A 33-year-old woman is referred to the endocrine clinic because her primary care physician is concerned about her levothyroxine replacement therapy. Five years ago, she underwent total thyroidectomy for relapsed Graves disease. Postoperatively, she was clinically and biochemically euthyroid while taking 150 mcg of levothyroxine daily.

However, over the last 6 months, despite treatment with up to 300 mcg of levothyroxine daily, she has had a persistently elevated TSH level.

Her pulse rate is 60 beats/min and regular, and blood pressure is 135/80 mm Hg. She is obese (BMI = 32.5 kg/m²) and has dry skin but is otherwise clinically euthyroid. There is no palpable thyroid remnant.

Laboratory test results:

Free T_4 = 1.3 ng/dL (0.8-1.6 ng/dL) (SI: 17.0 pmol/L [10.0-20.0 pmol/L])
TSH = 18.5 mIU/L (0.4-4.0 mIU/L)

There is no evidence of laboratory assay interference in either the free T_4 or TSH assay.

Which of the following is the most likely explanation for her TFT results?

A. Erratic adherence to her levothyroxine regimen

B. Malabsorption of levothyroxine

C. Nonthyroidal illness (sick euthyroid syndrome)

D. Resistance to thyroid hormone due to *THRB* pathogenic variant

E. TSH-secreting pituitary adenoma (thyrotropinoma)

Answer: A) Erratic adherence to her levothyroxine regimen

This patient has previously achieved clinical and biochemical euthyroidism while taking levothyroxine, 150 mcg daily (ie, not requiring supraphysiologic dosages), which argues strongly against an underlying diagnosis of *THRB*-related resistance to thyroid hormone (Answer D). However, in the absence of such information, and without historical TFT results outside the context of untreated acute Graves disease, the possibility of coexistent autoimmune thyroid disease and resistance to thyroid hormone would otherwise need to be considered. Similarly, and assuming the original TFT results at the time of her presentation with Graves disease were correctly interpreted (ie, the TSH was appropriately fully suppressed) then, although the patient could have subsequently developed a thyrotropinoma (Answer E), this would be less likely than the other options listed. The development of a malabsorption syndrome (eg, celiac disease) (Answer B) could lead to the development of hypothyroidism in a previously well-controlled patient, but the finding of a free T_4 level in the upper half of the reference range makes this option less likely. There is nothing specific in the clinical history to suggest nonthyroidal illness (Answer C). Erratic adherence to levothyroxine therapy (Answer A) could produce this pattern of results, especially if the patient takes a larger dosage of levothyroxine on the day(s) immediately before the blood test, which can be sufficient to produce serum T_4 levels within the laboratory reference range, but is inadequate to normalize a chronically raised TSH.

References

1. Gurnell M, Halsall DJ, Chatterjee VK. What should be done when thyroid function tests do not make sense. *Clin Endocrinol (Oxf)*. 2011;74(6):673-678. PMID: 21521292

2. Koulouri O, Moran C, Halsall D, Chatterjee K, Gurnell M. Pitfalls in the measurement and interpretation of thyroid function tests. *Best Pract Res Clin Endocrinol Metab*. 2013;27(6):745-762. PMID: 24275187

3. Després N, Grant AM. Antibody interference in thyroid assays: a potential for clinical misinformation. *Clin Chem*. 1998;44(3):440-454. PMID: 9510847

4. Stockigt JR, Lim CF. Medications that distort *in vitro* tests of thyroid function, with particular reference to estimates of serum free thyroxine. *Best Pract Res Clin Endocrinol Metab*. 2009;23(6):753-767. PMID: 19942151

5. Favresse J, Burlacu MC, Maiter D, Gruson D. Interferences with thyroid function immunoassays: clinical implications and detection algorithm. *Endocr Rev*. 2018;39(5):830-850. PMID: 29982406

6. Gurnell M, Visser T, Beck-Peccoz P, Chatterjee K. Resistance to thyroid hormone. In: Jameson JL, De Groot LJ, eds. *Endocrinology: Adult and Pediatric*. 7th ed. Philadelphia, PA: Saunders Elsevier, Philadelphia; 2015:1648-1665.

7. Gurnell M, Rajanayagam O, Barbar I, Jones MK, Chatterjee VK. Reversible pituitary enlargement in the syndrome of resistance to thyroid hormone. *Thyroid*. 1998;8(8):679-682. PMID: 9737363

8. Beck-Peccoz P, Persani L, Mannavola D, Campi I. Pituitary tumours: TSH-secreting adenomas. *Best Pract Res Clin Endocrinol Metab*. 2009;23(5):597-606. PMID: 19945025

9. Mannavola D, Persani L, Vannucchi G, et al. Different response to chronic somatostatin analogues in patients with central hyperthyroidism. *Clin Endocrinol (Oxf)*. 2005;62(2):176-181. PMID: 15670193

10. Koulouri O, Gurnell M. TSH-secreting pituitary adenomas. In: Huhtaniemi I, ed. *Encyclopedia of Endocrine Diseases*. 2nd ed, Vol 2. New York, NY: Elsevier; 2018:261-266.

Nonthyroidal Illness Syndrome in the Intensive Care Unit: Is There Ever a Case for Treatment?

Greet Van den Berghe, MD, PhD. Clinical Division and Laboratory of Intensive Care Medicine, KU Leuven University, Leuven, B-3000 Leuven, Belgium; E-mail: greet.vandenberghe@kuleuven.be

Learning Objectives

As a result of participating in this session, learners should be able to:

- Explain the pathophysiology of nonthyroidal illness syndrome as a biphasic stress response with different prognostic and possibly also different therapeutic implications.

- Distinguish iatrogenic from endogenous nonthyroidal illness syndrome and distinguish nonthyroidal illness syndrome from premorbid thyroid disease.

Main Conclusions

During acute severe illnesses requiring critical care, low plasma T_3 concentrations are present in the face of low-normal T_4, normal TSH, and high reverse T_3. This constellation of changes is referred to as nonthyroidal illness syndrome (NTIS) and is present across all ages.[1,2] Iatrogenic factors such a dopamine or glucocorticoid infusion or iodine intoxication via wound dressings or contrast agents[3,4] and the presence of premorbid thyroid disease further complicate the phenotype of NTIS and its clinical relevance. In the acute phase of illness, NTIS (noniatrogenic) is mostly brought about by peripheral inactivation of thyroid hormones in which reduced nutritional intake plays its part.[5,6] Recent indirect evidence has suggested that these acute, peripheral alterations are part of a beneficial adaptive response to reduce energy expenditure and to stimulate the innate immune response, important for survival. Hence, treatment is not indicated and could be harmful. In contrast, in more severely ill patients, with prolonged critical illness, an additional central suppression of the thyroid axis alters and further aggravates the NTIS. This central suppression may no longer be adaptive. Whether treatment of this central component of NTIS in patients with prolonged critical illness, with hypothalamic-releasing factors rather than with T_4 ($\pm T_3$), has the ability to improve outcomes remains to be investigated in randomized controlled trials. Clinicians should focus on diagnosing iatrogenic pathology and on identifying premorbid thyroid disease to avoid overlooking potentially lethal but tractable conditions.

Significance of the Clinical Problem

In response to critical illness, thyroid hormone parameters are altered. Patients with mild or moderate disease usually have normal plasma T_4 and TSH concentrations, but low T_3 and elevated reverse T_3 concentrations. Patients with more severe and prolonged illness also display low serum T_4 and TSH concentrations. Indirect evidence has suggested that the acute changes are brought about by altered thyroid hormone metabolism and are likely adaptive and beneficial, whereas the central thyroid axis suppression that follows later could be harmful. Although pathophysiologically and prognostically distinct, these constellations are usually grouped under the term NTIS, a name that highlights the importance of differentiating from typical primary thyroid diseases, which is a complicated issue. Iatrogenic factors further complicate interpretation of adaptation vs maladaptation.

Barriers to Optimal Practice

The biphasic nature of NTIS and the interference exerted by fasting and feeding, by drugs, and by premorbid thyroid diseases together explains why clinicians are often left in the dark regarding the need and modality for diagnosis and treatment. This may evoke a nihilistic approach that could overlook potentially dangerous pathology that is left undiagnosed and untreated.

Strategies for Diagnosis, Therapy, and/or Management

In critical illness, following a brief transient rise in plasma T_4 and TSH, most patients present with low plasma T_3 concentration and low or low-normal T_4 concentration, without a concomitant rise in TSH. In contrast, plasma concentrations of the inactive hormone reverse T_3 increase. This constellation of changes is referred to as NTIS. Patients with mild or moderate NTIS usually have normal plasma T_4 and TSH concentrations, whereas patients with more severe and prolonged illness also display low serum T_4 and TSH concentrations, both indicative of a poor prognosis.[1,2]

The expression of the inactivating outer-ring deiodinase D3, responsible for conversion of T_4 to inactive reverse T_3, is upregulated in liver and skeletal muscle. Also, within granulocytes, critical illness upregulates D3 activity, where it contributes to the bacterial killing capacity of these cells. However, increased D2 expression has also been reported in activated macrophages, which could activate phagocytosis and release of cytokines. In contrast, hepatic activity of the activating inner-ring deiodinase D1 is suppressed by critical illness, which results in decreased deiodination of T_4 into T_3. Cytokines and hypoxia are among the possible drivers of such peripherally altered thyroid hormone metabolism, and low levels of thyroid hormone–binding globulin and albumin contribute to altered peripheral thyroid hormone availability at target tissues.

When patients require prolonged intensive care, plasma T_3 remains low and plasma T_4 and TSH concentrations are also decreased. Suppressed expression of thyrotropin-releasing hormone in the hypothalamus drives these more chronic changes. In prolonged critical illness, peripheral tissues such as muscle show signs of compensatory attempts to restore T_3 availability; for example, by upregulating D2 activity. Also, the thyroid hormone transporter monocarboxylate transporter 8 has been found to be upregulated in muscle and liver of patients with prolonged critical illness. At onset of recovery from illness, a brisk rise in TSH and T_4 has been observed, suggestive of reactivation of thyrotropin-releasing hormone, changes that are assumed to normalize again upon full recovery.

The changes within the thyroid axis are only one part of a broader orchestrated neuroendocrine response to illness, encompassing all major endocrine axes, together altering the balance between anabolism and catabolism. Whereas the changes that occur acutely in response to critical illness are considered beneficial, reflecting an attempt to provide energy and limit unnecessary energy expenditure to promote survival, the changes that occur in prolonged critical illness may be harmful, with potentially detrimental consequences such as wasting, organ dysfunction, and impaired cognition. Such differences may explain the controversy about whether to treat

NTIS with T_4 and/or T_3 with the intention to improve the outcome of critical illness. There may be positive impact on the heart, for example, as shown in patients after cardiac surgery, but patient-centered clinical outcomes have not been beneficially affected. In fact, in patients with low serum T_4 levels, T_4 treatment may also be harmful. The often supraphysiological dosages of T_4 or T_3 that were tested further exert negative feedback inhibition, which could hamper the recovery of TSH secretion. Interestingly, a proof-of-concept study of patients with prolonged critical illness investigated the impact of a continuous infusion of thyrotropin-releasing hormone combined with a growth hormone secretagogue and found that this strategy not only normalized thyroid hormone levels, but also reduced catabolism and increased anabolism. Larger studies investigating clinical outcomes are currently lacking.

Several iatrogenic and nutritional factors interfere with the pathophysiology and impact of NTIS.[3-7] Critically ill patients often receive high doses of glucocorticoids, which can lower serum TSH. Also, dopamine infusion, prescribed as an inotrope and/or vasopressor for the critically ill, suppresses TSH secretion in adults, children, and infants, causing iatrogenic hypothyroidism, which quickly reverses upon discontinuation of dopamine.[3] Although no longer a preferred drug for adults, dopamine is still extensively used in pediatric and neonatal intensive care units. Less commonly used drugs such as anticonvulsant medications, certain antiarrhythmic drugs, and lithium can also affect the hypothalamus-pituitary-thyroid axis. Importantly, an often overlooked problem is iatrogenic iodine intoxication, through the use of iodine-containing contrast fluids or antiseptic dressings, which can affect thyroid hormone availability.[4]

Fasting in healthy individuals induces changes in the thyroid axis that are similar to those in NTIS: plasma T_3 decreases, whereas plasma reverse T_3 concentrations rise, changes that rapidly return to baseline upon refeeding. Recently, 2 large multicenter studies, the EPaNIC and the PEPaNIC randomized controlled trials performed in critically ill adults and children, respectively, showed that accepting poor enteral feeding during the first week of critical illness, as compared with the early administration of supplemental parenteral nutrition, resulted in fewer infections, fewer complications, and accelerated recovery.[5,6] While restricting macronutrient administration in the first week of critical illness improved the outcomes of these patients suffering from NTIS, it further aggravated NTIS by lowering TSH, total T_4, T_3, and the T_3-to-reverse T_3 ratio. Importantly, the clinical benefit of accepting virtual fasting during week 1 of critical illness was statistically explained, in part, by the early further suppression of T_3 and the T_3-to-reverse T_3 ratio in both the adult and pediatric populations, suggesting that the acute peripheral changes of NTIS most likely represent a beneficial adaptation to illness. Such an effect on the peripheral component of NTIS was also shown to be evoked by targeting normal fasting blood glucose levels in critically ill children. This further suppression of T_3 and the T_3-to-reverse T_3 ratio also explains, in part, the mortality benefit of tight blood glucose control in this population.[7] The further aggravation of the central component of NTIS, with suppression of TSH-induced T_4 release, in critically ill adults and children evoked by not forcefully feeding early appeared to counteract the outcome benefits of the intervention. The central component of NTIS, unlike the acute peripheral component, overt in the more chronic phase of illness may thus no longer be adaptive and could be deleterious. This indirect evidence thus suggests the potential of treatment with hypothalamic-releasing factors, which could also be safer than treatment with T_4 and/or T_3 given the normal negative feedback exerted by thyroid hormones at the pituitary level, which would be maintained, whereby excessively elevated thyroid hormone levels could be avoided.[1,2]

Distinguishing NTIS from premorbid thyroid disease is also challenging. Indeed, diagnosis of hypothyroidism during critical illness can be very difficult because of the superimposed NTIS. High plasma TSH and low plasma T_4 are indicative, but absence of elevated TSH does not exclude hypothyroidism in the context of critical illness. It is generally accepted that patients with premorbid hypothyroidism, present in about 7% of the elderly population, should continue to receive T_4 replacement while in the intensive care unit. Hyperthyroidism is characterized by suppressed plasma TSH in the face of high plasma free T_4 and T_3, but this constellation can be altered by superimposed NTIS during critical illness. Physical examination and measurement of thyroid antibodies can provide further information to help distinguish thyroid diseases from NTIS.

Clinical Case Vignettes

Case 1

A 68-year-old woman with a history of subclinical hypothyroidism (currently on no treatment) is admitted to the intensive care unit with a diagnosis of pneumonia-induced septic shock. She is intubated and is hemodynamically difficult to manage (mean arterial pressure, 68 mm Hg; pulse rate, 83 beats/min; cardiac output, 4.6 L/min). She receives norepinephrine (0.8 mcg/kg per min). Because of her clinical history, the attending physician has ordered measurement of TSH, total T_4, T_3, and reverse T_3.

> TSH = 4.0 mIU/L (0.5-6.0 mIU/L)
> Total T_4 = 11 µg/dL (4.3-12.0 µg/dL)
>   (SI: 141.6 nmol/L [55.3-154.4 nmol/L])
> T_3 = 40 ng/dL (70-204 ng/dL) (SI: 0.6 nmol/L
>   [1.1-3.1 nmol/L])
> Reverse T_3 = 100 ng/dL (30-80 ng/dL)
>   (SI: 1.5 nmol/L [0.5-1.2 nmol/L])

Regarding treatment, which of the following do you conclude?

A. This patient has hypothyroidism that requires treatment

B. This is "normal," and no treatment is required

Answer: B) This is normal, and no treatment is required

This vignette represents the acute presentation of the NTIS, and these acute changes are adaptive. Therefore, no treatment is needed.

Case 1 (Continued)

Twenty days later, the same patient is still in the intensive care unit. She is unresponsive, remains vasopressor dependent, and is hypothermic. She cannot be weaned from the ventilator.

> TSH = 0.2 mU/L (0.5-6.0 mIU/L)
> Total T_4 = 2.0 µg/dL (4.3-12.0 µg/dL)
>   (SI: 25.7 nmol/L [55.3-154.4 nmol/L])
> T_3 = 23 ng/dL (70-204 ng/dL) (SI: 0.4 nmol/L
>   [1.1-3.1 nmol/L])
> Reverse T_3 = 70 ng/dL (30-80 ng/dL) (SI: 1.1 nmol/L
>   [0.5-1.2 nmol/L])

Regarding treatment, which of the following do you conclude?

A. This patient may have central hypothyroidism of prolonged critical illness, which may need treatment

B. This is "normal," and no treatment is required

Answer: A) This patient may have central hypothyroidism of prolonged critical illness, which may need treatment

These thyroid abnormalities are typical of those present in the protracted phase of critical illness, which may be maladaptive, particularly when the patient has symptoms that may respond to treatment with levothyroxine.

Case 2

A 70-year-old man is admitted to the intensive care unit with acute respiratory distress syndrome, a serious complication after thyroidectomy. Because of his clinical history, the attending physician has ordered measurement of TSH, total T_4, and T_3.

> TSH = 11.5 mIU/L (0.5-6.0 mIU/L)
> Total T_4 = 4.0 µg/dL (4.3-12.0 µg/dL)
>   (SI: 51.5 nmol/L [55.3-154.4 nmol/L])
> T_3 = 49 ng/dL (70-204 ng/dL) (SI: 0.8 nmol/L
>   [1.1-3.1 nmol/L])

Does this patient need to be treated?

A. Yes

B. No

Answer: A) Yes

Given that this patient has no thyroid gland, he will need substitution therapy.

Case 3

A 4-week-old infant is admitted to the pediatric intensive care unit with extensive severe burn injuries and is treated for 14 days with iodine wound dressings. The baby appears to be unconscious without obvious cause, is hypothermic, and has bradycardia. Given this context, the attending physician has ordered measurement of TSH, total T_4, T_3, reverse T_3, and urinary iodine.

TSH = 9.5 mIU/L (0.5-6.5 mIU/L)
Total T_4 = 2.0 μg/dL (5.9-16.0 μg/dL)
 (SI: 25.7 nmol/L [75.9-205.9 nmol/L])

T_3 = 50.0 ng/dL (100-250 ng/dL) (SI: 0.8 nmol/L [1.5-3.6 nmol/L])
Reverse T_3 = 20 ng/dL (11-129 ng/dL) (SI: 0.3 nmol/L [0.2-2.0 nmol/L])
Urinary iodine = >10.000 μg/L

Which of the following do you conclude?

A. This is normal

B. This patient has iodine-induced hypothyroidism and NTIS and treatment is necessary

Answer: B) This patient has iodine-induced hypothyroidism and NTIS and treatment is necessary

This case represents iodine intoxication-induced hypothyroidism in a newborn and treatment is necessary.

References

1. Van den Berghe G. Non-thyroidal illness in the ICU: a syndrome with different faces. *Thyroid.* 2014;24(10):1456-1465. PMID: 24845024

2. Langouche L, Jacobs A, Van den Berghe G. Nonthyroidal illness syndrome across the ages. *J Endocr Soc.* 2019;3(12):2313-2325. PMID: 31745528

3. Van den Berghe G, de Zegher F. Anterior pituitary function during critical illness and dopamine treatment. *Crit Care Med.* 1996;24(9):1580-1590. PMID: 8797634

4. Markou K, Georgopoulos N, Kyriazopoulou V, Vagenakis AG. Iodine-induced hypothyroidism. *Thyroid.* 2001;11(5):501-510. PMID: 11396709

5. Langouche L, Vander Perre S, Marques M, et al. Impact of early nutrient restriction during critical illness on the nonthyroidal illness syndrome and its relation with outcome: a randomized, controlled clinical study. *J Clin Endocrinol Metab.* 2013;98(3):1006-1013. PMID: 23348400

6. Jacobs A, Derese I, Vander Perre S, et al. Non-thyroidal illness syndrome in critically ill children: prognostic value and impact of nutritional management. *Thyroid.* 2019;29(4):480-492. PMID: 30760183

7. Gielen M, Mesotten D, Wouters PJ, et al. Effect of tight glucose control with insulin on the thyroid axis of critically ill children and its relation with outcome. *J Clin Endocrinol Metab.* 2012;97(10): 3569-3576. PMID: 22872689

Moderate to Severe Active Thyroid Eye Disease

Chrysoula Dosiou, MD, MS. Stanford University School of Medicine, Stanford, CA; E-mail: cdosiou@stanford.edu

Andrea L. Kossler, MD, FACS. Stanford University School of Medicine, Stanford, CA; E-mail: akossler@stanford.edu

Learning Objectives

As a result of participating in this session, learners should be able to:

- Perform a basic ophthalmologic clinical assessment and evaluation.

- Recognize the signs and symptoms of thyroid eye disease (TED).

- Distinguish between mild vs moderate/severe TED and inactive vs active TED.

- Determine when to refer patients for ophthalmologic evaluation and subspecialized care.

- Educate patients about their treatment options.

Main Conclusions

The initial evaluation of all patients with Graves disease should include an evaluation for TED. When TED is present, particular attention should be paid to disease activity, disease severity, and the impact on the patient's quality of life. These elements will shape the therapeutic approach, which should be pursued in a multidisciplinary manner, with the endocrinologist and the ophthalmologist. This team can work together to modify risk factors, normalize thyroid function, and recommend treatments. Patients with mild disease generally benefit from local therapies and selenium, while patients with moderate to severe disease usually require the addition of intravenous glucocorticoids. If there is an inadequate response to glucocorticoid therapy, several second-line therapies have been investigated for use, including orbital radiation, rituximab, cyclosporine, mycophenolate mofetil, methotrexate, and azathioprine. New biologic agents, including teprotumumab and tocilizumab, have demonstrated impressive reductions in disease activity and severity and improvement in quality of life. Teprotumumab is currently awaiting FDA approval for treatment of moderate to severe active TED. A decision is expected in early 2020. As new treatment options emerge, the treatment paradigm for TED will continue to evolve.

Significance of the Clinical Problem

Thyroid eye disease, also known as Graves ophthalmopathy, is an autoimmune, inflammatory disorder of the orbit and represents the most common extrathyroidal manifestation of Graves disease, present in 50% to 70% of cases.[1] While most cases of TED are associated with hyperthyroidism, a minority of patients (about 10%) may be hypothyroid or remain euthyroid.[2] The onset and progression of TED are influenced by factors that are potentially controllable such as cigarette smoking, thyroid dysfunction, and choice of treatment modalities for hyperthyroidism. Although most patients have mild disease, approximately one-third of patients with TED have moderate to severe disease and 5% develop sight-threatening disease, such as dysthyroid optic neuropathy or exposure keratopathy (when the cornea is exposed due to inability to completely close the eyes).

Typically, the natural history of the disease is biphasic. It begins with an active inflammatory stage, lasting on average 18 months, where ocular manifestations can quickly worsen, followed by an inactive phase, characterized mainly by fibrosis often without return of normal ocular function (Rundle curve). Treatment of TED early during the active phase is crucial to stop disease progression and minimize ocular sequelae. Timely and effective management of TED is often based on the endocrinologist's familiarity with the manifestations of orbital disease and their grading. All patients diagnosed with Graves disease should be evaluated clinically for the presence or absence of ocular symptoms. If symptoms are present, the patient should be referred to an oculoplastic surgeon or ophthalmologist familiar with the management of TED for a complete eye exam. Hence, it is important that the endocrinologist assess for TED in all patients with Graves disease and refer for ophthalmologic evaluation if symptoms are present to ensure the opportunity for timely treatment, ideally in a multidisciplinary setting.

The European Group on Graves Orbitopathy (EUGOGO) published a set of guidelines in 2008 (updated in 2016) that outline the recommended management for these patients.[3] Since then, a number of randomized controlled trials have been published that offer promising alternatives to the traditional treatment approaches. Despite those guidelines, there are still gaps in physician knowledge regarding this disease that translate into delay in diagnosis and treatment. In a recent EUGOGO study, time from the first symptom of TED to diagnosis was on average 9 months and time from diagnosis of TED by physician to tertiary referral center was 6 months.[4] In a 2009 United Kingdom survey, 58% of patients with TED were initially given the wrong diagnosis.[5]

Suboptimal management and delays to treatment of TED appear to be widespread. The objective of this session is to provide practical information for TED diagnosis and management for endocrinologists.

Barriers to Optimal Practice

- Patient, public, and medical community awareness of this condition is lacking. Many patients with symptoms of TED are told they have dry eyes or aging changes, leading to a delay in diagnosis and treatment.

- Endocrinologists and primary care physicians are unsure when to refer a patient for ophthalmologic examination or do not have a relationship with an ophthalmologist or a multidisciplinary care setting that treats TED.

- Current therapies for active TED only stop disease progression but do not reverse the eye changes. Therefore, patients must be diagnosed early in order to treat the disease during the active phase to minimize the severity of eye disease. Once eye findings have occurred, patients often need surgical rehabilitation to reverse the functional and aesthetic changes to the eye.

- Steroid-refractory disease or recurrence of disease is common; however, there is a lack of effective second-line options or consensus regarding the best second-line treatments.

- Delays or denial with insurance approval for off-label treatment can compromise efficient patient care.

Strategies for Diagnosis, Therapy, and/or Management

Initial evaluation of patients with Graves disease should also include clinical evaluation for eye symptoms. If eye symptoms are present, patients should be referred to an ophthalmologist who treats TED for evaluation, as other diseases can mimic TED. Patients with TED are best managed by a multispecialty team including an endocrinologist and an ophthalmologist. A simple tool for assessing patients with TED is provided by EUGOGO (*Table*).[6]

Patients with TED should also be evaluated for: (1) degree of activity, (2) degree of severity, and (3) impact on the patient's quality of life. This will help classify patients into 1 of 4 groups: mild active, mild inactive, moderate/severe active, moderate/severe inactive.

Activity of the disease is assessed through the Clinical Activity Score (CAS), checking for the presence of 7 features, with a score ≥3/7 representing active disease. The 7 features are retroorbital pain at rest, pain with eye movement, inflammatory lid edema, lid erythema, conjunctival injection, chemosis, caruncle/plica inflammation. In follow-up visits, a modified CAS score is used, which includes points for worsening visual acuity, worsening proptosis (2 mm or more), or worsening diplopia (8 degrees or more). A score of ≥4/10 is active disease.

Severity of the disease is defined by the impact of different aspects of TED on the patient's quality of life. Per EUGOGO guidelines:[3]

1. Sight-threatening TED: Patients with dysthyroid optic neuropathy and/or corneal breakdown. This category warrants immediate intervention.

2. Moderate to severe TED: Patients without sight-threatening TED whose eye disease has sufficient impact on daily life to justify the risks of immunosuppression (if active) or surgical intervention (if inactive). Patients with moderate-to-severe TED usually have 1 or more of the following: lid retraction >2 mm, moderate or severe soft-tissue involvement, exophthalmos >3 mm above normal for race and gender, and inconstant or constant diplopia.

Table. Tool for Assessing Patients With TED

• Patients with a history of Graves disease, who have neither symptoms nor signs of TED, require no further ophthalmological assessments and do not need to be referred for ophthalmologic evaluation.
• Patients with unusual presentations (unilateral Graves ophthalmopathy or euthyroid Graves ophthalmopathy) should be referred, regardless of how mild their symptoms or signs are, in order to make an accurate diagnosis.
All other patients should be screened according to the following protocol:
Refer urgently if any of the following symptoms or signs are present: • Unexplained deterioration in vision   • Awareness of change in intensity or quality of color vision in one or both eyes   • History of eye(s) suddenly "popping out" (globe subluxation)   • Obvious corneal opacity   • Optic disc swelling
Refer nonurgently if any of the following symptoms or signs are present: • Eyes abnormally sensitive to light: troublesome or deteriorating over the past 1 to 2 months   • Eyes excessively gritty and not improving after 1 week of topical lubricants   • Pain in or behind the eyes: troublesome or deteriorating over the past 1 to 2 months   • Progressive change in appearance of the eyes and/or eyelids over the past 1 to 2 months   • Appearance of the eyes has changed causing concern to the patient   • Seeing 2 separate images when there should only be 1   • Troublesome eyelid retraction   • Abnormal swelling or redness of eyelid(s) or conjunctiva   • Restriction of eye movements or double vision   • Tilting of the head to avoid double vision

3. Mild TED: Patients whose features of TED have only a minor impact on daily life insufficient to justify immunosuppressive or surgical treatment. They usually have only 1 or more of the following: minor lid retraction (<2 mm), mild soft-tissue involvement, exophthalmos <3 mm above normal for race and gender, no or intermittent diplopia, and corneal exposure responsive to lubricants.

Quality of Life

Several questionnaires have been validated for patients with TED. While specific questions vary among questionnaires, key concepts of importance include impact of TED on daily visual functioning, impact on appearance and self-perception, and impact on mood and overall perceptions of wellness. EUGOGO has developed GOQoL, a short, validated, TED-specific quality-of-life questionnaire that has been translated into multiple languages.

Treatment

Mild TED

Treatment is focused on low-risk measures to help with symptom management.

- Corneal protection (artificial tears, ointments, taping lids)

- Prisms or eye patching for diplopia

- Tobacco avoidance

- Selenium, 100 mcg twice daily, for mild active TED[7]

- Restoration of euthyroidism

Moderate to Severe TED

Intravenous steroids have been the mainstay of treatment for TED. The initial regimen was with oral steroids, but after 2 randomized controlled trials showed the benefit of intravenous steroids vs oral steroids with fewer adverse effects,[8,9] intravenous steroids are now preferred. The study by Kahaly and colleagues randomly assigned 70 patients with severe and active TED to intravenous steroids (total dose of 4.5 g) vs oral steroids (total dose of 4 g) over 12 weeks. Seventy-seven percent of patients receiving the intravenous regimen responded compared with 51% of the patients on oral steroids.[8] The traditional regimen is methylprednisolone, 500 mg intravenously weekly for 6 weeks, followed by 250 mg intravenously weekly for 6 weeks. Baseline laboratory tests should be obtained to rule out recent hepatitis or the presence of hepatic dysfunction, and a comprehensive metabolic panel should be followed monthly. Bone prophylaxis with bisphosphonates and gastrointestinal prophylaxis with a proton-pump inhibitor should be considered. A recent meta-analysis confirmed the benefit of intravenous steroids over oral steroids with a risk ratio of 1.51.[10] A study that treated patients with 3 different intravenous steroid regimens showed that even though 50% to 60% of patients respond to intravenous steroids, around 10% of patients deteriorate while on treatment and 30% of responders progress after therapy withdrawal.[11]

In the past, for patients with refractory disease, repeated steroids + orbital radiation (XRT), cyclosporine, or rituximab (anti-CD20 antibody) were used. Oral steroids + XRT have been shown to be more effective than either modality alone.[12,13] The efficacy of intravenous steroids + XRT has not yet been evaluated in a randomized controlled trial. There have been 2 randomized controlled trials of rituximab: one with positive results from Italy and one with negative results from the Mayo clinic.[14,15] Different timing of intervention might explain incongruent results, with responders seen in the trial that had early treatment (4.5 months from onset of disease in the Italian study vs 11.2 months in the US study).

Novel Immunomodulatory Therapies

Therapies Studied Already in Randomized Controlled Trials:

- Intravenous steroids plus mycophenolate vs only intravenous steroids[16]

  □ 164 patients were randomly assigned to intravenous steroids (12-week course) plus mycophenolate 360 mg twice daily for 24 weeks vs intravenous steroids alone. The addition of mycophenolate to intravenous steroids improved the rate of response to therapy by 24 weeks from 53% to 71%.

- Teprotumumab (IGF-1 receptor antagonist),[17] which is waiting for FDA approval, expected in 2020

  □ Teprotumumab is a human monoclonal blocking antibody that binds to the extracellular portion of the IGF-1 receptor. IGF-1 normally forms a signaling complex with the thyrotropin receptor, through which it is transactivated. In this multicenter, double-blind, placebo-controlled randomized controlled trial, 88 patients were randomly assigned to 8 infusions of teprotumumab, every 3 weeks, vs placebo. Sixty-nine percent of the teprotumumab group had a response at week 24 compared with 20% of the placebo group, with response defined as a decrease of at least 2 points in the CAS score and a reduction of 2 mm or more in proptosis.

- Tocilizumab (IL-6 receptor antagonist)[18]

  □ Tocilizumab is a recombinant humanized monoclonal antibody directed against the IL-6 receptor. IL-6 is a proinflammatory cytokine, which is also overexpressed in TED orbital tissues. In this randomized controlled trial, 32 patients with moderate to severe corticosteroid-resistant TED were randomly assigned to 4 monthly cycles of tocilizumab at 8 mg/kg vs placebo. The percentage of patients who improved their CAS score by at least 2 points by week 16 was 93.3% in the tocilizumab group and 58.8% in the placebo group.

Therapies Under Investigation

- TSH receptor small molecule antagonists
- TSH receptor monoclonal blocking antibodies
- Fingolimod
- Belimumab (anti-BAFF monoclonal antibody)
- Microbiome manipulation

Clinical Case Vignettes
Case

A 51-year-old man presents with eye symptoms of redness, pain, swelling, and diplopia over the last 3 months. He has no symptoms of hyperthyroidism or other symptoms. Medications include a statin. He smokes cigarettes. He has normal vital signs. Findings on eye examination are notable for periorbital edema and erythema, conjunctival injection and chemosis, retroorbital pain with movement, and diplopia in all directions of gaze with marked left hypotropia. Hertel measurements are 23 mm on the right side and 24 mm on the left side. The rest of the examination findings, including those on thyroid exam, are normal.

Which of the following is the best initial treatment?

A. Oral steroids

B. Intravenous steroids

C. Orbital radiation

D. Rituximab

E. Orbital decompression

Answer: B) Intravenous steroids

This patient has active moderate/severe TED. The first-line treatment, in the absence of contraindications, is a 12-week course of intravenous steroids (Answer B) (methylprednisolone, 500 mg intravenously weekly for 6 weeks, followed by 250 mg intravenously weekly for 6 weeks).

Oral steroids (Answer A) are only effective in 50% of patients and require a high starting dosage with a long taper resulting in significant adverse effects. Intravenous steroids have better efficacy with a lower adverse effect profile. Orbital radiation (Answer C) is a reasonable option, mostly effective in improving diplopia. However, studies show that it is effective in 60% of patients with active eye disease, whereas the intravenous steroid protocol is 80% effective. Orbital decompression (Answer E) would not be indicated at this time, as the patient does not have evidence of optic nerve compression and instead has active TED symptoms. It is better to control active TED before surgery, if there is no sight-threatening disease. Rituximab (Answer D) is a third-line option if intravenous steroids and orbital radiation are not effective; however, there are other options that could be considered before rituximab such as tocilizumab or teprotumumab.

Case (Continued)

The patient has a good initial response to this regimen. Two months later, he returns with decreased color perception and blurry vision. During the eye evaluation, decreased visual acuity and a right relative afferent pupillary defect are noted.

Which of the following is the best next step?

A. Urgently refer to ophthalmology
B. Check thyroid function tests and adjust medications if needed
C. Refer to ophthalmology within the next few months
D. Start oral steroids

Answer: A) Urgently refer to ophthalmology

This patient's symptoms and examination findings raise concern for dysthyroid optic neuropathy. He needs an urgent comprehensive ophthalmologic evaluation (Answer A) followed usually by a 3-day pulse of intravenous steroids and possible orbital decompression if there is no response to medical management.

Adjusting thyroid medications (Answer B) would not address the vision symptoms. Referral to ophthalmology in a few months (Answer C) could result in vision loss due to delay in diagnosis. Starting oral steroids (Answer D) could be done in addition to the urgent referral to ophthalmology, but this would be insufficient to diagnose and treat the vision symptoms. Therefore, urgent ophthalmology evaluation should be the first step.

Case (Continued)

He is evaluated by an ophthalmologist, and compressive optic neuropathy is diagnosed. He is treated with methylprednisolone, 500 mg intravenously every day for 3 days, without vision improvement. He undergoes right orbital decompression with improvement of his vision and decrease in proptosis from 24 to 21 mm. He then continues intravenous steroids (500 mg weekly for 6 weeks followed by 250 mg weekly for 6 weeks), with the addition of orbital XRT in weeks 3 and 4, resulting in improvement in disease activity. Two months after the second steroid course, his disease reactivates with a CAS of 4/7. There is no evidence of optic neuropathy or exposure keratopathy.

Which of the following is the best step now?

A. Repeated orbital XRT and intravenous steroids
B. Tocilizumab or other targeted therapy
C. Observation and evaluation in 2 to 3 months
D. Further orbital decompression

Answer: B) Tocilizumab or other targeted therapy

This patient has failed 2 courses of intravenous steroids and orbital radiation. A second round of orbital XRT could have significant ocular adverse effects, so additional orbital XRT and intravenous steroids (Answer A) is not the best option. He continues to have active, moderate/severe TED and would therefore benefit from more immunosuppression. Tocilizumab or another immunomodulatory agent (Answer B) would be his best next choice. Further decompression (Answer D) is not necessary because the patient does not have evidence of compressive optic neuropathy or exposure keratopathy. Observation and evaluation in 2 to 3 months (Answer C) would be insufficient care of his eye disease.

Case (Continued)

He is treated with tocilizumab, 8 mg/kg monthly for 6 doses, with subsequent inactivation of his disease and normalization of thyroid-stimulating immunoglobulin. He develops no adverse effects. Now, 2 months after his last tocilizumab dose, his TED is no longer active and he is euthyroid. However, his quality of life is still significantly compromised given the constant diplopia. He inquires about further treatment options.

Which of the following is the best recommendation?

A. Orbital decompression followed by extraocular muscle surgery and possible lid surgery now

B. Supportive care with prisms with no plans for surgery

C. Another course of tocilizumab

D. Close monitoring and prisms for now until his disease remains inactive and stable for at least 6 months, then rehabilitative orbital/ocular surgery

Answer: D) Close monitoring and prisms for now until his disease remains inactive and stable for at least 6 months, then rehabilitative orbital/ocular surgery

This patient has most likely entered the inactive, chronic phase of his disease but continues to have moderate/severe disease, interfering with his quality of life. He would benefit from reconstructive orbital/ocular surgery after he has remained euthyroid with stable, inactive disease for at least 6 months (Answer D).

Supportive care with prisms (Answer B) would not give him adequate relief of his ocular symptoms. Immediate orbital decompression followed by extraocular muscle surgery (Answer A) is not indicated, as it is important to ensure stable eye and thyroid disease for at least 6 months before initiating rehabilitative orbital surgery. Another course of tocilizumab (Answer C) is not indicated at this time, as his eye disease is no longer active.

References

1. Bahn RS. Graves' ophthalmopathy. *N Engl J Med.* 2010;362(8):726-738. PMID: 20181974

2. Eckstein AK, Lösch C, Glowacka D, Schott M, Mann K, Esser J, Morgenthaler NG. Euthyroid and primarily hypothyroid patients develop milder and significantly more asymmetrical Graves' ophthalmopathy. *Br J Ophthalmol.* 2009;93(8):1052-1056. PMID: 19221109

3. Bartalena L, Baldeschi L, Boboridis K, et al; European Group on Graves' Orbitopathy (EUGOGO). The 2016 European Thyroid Association/European Group on Graves' Orbitopathy guidelines for the management of Graves' orbitopathy. *Eur Thyroid J.* 2016;5(1):9-26. PMID: 27099835

4. Perros P, Zarkovic M, Azzolini C, et al. PREGO (presentation of Graves' orbitopathy) study: changes in referral patterns to European Group on Graves' Orbitopathy (EUGOGO) centres over the period from 2000 to 2012. *Br J Ophthalmol.* 2015;99(11):1531-1532. PMID: 25953846

5. Estcourt S, Hickey J, Perros P, Dayan C, Vaidya B. The patient experience of services for thyroid eye disease in the United Kingdom: results of a nationwide survey. *Eur J Endocrinol.* 2009;161(3):483-487. PMID: 19542244

6. European Group on Graves' Orbitopathy (EUGOGO), Wiersinga WM, Perros P, et al. Clinical assessment of patients with Graves' orbitopathy: the European Group on Graves' Orbitopathy recommendations to generalists, specialists and clinical researchers. *Eur J of Endocrinol.* 2006;155(3):387-389. PMID: 16914591

7. Marcocci C, Kahaly GJ, Krassas GE, et al; European Group on Graves' Orbitopathy. Selenium and the course of mild Graves' orbitopathy. *N Engl J Med.* 2011;364(20):1920-1931. PMID: 21591944

8. Kahaly GJ, Pitz S, Hommel G, Dittmar M. Randomized, single blind trial of intravenous versus oral steroid monotherapy in Graves' orbitopathy. *J Clin Endocrinol Metab.* 2005;90(9):5234-5240. PMID: 15998777

9. Marcocci C, Bartalena L, Tanda ML, et al. Comparison of the effectiveness and tolerability of intravenous or oral glucocorticoids associated with orbital radiotherapy in the management of severe Graves' ophthalmopathy: results of a prospective, single-blind, randomized study. *J Clin Endocrinol Metab.* 2001;86(8):3562-3567. PMID: 11502779

10. Zhao L, Yu D, Cheng J. Intravenous glucocorticoids therapy in the treatment of Graves' ophthalmopathy: a systemic review and meta-analysis. *Int J Ophthalmol.* 2019;12(7):1177-1186. PMID: 31341811

11. Bartalena L, Krassas GE, Wiersinga W, et al; European Group on Graves' Orbitopathy. Efficacy and safety of three different cumulative doses of intravenous methylprednisolone for moderate to severe and active Graves' orbitopathy. *J Clin Endocrinol Metab.* 2012;97(12):4454-4463. PMID: 23038682

12. Bartalena L, Marcocci C, Chiovato L, et al. Orbital cobalt irradiation combined with systemic corticosteroids for Graves' ophthalmopathy: comparison with systemic steroids alone. *J Clin Endocrinol Metab.* 1983;56(6):1139-1144. PMID: 6341388

13. Marcocci C, Bartalena L, Bogazzi F, Bruno-Bossio G, Lepri A, Pinchera A. Orbital radiotherapy combined with high dose systemic glucocorticoids for Graves' ophthalmopathy is more effective than radiotherapy alone: results of a prospective randomized study. *J Endocrinol Invest*. 1991;14(10):853-860. PMID: 1802923

14. Salvi M, Vannucchi G, Curro N, et al. Efficacy of B-cell targeted therapy with rituximab in patients with active moderate-severe Graves' orbitopathy: a randomized controlled study. *J Clin Endocrinol Metab*. 2015;100(2):422-431. PMID: 25494967

15. Stan MN, Garrity JA, Carranza Leon BG, Prabin T, Bradley EA, Bahn RS. Randomized controlled trial of rituximab in patients with Graves' orbitopathy. *J Clin Endocrinol Metab*. 2015;100(2):432-441. PMID: 25343233

16. Kahaly GJ, Riedl M, König J, et al; European Group on Graves' Orbitopathy (EUGOGO). Mycophenolate plus methylprednisolone versus methylprednisolone alone in active, moderate-to-severe Graves' orbitopathy (MINGO): a randomized, observer-masked, multicenter trial. *Lancet Diabetes Endocrinol*. 2018;6(4):287-298. PMID: 29396246

17. Smith TJ, Kahaly GJ, Ezra DG, et al. Teprotumumab for thyroid-associated ophthalmopathy. *N Engl J Med*. 2017;376(18):1748-1761. PMID: 28467880

18. Perez-Moreiras JV, Gomez-Reino JJ, Maneiro JR, et al; Tocilizumab in Graves' Orbitopathy Study Group. Efficacy of tocilizumab in patients with moderate-to-severe corticosteroid-resistant Graves' orbitopathy: a randomized clinical trial. *Am J Ophthalmol*. 2018;195:181-190. PMID: 30081019

19. Faggiano M, Criscuolo T, Perrone L, Quarto C, Sinisi AA. Sexual precocity in a boy due to hypersecretion of LH and prolactin by a pituitary adenoma. *Acta Endocrinol (Copenh)*. 1983;102(2):167-172. PMID: 6681924

20. Ambrosi B, Bassetti M, Ferrario R, Medri G, Giannattasio G, Faglia G. Precocious puberty in a boy with a PRL-, LH- and FSH-secreting pituitary tumour: hormonal and immunocytochemical studies. 1990;122(5):569-576. PMID: 2112813

21. Chanson P, Maiter D. The epidemiology, diagnosis and treatment of prolactinomas: the old and the new. *Best Pract Res Clin Endocrinol Metab*. 2019;33(2):101290. PMID: 31326373

22. Briet C, Salenave S, Bonneville JF, Laws ER, Chanson P. *Pituitary apoplexy*. *Endocr Rev*. 2015;36(6):622-645. PMID: 26414232

23. Chanson P, Brochier S. Non-functioning pituitary adenomas. *J Endocrinol Invest*. 2005;28(11 Suppl International):93-99. PMID: 16625856

24. Raverot G, Assie G, Cotton F, et al. Biological and radiological exploration and management of non-functioning pituitary adenoma. *Ann Endocrinol (Paris)*. 2015;76(3):201-209. PMID: 26122495

25. Cooper O, Geller JL, Melmed S. Ovarian hyperstimulation syndrome caused by an FSH-secreting pituitary adenoma. *Nat Clin Pract Endocrinol Metab*. 2008;4(4):234-238. PMID: 18268519

26. Chanson P, Dormoy A, Dekkers O. Use of radiotherapy after pituitary surgery for non-functioning pituitary adenomas. *Eur J Endocrinol*. 2019;181(1):D1-D13. PMID: 31048560

27. Knoepfelmacher M, Danilovic DL, Rosa Nasser RH, Mendonca BB. Effectiveness of treating ovarian hyperstimulation syndrome with cabergoline in two patients with gonadotropin-producing pituitary adenomas. *Fertil Steril*. 2006;86(3):719.e15-e18. PMID: 16952513

28. Paoletti AM, Depau GF, Mais V, Guerriero S, Ajossa S, Melis GB. Effectivenesses of cabergoline in reducing follicle-stimulating hormone and prolactin hypersecretion from pituitary macroadenoma in an infertile woman. *Fertil Steril*. 1994;62(4):882-885. PMID: 7926104

29. Chanson P, Schaison G. Pituitary apoplexy caused by GnRH-agonist treatment revealing gonadotroph adenoma. *J Clin Endocrinol Metab*. 1995;80(7):2267-2268. PMID: 7608291

Surveillance of the Patient Who Has Had Therapeutic Hemithyroidectomy for Thyroid Cancer

Whitney Goldner, MD. Department of Internal Medicine, Division of Diabetes, Endocrinology, and Metabolism, University of Nebraska Medical Center, Omaha, NE; E-mail: wgoldner@unmc.edu

Learning Objectives

As a result of participating in this session, learners should be able to:

- List the indications for hemithyroidectomy for well-differentiated thyroid cancer.

- Describe imaging and biochemical surveillance of well-differentiated thyroid cancer following hemithyroidectomy.

- Explain the modified dynamic risk stratification criteria following hemithyroidectomy for well-differentiated thyroid carcinoma.

- Describe the role of thyroid hormone therapy in the treatment and surveillance of well-differentiated thyroid cancer.

Main Conclusions

- Hemithyroidectomy as definitive therapy for well-differentiated thyroid cancer is recommended for low- and some intermediate-risk thyroid cancers that do not need radioactive iodine therapy. If a patient meets criteria for radioactive iodine, then completion thyroidectomy ± central neck dissection is recommended.

- Imaging surveillance after hemithyroidectomy is primarily with neck ultrasonography. Optimal frequency of follow-up is unknown.

- Dynamic risk stratification after hemithyroidectomy has different thyroglobulin thresholds that define response to therapy as compared with thresholds of persons who have undergone total thyroidectomy.

- Many patients need thyroid hormone following hemithyroidectomy to achieve goal TSH.

- It is important to discuss all of these issues preoperatively to determine the best treatment for the patient.

Significance of the Clinical Problem

Hemithyroidectomy (thyroid lobectomy ± isthmusectomy) is acceptable and often preferred for thyroid nodules with Bethesda 3 and 4 indeterminate cytopathology (follicular lesion of undetermined significance, follicular neoplasm, Hurthle-cell neoplasm) on preoperative FNA.[1] This approach is also acceptable for many low- and intermediate-risk well-differentiated thyroid carcinomas.[1,2] There are defined histologic criteria that influence whether a tumor is categorized as having a low, intermediate, or high risk of recurrence, which in turn influences the decision regarding whether a person needs completion thyroidectomy and adjuvant therapy with radioactive iodine.[1,2] The decision to pursue hemithyroidectomy vs total thyroidectomy ± lymph node dissection is an individual decision based on preoperative imaging, FNA results, risk factors, and patient preference. Ideally, the discussion of pros and cons of hemithyroidectomy vs total thyroidectomy and indications for completion thyroidectomy occurs preoperatively. However, many of the details that will inform decision-making are not known until final histopathology is obtained. Historically, it was common for all patients to undergo completion thyroidectomy if histopathology revealed malignancy, given that most patients underwent adjuvant radioactive iodine therapy.[3] However, current guidelines do not recommend radioactive iodine in all patients. American Thyroid Association and National Comprehensive Cancer Network guidelines recommend radioactive iodine in select patients with intermediate risk of recurrence and in all patients at high risk.[1,2] Hence, completion thyroidectomy is not indicated in most low- and select intermediate-risk thyroid malignancies.

Follow-up and surveillance of well-differentiated thyroid cancer consists of imaging, serum thyroglobulin concentration as a tumor marker, thyroglobulin antibodies to ensure accuracy of the thyroglobulin measurement, and evaluation of thyroid hormone levels to optimize TSH levels. Since thyroglobulin is produced by both normal and malignant thyroid tissue, it can be detectable or elevated in patients who have undergone total thyroidectomy without radioactive iodine or hemithyroidectomy. Detectable thyroglobulin does not always indicate recurrence of thyroid cancer, and it may indicate the presence of normal thyroid tissue. A dynamic risk stratification system has been developed to predict risk of recurrence over time for those who have undergone total thyroidectomy + radioactive iodine (Table).[4] This assessment is designed to be performed at each follow-up visit and is categorized into excellent, indeterminate, biochemically incomplete, and structurally incomplete response to therapy.[4] The same criteria to assess recurrence risk cannot be applied to those who have undergone hemithyroidectomy, hence a modified dynamic risk stratification has been developed,[5,6] which has a thyroglobulin threshold of less than 30 ng/mL (<30 µg/L) to define an excellent response to therapy (Table). Unfortunately, the absolute thyroglobulin cutoffs for indicating recurrence are still unknown and the thyroglobulin concentration at a single time point is less predictive than the overall trend of the thyroglobulin level. American Thyroid Association guidelines recommend considering

Table. Thyroglobulin Thresholds for Response to Therapy and TSH Targets for Each Category[1,4-6]

Response to Therapy	Post Total Thyroidectomy + Radioactive Iodine	Post Hemithyroidectomy	TSH Goals
Excellent	Nonstimulated thyroglobulin <0.2 ng/mL (SI: <0.2 µg/L) Stimulated thyroglobulin <2 ng/mL (SI: <2 µg/L)	Nonstimulated thyroglobulin <30 ng/mL (SI: <30 µg/L)	0.5-2.0 mIU/L
Indeterminate	Nonstimulated thyroglobulin 0.2-1.0 ng/mL (SI: 0.2-1.0 µg/L) Stimulated thyroglobulin 2-10 ng/mL (SI: 2-10 µg/L)	Stable or declining thyroglobulin antibody levels	0.1-0.5 mIU/L
Biochemically Incomplete	Nonstimulated thyroglobulin >1.0 ng/mL (SI: >0.1 µg/L) Stimulated thyroglobulin >10 ng/mL (SI: >10 µg/L)	Nonstimulated thyroglobulin >30 ng/mL (SI: >30 µg/L)	0.1-0.5 mIU/L
Structurally Incomplete	Thyroglobulin and thyroglobulin antibodies do not define; based on imaging	Thyroglobulin and thyroglobulin antibodies do not define; based on imaging	<0.1 mIU/L

checking serum thyroglobulin after lobectomy and then checking it every 12 to 24 months.[1] A rising thyroglobulin level over time is more predictive of recurrence than one that is stable or dropping. Recently, however, Park et al showed that thyroglobulin levels increase gradually by about 10% per year following lobectomy without evidence of recurrence.[7] The thyroglobulin-to-TSH ratio also did not differ between those with and without proven disease recurrence. Overall, the risk of recurrence in low- and intermediate-risk tumors is low and the misinterpretation of detectable thyroglobulin levels may lead to unnecessary surveillance or intervention.

Thorough preoperative imaging of both the thyroid and central and lateral neck compartments is essential when evaluating persons with suspicious thyroid nodules, especially with indeterminate or malignant cytology, and when surgery is planned.[8] Preoperative imaging guides the extent of initial surgery and serves as a baseline for postoperative follow-up imaging. If a patient has undergone hemithyroidectomy and there is no preoperative assessment of the contralateral lobe and central/lateral neck compartments, this should be done postoperatively to determine next steps in therapy. The presence of contralateral nodules and/or abnormal lymph nodes prompts further workup and possible therapy. If preoperative imaging is otherwise negative and hemithyroidectomy is performed for definitive therapy, then surveillance consists of serial ultrasonography (with or without thyroglobulin as discussed above). However, studies have shown that false-positive findings on surveillance ultrasonography can occur in 57% to 67% of patients with low and intermediate risk of recurrence.[9,10] Hence, the potential for over-monitoring and unnecessary procedures exists, and the optimal frequency of long-term follow-up imaging is still unknown.

Guidelines recommend a TSH goal based on the dynamic response to therapy categories (*Table*).[1] Many patients choose to have hemithyroidectomy to avoid long-term thyroid hormone therapy. However, studies have shown

that in order for patients to attain goal TSH (<2.0 mIU/L for most patients based on response to therapy), 50% to 71% of patients require some amount of thyroid hormone therapy. Predictors of not requiring postoperative thyroid hormone include lower preoperative TSH, male gender, and normal thyroid parenchyma (no autoimmunity).[11-13] However, there are no absolute preoperative predictors of the need for thyroid hormone therapy.

Barriers to Optimal Practice

- Thyroglobulin

  □ Thyroglobulin can be elevated in benign and malignant disease. Thyroglobulin thresholds to predict recurrence are not absolute. Thyroglobulin values can vary between assays, so they must be evaluated using the same assay every time.

  □ Thyroglobulin thresholds following hemithyroidectomy are individualized. Each patient serves as their own baseline. However, thyroglobulin levels may rise over time without recurrence, which can lead to increased surveillance and patient anxiety.

- Imaging

  □ Preoperative imaging is essential. Often, endocrinologists first meet patients postoperatively.

  □ Optimal frequency of imaging surveillance is unknown.

- Thyroid Hormone Therapy

  □ Many patients require thyroid hormone postoperatively to achieve optimal TSH. There are no definite predictors of patients who will require postoperative thyroid hormone therapy.

  □ If a patient does not take thyroid hormone, this may cause a rise in thyroglobulin without recurrence.

Strategies for Diagnosis, Therapy, and/or Management

Preoperatively, clinicians should fully evaluate the thyroid and both central and lateral neck lymph nodes with ultrasonography. If there is bilateral thyroid nodularity, abnormal lymph nodes, or suspicion of extracapsular extension, this must be considered when discussing possibilities of total thyroidectomy vs hemithyroidectomy. If cytopathology is Bethesda 3 or 4 and no other worrisome features are present, or cytopathology is Bethesda 5 or 6 and the patient is determined to be at low or intermediate risk by imaging, then clinicians should discuss the pros and cons of hemithyroidectomy and indications for completion thyroidectomy. Size should also be factored into the discussion when determining the appropriate surgery. Both the American Thyroid Association and National Comprehensive Cancer Network guidelines recommend consideration of hemithyroidectomy for nodules smaller than 4 cm without other worrisome features.[1,2] Additionally, one should discuss expectations for postoperative surveillance, including imaging and thyroglobulin monitoring (especially if the patient has bilateral nodules). There should also be discussion regarding preference for thyroid hormone therapy. Many patients assume they will not need thyroid hormone if they have a hemithyroidectomy. It is important to discuss the possibility of postoperative thyroid hormone therapy (taking into account baseline autoimmunity, baseline TSH, and remnant thyroid volume), TSH goals, and threshold for starting therapy. Ultimately, all of these issues should be addressed preoperatively to gauge patient comfort with both treatment and the long-term surveillance plan. It is equally important to communicate with the surgeon to ensure consistency of expectations from all members of the medical team and with the patient. The surgeon must also consider the patient's operative risk profile to determine whether a potential second operation for completion thyroidectomy would be risk prohibitive compared with total thyroidectomy as the index operation. Ideally, this decision should be made in a multidisciplinary forum.

If the clinician first meets the patient after they have already undergone hemithyroidectomy, then the overall risk of recurrence should be evaluated. If adequate preoperative imaging was not done, this should be completed postoperatively. If there is concern for contralateral disease or abnormal lymph nodes, further evaluation should proceed with FNA of the suspicious areas. If staging and recurrence risk indicate the need for radioactive iodine therapy, then completion thyroidectomy ± appropriate lymph node dissection is indicated, and when appropriate, adjuvant therapy with radioactive iodine.

If the recurrence risk is low or intermediate and hemithyroidectomy is appropriate, one should proceed with surveillance imaging, consideration of thyroglobulin monitoring, and evaluation of the need for thyroid hormone therapy. On ultrasonography, if there are no abnormalities in the remaining lobe and no pathologic-appearing lymphadenopathy, one can check yearly ultrasonography and reduce the frequency after 2 to 5 years. If there is a nodule in the remaining lobe, the clinician should determine whether the patient needs to be monitored closely or if FNA should be performed if the nodule meets criteria based on American Thyroid Association Thyroid Nodule Guidelines.[1] If thyroid ultrasonography shows a new nodule or increasing size of nodule or abnormal lymph node, then FNA should be performed (+thyroglobulin washings if it is a lymph node).

The clinician must determine whether to follow thyroglobulin levels postoperatively. Not all clinicians routinely check thyroglobulin in patients who have undergone hemithyroidectomy. If a baseline thyroglobulin concentration was documented postoperatively, then thyroglobulin can be included with yearly labs along with periodic ultrasonography. If thyroglobulin is rising, the neck should be imaged with ultrasonography. One should also consider levothyroxine therapy if the patient is not already taking it, to achieve a goal TSH level of 0.1 to

0.5 mIU/L (indeterminate response to therapy). If the thyroglobulin is higher than expected or increases dramatically, one should evaluate for other areas of recurrence (chest) if neck imaging is negative.

Clinical Case Vignettes

Case 1

A 35-year-old woman seeks evaluation of newly diagnosed papillary thyroid cancer. She has a 1.2-cm nodule in the left thyroid lobe. There is also a small 5-mm spongiform nodule in the right thyroid lobe. No abnormal lymph nodes are seen on ultrasonography in the central or lateral neck. She undergoes left lobectomy and isthmusectomy. Pathology documents a 1.2-cm classic papillary thyroid carcinoma (pT1bNxMx). She understands that her right thyroid lobe nodule needs surveillance. She underwent hemithyroidectomy because she did not want to take thyroid hormone. Three months postoperatively, her thyroglobulin level is 35 ng/mL (35 µg/L) with negative thyroglobulin antibodies.

She is now 1 year out from surgery and would like your recommendations.

Neck ultrasonography shows a small 4-mm spongiform nodule in the right lobe, which is very low risk sonographically. There is no cervical lymphadenopathy.

Laboratory test results:

> TSH = 2.7 mIU/L
> Thyroglobulin (different assay) = 75 ng/mL
>   (SI: 75 µg/L)
> Thyroglobulin antibodies = <20 IU/mL
>   (SI: <20 kIU/L)

Which of the following is the best next step?

A. Chest CT to evaluate for metastatic disease

B. FNA of the right thyroid nodule

C. Initiation of levothyroxine, 50 mcg daily

D. Continued observation and repeated ultrasonography; measurement of thyroglobulin, thyroglobulin antibodies, and thyroid function in 6 months

E. Completion thyroidectomy followed by radioactive iodine

Answer: C or D) Initiation of levothyroxine, 50 mcg daily or *continued observation and repeated ultrasonography. measurement of thyroglobulin, thyroglobulin antibodies, and thyroid function in 6 months*

This patient's neck imaging is negative, her TSH concentration is above the goal of 0.5 to 2.0 mIU/L, and she is not currently on levothyroxine replacement. Therefore, starting low-dosage levothyroxine (Answer C) is recommended, with follow-up measurement of TSH, thyroglobulin, and thyroglobulin antibodies. If thyroglobulin remains high and continues rising on levothyroxine, then additional imaging of the chest (Answer A) would be warranted.

Ultrasonography does not show any abnormalities in the neck and the nodule in the right lobe is stable. Thyroglobulin was measured using a different assay, making it difficult to directly compare, but it is much higher than previous measurements. This patient chose hemithyroidectomy because she wanted to avoid long-term levothyroxine therapy. If she is opposed to taking thyroid hormone, continued surveillance at a short interval (6 months) (Answer D) with the same thyroglobulin and thyroglobulin antibody assays is reasonable. If the thyroglobulin rises, then additional imaging should be pursued.

This is a low-risk nodule sonographically and it is subcentimeter in size. Hence, FNA (Answer B) would not be recommended.

It is reasonable to consider completion thyroidectomy (Answer E) as one of the options; however, empirically treating with radioactive iodine before evaluating the pathology results and postoperative thyroglobulin would not be recommended.

Case 2

A 42-year-old man presents for evaluation and continued management of his thyroid cancer. Follicular thyroid carcinoma was diagnosed 1 year ago at an outside hospital. His 1.5-cm tumor was in the right thyroid lobe, and no lymph nodes were removed. Postoperative ultrasonography showed no nodules in the remaining left thyroid lobe. There was no cervical lymphadenopathy.

You obtain his outside pathology reports, which reveal extensive vascular invasion (more than 4 foci of vascular invasion) in his primary tumor.

Laboratory test results:

Thyroglobulin = 20 ng/mL (SI: 20 μg/L)
Thyroglobulin antibodies = <20 IU/mL
    (SI: <20 kIU/L)
TSH = 2.1 mIU/L

Current ultrasonography shows a normal left thyroid lobe and no cervical lymphadenopathy.

Which of the following is the best recommendation?

A. Continued surveillance with ultrasonography and measurement of thyroglobulin, thyroglobulin antibodies, and TSH yearly

B. Completion thyroidectomy and consideration of radioactive iodine

C. Initiation of levothyroxine, 50 mcg daily, for goal TSH of 0.5 to 2.0 mIU/L

D. ^{131}I whole-body scan

E. Chest CT to evaluate for metastatic disease

Answer: B) Completion thyroidectomy and consideration of radioactive iodine

This patient has angioinvasive (>4 vessels) follicular thyroid carcinoma (American Joint Committee on Cancer [AJCC] 8th ed pT1bNxMx, stage 1). More than 4 vessels of angioinvasion predicts a high recurrence risk according to the American Thyroid Association risk of recurrence classification.[1] These tumors are also at higher risk for distant metastatic disease. High-risk angioinvasive follicular thyroid

carcinoma is an indication for adjuvant radioactive iodine therapy at the time of diagnosis.[1,2] In this situation, many clinicians would choose completion thyroidectomy with adjuvant radioactive iodine (Answer B), which would have been the appropriate therapy at the time of diagnosis. Initiation of levothyroxine (Answer C) to attain goal TSH is appropriate. However, the TSH treatment goal should be 0.1 to 0.5 mIU/L, rather than 0.5 to 2.0 mIU/L. Continued surveillance alone (Answer A) is not preferred, but chest CT (Answer E) to evaluate for other sites of disease would be reasonable if the patient does not agree to surgery and radioactive iodine and has a rising thyroglobulin and negative neck imaging. With a remaining thyroid lobe in place, ^{131}I whole-body scan (Answer D) would not be recommended before completion thyroidectomy.

Case 3

A 23-year-old woman presents for evaluation of a sonographically intermediate-risk solitary thyroid nodule that measures 1.8 cm. FNA of the nodule determines that it is a follicular neoplasm. Results of molecular testing are suspicious. The contralateral lobe does not have any abnormalities, and there are no pathologic-appearing lymph nodes on ultrasonography. She does not have a history of preexisting autoimmune thyroid disease or radiation exposure. Her TSH concentration is 0.9 mIU/L.

She opts for hemithyroidectomy for definitive diagnosis. Histopathology shows a follicular variant of papillary thyroid carcinoma, partially encapsulated, 1.8 cm. The margins are negative and there is no vascular invasion.

It is now is 6 months after surgery. Which of the following do you recommend? (select all that apply)

A. TSH measurement and thyroid hormone therapy if TSH is >2.0 mIU/L

B. Neck ultrasonography

C. Measurement of thyroglobulin and thyroglobulin antibodies

D. Chest CT to evaluate for metastatic disease

E. Completion thyroidectomy and consideration of radioactive iodine

Answer: A, B, and possibly C) TSH measurement and thyroid hormone therapy if TSH is >2.0 mIU/L, neck ultrasonography, and possibly measurement of thyroglobulin and thyroglobulin antibodies

This patient has a follicular variant of papillary thyroid carcinoma (AJCC 8th ed pT1bNxMx, stage 1). According to the American Thyroid Association, the tumor has a low risk of structural recurrence.[1] Her contralateral lobe is normal and there are no abnormal-appearing lymph nodes. Therefore, completion thyroidectomy or radioactive iodine therapy (Answer E) would not be recommended. There is no reason to suspect a high risk for metastatic disease, so CT chest (Answer D) is not indicated. Postoperative neck ultrasonography (Answer B) at 6 months should be performed as a baseline to evaluate for suspicious lesions in the contralateral lobe or lymph nodes. TSH should also be measured and levothyroxine therapy should be started if her TSH is not at goal (0.5-2.0 mIU/L) (Answer A). There is controversy about routine measurement of thyroglobulin and thyroglobulin antibodies (Answer C) in patients with low recurrence risk who have undergone hemithyroidectomy. Thyroglobulin can rise slowly over time even without evidence of recurrence.[7] In select patients, some clinicians check thyroglobulin and thyroglobulin antibodies postoperatively and use the response to therapy thyroglobulin thresholds in the table above.

Case 3 (Continued)

Would your recommendations change if the pathology showed:

A. Noninvasive follicular thyroid neoplasm with papillary-like nuclear features (NIFT-P)?

   NIFT-P has been reclassified as its own entity with a very low malignant potential.[14] Given that the contralateral lobe was normal and there were no abnormal lymph nodes, most clinicians should not recommend thyroglobulin or thyroglobulin antibody measurement, CT chest, or completion thyroidectomy. TSH should be measured, and a normal TSH level should be maintained, but treating with levothyroxine for a goal TSH less than 2.0 IU/L is not necessary. Routine follow-up postoperative ultrasonography is not required, but imaging should be done if there are other clinical indications.

B. Vascular invasion?

   If the tumor had vascular invasion, then it would be classified at intermediate risk of structural recurrence according to the American Thyroid Association classification (approximately 15%-30%).[1] However, with a normal contralateral lobe and no abnormal lymph nodes, completion thyroidectomy would not be recommended based on the pathologic staging alone. The patient could be followed with ultrasonography and also be treated with levothyroxine for a goal TSH less than 2.0 mIU/L. In contrast to the original case, there is reason to more strongly consider checking thyroglobulin and thyroglobulin antibodies postoperatively to potentially identify occult metastatic disease. If the thyroglobulin is much higher than expected or if it rises significantly over time, that would prompt additional imaging, workup, and additional therapy.

C. Microscopic positive margins on the tumor?

   There is conflicting evidence regarding positive margins as a predictor of local recurrence and the need for adjuvant radioactive iodine therapy. Some studies report no association between microscopically positive surgical margins and local recurrence, especially anterior positive margins.[15,16] However, posterior microscopically positive margins have been associated with higher rates of local recurrence.[15] In this case, completion thyroidectomy is reasonable to allow the clinician to further evaluate with postoperative thyroglobulin and thyroglobulin antibodies and determine the need for adjuvant radioactive iodine. If there was a positive posterior margin, many clinicians would recommend adjuvant radioactive iodine therapy. If there was a positive anterior margin, then thyroglobulin and thyroglobulin antibodies should be evaluated 6 weeks postoperatively, and if the thyroglobulin is elevated, adjuvant radioactive iodine would be recommended. If the thyroglobulin is undetectable, the clinician should have a discussion with the patient about pros and cons of watching vs proceeding with radioactive iodine therapy.

References

1. Haugen BR, Alexander EK, Bible KC, et al. 2015 American Thyroid Association Management guidelines for adult patients with thyroid nodules and differentiated thyroid cancer: the American Thyroid Association Guidelines Task Force on Thyroid Nodules and Differentiated Thyroid Cancer. *Thyroid.* 2016;26(1):1-133. PMID: 26462967

2. National Comprehensive Cancer Network. NCCN Thyroid Carcinoma Guidelines Version 2.2019. Available at: www.NCCN.org. Accessed for verification November 2019.

3. American Thyroid Association (ATA) Guidelines Taskforce on Thyroid Nodules and Differentiated Thyroid Cancer, Cooper DS, Doherty GM, et al. Revised American Thyroid Association management guidelines for patients with thyroid nodules and differentiated thyroid cancer. *Thyroid.* 2009;19(11):1167-1214. PMID: 19860577

4. Tuttle RM, Tala H, Shah J, et al. Estimating risk of recurrence in differentiated thyroid cancer after total thyroidectomy and radioactive iodine remnant ablation: using response to therapy variables to modify the initial risk estimates predicted by the new American Thyroid Association staging system. *Thyroid.* 2010;20(12):1341-1349. PMID: 21034228

5. Momesso DP, Tuttle RM. Update on differentiated thyroid cancer staging. *Endocrinol Metab Clin N Am.* 2014;43(2):401-421. PMID: 24891169

6. Momesso DP, Vaisman F, Yang SP, et al. Dynamic risk stratification in patients with differentiated thyroid cancer treated without radioactive iodine. *J Clin Endocrinol Metab.* 2016;101(7):2692-2700. PMID: 27023446

7. Park S, Jeon MJ, Oh HS, et al. Changes in serum thyroglobulin levels after lobectomy in patients with low-risk papillary thyroid carcinoma. *Thyroid.* 2018;28(8):997-1003. PMID: 29845894

8. Yeh MW, Bauer AJ, Bernet VA, et al; American Thyroid Association Surgical Affairs Committee Writing Task Force. American Thyroid Association statement on preoperative imaging for thyroid cancer surgery. *Thyroid.* 2015;25(1):3-14. PMID: 25188202

9. Peiling Yang S, Back AM, Tuttle RM, Fish SA. Frequent screening with serial neck ultrasound is more likely to identify false-positive abnormalities than clinically significant disease in the surveillance of intermediate risk papillary thyroid cancer patients without suspicious findings on follow-up ultrasound evaluation. *J Clin Endocrinol Metab.* 2015;100(4):1561-1567. PMID: 25632970

10. Yang SP, Bach AM, Tuttle RM, Fish SA. Serial neck ultrasound is more likely to identify false-positive abnormalities than clinically significant disease in low-risk papillary thyroid cancer patients. *Endocr Pract.* 2015;21(12):1372-1379. PMID: 26372300

11. Lee MC, Kim MU, Choi HS, et al. Postoperative thyroid-stimulating hormone levels did not affect recurrence after thyroid lobectomy in patients with papillary thyroid cancer. *Endocrinol Metab (Seoul).* 2019;34(2):150-157. PMID: 31099202

12. Ha TK, Kim DW, Park HK, Lee YJ, Jung SJ, Baek HJ. Factors influencing the successful maintenance of euthyroidism after lobectomy in patients with papillary thyroid microcarcinoma: a single-center study. *Endocr Pract.* 2019;25(10):1035-1040. PMID: 31241363

13. Lee YM, Jeon MJ, Kim WW, et al. Optimal thyrotropin suppression therapy in low-risk thyroid cancer patients after lobectomy. *J Clin Med.* 2019;8(9):E1279. PMID: 31443521

14. Nikiforov YE, Seethala RR, Tallini G, et al. Nomenclature revision for encapsulated follicular variant of papillary thyroid carcinoma: a paradigm shift to reduce overtreatment of indolent tumors. *JAMA Oncol.* 2016;2(8):1023-1029. PMID: 27078145

15. Lang BH, Shek TW, Wan KY. Does microscopically involved margin increase disease recurrence after curative surgery in papillary thyroid carcinoma? *J Surg Oncol.* 2016;113(6):635-639. PMID: 26843438

16. Sanabria A, Rojas A, Arevalo J, Kowalski L, Nixon I. Microscopically positive surgical margins and local recurrence in thyroid cancer. A meta-analysis. *Eur J Surg Oncol.* 2019;45(8):1310-1316. PMID: 30795955

Management of Thyroid Dysfunction Before and During Pregnancy

Kristien Boelaert, MD, PhD, FRCP. Institute of Applied Health Research, School of Medical and Dental Sciences, University of Birmingham, Birmingham, United Kingdom; E-mail: k.boelaert@bham.ac.uk

Learning Objectives

As a result of participating in this session, learners should be able to:

- Discuss the evidence of benefits and risks of treatment of mild thyroid hypofunction before and during pregnancy in relation to obstetric and child neurodevelopmental outcomes.

- Review what is known about the relationship between thyroid autoimmunity and pregnancy outcomes, as well as the effects of levothyroxine therapy in this setting.

- Articulate the optimal management of hyperthyroidism before and during pregnancy.

Main Conclusions

Significant controversy continues to surround the management of thyroid dysfunction before and during pregnancy and indications for treatment are not adopted in a universally uniform manner. The physiological changes to thyroid function associated with pregnancy make the interpretation of thyroid function tests difficult, and ideally population- and pregnancy-specific reference ranges should be used. The previous upper limit for TSH concentrations of 2.5 mIU/L has been revised in view of accumulating evidence that levothyroxine replacement for women with serum TSH concentrations below 4 mIU/L does not necessarily result in improved obstetric or neurocognitive outcomes and may in fact be associated with a degree of harm. While there are clear links between thyroid autoimmunity and increased risks of miscarriage and preterm delivery, a number of well-conducted clinical trials have failed to demonstrate beneficial effects on obstetric outcomes with levothyroxine replacement in euthyroid women who have raised concentrations of autoimmune antibodies. Uncontrolled hyperthyroidism during pregnancy is associated with significant risks of adverse outcomes and should be distinguished from transient rises in circulating thyroid hormones. Specific consideration is required as to the choice of antithyroid drugs to be used, especially before and during early pregnancy, aiming to use the lowest possible dosages with regular monitoring of thyroid function.

The field currently lacks clinical trial data, which are necessary to prove beneficial effects but also to evaluate the potential risk associated with treatment and overtreatment with levothyroxine and antithyroid drugs.

Significance of the Clinical Problem

Thyroid hormones are essential for normal pregnancy and optimal fetal growth and development.[1] Pregnancy directly affects thyroid function, and the fetal thyroid gland is not functionally mature until 18 to 20 weeks' gestation. Early pregnancy is therefore a critical period during which maternal thyroid dysfunction may have deleterious effects on the health of the mother and fetus.[2] Careful and pragmatic preconception planning and management of thyroid function is key to ensuring optimal outcomes, aiming to mirror normal physiological adaptive changes during pregnancy and minimize potential unwanted effects of the treatment administered.[3]

Overt hypothyroidism affects 0.2% to 0.6% of pregnancies, whereas subclinical hypothyroidism occurs in 3.5% to 18%, depending on the definition used.[4] Thyroid autoimmunity, characterized by the presence of elevated TPO antibodies, is the main risk factor for maternal hypothyroidism and occurs in up to 30% of women with recurrent miscarriage and subfertility.[5] Isolated hypothyroxinemia may reflect a state of mild iodine deficiency but is likely multifactorial and may, in part, be explained by assay interference due to changes in binding proteins as a result of pregnancy. There is continued debate regarding what constitutes overt and subclinical hypothyroidism in pregnancy and which cutoffs should be used to identify high-risk pregnancies requiring levothyroxine replacement therapy, especially in view of emerging evidence of potential risks associated with overtreatment.[1]

Hyperthyroidism in pregnancy may be due to Graves disease or may be caused by transient elevations of thyroid hormone concentrations due to high levels of hCG in early pregnancy. The former requires active management with antithyroid drugs, whereas the latter is usually treated conservatively. The goal of therapy is to control hyperthyroidism while avoiding unwanted adverse effects of medication, as well as overzealous induction of hypothyroidism.[1,3]

The current state of knowledge leaves physicians managing women before and during pregnancy uncertain regarding the indications for treatment of thyroid dysfunction and autoimmunity, as well as the choice of treatment to be administered to optimize fetal and maternal outcomes.

Barriers to Optimal Practice

- Uncertainty regarding optimal reference ranges for determination of thyroid dysfunction, taking into account factors affecting thyroid physiology before and during pregnancy.

- A lack of large randomized controlled trials evaluating outcomes in mothers with mild thyroid hypofunction and their offspring following therapy started before or during early gestation.

- The demonstration that levothyroxine therapy is ineffective in optimizing live births in women with previous miscarriage who have raised TPO antibody concentrations.

- Emerging data demonstrating teratogenic effects of antithyroid drugs and deleterious effects of high levels of circulating thyroid hormones on pregnancy outcomes.

Strategies for Diagnosis, Therapy, and/or Management
Definition of Thyroid Dysfunction Before and During Pregnancy

Pregnancy affects thyroid physiology dramatically. Fetal consumption of maternal thyroid hormones, increased concentrations of thyroxine-binding globulin, increased urinary iodine clearance, and increasing degradation of thyroid hormone by placental type 3 deiodinase require enhanced maternal thyroid hormone production to ensure adequate availability for the mother and fetus. High concentrations of hCG stimulate the pituitary TSH receptor resulting in increased thyroid hormone production, which is usually associated with reduced serum TSH concentrations reaching a trough at 10 to 12 weeks of pregnancy.[1,3] A number of additional factors affect thyroid function during pregnancy. These include the population iodine status, ethnicity, BMI, age, parity, and cigarette smoking. Importantly, the usual physiological response to hCG stimulation during pregnancy is impaired in women with high concentrations of thyroid autoantibodies.[6]

As a result of these changes, thyroid dysfunction is best defined according to pregnancy-specific reference ranges that are calculated in a population of euthyroid, iodine-sufficient pregnant women free of major factors that interfere with thyroid function. If such ranges are not available, then the adoption of pregnancy-specific ranges determined in a population with similar characteristics is recommended. If no suitable generalizable ranges can be found, then current guidance suggests the use of 4 mIU/L as the cutoff for TSH concentrations during pregnancy. The previous pragmatic upper limit of normal of 2.5 mIU/L is now deemed too low.[7]

Most laboratories use free T_4 immunoassays, but due to changes in thyroid hormone–binding proteins, the interpretation of free T_4 concentrations is difficult and ideally this should be determined using liquid chromatography/mass spectrometry or equilibrium dialysis. The use of total T_4 concentrations has also been proposed as an alternative, but since there is large variation in thyroxine-binding globulin concentrations, especially during early pregnancy, these provide only relatively crude measures.[1]

Management of Hypothyroidism Before and During Pregnancy

Overt hypothyroidism—raised serum TSH and below-normal free T_4 concentration—is usually caused by autoimmune Hashimoto thyroiditis or following previous thyroidectomy or radioiodine ablation in iodine-replete areas. When uncorrected during pregnancy, it is associated with adverse outcomes, including miscarriage, preeclampsia, low birth weight, and preterm birth. In addition, maternal hypothyroidism has been associated with detrimental effects of child neurodevelopment, illustrating the importance of timely levothyroxine administration. The preconception and first trimester of pregnancy TSH target is between the lower reference limit and 2.5 mIU/L. An empirical increase in the dosage of levothyroxine upon finding of a positive pregnancy test is appropriate, and often women are advised to double the dose on 2 days of the week. Regular tests of thyroid function (every 4 weeks) are recommended, especially during the first 20 weeks of gestation.[8]

The definition of subclinical hypothyroidism and the cutoffs to be used for starting levothyroxine replacement are much less clear. Progression rates to overt hypothyroidism are 2% to 5% per year and are higher in women with raised TPO antibodies and with TSH concentrations greater than 10 mIU/L. Pregnancy risks associated with subclinical hypothyroidism have been demonstrated in large retrospective studies, although TSH thresholds have not been consistently defined and the largest effect sizes are seen when population-based reference ranges are used. A recent large individual patient data meta-analysis (IPDM), including 47,045 pregnant women from 35 cohorts with a mean age of 29 years who had gestational blood sampling at a median of 12.9 weeks of pregnancy, identified 1234 women (3.1%) with subclinical hypothyroidism (increased TSH concentration with normal free T_4 concentration). The risk of preterm birth was higher for women with subclinical hypothyroidism than for euthyroid women (6.1% vs 5.0%, respectively; absolute risk difference, 1.4% [95% confidence interval (CI), 0%-3.2%]; odds ratio, 1.29 [95% CI, 1.01-1.64]).[9]

Thyroid autoimmunity is a major risk factor for subclinical hypothyroidism, and approximately one-third of women with subclinical hypothyroidism are TPO positive. The risk of adverse pregnancy outcomes is higher in women with combined thyroid autoimmunity and serum TSH concentrations greater than 2.5 mIU/L. In recent years, a number of studies have evaluated the effects of levothyroxine treatment on obstetric outcomes in pregnant women with subclinical hypothyroidism. A large observational study found that a median levothyroxine dosage of 50 mcg daily in pregnant women with serum TSH values of 2.5 to 10.0 mIU/L was associated with a lower risk of pregnancy loss but increased risks of premature delivery, gestational diabetes, and preeclampsia compared with nontreatment. Importantly. the beneficial effects of levothyroxine replacement were predominantly present in the subgroup of women with TSH values greater than 4.0 mIU/L. This study highlights that overzealous levothyroxine replacement in women with subclinical hypothyroidism may not be without risks and careful consideration should be given when considering the start of thyroid hormone therapy in this situation.[10]

In a small randomized controlled trial, preterm delivery rates but not premature labor were reduced following levothyroxine treatment of 65 women who were TPO positive and had mild thyroid dysfunction (TSH = 2.5-10 mIU/L) compared with those who did not receive thyroid hormone replacement. When 366 women, with TSH values between 2.5 and 4 mIU/L and negative for TPO antibodies, were randomly assigned to receive levothyroxine or not, there were no differences in preterm delivery rates. However, in those with TSH values greater than 4 mIU/L, beneficial effects of levothyroxine on preterm delivery were observed. In contrast, 2 clinical trials have shown beneficial outcomes with reduced adverse pregnancy events in women treated with levothyroxine for serum TSH concentrations between 2.5 and 10 mIU/L during pregnancy.[11,12]

Two large clinical trials have evaluated the benefits of maternal screening and levothyroxine therapy on child cognition. The controlled antenatal thyroid screening study (CATS) randomly assigned 21,846 pregnant women to a screening or control group and treated the screened group with levothyroxine if they had subclinical hypothyroidism or hypothyroxinemia at a median gestational age of 13 weeks. At 3 years, IQ scores were not different in offspring from treated vs nontreated women.[13] A follow-up study of the CATS child cohort at 9 years also failed to demonstrated beneficial effects of levothyroxine treatment.[14] The other multicenter randomized controlled trial in the United States included 526 women with hypothyroxinemia and 677 women with subclinical hypothyroidism. They were randomly assigned to receive levothyroxine treatment or placebo starting at a mean of 17 to 18 weeks of gestation. No differences in child IQ were observed in offspring tested from 3 to 5 years of age.[15] Several explanations have been proposed, including late treatment initiation (median gestational age 13-18 weeks), possible overtreatment in the CATS trial, and high loss to follow-up (CATS study). Secondary analyses of obstetric outcomes did not identify beneficial effects of levothyroxine in either of these trials.

Taken together, there is insufficient evidence to universally treat pregnant women with serum TSH values between 2.5 and 4 mIU/L regardless of TPO antibody status. Levothyroxine should be considered in women who are TPO positive and have serum TSH values greater than 4.0 mIU/L; TPO antibody–negative women with TSH values greater than 10 mIU/L, those with other risk factors for thyroid dysfunction, and those with infertility or recurrent pregnancy loss.[3,7]

Isolated Hypothyroxinemia During Pregnancy

Isolated hypothyroxinemia is the biochemical finding of a low serum free T_4 concentration in conjunction with a normal TSH concentration. Contributory factors include iodine deficiency; thyroid autoimmunity; assay techniques; and maternal characteristics including age, BMI, and coexistent diabetes. Its prevalence ranges from 1% to 10% in iodine-sufficient countries and 20% to 30% in areas of iodine deficiency. Maternal hypothyroxinemia has been predominantly linked to adverse neurobehavioral outcomes in offspring, including reduced IQ, increased risk of autism spectrum disorder, attention deficit–hyperactivity disorder, schizophrenia, and lower grey matter and cortical volumes.[1,3] The randomized controlled trials investigating potential benefits of levothyroxine in women with hypothyroxinemia have not shown beneficial effects on child neurocognition.[13,15]

Many studies have focused on the effects of maternal thyroid hypofunction on child neurodevelopment. However, analysis of outcomes in offspring of children in the generation R study indicate that high maternal free T_4 concentrations are also associated with lower IQ scores, reduced grey matter, and lower cortical volume.[16] Importantly, offspring from mothers "overtreated" in the CATS trial when high levothyroxine dosages were used had higher rates of attention deficit–hyperactivity disorder compared with offspring from mothers whose thyroid function was treated suboptimally.[14] Since there is no clear evidence of benefits of treating gestational hypothyroxinemia with levothyroxine and in the presence of studies indicating potential harm, this approach is generally not recommended,[7] although some guidelines suggest consideration of treatment in early pregnancy.[17]

Levothyroxine Replacement in Euthyroid TPO-Positive Women Before and During Pregnancy

Women who have thyroid autoimmunity, evidenced by raised concentrations of TPO antibodies, are at increased risk of miscarriage and preterm delivery even when they are biochemically euthyroid.[5] Approximately one-fifth of untreated TPO antibody–positive women develop elevated serum TSH during the course of pregnancy. Two major hypotheses have been proposed: (1) TPO antibody positivity reflects a general diffuse autoimmune process potentially resulting in rejection of the fetal allograft or (2) TPO antibody positivity drives thyroid dysfunction and subsequently results in poor obstetric outcomes.

Previous studies have shown reduced miscarriage rates following levothyroxine treatment in TPO antibody–positive euthyroid women.[18,19] A recent prospective study of 825 women with recurrent pregnancy loss (≥3 pregnancy losses) found that TPO antibody positivity was associated reduced live birth rate (51.3% vs 65.2% in TPO antibody–negative

women; $P = .001$) and treatment with levothyroxine increased live birth rates significantly (adjusted odds ratio, 3.7 [95% CI, 1.4-9.8]; $P = .007$).[20]

In contrast, a randomized clinical trial of 600 women undergoing in vitro fertilization and embryo transfer found similar rates of miscarriage (10.3% vs 10.6%, $P = $ NS) in women treated with levothyroxine compared with those who were not treated. Furthermore, there were no differences in live birth rates or intrauterine pregnancy rates when comparing the intervention group with the control group.[21] The TABLET trial randomly assigned 952 women with raised TPO antibodies and biochemical euthyroidism to receive 50 mcg of levothyroxine or placebo across 49 United Kingdom centers. The live birth rate at 34 weeks' gestation was 37.4% in the levothyroxine group and 37.9% in the placebo group (relative risk, 0.97 [95% CI, 0.83-1.14]; $P = .74$). There were no significant between-group differences in other pregnancy outcomes, including pregnancy loss or preterm birth, or in neonatal outcomes. Serious adverse events occurred in 5.9% of women in the levothyroxine group and 3.8% in the placebo group ($P = .14$).[22]

Overall, current evidence does not demonstrate that the use of levothyroxine results in beneficial pregnancy outcomes in women with thyroid autoimmunity and normal thyroid function, indicating that the effects of TPO antibodies may not be related through thyroid dysfunction but rather reflect a generalized adverse autoimmune state.

Management of Hyperthyroidism Before and During Pregnancy

The main subtypes of thyrotoxicosis during pregnancy are Graves disease and transient gestational thyrotoxicosis caused by high hCG concentrations stimulating the TSH receptor. Preexisting Graves disease is present in about 0.5% to 1.3% of pregnancies and new-onset autoimmune hyperthyroidism occurs in 0.05%. When thyrotoxicosis develops newly during early pregnancy, it is important to distinguish the small minority of women with pathological hyperthyroidism from those who have gestational thyrotoxicosis. Measurement of TSH-receptor antibodies (TRAb) and free T_3 concentrations are informative, as they will be raised in the former but not in the latter. Transient rises in circulating thyroid hormones are usually treated in a supportive manner, as these patients often have hyperemesis gravidarum.[1,3]

Uncontrolled overt hyperthyroidism before and during pregnancy is associated with increased risks of miscarriage, stillbirth, intrauterine growth retardation, maternal hypertension, and heart failure, whereas subclinical hyperthyroidism has not been associated with adverse pregnancy outcomes. If Graves disease is newly diagnosed during pregnancy, antithyroid drug treatment is usually required. Outside pregnancy, methimazole is the most commonly used antithyroid drug, but since this is associated with a higher risk of teratogenicity than propylthiouracil,[23,24] the latter is usually preferred before and during the first 16 weeks of pregnancy. The highest risk window for birth defects is from gestation weeks 6 to 10,[25] and some practitioners prefer to avoid antithyroid drugs altogether during this period. Propylthiouracil has been associated with increased risks of liver dysfunction and liver failure both within and outside pregnancy.[26] Block-and-replace regimens are not advisable during pregnancy since antithyroid drugs preferentially cross the placenta, resulting in increased risk of fetal hypothyroidism.

The aim of treatment of gestational hyperthyroidism is to control hyperthyroidism and to limit fetal-maternal drug exposure, using the lowest possible dosage to maintain normal thyroid status. Thyroid function can change relatively quickly during early pregnancy, and regular testing every 2 to 4 weeks is advisable. Preexisting Graves disease often goes into remission during pregnancy as a result of decline in thyroid autoimmunity (TRAb concentrations) and often antithyroid drugs can be discontinued. Usually methimazole is switched to propylthiouracil before or during early pregnancy and if antithyroid drugs are still required beyond 16 weeks' gestation, then often propylthiouracil is switched to methimazole, although not all studies indicate that this approach is associated with improved outcomes.[23,24]

Women of childbearing age with active hyperthyroidism should be counseled on the risk of fetal harm from uncontrolled hyperthyroidism and advised to delay pregnancy with effective contraception until a stable euthyroid state has been achieved. Definitive treatment with radioiodine or surgery is an option since this will avoid exposure to the risks of antithyroid drugs during pregnancy, as well as the risk of relapse of Graves disease following delivery. Pregnancy should be avoided during the 6 months following radioiodine administration. Circulating maternal TRAbs cross the placenta and may induce fetal hyperthyroidism and goiter.[1,3] An important consideration is that pregnant women with Graves disease who were rendered hypothyroid by radioiodine therapy or surgery may continue to harbor high levels of TRAbs, thereby placing the fetus at risk of thyroid dysfunction. Persistence of TRAbs well beyond 18 months following treatment has been documented in 75% of those who received radioiodine vs only 30% of patients treated with surgery and 3% of those treated with antithyroid drugs.[27] Measurement of TRAbs in early pregnancy is indicated in those with preexisting Graves disease and is often repeated around 20 weeks' gestation. Regular monitoring with assessment of fetal heart rate, fetal growth, and fetal thyroid is appropriate in those with significantly elevated TRAb concentrations.

Clinical Case Vignettes
Case 1

A 32-year-old woman presents for her first antenatal appointment at 8 weeks' gestation. She has had 3 first-trimester miscarriages. She reports tiredness and some abdominal bloating. Physical examination suggests she is clinically euthyroid. Her BMI is 25 kg/m².

Laboratory test results:

> TSH = 4.2 mIU/L (0.4-4.0 mIU/L)
> Free T_4 = 0.9 ng/dL (0.8-1.8 ng/dL) (SI: 11.6 pmol/L [10.30-23.17 pmol/L])
> TPO antibodies = 350 IU/mL (<50 IU/mL)

Which of the following should be advised?

A. Reassure patient and discharge to routine antenatal care

B. Repeat thyroid function tests after 4 weeks

C. Repeat thyroid function tests at 20 weeks' gestation

D. Start levothyroxine, 1.6 mcg/kg daily

E. Start levothyroxine, 25 to 50 mcg daily

Answer: B or E) Repeat thyroid function tests after 4 weeks or start levothyroxine, 25 to 50 mcg daily

This patient has a history of recurrent miscarriage and has evidence of thyroid autoimmunity and very mild subclinical hypothyroidism. While the evidence supporting levothyroxine use in patients with thyroid autoimmunity who are euthyroid is not convincing, the finding of a serum TSH concentration greater than 4 mIU/L in association with raised TPO antibodies represents a reasonable indication to start low-dosage levothyroxine (Answer E). Repeating thyroid function testing after 4 weeks (Answer B) is appropriate regardless of whether levothyroxine is started.

Case 2

You are asked for advice regarding a 29-year-old woman who is 13 weeks pregnant in her third pregnancy. She conceived spontaneously. Her first child was born prematurely at 33 weeks' gestation, and she underwent cesarean delivery at 38 weeks' gestation with her second child. Her second pregnancy was complicated by gestational diabetes. She is clinically euthyroid and has no palpable goiter. Her BMI is 29 kg/m^2.

Laboratory test results:

> TSH = 1.4 mIU/L (0.4-4.0 mIU/L)
> Free T_4 = 0.6 ng/dL (0.8-1.8 ng/dL) (SI: 7.7 pmol/L [10.30-23.17 pmol/L])
> TPO antibodies = 40 IU/mL (<50 IU/mL)

Which of the following should be advised?

A. Measure free T_3 concentration and start levothyroxine if this is low

B. Urgently measure 9-AM cortisol concentration

C. Repeat thyroid function tests after 4 weeks

D. Start levothyroxine, 1.6 mcg/kg daily

E. Start levothyroxine, 25 to 50 mcg daily

Answer: C or E) Repeat thyroid function tests after 4 weeks or start levothyroxine, 25 to 50 mcg daily

This patient has isolated hypothyroxinemia. Since she conceived spontaneously, it seems unlikely that she has significant pituitary dysfunction, and measurement of a 9-AM cortisol concentration (Answer B) is not required. Clinical trials of levothyroxine replacement in this setting have not indicated significantly improved obstetric or neurocognitive outcomes. Current American Thyroid Association guidelines[7] do not recommend treatment of this condition, whereas European guidance suggests that treatment may be considered in the first trimester of pregnancy.[17] Repeating thyroid function tests after 4 weeks (Answer C) seems a reasonable option, although some practitioners may favor starting levothyroxine, 25 to 50 mcg daily (Answer E). Measurement of free T_3 (Answer A) is usually not indicated in the management of hypothyroidism either during or outside of pregnancy.

Case 3

A 28-year-old woman with Graves disease attends a follow-up appointment and states that she wishes to become pregnant. Graves disease was diagnosed 18 months ago and TRAbs were raised at presentation (5.2 IU/L [<1.0 IU/L]). She is taking methimazole, 30 mg daily. She has not been pregnant before. She is clinically euthyroid and has a palpable small diffuse goiter. Her BMI is 23 kg/m^2.

Laboratory test results:

TSH = <0.01 mIU/L (0.4-4.0 mIU/L)
Free T$_4$ = 1.6 ng/dL (0.8-1.8 ng/dL) (SI: 20.6 pmol/L [10.30-23.17 pmol/L])
Total T$_3$ = 160 ng/dL (80-180 ng/dL) (SI: 2.5 nmol/L [1.2-2.8 nmol/L])

Which of the following should be advised?

A. Continue current dosage of methimazole

B. Change to propylthiouracil, 300 mg twice daily

C. Advise radioiodine therapy

D. Advise total thyroidectomy

E. Discontinue antithyroid drug treatment

Answer: B, C, or D) Change to propylthiouracil, 300 mg twice daily or advise radioiodine therapy or advise total thyroidectomy

This patient has treated Graves disease that is controlled, although serum TSH remains fully suppressed. Discontinuation of antithyroid drugs (Answer E) would be inappropriate. In view of risks of teratogenicity, many practitioners and current guidelines[7] recommend changing methimazole to propylthiouracil (Answer B), and continuation of methimazole (Answer A) is a less preferred option. Consideration of definitive treatment with radioiodine (Answer C) or surgery (Answer D) would also be appropriate.

References

1. Korevaar TIM, Medici M, Visser TJ, Peeters RP. Thyroid disease in pregnancy: new insights in diagnosis and clinical management. *Nat Rev Endocrinol.* 2017;13(10):610-622. PMID: 28776582

2. Moog NK, Entringer S, Heim C, Wadhwa PD, Kathmann N, Buss C. Influence of maternal thyroid hormones during gestation on fetal brain development. *Neuroscience.* 2017;342:68-100. PMID: 26434624

3. Okosieme OE, Khan I, Taylor PN. Preconception management of thyroid dysfunction. *Clin Endocrinol (Oxf).* 2018;89(3):269-279. PMID: 29706030

4. Dong AC, Stagnaro-Green A. Differences in diagnostic criteria mask the true prevalence of thyroid disease in pregnancy: a systematic review and meta-analysis. *Thyroid.* 2019;29(2):278-289. PMID: 30444186

5. Thangaratinam S, Tan A, Knox E, Kilby MD, Franklyn J, Coomarasamy A. Association between thyroid autoantibodies and miscarriage and preterm birth: meta-analysis of evidence. *BMJ.* 2011;342:d2616. PMID: 21558126

6. Korevaar TI, Steegers EA, Pop VJ, Broeren MA, Chaker L, de Rijke YB, et al. Thyroid autoimmunity impairs the thyroidal response to human chorionic gonadotropin: two population-based prospective cohort studies. *J Clin Endocrinol Metab.* 2017;102(1):69-77. PMID: 27754809

7. Alexander EK, Pearce EN, Brent GA, Brown RS, Chen H, Dosiou C, et al. 2017 Guidelines of the American Thyroid Association for the diagnosis and management of thyroid disease during pregnancy and the postpartum. *Thyroid.* 2017;27(3):315-389. PMID: 28056690

8. Chan S, Boelaert K. Optimal management of hypothyroidism, hypothyroxinaemia and euthyroid TPO antibody positivity preconception and in pregnancy. *Clin Endocrinol (Oxf).* 2015;82(3):313-326. PMID: 25200555

9. Consortium on Thyroid Pregnancy--Study Group on Preterm Birth, Korevaar TIM, Derakhshan A, et al. Association of thyroid function test abnormalities and thyroid autoimmunity with preterm birth: a systematic review and meta-analysis. *JAMA.* 2019;322(7):632-641. PMID: 31429897

10. Maraka S, Mwangi R, McCoy RG, et al. Thyroid hormone treatment among pregnant women with subclinical hypothyroidism: US national assessment. *BMJ.* 2017;356:i6865. PMID: 28122781

11. Negro R, Schwartz A, Gismondi R, Tinelli A, Mangieri T, Stagnaro-Green A. Universal screening versus case finding for detection and treatment of thyroid hormonal dysfunction during pregnancy. *J Clin Endocrinol Metab.* 2010;95(4):1699-1707. PMID: 20130074

12. Ma L, Qi H, Chai X, et al. The effects of screening and intervention of subclinical hypothyroidism on pregnancy outcomes: a prospective multicenter single-blind, randomized, controlled study of thyroid function screening test during pregnancy. *J Matern Fetal Neonatal Med.* 2016;29(9):1391-1394. PMID: 26181769

13. Lazarus JH, Bestwick JP, Channon S, et al. Antenatal thyroid screening and childhood cognitive function [published correction appears in *N Engl J Med.* 2012;366(17):1650]. *N Engl J Med.* 2012;366(6):493-501. PMID: 22316443

14. Hales C, Taylor PN, Channon S, et al. Controlled antenatal thyroid screening II: effect of treating maternal sub-optimal thyroid function on child behaviour. *J Clin Endocrinol Metab.* [Epub ahead of print]

15. Casey BM, Thom EA, Peaceman AM, et al. Treatment of subclinical hypothyroidism or hypothyroxinemia in pregnancy. *N Engl J Med.* 2017;376(9):815-825. PMID: 28249134

16. Korevaar TI, Muetzel R, Medici M, et al. Association of maternal thyroid function during early pregnancy with offspring IQ and brain morphology in childhood: a population-based prospective cohort study. *Lancet Diabetes Endocrinol.* 2016;4(1):35-43. PMID: 26497402

17. Lazarus J, Brown RS, Daumerie C, Hubalewska-Dydejczyk A, Negro R, Vaidya B. 2014 European Thyroid Association guidelines for the management of subclinical hypothyroidism in pregnancy and in children. *Eur Thyroid J.* 2014;3(2):76-94. PMID: 25114871

18. Negro R, Formoso G, Mangieri T, Pezzarossa A, Dazzi D, Hassan H. Levothyroxine treatment in euthyroid pregnant women with autoimmune thyroid disease: effects on obstetrical complications. *J Clin Endocrinol Metab.* 2006;91(7):2587-2591. PMID: 16621910

19. Nazarpour S, Ramezani Tehrani F, Simbar M, Tohidi M, Alavi Majd H, Azizi F. Effects of levothyroxine treatment on pregnancy outcomes in pregnant women with autoimmune thyroid disease. *Eur J Endocrinol.* 2017;176(2):253-265. PMID: 27879326

20. Bliddal S, Feldt-Rasmussen U, Rasmussen AK, et al. Thyroid peroxidase antibodies and prospective live birth rate: a cohort study of women with recurrent pregnancy loss. *Thyroid.* 2019;29(10):1465-1474. PMID: 31407629

21. Wang H, Gao H, Chi H, et al. Effect of levothyroxine on miscarriage among women with normal thyroid function and thyroid autoimmunity undergoing in vitro fertilization and embryo transfer: a randomized clinical trial. *JAMA.* 2017;318(22):2190-2198. PMID: 29234808

22. Dhillon-Smith RK, Middleton LJ, Sunner KK, Cheed V, Baker K, Farrell-Carver S, et al. Levothyroxine in women with thyroid peroxidase antibodies before conception. *N Engl J Med.* 2019;380(14):1316-1325. PMID: 30907987

23. Andersen SL, Olsen J, Wu CS, Laurberg P. Birth defects after early pregnancy use of antithyroid drugs: a Danish nationwide study. *J Clin Endocrinol Metab.* 2013;98(11):4373-4381. PMID: 24151287

24. Seo GH, Kim TH, Chung JH. Antithyroid drugs and congenital malformations: a nationwide Korean cohort study. *Ann Intern Med.* 2018;168(6):405-413. PMID: 29357398

25. Laurberg P, Andersen SL. Therapy of endocrine disease: antithyroid drug use in early pregnancy and birth defects: time windows of relative safety and high risk? *Eur J Endocrinol.* 2014;171(1):R13-R20. PMID: 24662319

26. Taylor PN, Vaidya B. Side effects of anti-thyroid drugs and their impact on the choice of treatment for thyrotoxicosis in pregnancy. *Eur Thyroid J.* 2012;1(3):176-185. PMID: 24783017

27. Laurberg P, Wallin G, Tallstedt L, Abraham-Nordling M, Lundell G, Torring O. TSH-receptor autoimmunity in Graves' disease after therapy with anti-thyroid drugs, surgery, or radioiodine: a 5-year prospective randomized study. *Eur J Endocrinol.* 2008;158(1):69-75. PMID: 18166819

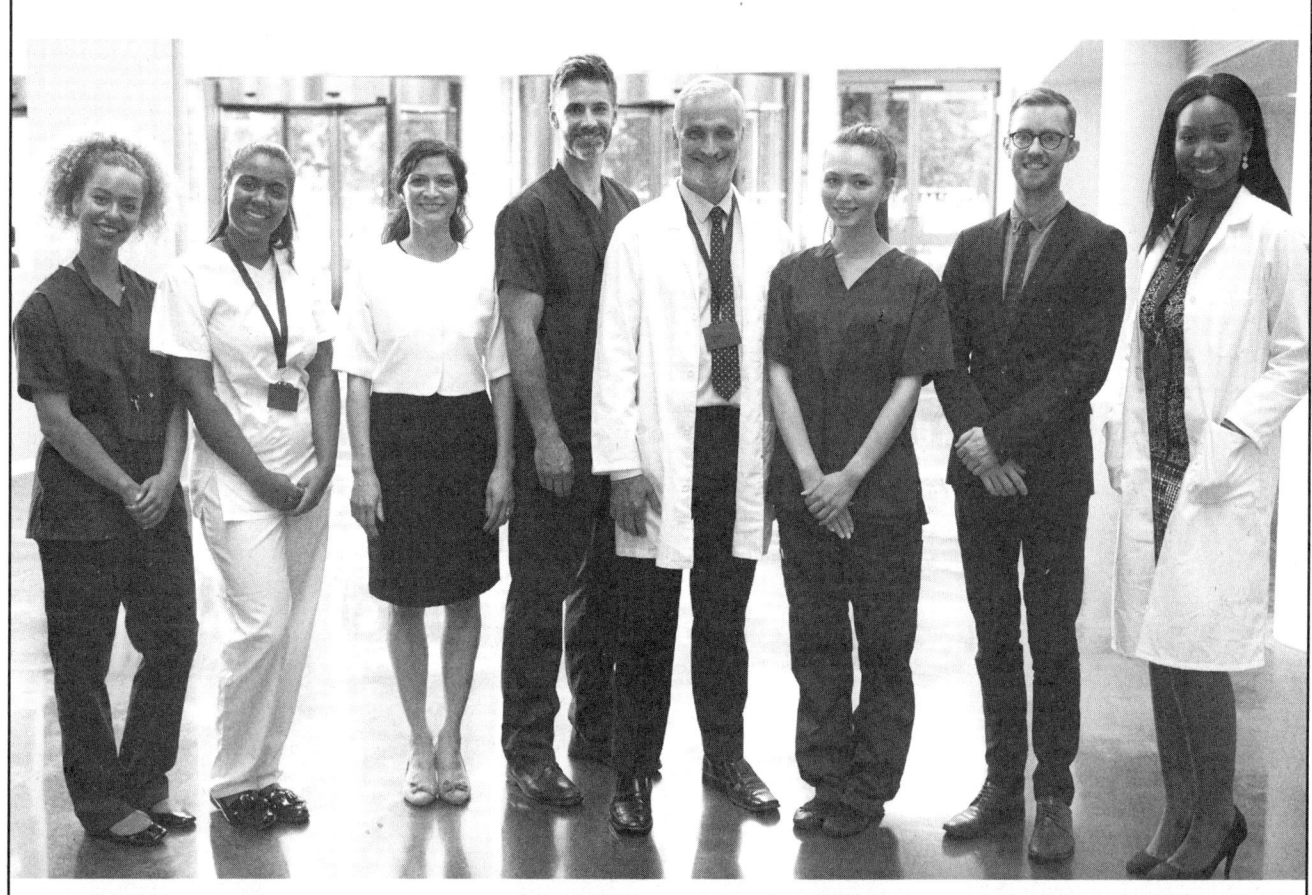

MISCELLANEOUS

Endocrine Assays and Interfering Substances

Carole Spencer, PhD. Department of Medicine, University of Southern California, Los Angeles, CA; E-mail: cspencer@usc.edu

Learning Objectives

As a result of participating in this session, learners should be able to:

- Recognize when to suspect that interference may be compromising an endocrine test result.

- Explain the causes of non–analyte-related and analyte-specific interferences.

Main Conclusions

Endocrine tests use immunoassay methodology that is prone to interferences (estimated incidence 0.1%-2%). Failure to recognize test interference has led to misdiagnoses and inappropriate management in approximately 50% of cases. The hallmark of interference is discordance between the test result and the clinical presentation of the patient. In addition, interference is suggested by discordance between test results reported by different instruments or an unexplained change in the test result. Usually only the physician can suspect interference because the laboratory rarely receives clinical information with the specimen. Interferences can be unrelated or related to the test analyte. Non–analyte-related serum factors can interfere by interacting with test reagents, causing a false-high or false-low test result. Tests that use biotin in their separation systems are prone to interference by the high-dosage dietary biotin contained in hair and nail products. Paraproteins and mutant hormone-binding protein variants are sources of interference with tests. Immunoassays use monoclonal antibody reagents that target specific epitopes on the test analyte. Analyte-specific interferences are caused by unusual molecular variants of the analyte or autoantibodies that bind the analyte. The multiplicity of nonspecific and analyte-specific interferences mandates collaboration between physicians and the laboratory to confirm the presence of interference and mitigate any clinical impact on patient care. Since many interferences are unique to the patient, can persist over time, and affect multiple tests, a warning in the electronic medical record regarding the type of interference, the tests affected, and the instrument used would be advisable.

Significance of the Clinical Problem

The estimated incidence of interferences affecting immunoassay methodology ranges from 0.1% to 2%.[1,2] It follows that physicians should be vigilant and suspect interference whenever a test result is clinically unexpected or inconsistent with other clinical correlates or biochemical tests, when there is a significant or unexplained change from a previous test result, or when there is discordance between tests reported by different instruments.[3] Patients with autoimmune or chronic diseases, recent immunizations, blood transfusions, monoclonal antibody therapy,[4] or exposure to animals are more prone to test interferences.[3] Discordance between the test result and the patient's clinical presentation is typically the hallmark of interference. Since laboratories generally have to report test results in the absence of clinical information, the laboratory cannot proactively identify interference without first being alerted by the physician. When interference is suspected, it is critical that the laboratory and physician work collaboratively to confirm the source of the interference.[5] This may necessitate drawing another blood specimen to test on a different manufacturer's instrument or to use for laboratory investigations involving blockers, precipitating the IgG fraction with polyethylene glycol, or performing a column chromatographic separation to assess whether the hormone is measured as a high molecular weight aggregate.[3,5] It is critical to identify the source of interference. Some interferences can be eliminated (high-dosage dietary biotin), whereas others, such as heterophile antibodies (HAb), tend to be patient-specific, persist for long periods (years), and affect multiple test analytes from different endocrine systems. Therefore, it would be prudent to update the patient's electronic medical record with the type of interference identified, the tests affected, and the instrument used.

Laboratories use different manufacturers' instrument platforms to measure endocrine analytes. Each platform uses proprietary reagents that differ in their propensity for both non–analyte-related and analyte-specific interferences. Most physicians do not know which platform their laboratory uses, or the profile of interferences likely to affect that platform. Insurance companies compound this problem by often requiring physicians to use a designated commercial laboratory for the testing. A change in the patient's insurance can prompt a mandated change in laboratory, leading to a significant change in test results as a consequence of changing methods. Changing the test platform is especially problematic when monitoring trends in tumor markers that are typically monitored over long periods as trends.

Barriers to Optimal Practice

- Laboratories typically select the instrument platform used for endocrine testing based on cost and convenience, not necessarily test sensitivity or specificity. Often laboratories change methods without first notifying physicians.

- Endocrinologists must make clinical judgments without knowing which instrument platform their laboratory uses, or the propensity of that instrument for interferences with the potential to compromise diagnosis and clinical management.

Strategies for Diagnosis, Therapy, and/or Management

The potential for interference is specific to the platform, test, and patient. A test result reported by different instruments can differ as a consequence of inherent differences in test specificity. Typically, such between-method differences are small, clinically inconsequential, and reflected by minor differences in the reference range of the test on that instrument.[6] In contrast, interferences are typically characterized by a false-high or false-low test result that is outside the test reference range.[1]

The propensity for test interference is multifactorial. Many interferences are unique to the patient and may persist or change over time. Immunoassays are based on a noncompetitive (2-site immunometric assay [IMA]) or competitive immunoassay format.[2] Both formats use the specificity of interactions between antibodies, usually monoclonal antibody (MAb) reagents, and a target epitope(s) on the test antigen.[2,3] Both immunoassay formats are prone to interferences. An interfering substance in a patient's serum may persist over time (years), is often patient-specific, and may affect a range of tests on different instrument platforms. These interfering substances are often nonspecific antibodies that bind components of the assay system and either mimic the presence of antigen causing a false-high test result, or less commonly block the action of a critical assay component causing a false-low test result. Some patients take drugs, such as high-dosage dietary biotin, that interfere with assay components. Such interferences produce false-low or false-high test results depending on the instrument, test, and immunoassay format.

Analyte-specific interferences only affect that test analyte, but they may affect that same test measured on a different manufacturer's instrument. Molecular variants of the analyte can cause interference when the target epitopes needed for assay detection are masked, resulting in a false-low test value, or when the analyte has unusual epitopes exposed that interact abnormally with test reagents, producing a false-high test value. Autoantibodies targeting the analyte are another source of analyte-specific interference. These autoantibodies can be relatively common (~1.8% of TSH tests[7,8]). Patients with underlying autoimmune conditions are most prone to autoantibody interferences.

Non–Specific-Related Interferences: Interferences Unrelated to the Test Analyte

Heterophilic Antibodies

The term heterophile antibodies (HAb) encompasses a diverse group of interfering immunoglobulins with a lexicon of abbreviations: human antianimal antibodies (HAAA) described as monospecific, high-affinity antibodies targeting animal epitopes from rabbits, sheep, horses, and goats.[9] Human antimouse antibodies (HAMA) have been identified most frequently. It should be noted that rheumatoid factor is also considered to be an HAb. Rheumatoid factor cross-reacts with animal antibodies and reacts against the Fc region of human immunoglobulins causing interference in some tests.[10,11]

The incidence of HAb is significant and highly variable (0.05% to >6%[1]) depending on the analyte and the instrument platform. Clearly, the concentration of HAb in some sera is high enough

to overcome the blockers that the manufacturers add to their tests to minimize HAb effects. Typically, HAb interference causes false-high test results, although false-low test results have occasionally been described.[11,12] The literature contains multiple reports of HAb interference, most commonly with thyroid tests such as TSH measurement.[1] However, HAb interference has been reported to affect a diverse range of analytes, including, but not limited to, ACTH, α-fetoprotein, creatine kinase-MB, hCG, cancer antigen 125, carcinoembryonic antigen, calcitonin, cardiac troponin, free T_4, free T_3, FSH, gastrin, PSA, TSH, and thyroglobulin. In some case reports, the HAb in the specimen interferes with multiple analytes.[10,13]

Antireagent Interferences

Each test contains reagents unrelated to the test analyte. These reagents are used in the separation and signaling systems.[2] Some patient sera contain exogenous sources of interference (ie, biotin). Alternatively, there can be endogenous interferences from antibodies that target test reagents, such as alkaline phosphatase antibodies, streptavidin antibodies, and ruthenium antibodies.

High-Dosage Dietary Biotin

Approximately 50% of endocrine tests have been developed using biotin in their separation step.[1,14] It follows that that high doses of dietary biotin have the potential to interfere with any test using biotin as a reagent. Biotin interference causes false-high or false-low test results, depending on the immunoassay format. Over the last 10 years, there has been increasing recognition of biotin interference in the wake of aggressive marketing of biotin-containing hair and nail products and the use of high-dosage biotin treatment for various neuropathies and multiple sclerosis.[15,16] A Mayo Clinic study recently found that approximately 8% of outpatients used higher doses of biotin (0.5-20 mg daily) than are typically found in multivitamins, and that biotin use was rarely listed in the electronic medical record.[17] The threshold for biotin interference is test and platform dependent. In general, a biotin intake greater than 5 mg daily is thought to increase the risk for biotin interference. Recommendations are to withhold biotin for 2 to 3 days before drawing the blood specimen. Biotin is cleared by the kidney, necessitating a longer washout period for patients with impaired renal function. Typically, a high biotin intake causes false-LOW interference when measuring large molecules by noncompetitive IMA methodology. Examples include C-peptide, FSH, LH, prolactin, TSH, troponin, and thyroglobulin. In contrast, high dietary biotin causes false-HIGH interference when measuring small molecules by competitive immunoassay methodology. Examples include progesterone, steroid hormones, thyroid hormones, and vitamin D.[18] Since the direction for biotin interference is different for TSH (false-low) vs thyroid hormones (false high), it is not surprising that there are many reports of biotin interference leading to a false diagnosis of Graves hyperthyroidism that in some cases has prompted appropriate treatment.[1] Physicians should ask patients regarding their use of hair and nail products likely to contain high biotin doses and recommend withholding the product for 2 to 3 days before their blood draw. Once the physician alerts the laboratory that biotin interference could be the cause of interference, the laboratory can treat the specimen with streptavidin beads or use other approaches to confirm that biotin was interfering with the test result.[18]

Streptavidin Antibodies

Streptavidin is a reagent often used together with biotin in the separation system of many endocrine tests. There are a number of case reports of streptavidin antibody interference but there are no formal studies on the prevalence of this source of interference.[1,2,19] Streptavidin antibodies have the potential to interfere with a wide range of endocrine tests on different platforms that use streptavidin in their separation system.[20] Streptavidin interference usually produces a similar profile as biotin (false-low for noncompetitive IMA methods/false-high

for competitive immunoassay methods). It is difficult for a physician to know whether a test reported by their laboratory instrument would be affected by biotin or streptavidin antibody interference. However, after the physician alerts the laboratory that interference is suspected, based on discordance between the test result and the patient's clinical presentation, the laboratory should be able to arrange a remeasurement on a different instrument platform that does not use biotin or streptavidin.

Ruthenium Antibodies

Ruthenium (^{44}Ru) is a chemical element that is used as a reagent in the electrochemiluminescence signaling systems of many endocrine tests (primarily on Roche analyzers). Ruthenium antibody interference typically causes false-high values for endocrine tests.[1,3,21] The prevalence of ruthenium antibody interference is thought to be low (<0.1%-0.24%).[1] However, over the last 10 years, there have been a number of reports of ruthenium interference, primarily with thyroid tests (false-high TSH and thyroid hormones).[1] When the physician questions an unexpectedly high result, it would be useful to know whether the test was reported by a Roche instrument, associated with the propensity for ruthenium antibody interference. The physician should be able to work with the laboratory to remeasure the test on a non-Roche analyzer. The laboratory should be able to communicate with Roche to determine whether the interference is related to ruthenium antibodies.

Paraprotein Interferences

Paraproteins have the potential to interfere by binding the test reagents of endocrine and nonendocrine tests on different instrument platforms.[22] Patients with multiple myeloma and monoclonal gammopathies are especially prone to such interferences. The mechanism for these interferences may relate to the increased turbidity of these types of specimens.

Mutant Analyte-Binding Proteins

Mutations in hormone-binding proteins, as well as drug effects, can disrupt hormone binding to its carrier protein(s) and produce test interference. Variants of thyroid hormone–binding protein are the most studied.[1] Whether binding protein variants interfere with a free hormone test depends on the test and instrument platform. Thyroid hormones primarily circulate bound to thyroxine-binding globulin and to a lesser extent transthyretin and albumin. Many thyroid hormone–binding protein variants have been described. These typically influence total hormone levels while free hormone and metabolic status remain normal.[23] Most laboratories use automated hormone immunoassays that are only estimate tests and not direct free hormone measurements. Direct free hormone measurement can be made by expensive, labor-intensive techniques such as equilibrium dialysis, ultrafiltration, and tandem mass spectrometry. These direct hormone tests are typically reserved for patients who present as diagnostic dilemmas—discordance between the hormone estimate test result and clinical status. For example, familial dysalbuminemic hyperthyroxinemia is caused by a spectrum of thyroid hormone (T_4 and/or T_3) binding albumin variants. These albumin variants interfere with most free T_4 and/or free T_3 immunoassays, producing false-high values in a patient-, test-, and instrument-specific manner.[23,24]

Analyte-Specific Interferences: Interferences Related to the Test Analyte

There are primarily 2 categories of analyte-specific interferences: interferences caused by molecular variants of the analyte and autoantibodies targeting the analyte.

Molecular Variants of the Test Analyte

Many endocrine analytes are complex proteins that circulate as heterogeneous molecular variants. Examples include, but are not limited to, ACTH, calcitonin, hCG, prolactin, PTH, TSH, thyroglobulin, and autoantibodies. These endocrine analytes are typically measured using IMA or immunoassay methodology that relies on the specificity of the interactions between target epitopes on the protein structure and MAb reagent(s).[2] The MAbs developed for each test are proprietary to that test and that manufacturer's instrument and are designed to recognize an epitope(s) on the most common (normal) variant of the test protein. The specificity of the MAb for target epitopes on the analyte may differ from those for the same analyte measured using a different instrument platform, giving rise to significant between-method variability.[25-27] This between-method variability is sometimes evident from differences in the test reference range on different instrument platforms.[25] Clinical care can be disrupted by these test specificity differences, especially when heterogeneous isoforms of the analyte circulate that differ in biologic vs immunologic activity. This is the case for TSH. Some patients are euthyroid but have a genetically abnormal TSH variant that is biologically active but not detected by some of the TSH tests (false-low results).[28] Other euthyroid patients secrete TSH genetic variants that are bioinactive but are recognized as "normal TSH" by test reagents, resulting in a false-high TSH result.[29] Discordance between bioactive and bioinactive TSH is common with hypothalamic-pituitary dysfunction. Because the MAb reagents of most TSH tests cannot distinguish between normal bioactive TSH isoforms and bioinactive TSH variants, a paradoxically normal or low TSH is reported when the bioinactive TSH isoforms secreted in central hypothyroidism are detected as "normal TSH."[30] Conversely, TSH isoforms with enhanced bioactivity are secreted by some TSH-secreting pituitary tumors, and these are recognized as "normal TSH" by test reagents, giving rise to a paradoxically normal/high TSH in the face of clinical hyperthyroidism.[31]

It should be noted that specificity differences in tumor-marker tests are especially problematic, because tumors often secrete abnormal molecular variants that may, or may not be, detected as normal analyte by test reagents. The reference range for a tumor-marker analyte is typically established using the nonneoplastic form of the analyte. Tumor-derived variants of the analyte may have abnormal conformations that mask the epitopes needed for detection (false-low test result),[32] or have unusual epitopes exposed that react abnormally with test reagents, producing a false-high test result. It follows that tumor-marker results are to some extent patient-specific and the trend or doubling time of the patient's test value may be more clinically relevant than the numeric test value or the reference range of the test.[33,34] Tumor-marker heterogeneity leading to between-method differences can be clinically disruptive when the laboratory changes instruments without notifying physicians who may need time to re-baseline critical patients. Significant differences in the numeric thyroglobulin values reported for the same serum measured by different methods are seen even in the absence of interfering thyroglobulin antibodies.[35] Thyroglobulin heterogeneity can cause a 2-fold difference in the thyroglobulin level when the same serum is measured by different methods.[26] These differences appear related to thyroglobulin heterogeneity and not necessarily the different methodologies (radioimmunoassay, IMA, and liquid-chromatography/tandem mass spectrometry) currently used to measure serum thyroglobulin.[35]

Autoantibodies Targeting the Test Analyte
There are many reports of autoantibodies interfering with endocrine test analytes. These include, but are not limited to, antibodies to ACTH, calcitonin, cardiac troponin, FSH, LH, insulin, prolactin (macroprolactin), thyroglobulin, TSH (macroTSH), T_4, and T_3. Patients with autoimmune conditions are most prone to autoantibody interferences. It should be noted that as with other antibodies, maternal autoantibodies cross the placenta and can impact neonatal testing.[36] Autoantibodies form high molecular weight analyte-IgG complexes in the circulation and are often considered "macro" forms of the hormone. However, these large hormone-IgG complexes are typically not bioactive.[7,8] Most assays cannot distinguish between the bioactive hormone monomer and a bioinactive hormone-IgG complex. It follows that a characteristic of autoantibody interference is a diagnostically inappropriate and false-high test result.[37] When autoantibody interference is suspected, the physician should alert the laboratory of the need to confirm the problem by precipitating the immunoglobulins in the specimen with polyethylene glycol and remeasuring analyte in the supernatant.[1,3] A lower test result in the polyethylene glycol supernatant is a presumptive positive test for autoantibodies.[3] Alternatively, column chromatography can be used to identify hormone immunoactivity in the high molecular weight fraction.[3] Although the prevalence of autoantibodies varies with the test analyte and the clinical setting, this source of interference is not inconsequential. For example, the prevalence of TSH antibodies has been estimated to be 0.6% to 1.6%.[7,8]

Thyroglobulin Autoantibodies
It should be noted that the prevalence of thyroglobulin antibodies is as high as 25% in patients with differentiated thyroid cancer—twice that of the normal population.[38,39] Thyroglobulin antibody interference with thyroglobulin IMA tests differs from other hormone autoantibody interferences by producing false-low/undetectable thyroglobulin IMA results.[35] The mechanism appears to involve masking the epitopes needed for IMA detection. Thyroglobulin antibody interference with thyroglobulin measurement is the major factor limiting the clinical utility of the dominant methodology used for thyroglobulin testing—automated IMA. It should be noted that the problem of thyroglobulin antibody interference with thyroglobulin measurement has not been overcome by using a thyroglobulin mass spectrometry test (liquid chromatography/tandem mass spectrometry).[35,40,41] Specifically, several studies now report paradoxically undetectable serum thyroglobulin for a significant percentage of thyroglobulin antibody–positive patients with

differentiated thyroid cancer who have structural disease.[35,40,41] Currently, it appears as if the thyroglobulin radioimmunoassay methodology remains the most reliable way to detect thyroglobulin in the presence of thyroglobulin antibodies.[35] One mitigating factor is that recently the trend in thyroglobulin antibody concentrations has become a useful prognostic indicator that is independent of the thyroglobulin measurement, provided the same thyroglobulin antibody test is used.[26]

In patients with differentiated thyroid cancer, thyroglobulin antibody measurement serves a dual purpose. Most laboratories measure antibodies as part of a thyroglobulin + thyroglobulin antibody panel. The presence of thyroglobulin antibodies is considered a risk factor for interference with IMA methodology.[35] Most laboratories consider IMA methodology to be contraindicated when thyroglobulin antibodies are detected. Instead, the trend in thyroglobulin antibody concentrations is now considered a more useful prognostic indicator than thyroglobulin IMA measurement.[26] Specifically, decreasing thyroglobulin antibodies is generally a good prognostic sign, whereas a rising or de novo appearance of thyroglobulin antibodies suggests clinical correlations.[26] Unfortunately, the sensitivity and specificity of thyroglobulin antibody tests are dependent on method and instrument.[27] Failure to use a sensitive method risks the reporting of a falsely low/undetectable thyroglobulin IMA test result.[35] Over recent years, epitope mapping studies have found different thyroglobulin antibody epitope profiles relating to the underlying pathology such as autoimmune thyroid disease (Hashimoto thyroiditis and Graves disease), non-autoimmune thyroid disease (nontoxic multinodular goiter), and papillary thyroid carcinoma (papillary thyroid carcinoma with or without associated histological thyroiditis).[42,43] The specificity of the thyroglobulin antibody test differs among instruments because proprietary MAb reagents target different epitopes on thyroglobulin antibody molecules. As a result, the same serum can have a 100-fold difference in numeric antibody values reported for the same serum measured by different methods.[27] This between-method variability compromises the value of using the thyroglobulin antibody trend as a prognostic indicator should there be a change in method. The epitope specificity of the thyroglobulin antibodies secreted by each patient differs. Despite the differences in numeric values reported for the same serum measured by different methods, the ratio between the numeric values of 2 different tests remains a constant, despite changes in the thyroglobulin antibody concentration per se.[44] This is evidence of patient-related thyroglobulin antibody specificity that can be used to re-baseline a patient to a new method should a method change be necessary.

Clinical Case Vignettes
Case 1

A 28-year-old woman has a preemployment health screen, which documents an elevated TSH level and a normal free T_4 level. Her serum shows other endocrine abnormalities despite no evidence of an endocrine problem. She has regular monthly menses and a BMI of 29.5 kg/m². Other than a desire for weight loss, she has no concerns.

Thyroid panel test results (instrument #1):

> TSH = 25.8 mIU/L (0.4-4.0 mIU/L)
> Free T_4 = 0.9 ng/dL (0.8-1.8 ng/dL)
>   (SI: 11.6 pmol/L [10.3-23.2 pmol/L])
> TPO antibodies = negative (<1 kIU/L)
> Prolactin = 54 ng/mL (5-23 ng/mL)
>   (SI: 2.3 nmol/L [0.2-1.0 nmol/L])
> FSH = 3.1 mIU/mL (3.5-12.5 mIU/mL)
>   (SI: 3.1 IU/L [3.5-12.5 IU/L])
> β-hCG = 0.1 mIU/mL (<0.5 mIU/mL)
>   (SI: 0.1 IU/L [<0.5 IU/L])
> PTH = 85 pg/mL (7-63 pg/mL) (SI: 85 ng/L [7-63 ng/L])

Heterophile antibody interference is suspected. The tests are conducted again in a HAb blocker tube. The blocker tube treatment significantly lowers TSH, but it does not normalize. The blocker tube treatment normalizes the prolactin and PTH:

> TSH = 8.7 mIU/L (0.4-4.0 mIU/L)
> Free T_4 = 1.0 ng/dL (0.8-1.8 ng/dL)
>   (SI: 12.9 pmol/L [10.3-23.2 pmol/L])

Prolactin = 19 ng/mL (5-23 ng/mL)
(SI: 0.8 nmol/L [0.2-1.0 nmol/L])
FSH = 2.9 mIU/mL (3.5-12.5 mIU/mL)
(SI: 2.9 IU/L [3.5-12.5 IU/L])
β-hCG = 0.4 mIU/mL (<0.5 mIU/mL)
(SI: 0.4 IU/L [<0.5 IU/L])
PTH = 51 pg/mL (7-63 pg/mL)
(SI: 51 ng/L [7-63 ng/L])

A fresh specimen is drawn to repeat the tests using a different instrument platform. A different profile of abnormalities is reported by the second instrument:

Laboratory test results (instrument #2):

TSH = 1.1 mIU/L (0.4-5.3 mIU/L)
Free T_4 = 1.3 ng/dL (0.8-1.8 ng/dL)
(SI: 16.7 pmol/L [10.3-23.2 pmol/L])
Prolactin = 45 ng/mL (3-27 ng/mL)
(SI: 2.0 nmol/L [0.1-1.2 nmol/L])
FSH = 22.5 mIU/mL (3.5-12.5 mIU/mL)
(SI: 22.5 IU/L [3.5-12.5 IU/L])
β-hCG = 265 mIU/mL (<0.5 mIU/mL)
(SI: 265 IU/L [<0.5 IU/L])
PTH = 53 pg/mL (12-88 pg/mL)
(SI: 53 ng/L [12-88 ng/L])

Question 1: Which of the following was the primary indication of test interference in this case?

A. Unexpected test abnormalities for a young patient without evidence of an endocrine problem

B. Discordant TSH and free T_4 relationship—the degree of TSH elevation was incompatible with the normal free T_4 (expect a log/linear relationship)

C. Negative TPO antibodies—an additional indicator that the elevated TSH was not due to subclinical hypothyroidism

Answer: A) Unexpected test abnormalities for a young patient without evidence of an endocrine problem

Question 2: When investigating for interference, why is repeating the tests on a new specimen useful?

A. Potential contamination of the original specimen by carryover from another specimen

B. Potential mislabeling of the specimen at some stage of the testing process

C. Potential instrument malfunction leading to an erroneous result

Answer: B) Potential mislabeling of the specimen at some stage of the testing process

This case illustrates HAb interference. Discordance between the clinical presentation and the test result is the hallmark of interference. Lowering of the test result by greater than 20% when re-measured in a HAb blocker tube is presumptive evidence of HAb interference. However, the lower blocker tube test result is not considered clinically reliable and should not be reported or used clinically. Most reported cases of HAb interference have involved a single analyte (usually a thyroid analyte). This case illustrates how HAb interference can affect multiple tests from different endocrine systems and shows that the abnormality profile is instrument dependent. It is not unusual for errors to arise from the processing and labeling of specimens before testing. Internal laboratory checks should make the possibility of carryover and instrument malfunction less likely.

Once HAb has been identified as affecting one analyte, there is a risk that analytes from other endocrine systems could be affected. Therefore, it would be prudent to update the patient's electronic medical record with the likely cause of the interference (HAb in this case), the test(s) affected, and the instrument used for the testing. Disseminating this information could help prevent misdiagnoses should the interference affect other tests from different endocrine systems.

Case 2

A 23-year-old woman presents with fatigue. Her BMI is 23 kg/m², and her menses are normal. Because the patient has a sister with Hashimoto thyroiditis, a thyroid evaluation is initiated. The thyroid gland appears normal on palpation, and the patient takes no prescription or over-the-counter drugs or vitamins. TSH is very elevated but free T_4 is within normal limits. The TSH exhibits nonparallelism on dilution. TPO antibodies are mildly positive at 2 kIU/L (>1 kIU/L).

Laboratory test results (instrument #1):

> TSH = 110 mIU/L (0.4-4.0 mIU/L) and 150 mIU/L using a 1:10 dilution
> Free T_4 = 0.8 ng/dL (0.8-1.8 ng/dL) (SI: 10.3 pmol/L [10.3-23.2 pmol/L])

TSH is not significantly lowered by re-measurement in a HAb blocker tube—a contraindication but not an elimination of the possibility of HAb interference. The possibility of a pituitary TSH-secreting tumor is excluded by finding an undetectable TSH α subunit (<0.2 ng/mL). A new specimen is drawn and sent to a different laboratory for TSH measurement using a different instrument platform.

Laboratory test results (instrument #2):

> TSH = 16.7 mIU/L and 87 mIU/L (0.4-5.3 mIU/L) using a 1:10 dilution
> Free T_4 = 0.7 ng/dL (0.6-1.2 ng/dL) (SI: 9.0 pmol/L [7.7-15.4 pmol/L])

Question 1: Which of the following is/are the primary factor(s) suggesting TSH interference in this patient using instrument #1?

A. High TSH discordant with the euthyroid clinical presentation; thyroid gland appeared normal, despite a family history of thyroid disease; and TPO antibodies were only mildly positive

B. TSH disproportionately high relative to free T_4—higher than would be expected for subclinical hypothyroidism (expect a log/linear TSH/free T_4 relationship)

C. Significant discordance in the TSH levels reported by the 2 different instrument platforms

D. TSH dilutions were nonparallel on both instruments

E. TSH discordance observed with 2 separate blood draws (eliminates the possibility that carryover from a previously high specimen contaminated the patient's first test, or that there was a random technical malfunction with the instrument)

Answers: A and B) High TSH discordant with the euthyroid clinical presentation, thyroid gland appeared normal, despite a family history of thyroid disease, and TPO antibodies were only mildly positive and TSH disproportionately high relative to free T_4—higher than would be expected for subclinical hypothyroidism (expect a log/linear TSH/free T_4 relationship)

All these factors, however, are consistent with TSH interference. Had instrument #2 been used first, the TSH was only mildly affected by the interference and would not have been high enough to prompt a dilution that would have detected nonparallelism in the TSH test. In the case of instrument #2, there could have been an erroneous diagnosis of subclinical hypothyroidism prompting initiation of levothyroxine treatment. Note the differences in reference ranges between the 2 instruments. The free T_4 value of 0.7 ng/dL (9.0 pmol/L) reported by instrument #2 was low relative to the free T_4 reference range of instrument #1.

Question 2: Which of the following is the most likely cause of the TSH interference in this patient?

A. HAb interference

B. TSH autoantibody (TSH antibody, macro TSH) interference

Answer: B) TSH autoantibody (TSH antibody, macro TSH) interference

The HAb blocker tube test did not lower this patient's TSH. Although the HAb blocker does not detect all cases of HAb interference, the failure of the HAb blocker tube treatment to lower the TSH to *any* degree suggests that the cause of the TSH interference is not HAb but is more likely due to TSH antibodies.

The TSH reported by both platforms was considered to be falsely high due to interference. The negative HAb blocker tube test suggested the interference was not caused by HAb but was more likely due to TSH antibodies. Hormone autoantibodies can only be confirmed by laboratory studies. A polyethylene glycol precipitation of IgG complexes from the serum, and finding a lower test result in the polyethylene glycol supernatant is a test for autoantibodies. Alternatively, the serum could be subjected to column chromatography to confirm the presence of immunoactivity in the high molecular weight region, indicating the presence of a TSH-IgG complex. Because most laboratories are not equipped to do these studies, in this case TSH antibodies would have to be a *presumptive* cause of the interference in this patient. Since the patient was judged to be euthyroid and the interference affected different instruments, a recommendation was made that any future thyroid tests should rely on free T_4 and not TSH.

Case 3

A 52-year-old man had thyroid tests performed during evaluation of a goiter. There is no history of thyroid treatment. The patient appears euthyroid.

Laboratory test results:

> TSH = 1.5 mIU/L (0.4-5.3 mIU/L)
> Free T_4 = 0.8 ng/dL (0.6-1.2 ng/dL)
>   (SI: 10.3 pmol/L [7.7-15.4 pmol/L])
> Serum thyroglobulin
>   (IMA method) = 1.1 ng/mL
>   (4-40 ng/mL)(SI: 1.1 µg/L [4-40 µg/L])
> Thyroglobulin antibodies (IMA method), not
>   detected

Serum thyroglobulin measured by radioimmunoassay methodology is discordant with the thyroglobulin IMA result, but is more appropriate for the clinical status of the patient (thyroglobulin by radioimmunoassay = 12.5 ng/mL [12.5 µg/L]).

Usually HAb interference is expected to cause false-high thyroglobulin IMA test results. However, false-low thyroglobulin IMA results have been reported to result from HAb.[12] Remeasurement of the patient's serum in a HAb blocker tube fails to raise the thyroglobulin IMA value, so HAb is not considered the cause of the low thyroglobulin IMA discrepancy.

Goiters are known to sometimes secrete thyroglobulin variants. The possibility that the low thyroglobulin IMA is a result of a thyroglobulin variant with an abnormal molecular conformation in which the target epitopes needed for IMA detection are masked is investigated by remeasuring thyroglobulin by liquid chromatography–tandem mass spectrometry (10.1 ng/mL [10.1 µg/L]), which is in agreement with the thyroglobulin radioimmunoassay result (12.5 ng/mL [12.5 µg/L]) and clinical status. This suggests the possibility of a thyroglobulin variant that is not being detected by the thyroglobulin IMA test.

At this point, the laboratory receives some additional clinical information. The patient has multiple sclerosis and is being treated with high-dosage biotin as one of his medications.[16] Interference by exogenous high-dosage biotin is a likely source of interference with the thyroglobulin IMA test since biotin is used as a reagent in the separation system on this instrument.

When the laboratory repeats the thyroglobulin IMA test after adding streptavidin beads to the serum to adsorb excess biotin,[18] the thyroglobulin IMA result measured in the streptavidin supernatant normalizes to 11.2 ng/mL (11.2 µg/L)—in agreement with the thyroglobulin radioimmunoassay, thyroglobulin liquid chromatography–tandem mass spectrometry, and clinical status.

Question 1: Which of the following suggested that the thyroglobulin IMA result was inappropriately low in this patient?

A. TSH and free T_4 within normal limits

B. Negative thyroglobulin antibodies

C. The presence of goiter

Answer: C) The presence of goiter

Thyroid tissue mass, thyroid damage, and the degree of TSH stimulation are the major physiologic factors determining the serum thyroglobulin level. In this case, there was increased tissue mass (goiter) (Answer C), no surgical history, and a normal TSH value.

Question 2: Could thyroglobulin antibody interference be the cause of a false-low thyroglobulin IMA test result?

A. No; thyroglobulin antibodies were absent

B. Yes; the thyroglobulin antibody result could be a false negative

Answer: B) Yes, the thyroglobulin antibody result could be a false negative

There is considerable variability among thyroglobulin antibody testing methods—both in terms of the numeric values they report (can vary 100-fold when measuring the same specimen) and the fact that laboratories often select an inappropriately high cutoff value to determine thyroglobulin antibody "positivity." There can be serum specimens that are reported as thyroglobulin antibody positive by one method and thyroglobulin antibody negative by another. Even very low levels of thyroglobulin antibodies can interfere with a thyroglobulin IMA result, causing a falsely low/undetectable thyroglobulin IMA result. Biotin interference also has the potential to cause a false-low thyroglobulin antibody measurement had the test used IMA methodology and used biotin as a reagent in the separation system.

High-dosage biotin intake can affect any test that uses biotin as a test reagent. The direction of interference depends on the methodology—false-low with noncompetitive IMA tests (such as thyroglobulin and TSH) and false-high for competitive immunoassay tests (such as free T_4 and some autoantibody methods). On a different instrument, the profile of biotin-related abnormalities might have been different.

This case illustrates the need to supply clinical and medication information to the laboratory along with the specimen. There is increasing patient and physician awareness that some tests are prone to interference by high-dosage dietary biotin. Currently, instrument manufacturers are attempting to reformat tests to remove the biotin components. However, it could take years to eliminate the biotin interference problem. In the meantime, physicians should ask patients whether they use hair and nail products likely to contain high-dosage biotin and recommend a 2- to 3-day biotin hold before their blood draw.

References

1. Favresse J, Burlacu MC, Maiter D, Gruson, D. Interferences with thyroid function immunoassays: clinical implications and detection algorithm. *Endocr Rev.* 2018;39(5):830-850. PMID: 29982406

2. Haddad RA, Giacherio D, Barkan AL. Interpretation of common endocrine laboratory tests: technical pitfalls, their mechanisms and practical considerations. *Clin Diabetes Endocrinol.* 2019;5:12. PMID: 31367466

3. Ward G, Simpson A, Boscato L, Hickman PE. The investigation of interferences in immunoassay. *Clin Biochem.* 2017;50(18):1306-1311. PMID: 28847718

4. Nakano K, Yasuda K, Shibuya H, Moriyama T, Kahata K, Shimizu C. Transient human anti-mouse antibody generated with immune enhancement in a carbohydrate antigen 19.9 immunoassay after surgical resection of recurrent cancer. *Ann Clin Biochem.* 2016;53(Pt 4):511-515. PMID: 26744502

5. Sturgeon C, Viljoen A. Analytical error and interference in immunoassay: minimizing risk. *Ann Clin Biochem.* 2011;48(Pt 5):418-432. PMID: 21750113

6. Thienpont LM, Van Uytfanghe K, Beastall G, et al; IFCC Working Group on Standardization of Thyroid Function Tests. Report of the IFCC Working Group for Standardization of Thyroid Function Tests; part 3: total thyroxine and total triiodothyronine. *Clin Chem.* 2010;56(6):921-929. PMID: 20395622

7. Hattori N, Ishihara T, Yamagami K, Shimatsu A. Macro TSH in patients with subclinical hypothyroidism. *Clin Endocrinol (Oxf).* 2015;83(6):923-930. PMID: 25388002

8. Hattori N, Ishihara T, Shimatsu A. Variability in the detection of macro TSH in different immunoassay systems. *Eur J Endocrinol.* 2016;174(1):9-15. PMID: 26438715

9. Bolstad N, Warren D, Nustad K. Heterophilic antibody interference in immunometric assays. *Best Pract Res Clin Endocrinol Metab.* 2013;27(5):647-661. PMID:24094636

10. Mongolu S, Armston AE, Mozley E, Nasruddin A. Heterophilic antibody interference affecting multiple hormone assays: is it due to rheumatoid factor? *Scand J Clin Lab Invest.* 2016;76(3):240-242. PMID: 26924790

11. Wang H, Bi X, Xu L, Li Y. Negative interference by rheumatoid factor in alpha-fetoprotein chemiluminescent microparticle immunoassay. *Ann Clin Biochem.* 2017;54(1):55-59. PMID: 27073029

12. Giovanella L, Keller F, Ceriani L, Tozzoli R. Heterophile antibodies may falsely increase or decrease thyroglobulin measurement in patients with differentiated thyroid carcinoma. *Clin Chem Lab Med.* 2009;47(8):952-954. PMID: 19589101

13. Gulbahar O, Konca Degertekin C, Akturk M, et al. A case with immunoassay Interferences in the measurement of multiple hormones. *J Clin Endocrinol Metab*. 2015;100(6):247-253. PMID: 25897621

14. 14. Colon P, Green D. Biotin interference in clinical immunoassays. *J Am Lab Med*. 2018;2:941-951.

15. Bowen R, Benavides R, Colon-Franco J, et al. Best practices in mitigating the risk of biotin interference with laboratory testing. *Clin Biochem*.2019;74:1-11. PMID: 31473202

16. Tourbah A, Lebrun-Frenay C, Edan G, et al. MD1003 (high-dose biotin) for the treatment of progressive multiple sclerosis: A randomised, double-blind, placebo-controlled study. *Mult Scler*. 2016;22(13):1719-1731. PMID: 27589059

17. Katzman BM, Leuke AJ, Donato LJ, Jaffe AS, Baumann NA. Prevalence of biotin supplement usage in outpatients and plasma biotin concentrations in patients presenting to the emergency department. *Clin Biochem*. 2018;60:11-16. PMID: 30036510

18. Trambas C, Lu Z, Yen T, Sikaris K. Depletion of biotin using streptavidin-coated microparticles: a validated solution to the problem of biotin interference in streptavidin-biotin immunoassays. *Ann Clin Biochem*. 2018;55(2):216-226. PMID: 28406314

19. Favresse J, Lardinois B, Nassogne MC, Preumont V, Maiter D, Gruson D. Anti-streptavidin antibodies mimicking heterophilic antibodies in thyroid function tests. *Clin Chem Lab Med*. 2018;56(7):160-163. PMID: 29447115

20. Bayart LL, Favresse J, Melnik E, et al. Erroneous thyroid and steroid hormones profile due to anti-streptavidin antibodies. *Clin Chem Lab Med*. 2019;57(10):255-258. PMID: 30903751

21. Favresse J, Paridaens H, Pirson N, Maiter D, Gruson D. Massive interference in free T4 and free T3 assays misleading clinical judgment. *Clin Chem Lab Med*. 2017;55(4):84-86. PMID: 27665421

22. King RI, Florkowski CM. How paraproteins can affect laboratory assays: spurious results and biological effects. *Pathology*. 2010;42(5):397-401. PMID: 20632813

23. Cartwright D, O'Shea P, Rajanayagam O, et al. Familial dysalbuminemic hyperthyroxinemia: a persistent diagnostic challenge. *Clin Chem*. 2009;55(5):1044-1046. PMID: 19282355

24. Kragh-Hansen U, Galliano M, Minchiotti L. Clinical, genetic and protein structural aspects of familial dysalbuminemic hyperthyroxinemia and hypertriiodothyroninemia. *Front Endocrinol (Lausanne)*. 2017;8:29. PMID: 29163366

25. Faix JD, Miller WG. Progress in standardizing and harmonizing thyroid function tests. *Am J Clin Nutr*. 2016;104(Suppl 3):913S-917. PMID: 27534642

26. Spencer C, LoPresti J, Fatemi S. How sensitive (second-generation) thyroglobulin measurement is changing paradigms for monitoring patients with differentiated thyroid cancer, in the absence and presence of thyroglobulin autoantibodies. *Curr Opin Endocrinol Diab Obes*. 2014;21(5):394-340. PMID: 25122493

27. Spencer C, Petrovic I, Fatemi S. Current thyroglobulin autoantibody (TgAb) assays often fail to detect interfering TgAb that can result in the reporting of falsely low/undetectable serum Tg IMA values for patients with differentiated thyroid cancer. *J Clin Endocrinol Metab*. 2011;96(5):1283-1291. PMID: 21325460

28. Pappa T, Johannesen J, Scherberg N, Torrent M, Dumitrescu A, Refetoff S. TSHb variant with impaired immunoreactivity but intact biological activity and its clinical implications. *Thyroid*. 2015;25(8):869-87. PMID: 25950606

29. Partsch CJ, Riepe FG, Krone N, Sippell WG, Pohlenz J. Initially elevated TSH and congenital central hypothyroidism due to a homozygous mutation of the TSH beta subunit gene: case report and review of the literature. *Exp Clin Endocrinol Diabetes*. 2006;114(5):227-234. PMID: 16804796

30. Persani L, Ferretti E, Borgato S, Faglia G, Beck-Peccoz P. Circulating thyrotropin bioactivity in sporadic central hypothyroidism. *J Clin Endocrinol Metab*. 2000;85(10):3631-3635. PMID: 11061514

31. Beck-Peccoz P, Persani L, Mannavola D, Campi I. Pituitary tumours: TSH-secreting adenomas. *Best Pract Res Clin Endoc Metab*. 2009;23(5):597-605. PMID: 19945025

32. Chindris AM, Casler JD, Bernet VJ, et al. Clinical and molecular features of Hurthle cell carcinoma of the thyroid. *J Clin Endocrinol Metab*. 2015;100(1):55-62. PMID: 25259908

33. Miyauchi A, Kudo T, Miya A, et al. Prognostic impact of serum thyroglobulin doubling-time under thyrotropin suppression in patients with papillary thyroid carcinoma who underwent total thyroidectomy. *Thyroid*. 2011;21(7):707-716. PMID: 21649472

34. Ito Y, Miyauchi A, Kihara M, Kudo T, Miya A. Calcitonin doubling time in medullary thyroid carcinoma after the detection of distant metastases keenly predict patients' carcinoma death. *Endocr J*. 2016;63(7):663-667. PMID: 27097545

35. Spencer C, Petrovic I, Fatemi S, LoPresti J. Serum thyroglobulin (Tg) monitoring of patients with differentiated thyroid cancer using sensitive (second-generation) immunometric assays can be disrupted by false-negative and false-positive serum thyroglobulin autoantibody misclassifications. *J Clin Endocrinol Metab*. 2014;99(12):4589-4599. PMID: 25226290

36. Halsall DJ, Fahie-Wilson MN, et al. Macro thyrotropin-IgG complex causes factitious increases in thyroid-stimulating hormone screening tests in a neonate and mother. *Clin Chem*. 2006;52(10):1968-1969. PMID: 16998119

37. Hattori N, Aisaka K, Chihara K, Shimatsu A. Current thyrotropin immunoassays recognize macro-thyrotropin leading to hyperthyrotropinemia in females of reproductive age. *Thyroid*. 2018;28(10):1252-1260. PMID: 29943675

38. Spencer CA, Takeuchi M, Kazarosyan M, et al. Serum thyroglobulin autoantibodies: prevalence, influence on serum thyroglobulin measurement, and prognostic significance in patients with differentiated thyroid carcinoma. *J Clin Endocrinol Metab*. 1998;83(4):1121-1127. PMID: 9543128

39. Hollowell JG, Staehling NW, Flanders WD, et al. Serum TSH, T(4), and thyroid antibodies in the United States population (1988 to 1994): National Health and Nutrition Examination Survey (NHANES III). *J Clin Endocrinol Metab*. 2002;87(2):489-499. PMID: 11836274

40. Azmat U, Porter K, Senter L, Ringel MD, Nabhan F. Thyroglobulin liquid chromatography-tandem mass spectrometry has a low sensitivity for detecting structural disease in patients with antithyroglobulin antibodies. *Thyroid*. 2017;27(1):74-80. PMID: 27736322

41. Netzel BC, Grebe SK, Carranza Leon BG, et al. Thyroglobulin (Tg) testing revisited: Tg assays, TgAb assays, and correlation of results with clinical outcomes. *J Clin Endocrinol Metab*. 2015;100(8):1074-1083. PMID: 26078778

42. Latrofa F, Ricci D, Montanelli L, et al. Thyroglobulin autoantibodies in patients with papillary thyroid carcinoma: comparison of different assays and evaluation of causes of discrepancies. *J Clin Endocrinol Metab*. 2012;97(11):3974-3982. PMID: 22948755

43. Lupoli GA, Okosieme OE, Evans C, et al. Prognostic significance of thyroglobulin antibody epitopes in differentiated thyroid cancer. *J Clin Endocrinol Metab*. 2015;100(1):100-108. PMID: 25322272

44. Spencer C, Fatemi S. Thyroglobulin antibody (TgAb) methods - strengths, pitfalls and clinical utility for monitoring TgAb-positive patients with differentiated thyroid cancer. *Best Pract Res Clin Endocrinol Metab*. 2013;27(5):701-712. PMID: 24094640

A Little Help From My Friends: The Endocrinology–Oncology Interface—How Do We Help Each Other?

Claire Higham, DPhil, FRCP. Christie Hospital, Manchester, United Kingdom; E-mail: cehigham@doctors.org.uk

Sacha Howell, PhD, FRCP. Manchester University, Manchester, United Kingdom; E-mail: sacha.howell@manchester.ac.uk

Peter Trainer, MD, FRCPE. The Christie NHS Foundation Trust, Manchester, United Kingdom; E-mail: peter.trainer@manchester.ac.uk

Learning Objectives

- Explain why the initial clinical and biochemical assessment of patients with hyponatremia is crucial to optimal management.

- Recommend the correct management of endocrine complications of immune checkpoint inhibitor therapy to avoid discontinuation of this therapy.

- Anticipate the implications of systemic anticancer therapy for bone health and mitigate these adverse effects with lifestyle advice, bone density monitoring, and timely pharmacological intervention.

Main Conclusions

Endocrine complications of cancer and its treatment are common, varied in nature, and frequently complex, and some are all too frequently overlooked (eg, dexamethasone-induced diabetes). Endocrinologists are vital partners to oncologists in ensuring that the endocrinopathies do not delay or prohibit anticancer therapy.

Significance of the Clinical Problem

Improved survival and novel modalities of therapy mean that evermore patients with cancer will experience endocrine complications. In particular, immunotherapy with checkpoint inhibitors is improving outcomes in an increasing number of cancers, but at the expense of immune-mediated endocrinopathies such as hypophysitis, adrenalitis, thyroiditis, and diabetes mellitus, which can be serious, or even fatal. There has never been a greater need for endocrine input into the care of patients being treated for cancer.

Barriers to Optimal Practice

- Lack of patient education/awareness.

- Failure to anticipate endocrine complications of systemic anticancer therapy.

- Inadequate collaboration between oncologists and endocrinologists.

Strategies for Diagnosis, Therapy, and/or Management

Hyponatremia

Syndrome of inappropriate antidiuretic hormone secretion (SIADH) is common in patients with cancer, but incorrect diagnosis and subsequent incorrect management of hyponatremia increases the risk of mortality. The clinical presentation of hyponatremia depends on the severity, speed of onset, and underlying diagnosis.

Acute Life-Threatening Hyponatremia

Severe symptoms of acute life-threatening hyponatremia include vomiting, seizures, and reduced consciousness/coma.

Non–Life-Threatening Hyponatremia

Patients with non–life-threatening hyponatremia may be asymptomatic or experience moderately severe symptoms such as nausea without vomiting, confusion, and headache. Mild symptoms can include lethargy and irritability.

Hyponatremia can also be classified based on the serum sodium concentration:

> Mild: 130-135 mEq/L (SI: 130-135 mmol/L)
> Moderate: 126-129 mEq/L (SI: 126-129 mmol/L)
> Profound: ≤125 mEq/L (SI: ≤125 mmol/L)

Clinical Case Vignette 1

A 55-year-old man with small cell lung carcinoma presents with breathlessness, anorexia, sweats, and confusion.

Laboratory test results:

> Sodium = 110 mEq/L (136-142 mEq/L)
>   (SI: 110 mmol/L [136-142 mmol/L])
> Serum urea nitrogen = 12.6 mg/dL (8-23 mg/dL)
>   (SI: 4.5 mmol/L [2.9-8.2 mmol/L])
> Potassium = 4.6 mEq/L (3.5-5.0 mEq/L)
>   (SI: 4.6 mmol/L [3.5-5.0 mmol/L])
> Creatinine = 0.58 mg/dL (0.7-1.3 mg/dL)
>   (SI: 51 μmol/L [61.9-114.9 μmol/L])

He is euvolemic. Additional laboratory test results include the following:

> Serum osmolality = 226 mOsm/kg
>   (275-295 mOsm/kg)
> Urinary osmolality = 611 mOsm/kg
>   (150-1150 mOsm/kg)
> Urinary sodium = 42 mEq/L (SI: 45 mmol/L)
> Urinary potassium = 70 mEq/L (SI: 70 mmol/L)

Question 1: What is this patient's diagnosis?
Answer: SIADH

A diagnosis of SIADH requires 7 conditions to be met (in the untreated state):

- Clinical euvolemia
- Serum osmolality <275 mOsm/kg
- Urine osmolality ≥100 mOsm/kg
- Urinary sodium ≥20 mEq/L (≥20 mmol/L)
- Normal thyroid function
- Normal adrenal function
- Exclusion of drug-induced hyponatremia

Evaluation and differential diagnosis include exploring symptoms as a measure of severity and rapidity of onset. The medical history should be documented, including a timeline of change of serum sodium, comorbidities (eg, type and stage of malignancy, alcohol dependency, liver disease, heart failure), and drug history (especially new medications). Volume status should be determined (hypervolemia, hypovolemia, or euvolemia).

Investigations for the differential diagnosis of hyponatremia are shown in *Figure 1.*

- Measurement of serum osmolality, cortisol (document exogenous glucocorticoids), thyroid function, and glucose
- Measurement of urine osmolality and urine electrolytes (sodium and potassium)

Question 2: What is the best treatment?
Answer: Depends on the severity, speed of onset, and underlying diagnosis

Figure 1. Algorithm for the Differential Diagnosis of Hyponatremia

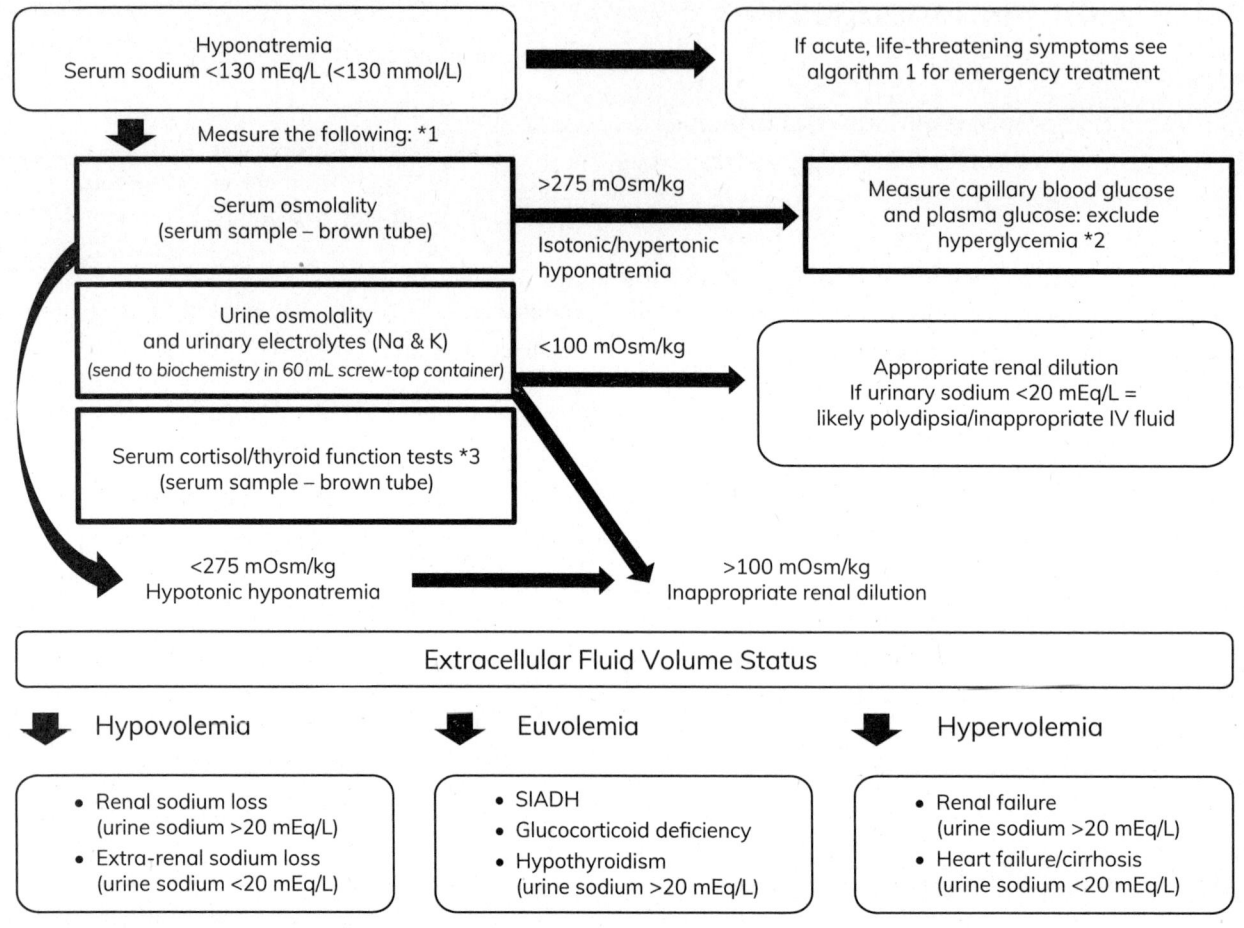

Treatment of SIADH

The cause of SIADH should be treated (eg, chemotherapy for small cell lung cancer). Fluid restriction is unlikely to be effective and has limited application in the oncology population. A high urine osmolality makes fluid restriction less likely to work. The urine to plasma electrolyte ratio is a useful guide for appropriate fluid restriction (*Table 1*).

Table 1. Fluid Restriction Guide Based on the Urine to Plasma Electrolyte Ratio

Ratio	Fluid Restriction
>1	unlikely to be effective
0.5-1.0	<0.5 L
<0.5	<1 L

The Furst formula =

$$\frac{\text{urinary sodium concentration} + \text{urinary potassium concentration}}{\text{serum sodium concentration}}$$

Demeclocycline is too slow to act and is of limited benefit. It induces nephrogenic diabetes insipidus and can take 2 to 14 days to be effective. The starting dosage is 150 mg twice daily, increased to a maximum dosage of 300 mg 4 times daily. Advantages are that it may be easier to tolerate than fluid restriction and can be initiated as an outpatient or inpatient. Cautions and disadvantages are that it may not be effective and it has slow onset of action. Adverse effects can include nausea, skin photosensitivity, and nephrotoxicity. Demeclocycline should not to be used in patients with renal impairment.

Figure 2. Safe Use of Tolvaptan

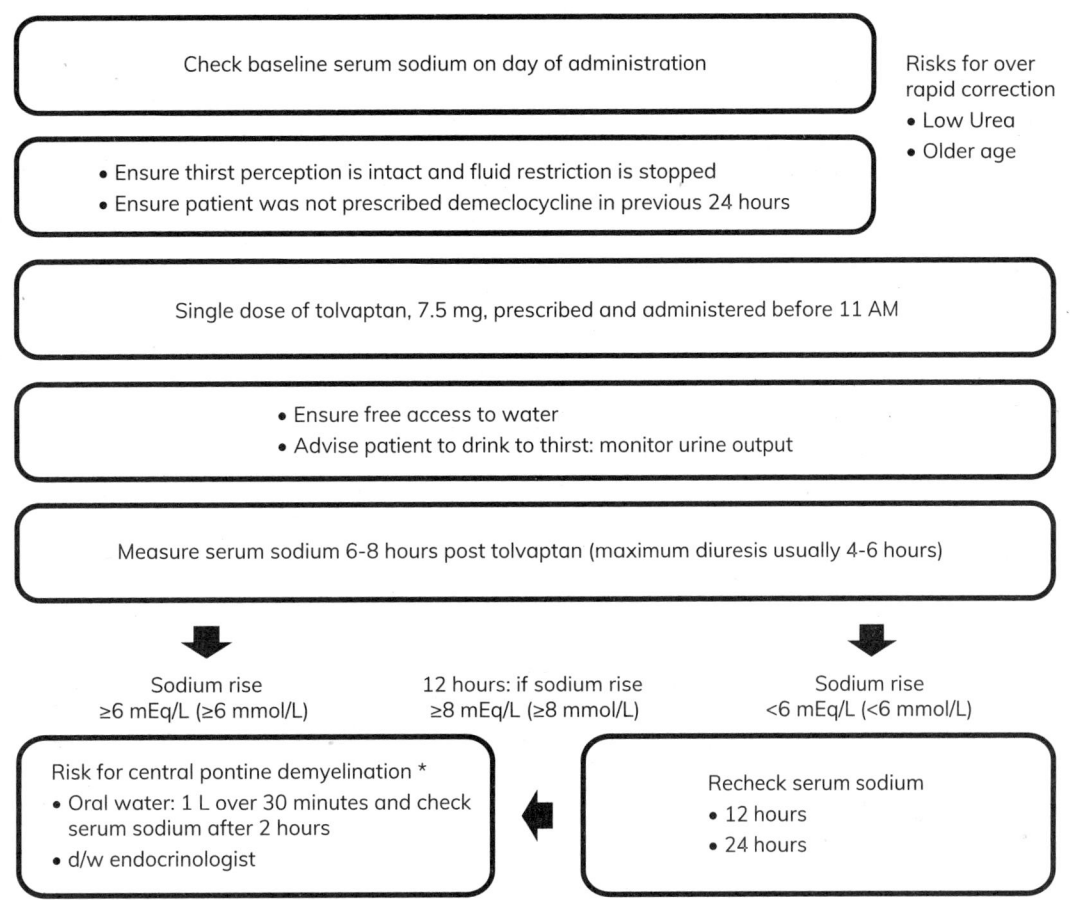

Check baseline serum sodium on day of administration

Risks for over rapid correction
• Low Urea
• Older age

• Ensure thirst perception is intact and fluid restriction is stopped
• Ensure patient was not prescribed demeclocycline in previous 24 hours

Single dose of tolvaptan, 7.5 mg, prescribed and administered before 11 AM

• Ensure free access to water
• Advise patient to drink to thirst: monitor urine output

Measure serum sodium 6-8 hours post tolvaptan (maximum diuresis usually 4-6 hours)

Sodium rise ≥6 mEq/L (≥6 mmol/L)   12 hours: if sodium rise ≥8 mEq/L (≥8 mmol/L)   Sodium rise <6 mEq/L (<6 mmol/L)

Risk for central pontine demyelination *
• Oral water: 1 L over 30 minutes and check serum sodium after 2 hours
• d/w endocrinologist

Recheck serum sodium
• 12 hours
• 24 hours

24 hours: if sodium rise ≥12 mEq/L (≥12 mmol/L)

Tolvaptan, when used appropriately, corrects sodium and permit chemotherapy to be started. The safe use of tolvaptan is depicted in *Figure 2.* Tolvaptan is a selective V_2-receptor antagonist in the renal collecting ducts and it increases water excretion. In the presence of hypovolemic hyponatremia and/or lack of appropriate monitoring of serum sodium and fluid balance, there can be a potentially life-threatening rapid rise in sodium. If switching from demeclocycline, it is ideal to wait 48 hours before administering the first dose of tolvaptan. Importantly, the patient must not be confused or fluid restricted and must have thirst perception. Initially, it is recommended to start with a single dose of tolvaptan of 7.5 mg (half the recommended dose). Subsequent doses should be prescribed and administered in accordance with serum sodium and symptoms. Following tolvaptan administration, serum sodium should be checked after 6 hours and 12 hours. If there is a 6 mEq/L or greater (≥6 mmol/L) rise in serum sodium within first 6 hours or an 8 mEq/L or greater (≥8 mmol/L) rise in 12 hours, hypotonic fluid may be required (oral water). Cautions and disadvantages include the risk of too rapid correction of sodium, which could potentially lead to osmotic demyelination. It should be used with caution in patients with chronic liver disease/cirrhosis.

Management of Acute, Life-Threatening Hyponatremia

The aim is to achieve a 5 mEq/L (5 mmol/L) rise in serum sodium within the first hour. If the clinical status of the patient does not improve after a 5 mEq/L (5 mmol/L) rise in serum sodium, then additional hypertonic saline may be required and further exploration of symptoms undertaken.

Figure 3. Management of Acute, Life-Threatening Hyponatremia

```
┌─────────────────────────────────────────────────────┐
│  Severe symptomatic hyponatremia — for hypertonic saline │
│  • Discuss with critical care/outreach —              │
│    *requires high monitoring environment*             │
│  • Baseline serum blood and urine samples as per algorithm 2 │
└─────────────────────────────────────────────────────┘
```

```
┌─────────────────────────────────────────────────────┐
│  Within first hour                                    │
│  • IV infusion 150 mL 3% hypertonic saline or *equivalent │
│    over 20 minutes                                    │
│  (* 2.7% 500 mL polyfuser available in Christie pharmacy/critical care) │
└─────────────────────────────────────────────────────┘
```

```
┌─────────────────────────────────────────────────────┐
│  Check serum sodium                                   │
│  • IV infusion 150 mL 3% hypertonic saline or *equivalent │
│    over 20 minutes while awaiting result              │
│  (* 2.7% 500 mL polyfuser available in Christie pharmacy/critical care) │
└─────────────────────────────────────────────────────┘
```

```
┌─────────────────────────────────────────────────────┐
│  • Repeat twice or until 5 mEq/L (5 mmol/L) increase in │
│    serum sodium                                       │
│  • Limit rise in serum sodium to 1 mEq/L (1 mmol/L) over 2 hours │
│    and <8 mEq/L (<8 mmol/L) over 24 hours             │
└─────────────────────────────────────────────────────┘
```

```
┌─────────────────────────────────────────────────────┐
│  Follow-up management after 5 mEq/L (5 mmol/L) increase │
│  in serum sodium and clinical improvement:            │
│  • Stop infusion of hypertonic saline                 │
│  • Keep IV line open (minimum volume of 0.9% saline)  │
│  • Start diagnosis-specific management (see algorithm 2) │
│  • Limit rise in serum sodium to 1 mEq/L (1 mmol/L) over 2 hours │
│    and <8 mEq/L (<8 mmol/L) over 24 hours             │
└─────────────────────────────────────────────────────┘
```

Ball S, Barth J, Levy M; Society for Endocrinology Clinical Committee. Society for Endocrinology Endocrine Emergency Guidance: emergency management of severe symptomatic hyponatraemia in adult patients. Endocr Connect. 2016;5(5):G4-G6.

The management of acute, life-threatening hyponatremia is depicted in *Figure 3*.

Immune Checkpoint Inhibitors

Immune checkpoint inhibitors are being used to treat an increasing number of cancers. Their use can be limited by immune-mediated complications, particularly with combination treatment. Immune-mediated endocrinopathies include hypophysitis, adrenalitis, thyroiditis, and diabetes mellitus. Deaths have been reported associated with checkpoint inhibitor–induced hypophysitis and adrenalitis. Diagnosis and management can be complicated by simultaneous multiorgan immune adverse effects (eg, colitis and hypophysitis).

Early recognition and appropriate management of endocrinopathies associated with immune checkpoint inhibitor therapy are essential. Patients should be educated about risk and symptoms of cortisol deficiency. Thyroid function should be checked with every cycle of immune checkpoint inhibitor therapy. Endocrine complications most commonly develop within 4 cycles of commencing treatment. However, endocrine complications are not a reason to discontinue immune checkpoint inhibitor therapy.

Thyroiditis

Thyroiditis in this setting tends to be transient, self-limiting hyperthyroidism that is often asymptomatic. Thionamide treatment (carbimazole/propylthiouracil) is of no value. Thyroiditis usually progresses to irreversible hypothyroidism. Cortisol deficiency must be excluded before levothyroxine is initiated. There have been reports of Graves hyperthyroidism and ophthalmopathy, thyroid storm, and myxedema.

Hypophysitis

Hypophysitis presents with mass effect and/or hormone deficiency, particularly hypoadrenalism. It inevitably results in permanent hypopituitarism. Hypophysitis frequently presents as isolated ACTH deficiency, and the differential diagnosis includes acute adrenalitis. A diagnostic pitfall is the use of exogenous glucocorticoid therapy (eg, inhaler), but in particular dexamethasone used as an antiemetic. Evaluation includes tests of basal pituitary function and pituitary MRI, with dynamic testing as indicated.

Management of hormone deficiency should be addressed as per standard protocols (except growth hormone therapy, which is likely contraindicated). Methylprednisolone may be beneficial for pressure effects such as optic chiasm compromise, visual field defects, cranial nerve palsies, and intractable headache. Methylprednisolone is not an appropriate treatment for acute cortisol deficiency secondary to ACTH deficiency alone. It is associated with worse long-term prognosis than physiological glucocorticoid replacement therapy.

Adrenalitis

Adrenalitis is rare and should be suspected if hyponatremia is present. If adrenalitis is suspected, ACTH, renin, and aldosterone should be measured. Fludrocortisone can be used in addition to glucocorticoid replacement therapy.

Clinical Case Vignette 2

A 43-year-old man with metastatic melanoma who has undergone 3 cycles of nivolumab therapy presents with a 4-week history of lethargy. His serum sodium concentration is 127 mEq/L (127 mmol/L). He is hypovolemic.

Other laboratory test results:

> Urinary sodium = 102 mEq/L (SI: 102 mmol/L)
> Random serum cortisol = 7.0 µg/dL (7.2-25.4 µg/dL)
>   (SI: 192 nmol/L [200-700 nmol/L])

A short cosyntropin-stimulation test gives the following results:

> 0 minutes   6.7 µg/dL (SI: 186 nmol/L)
> 30 minutes   5.7 µg/dL (SI: 157 nmol/L)
> 60 minutes   6.2 µg/dL (SI: 172 nmol/L)

He has no history of exogenous glucocorticoid use.

The working diagnosis is nivolumab-induced isolated ACTH deficiency. The patient continues nivolumab and starts hydrocortisone, 30 mg daily. Two weeks later, his condition is somewhat improved.

Laboratory test results:

> Serum sodium = 128 mEq/L (136-142 mEq/L)
>   (SI: 128 mmol/L [136-142 mmol/L])
> ACTH = 200 pg/mL (10-60 pg/mL)
>   (44.0 pmol/L [2.2-13.2 pmol/L])
> Renin activity = 19.8 nmol/L per h
>   (0.3-2.2 nmol/L per h)
> Aldosterone = <3.6 ng/dL (4-21 ng/dL)
>   (SI: <100 pmol/L [111.0-582.5 pmol/L])

What is this patient's diagnosis?
Answer: Nivolumab-induced primary adrenal failure, as evidenced by raised ACTH and renin

The patient's CT-PET imaging shows bilateral increased adrenal activity (*see image*).

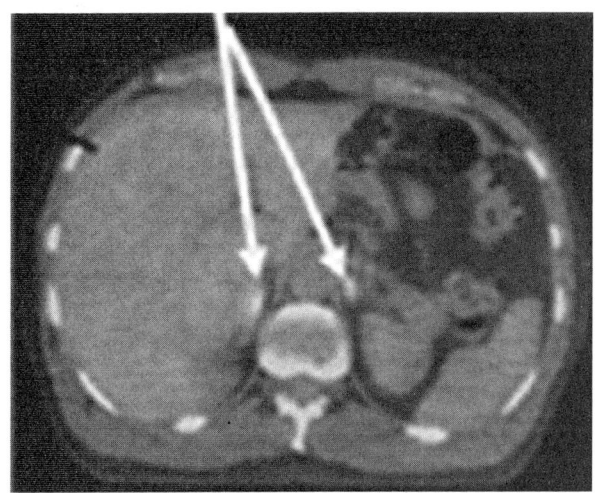

Fludrocortisone is started.

Laboratory test results:

> Serum sodium = 136 mEq/L (SI: 136 mmol/L)
> Renin activity = 1.6 nmol/L per h

Cancer Therapy–Related Bone Loss

Patients with nonmetastatic cancer are at risk for bone loss as a result of the disease process, local and systemic inflammation, and the treatment of the cancer (*Figure 4*). In particular, such therapy includes glucocorticoid and hormonal treatments (eg, GnRH agonists and chemotherapy-induced ovarian failure in premenopausal women, aromatase inhibitors in postmenopausal women, and antiandrogens in men with nonmetastatic prostate cancer).

Cancer therapy–related bone loss is more rapid than postmenopausal bone loss in women or normal age-related osteoporosis in men, with rates being up to 7-fold higher than that seen with normal aging.

Figure 4. Cancer Therapy–Related Bone Loss

At Risk

- Clinicians should be aware that patients with nonmetastatic cancer may have baseline risks for osteoporosis, as well as the added risks of treatment-related bone loss due to hypogonadism from endocrine therapy (ie, oophorectomy, GnRH agonists, chemotherapy-induced ovarian failure, aromatase inhibitors, anti-androgens), chemotherapy, or other cancer therapy-associated medications (ie, glucocorticoids).
- All patients should be counseled on intake of calcium and vitamin D, weight-bearing exercises, minimizing the risk of falls, and bone-healthy lifestyle and behaviors such as tobacco cessation and limiting alcohol consumption.
- Osteoporosis fracture risk assessment may include use of FRAX (www.sheffield.ac.uk/FRAX) or other tools.

Screening

When 1 or more risk factor for osteoporotic fracture is present, and there is consideration for use of a bone-modifying agent, then evaluate bone mineral density to further quantify fracture risk. The preferred assessment uses DXA of total spine, hip, and femoral neck.

All patients should be counseled on intake of calcium and vitamin D, weight-bearing exercises, minimizing the risk of falls, and bone-healthy lifestyle and behaviors such as tobacco cessation and limiting alcohol consumption.

Management

Deferral of Bone-Modifying Agent

If the bone density result does not demonstrate osteoporosis (or if there is not significant osteopenia with additional risk factors) and if FRAX calculation does not exceed 10-year risk of hip fracture of 3% or greater, or 10-year risk of non-hip fracture of 20%, and/or bone mineral density is not sufficiently low to trigger use of a bone-modifying agent, then repeat DXA in 2 years or in 1 year if medically indicated.

Initiation of Bone-Modifying Agent

Thresholds to initiate a bone-modifying agent include:

- FRAX (10-year risk of hip fracture of 3% or greater, or 10-year risk of non-hip fracture of 20%)
- The BMD (DXA) demonstrates osteoporosis or significant osteopenia with additional risk factors
- The clinical scenario indicates significant risk for osteoporotic fracture (such as history of prior osteoporotic fracture that has not been treated), then initiate a bone-modifying agent. Bisphosphonates (oral or IV) or denosumab are the preferred agents dosed for osteopenia or osteoporosis as clinically indicated.

Repeat DXA every 2 years or as clinically indicated.

Repeat DXA every 2 years or as clinically indicated.

Clinical Case Vignette 3

A woman has a history of breast cancer diagnosed at age 32 years (invasive ductal cancer with lymph node involvement; ER/PR+ve HER2 negative) treated with neoadjuvant chemotherapy (epirubicin, cyclophosphamide, docetaxel), mastectomy, axillary node clearance, and adjuvant radiotherapy. At age 33 years, she was amenorrheic after chemotherapy and started tamoxifen, 20 mg once daily. Her menstrual periods resumed.

Laboratory test results:

> Serum estradiol = 285 pg/mL (SI: 1047 pmol/L)
> LH = 12.0 mIU/mL (SI: 12.0 IU/L)
> FSH = 10.0 mIU/mL (SI: 10.0 IU/L)
> Serum estradiol measurement by liquid chromatography/tandem mass spectrometry = 297 pg/mL (SI: 1089 pmol/L)

Monthly goserelin is initiated at a dosage of 3.6 mg subcutaneously. Two months later, laboratory testing documents the following:

> Serum estradiol (immunoassay) = <19 pg/mL (SI: <70 pmol/L)
> Highly-sensitive estradiol by liquid chromatography/tandem mass spectrometry = 11 pg/mL (SI: 42 pmol/L)

Her regimen is switched from tamoxifen to exemestane, 25 mg once daily. Initial DXA scan is performed, and a second DXA is performed 2 years later (*see images and tables*).

The results of lumbar spine bone density from both DXA scans are shown (*see graph*), demonstrating that the patient's bone mineral density is worse now than at age 33 years.

FRAX is not applicable because she is younger than 40 years. She has no other risk factors for fracture.

Results of Initial DXA

Region	BMD, g/cm²	Z-Score
Anteroposterior spine (L1-L4)	0.971	−0.6
Femoral neck (left)	0.733	−0.9
Total hip (left)	0.901	−0.3

Results of Repeated DXA 2 Years Later

Region	BMD, g/cm²	Z-Score
Anteroposterior spine (L1-L4)	0.854	−1.7
Femoral neck (left)	0.685	−1.3
Total hip (left)	0.813	−1.0

Comparison of Both DXA Studies

Region	Exam Date	Age	BMD, g/cm²	T-Score	BMD Change vs Baseline	BMD Change vs Previous
Anteroposterior spine (L1-L4)	02.01.2019	35 years	0.854	−1.8	−12.1%*	−12.1%*
	08.11.2016	33 years	0.971	−0.7		
Total hip (left)	02.01.2019	35 years	0.813	−1.1	−9.8%*	−9.8%*
	08.11.2016	33 years	0.901	−0.3		

*Denotes significance at 95% confidence level; least significant change for anterioposterior spine = 0.022 g/cm²; least significant change for total hip = 0.027 g/cm².

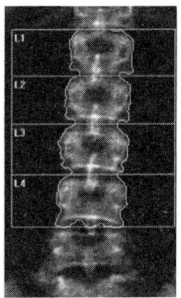 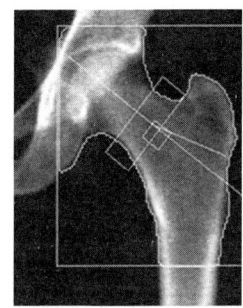

Initial DXA images.

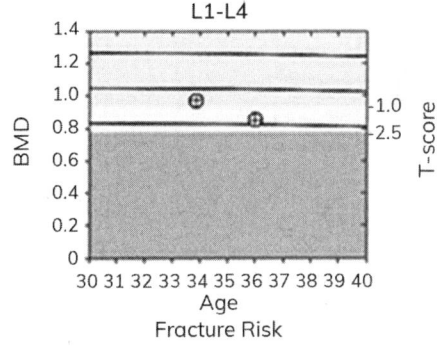

What is the best management for this patient?
Answer: Calcium, 700-1000 mg daily, and vitamin D, 800 IU daily

Lifestyle advice would include recommendations for exercise, smoking cessation (if applicable), and alcohol use. Screening for secondary causes is recommended. The risks and benefits of treatment with antiresorptive therapy (bisphosphonate vs denosumab) should be discussed with the patient, with particular emphasis on lack of data in young patients in this setting. Other issues to be discussed include the effects of tamoxifen on bone loss in premenopausal women and the measurement of serum estradiol levels in relation to tamoxifen, aromatase inhibitor, and fulvestrant by immunoassay and mass spectrometry.

References

1. Ball S, Barth J, Levy M; Society for Endocrinology Clinical Committee. Society for Endocrinology Endocrine Emergency Guidance: emergency management of severe symptomatic hyponatraemia in adult patients. *Endocr Connect*. 2016;5(5):G4-G6. PMID: 27935814

2. Higham CE, Olsson-Brown A, Carroll P, et al; Society for Endocrinology Clinical Committee. Society for Endocrinology Endocrine Emergency Guidance: acute management of the endocrine complications of checkpoint inhibitor therapy. *Endocr Connect*. 2018;7(7):G1-G7. PMID: 29930025

3. Shapiro CL, Van Poznak C, Lacchetti C, et al. Management of osteoporosis in survivors of adult cancers with nonmetastatic disease: ASCO clinical practice guideline. *J Oncol Pract*. 2019;37(3):2916-2946. PMID: 31532726

4. Owen LJ, Monaghan PJ, Armstrong A, et al. Oestradiol measurement during fulvestrant treatment for breast cancer. *Br J Cancer*. 2019;120(4):404-406. PMID: 30679781

Endocrine Effects of Immune Checkpoint Inhibitors: How to Screen and Treat

Simon H. S. Pearce, MD, FRCP. Translational and Clinical Research Institute, Newcastle University, United Kingdom; E-mail: simon.pearce@ncl.ac.uk

Learning Objectives

As a result of participating in this session, learners should be able to:

- Recognize and investigate the endocrine effects of immune checkpoint inhibitors.

- Manage the endocrine complications of immune checkpoint inhibitors.

Main Conclusions

Immune checkpoint inhibitors, including ipilimumab (anti-CTLA4), nivolumab, and pembrolizumab (anti-PD-1), are increasingly used to treat several advanced cancers: melanoma, non–small cell lung cancer, squamous cell head and neck cancer, renal and urothelial tumors, and Hodgkin lymphoma. Destructive thyroiditis, manifest as either transient hyperthyroidism or permanent hypothyroidism, is the most common endocrine adverse effect, typically seen after use of PD1/PD-L1 blockers. Hypophysitis, manifest as secondary hypoadrenalism and central hypothyroidism, is also relatively common with CTLA4 blockade. Fulminant type 1 diabetes, often with ketoacidosis, and primary adrenal insufficiency can also be observed but are more rare. Treatment is supportive with replacement of relevant hormones as clinically indicated. Recovery from endocrine dysfunction is not expected in most instances. Endocrine adverse effects should generally not lead to cessation of immune checkpoint inhibitor therapy, but a temporary pause may be appropriate if the patient is significantly unwell (eg, hypophysitis). Endocrinologists must liaise closely with oncologists to provide optimal care for this patient group.

Significance of the Clinical Problem

Ipilimumab, the first immune checkpoint inhibitor, was introduced to the market in 2011 and has revolutionized the prognosis of patients with disseminated malignant melanoma. Since then, 6 additional checkpoint inhibitors have been licensed. In addition to treating melanoma, this class of drugs is now indicated for advanced renal and urothelial cancer, advanced Hodgkin lymphoma, non–small cell lung cancer, squamous cell head and neck cancer, and mismatch repair/microsatellite instability tumors (ie, Lynch syndrome). These drugs inhibit a series of molecules that act as brakes on the normal immune activation process, including CTLA4 (cytotoxic T-lymphocyte antigen 4 [ipilimumab and tremelimumab]), PD-1 (programmed death-1 [nivolumab, pembrolizumab]), and PD-L1 (programmed death ligand-1 [atezolizumab, durvalumab, and avelumab]).[1,2] They are all human or humanized monoclonal antibodies and are generally administered in cycles, at 3-week intervals.

Cancer cells use positive molecular interactions with these lymphocyte cell-surface receptors to evade detection by the healthy immune system.

These checkpoint inhibitor monoclonal antibodies block these "evasive mechanisms," augmenting the natural immune responses against cancerous cells, thus harnessing the patient's endogenous immune response to attack the tumor and metastases. The transformative nature of these compounds as cancer therapy means that they are being increasingly used, and there are currently more than 200 open clinical trials with these agents. Therefore, the number of cancers for which they are indicated is certain to increase. Although initially used as sole agents, many trials now show that combination immune checkpoint inhibition (eg, nivolumab and ipilimumab) can lead to more complete and durable antitumor immune responses. As an adverse effect of this immune activation, immune-mediated endocrine dysfunction is observed in approximately 15% of patients treated with a single agent and in 20% to 30% of those treated with a combination of 2 checkpoint inhibitors.

While thyroid dysfunction is the most common problem that occurs during checkpoint inhibitor therapy, pituitary involvement, primary adrenal insufficiency, and type 1 diabetes may all cause acute and serious decompensation, requiring urgent intervention (*Table*). These toxicities may also be complicated by serious nonendocrine autoimmune disorders, including pneumonitis, colitis, hepatitis, encephalitis, myasthenia, and many others.

Barriers to Optimal Practice

- Close liaison is required between the oncologist and the endocrine team to first recognize that a deterioration is due to an immune-related endocrine complication and second to ensure optimal ongoing management.

- Affected patients often carry a high tumor burden, and nonspecific deterioration, including weight loss, poor appetite, lethargy, and hypotension may be misattributed to advancing cancer rather than to a readily treatable endocrinopathy, particularly primary or secondary adrenal insufficiency.

- The transformative nature of these treatments means that development of a treatable endocrine adverse effect should not routinely lead to discontinuation of the checkpoint inhibitor therapy.

Table. Prevalence of Endocrinopathies During Immune Checkpoint Inhibitor Therapy

Target	Drug	Hypothyroidism	Thyrotoxicosis	Pituitary Dysfunction	Primary Adrenal Insufficiency	Type 1 Diabetes
CTLA4	Ipilimumab	3.8%	1.4%	5.6%	1.4%	-
	Tremelimumab	-	-	1.8%	1.3%	-
PD-I	Nivolumab	8%	2.8%	0.5%	2.0%	2.0%
	Pembrolizumab	8.5%	3.7%	1.1%	0.8%	0.4%
PD-L1	Atezolizumab	6%	-	-	-	1.4%
	Durvalumab	4.7%	-	-	-	-
	Avelumab	5.5%	2.3%	-	1.1%	1.1%
CTLA4 + PD-1	Combination	10%-15%	10%	8%-10%	5%-7%	2.0%

Data adapted from de Filette J, Andreescu CE, Cools F, Bravenboer B, Velkeniers B. A systematic review and meta-analysis of endocrine-related adverse events associated with immune checkpoint inhibitors. *Horm Metab Res.* 2019;51(3):145-156.[1]

Strategies for Diagnosis, Therapy, and/or Management

Thyroid Dysfunction

Thyroid dysfunction is the most common endocrine adverse effect of immune checkpoint inhibitors. All patients should have serum TSH and free T_4 measured before starting checkpoint inhibitor treatment and with every cycle of therapy.

Thyrotoxicosis

Thyrotoxicosis occurs most frequently with the combination of either of the PD-1 blockers, nivolumab or pembrolizumab, with ipilimumab in approximately 10% of cases, compared with 3% to 4% with a PD-1 blocker alone. It is one of the earliest immune complications, with onset as soon as 3 weeks after treatment initiation, and it typically occurs during the third or fourth cycle of treatment (8-12 weeks). A rapid-onset painless thyroiditis occurs, characterized by 3 to 8 weeks of thyrotoxicosis followed by permanent hypothyroidism in approximately 50%, implying that this is frequently an irreversible destructive process.[2-5] The thyrotoxic phase is usually mild and best managed supportively with β-adrenergic blockers, as antithyroid drugs are not expected to work. A small number of patients presenting with thyroid storm have been reported and this should be managed with high-dosage glucocorticoids. Rarely, thyrotoxic patients are positive for TSH-receptor–stimulating antibodies and TSH-receptor antibody concentrations should be routinely measured to exclude Graves disease: these patients will have a prolonged course of hyperthyroidism unless they receive antithyroid drugs. Thyrotoxicosis is much less frequent with CTLA4 blockers than with PD-1/PD-L1 blockers, and Graves disease is as likely as transient thyroiditis in this situation.[5] In addition, many patients have received high loads of iodinated radiographic contrast media during staging CT imaging, and a transient iodine-induced thyroiditis may practically be indistinguishable from destructive thyroiditis in the acute phase. The initial management is identical, but a full recovery of thyroid function would be expected with the former, whereas long-term hypothyroidism is expected in the latter. Nuclide imaging is only warranted if there is a preexisting thyroid condition or clinically palpable thyroid nodules.

Hypothyroidism

Hypothyroidism is a later complication than thyrotoxicosis, typically occurring after 4 to 6 months of treatment. Primary, destructive thyroiditis is most common, but a significant proportion of affected patients develop central hypothyroidism as a result of hypophysitis. As in other situations, it is not necessary to treat patients with asymptomatic mild/subclinical primary hypothyroidism with serum TSH concentrations in the range of 4 to 10 mIU/L and normal serum free T_4 levels, but treatment is indicated once the TSH concentration rises to 10 mIU/L or higher. Primary hypothyroidism should be assumed to be permanent. Patients receiving CTLA4 blockade are at particular risk of central hypothyroidism due to hypophysitis, which presents with declining serum free T_4 concentrations in the context of normal or low TSH. It is important to recognize this, as it should immediately trigger testing for adrenocortical insufficiency, which may coexist with other pituitary insufficiencies. It is mandatory to screen for and treat hypoadrenalism before starting levothyroxine replacement. There can occasionally be diagnostic difficulty in distinguishing central hypothyroidism from sick euthyroid syndrome (nonthyroidal illness) in patients with high tumor burden. However, serum free T_4 tends to be relatively preserved in sick euthyroid syndrome and is likely to be lower in central hypothyroidism.

Pituitary Dysfunction

Pituitary dysfunction is most frequently seen with ipilimumab (~5%) and other CTLA4-blocking agents. Headache and fatigue are the earliest symptoms and are typically found after 3 to 5 cycles (9-16 weeks). It is more common in older men (male:female, 3:1) and with higher dosages of ipilimumab (10 mg/kg). Hormonal deficiencies owing to infiltrative hypophysitis are expected (85%-90%), but vision disturbance due to mass effect has very rarely been reported. ACTH deficiency leading to secondary adrenal insufficiency is the most common manifestation and requires urgent treatment. Central hypothyroidism and hypogonadotropic hypogonadism also occur in 70% to 80% of cases. The presentation of hormonal deficiency is typically nonspecific, with lethargy, weight loss, nausea, vomiting, poor appetite, hypotension, and hyponatremia.[2,4,7] Confusion or hallucinations may be prominent. Affected patients need pituitary MRI whether they present with mass effects or hormonal dysfunction, as other causes of pituitary failure (particularly metastasis) must be excluded. A moderately enlarged and bright pituitary is found and although stalk thickening is seen in 50% of cases, diabetes insipidus is very rare. In 20% of patients, the MRI shows no pituitary abnormality. Rarely, patients present with optic nerve compression causing visual disturbance, and they should be treated with high-dosage glucocorticoids such as methylprednisolone or dexamethasone until vision is restored. There is little evidence of benefit from high-dosage steroids in other circumstances. If the patient is unwell, a random cortisol concentration should be measured, and parenteral hydrocortisone, 100 mg, should immediately be administered and continued at a dosage of at least 50 mg every 6 hours. Replacement of levothyroxine and other anterior pituitary hormones should be undertaken as the patient recovers. Secondary adrenal insufficiency should be assumed to be permanent, although rare cases of recovery have been documented. Hypothyroidism and hypogonadism may recover in around 50% of patients and retesting after 6 months treatment is worthwhile.

Primary Adrenal Insufficiency

Primary adrenal insufficiency seems to be rare with single-agent checkpoint inhibition, but combination CTLA4/PD-1 blockade therapy multiplies the risks to encompass 5% to 7% of patients. It typically presents after 4 or more cycles of therapy (12 weeks onward) with fatigue, hypotension, loss of appetite, weight loss, nausea/vomiting, hyponatremia, and hyperkalemia. An early morning serum cortisol value can be diagnostic, with a formal cosyntropin-stimulation test only if the result is not clear. It is also important to measure ACTH to distinguish primary adrenal failure from central ACTH deficiency: first, because a primary adrenal insufficiency diagnosis heralds mineralocorticoid replacement, as well as glucocorticoid replacement, and second, because in the presence of a normal or low ACTH, investigations for hypophysitis (including testing of other pituitary axes and pituitary MRI) are needed. The differential diagnosis of primary adrenal insufficiency includes bilateral adrenal metastases, as well as hemorrhage and drug-induced adrenal insufficiency, so cross-sectional imaging (usually CT) should be undertaken. The adrenals may appear hyperplastic on scanning. Treatment with hydrocortisone, 15 to 20 mg daily, in divided doses and fludrocortisone, 50 to 300 mcg daily, is expected to be lifelong with no reports of recovery thus far.

Type 1 Diabetes Mellitus

Type 1 diabetes is rare and seems to be exclusively seen during PD-1/PD-L1 blockade. A "fulminant" pattern of type 1 diabetes is the rule with a short interval between the onset of symptoms and presentation with ketoacidosis, reflecting rapid destruction of insulin-secreting β cells, meaning that up to 70% of affected patients present with ketoacidosis. Onset can be very early, within 1 or 2 weeks of therapy, although the average is after 4 cycles (12 weeks). Plasma or urine C-peptide levels are low and islet-cell antibodies (glutamic acid decarboxylase, IA-2) are positive in approximately 50% of patients. Hyperglycemia is more severe than predicted by hemoglobin A_{1c} levels, reflecting the rapid onset of disease. It is good practice to warn patients about the possibility of developing polyuria and thirst, and that they must seek evaluation immediately if this occurs. Insulin must be started immediately to preempt ketoacidosis. Lifelong insulin dependence is the rule and the chances of recovery are negligible.

Parathyroid Dysfunction

There are a small number of case reports of hypoparathyroidism in patients receiving immune checkpoint inhibition. It is too early to be sure there is a real causative relation, but it remains a distinct possibility.

Nonendocrine Considerations

Several studies now show that the development of immune-related endocrine adverse events during checkpoint inhibitor therapy is associated with a positive survival advantage from the original tumor.[8] This stands to reason, in that a more aggressive autoimmune response is expected to correlate with a deeper antitumor immune response. With neat circularity, the development of vitiligo in patients with melanoma undergoing checkpoint blockade is associated with a better prognosis.[9] Many of these endocrine adverse effects are manageable with observation alone (thyrotoxicosis) or one or more hormone replacement therapies. Furthermore, the endocrine dysfunction is already irreversible at presentation and will not be worsened by ongoing checkpoint blockade therapy. This leads to the logic that in most patients experiencing endocrine adverse effects from checkpoint inhibitor therapy, the checkpoint blockade should be continued, either uninterrupted in the case of hypothyroidism, or following a short period to allow physical recuperation following a diagnosis of adrenal insufficiency, hypopituitarism, or type 1 diabetes. Close liaison between the endocrinologist and oncologist can often lead to early resumption of checkpoint blockade and ultimately improve the prognosis of this patient group.

Clinical Case Vignettes
Case 1

A 53-year-old man presents to the emergency department with an 18-hour history of nausea, 1 episode of vomiting, headache, and "nearly passing out" when moving from bed to the bathroom. His partner thinks he is now confused. Ten weeks ago, he started receiving combination ipilimumab and nivolumab therapy for advanced melanoma (this is now his third cycle). For the last 2 weeks, he has been feeling fatigued and "under the weather."

On physical examination, he is pale and drowsy. Glasgow Coma Scale score is 12. He has cool peripheries, blood pressure of 88/58 mm Hg, pulse rate of 102 beats/min and regular, temperature of 98.4°F (36.9°C), oxygen saturation of 95% on air, and respiratory rate of 22 breaths/min.

Neutropenic sepsis is suspected, and blood is drawn and cultures are sent. One liter of saline is administered stat, as well as intravenous tazocin, but 1 hour later he is still hypotensive with a Glasgow Come Scale score of 10.

Laboratory test results:

> White blood cell count =
> 12,300/μL (4500-11,000/μL)
> (SI: 12.3 × 10⁹/L [4.5-11.0 × 10⁹/L]) with mild neutrophilia
> C-reactive protein = 23 mg/L (0.8-3.1 mg/L)
> (SI: 219.05 nmol/L [7.62-29.52 nmol/L])
> Sodium = 126 mEq/L (136-142 mEq/L)
> (SI: 126 mmol/L [136-142 mmol/L])
> Potassium = 4.2 mEq/L (3.5-5.0 mEq/L)
> (SI: 4.2 mmol/L [3.5-5.0 mmol/L])

The endocrine fellow is called to advise about the hyponatremia and hypotension.

Which of the following is the immediate priority for management?

A. Measure serum cortisol, aldosterone, and ACTH

B. Measure serum cortisol and give intravenous hydrocortisone, 100 mg stat

C. Measure urine sodium and urine osmolality

D. Order pituitary MRI and measure pituitary antibodies

E. Perform a short 250-mcg cosyntropin-stimulation test

Answer: B) Measure serum cortisol and give intravenous hydrocortisone, 100 mg stat

This patient may have either primary or secondary adrenal insufficiency associated with checkpoint inhibitor therapy. Three to 6 cycles would be the typical time for this to present, and the associated headache and confusion (plus normal potassium) lead to a high index of suspicion that he has hypophysitis with secondary adrenal insufficiency. Measuring serum cortisol and giving intravenous hydrocortisone, 100 mg stat (Answer B) is correct because he is sick and should be treated immediately with parenteral hydrocortisone. Measure serum cortisol, aldosterone, and ACTH (Answer A), ordering MRI pituitary and measuring pituitary antibodies (Answer D), and performing a short 250-mcg cosyntropin-stimulation test (Answer E) might be correct if he was not ill. When he is better, a sample should be taken for matched cortisol and ACTH to elucidate whether the cause is primary or secondary adrenal insufficiency. Cosyntropin-stimulation testing would also be reasonable if the morning cortisol is equivocal. Additional testing for TSH, free T_4, and testosterone will be needed if ACTH is normal or low. Confusion is not unusual and might also lead to an early cranial MRI, which may disclose radiologic evidence of hypophysitis. Measuring urine sodium and urine osmolality (Answer C) is wrong because he is obviously hypotensive and hypovolemic, so you already know the answer (low urine sodium, high osmolality).

Case 2

A 64-year-old woman is found to have abnormal thyroid function (TSH = <0.05 mIU/L, free T_4 = 2.0 ng/dL [26 pmol/L]; free T_3 = 4.6 pg/mL [7.0 pmol/L]) on routine bloodwork before her fourth cycle of pembrolizumab for non–small cell lung cancer. She has been feeling well and reports no weight loss, palpitation, or heat intolerance. On physical examination, her pulse rate is 84 beats/min and regular and there is no goiter or eye signs.

What further action should be taken?

A. Cancel this cycle of pembrolizumab until further test results are available

B. Measure TSH-receptor antibodies and perform ^{99}Tc thyroid uptake scan

C. Start methimazole, 15 mg daily

D. Start propranolol, 80 mg daily

E. Order repeated thyroid function tests in 2 weeks with TSH-receptor antibodies

Answer: E) Order repeated thyroid function tests in 2 weeks with TSH-receptor antibodies

This patient had no symptoms and was only mildly thyrotoxic, so it is safe to monitor the situation (Answer E). Two weeks later, repeated tests showed TSH-receptor antibodies less than 1.0 U/L, TSH of 4.6 mIU/L, and free T_4 of 1.1 ng/dL (14.1 pmol/L) showing spontaneous improvement. Before her sixth cycle, her TSH was 39.0 mIU/L and free T_4 was 0.6 ng/dL (7.9 pmol/L). Levothyroxine, 75 mcg daily, was started. Thyrotoxicosis is frequently mild, and its natural history is spontaneous; permanent hypothyroidism occurs in approximately 50% of cases. Cancelling this cycle of pembrolizumab (Answer A) is wrong because she is not ill enough to interrupt the chemotherapy that is a life-prolonging treatment for her. Measuring TSH-receptor antibodies and performing a ^{99}Tc thyroid uptake scan (Answer B) is not wholly wrong, but it will be a waste of resources to order the scan because it would not distinguish between immune-mediated thyroiditis and iodine contrast load. It would be appropriate to measure TSH-receptor antibodies to rule out Graves disease. Starting methimazole (Answer C) is incorrect, as it will not improve thyrotoxicosis in thyroiditis; it will just make any rebound hypothyroidism more prolonged or severe. Starting propranolol (Answer D) is wrong because she is asymptomatic.

References

1. de Filette J, Andreescu CE, Cools F, Bravenboer B, Velkeniers B. A systematic review and meta-analysis of endocrine-related adverse events associated with immune checkpoint inhibitors. *Horm Metab Res.* 2019;51(3):145-156. PMID: 30861560

2. Chang LS, Barroso-Sousa R, Tolaney SM, Hodi FS, Kaiser UB, Min L. Endocrine toxicity of cancer immunotherapy targeting immune checkpoints. *Endocr Rev.* 2019;40(1):17-65. PMID: 30184160

3. Morganstein DL, Lai Z, Spain L, et al. Thyroid abnormalities following the use of cytotoxic T-lymphocyte antigen-4 and programmed death receptor protein-1 inhibitors in the treatment of melanoma. *Clin Endocrinol (Oxf).* 2017;86(4):614-620. PMID: 28028828

4. Ryder M, Callahan M, Postow MA, Wolchok J, Fagin JA. Endocrine-related adverse events following ipilimumab in patients with advanced melanoma: a comprehensive retrospective review from a single institution. *Endocr Relat Cancer.* 2014;21(2):371-381. PMID: 24610577

5. Higham CE, Olsson-Brown A, Carroll P, et al; Society for Endocrinology Clinical Committee. Society for Endocrinology Endocrine Emergency Guidance: acute management of the endocrine complications of checkpoint inhibitor therapy. *Endocr Connect.* 2018;7(7):G1-G7. PMID: 29930025

6. Gan EH, Mitchell AL, Plummer R, Pearce S, Perros P. Tremelimumab-induced Graves hyperthyroidism. *Eur Thyroid J.* 2017;6(3):167-170. PMID: 28785544

7. Joshi MN, Whitelaw BC, Palomar MT, Wu Y, Carroll PV. Immune checkpoint inhibitor-related hypophysitis and endocrine dysfunction: clinical review. *Clin Endocrinol (Oxf).* 2016;85(3):331-339. PMID: 26998595

8. Osorio JC, Ni A, Chaft JE, et al. Antibody-mediated thyroid dysfunction during T-cell checkpoint blockade in patients with non-small-cell lung cancer. *Ann Oncol.* 2017;28(3):583-589. PMID: 27998967

9. Nakamura Y, Tanaka R, Asami Y, et al. Correlation between vitiligo occurrence and clinical benefit in advanced melanoma patients treated with nivolumab: a multi-institutional retrospective study. *J Dermatol.* 2017;44(2):117-122. PMID: 27510892

A Little Help From My Friends: The Endocrinology–Psychiatry Interface—How Do We Help Each Other?

Elizabeth J. Murphy, MD, DPhil. Department of Medicine, Division of Endocrinology UCSF and San Francisco General Hospital, San Francisco, CA; E-mail: lisa.murphy@ucsf.edu

Erick Hung, MD. Department of Psychiatry, UCSF, San Francisco, CA; E-mail: erick.hung@ucsf.edu

Learning Objectives

As a result of participating in this session, learners should be able to:

- Develop an approach to addressing hyperprolactinemia in psychiatric patients.

- Develop an approach to addressing the metabolic effects of antipsychotic medications.

- Describe the potential risks and benefits of the use of liothyronine (T_3) for refractory severe depression.

- Engage in meaningful communication with psychiatric colleagues around common areas of clinical overlap.

Main Conclusions

Hyperprolactinemia is commonly seen in patients taking antipsychotic medications. In most cases, the patient has no underlying pituitary disorder. Treatment with a dopamine agonist with a sole focus of reducing the prolactin concentration may result inadvertent worsening of the patient's psychiatric condition. Careful consideration should be given in these situations to the psychiatric needs of the patient, clinical manifestation of the high prolactin that needs to be addressed (eg, galactorrhea or hypogonadism), and whether or not there is underlying pituitary pathology.

Weight gain, glucose abnormalities, and dyslipidemia are common adverse effects of antipsychotic medication use. Providers need to be on the lookout and monitor for these effects in patients started on a new medication. Treatment focuses on managing the various risk factors and changing the antipsychotic treatment if feasible.

Depression is a life-threatening condition. Despite limited data on its clinical efficacy, liothyronine (T_3) remains a popular add-on treatment in combination with traditional antidepressants for refractory depression. Monitoring its use with appropriate thyroid function and DXA testing is a crucial safety consideration.

Significance of the Clinical Problem

The complex interplay between endocrine hormones and psychiatric disease has been recognized for more than a century, dating back to the original descriptions of disorders such as hypothyroidism and Cushing syndrome. Prior to surgical options, the leading cause of death for patients with Cushing syndrome was suicide. The wide range of psychiatric manifestations of both hypothyroidism and hyperthyroidism is well known, and approximately 1 in 20 adults in the United States has some abnormality in thyroid function.

The complexity of these relationships has been further exacerbated by medication adverse effects. It is estimated that 1 in 6 adults in the United States is taking a psychiatric medication or sedative. These medications can lead to a host of adverse endocrine effects including weight gain, insulin resistance, pancreatic failure, diabetes mellitus, and hyperprolactinemia. Moreover, there is a strong association between depression and obesity and diabetes complicating treatment.

It is critical for optimal management in these overlap situations to understand the risks and benefits for both psychiatric and endocrine outcomes. During this session, several common medical scenarios from both an endocrine and psychiatric perspective will be discussed, and suggestions will be provided regarding optimal provider communication to allow for thoughtful clinical decision making.

Barriers to Optimal Practice

- There is a shortage of both mental health providers and endocrinologists.

- Opportunities are often rare for easy communication between endocrinologists and psychiatrists, which makes collaborative decision making around treatment difficult.

- Widespread use and, at times, overuse of atypical antipsychotic medications for non–FDA-approved indications leads to unnecessary adverse events.

Strategies for Diagnosis, Therapy, and/or Management

Antipsychotic Therapy Overview

In 2013, it was estimated that 1 in 6 adults in the United States was taking a psychiatric medication or sedative, speaking both to the prevalence of psychiatric disorders, but also to the opportunity for unintended adverse events related to their treatment. One of the classes of medications with the most significant adverse effect profile is the antipsychotics. These medications, available since the 1950s, are the mainstay treatment for schizophrenia, but are also used to treat a host of other disorders. The atypical or second-generation antipsychotic agents became available starting in the 1970s with clozapine, which was found to cause agranulocytosis. During the 1990s and 2000s, olanzapine, risperidone, quetiapine, ziprasidone, aripiprazole, and paliperidone were introduced with the promise of reduced extrapyramidal adverse effects and improved clinical efficacy.

Most antipsychotic agents work in part as dopamine receptor (D_2) antagonists. Thus, it is not surprising that hyperprolactinemia is a common adverse effect. The second-generation drugs were designed to also target 5-HT_2, histamine, and acetylcholine receptors. It is these actions that are thought to contribute to the significant metabolic adverse effects seen with these agents. These effects include weight gain, metabolic syndrome, type 2 diabetes, diabetic ketoacidosis, pancreatic failure, and dyslipidemia.

Antipsychotic Agents and Hyperprolactinemia

The potency of antipsychotic medications blocking the D_2 receptor is highly variable, resulting in significant variation in inducing hyperprolactinemia. First-generation antipsychotics and some second-generation agents such as risperidone and paliperidone result in frequent prolactin elevation in 90% or more of patients, while other second-generation agents such as aripiprazole and quetiapine have a minimal effect on prolactin concentrations.[1-3] These effects on prolactin secretion are seen in patients without underlying prolactinomas.

In addition to galactorrhea in women, the primary adverse effects of hyperprolactinemia are related to subsequent hypogonadism. This includes amenorrhea in premenopausal women and low testosterone and libido in men, which importantly contribute to bone loss. While there have been other postulated effects of hyperprolactinemia, none have been firmly established in human studies. Therefore, while it is important to monitor patients for symptoms of hyperprolactinemia such as galactorrhea, amenorrhea, and decreased libido, we do not recommend routinely checking prolactin levels in patients on these medications.

The Endocrine Society guidelines[4] recommend that patients with suspected drug-induced hyperprolactinemia stop the offending medication and recheck prolactin after 3 days. If prolactin has not normalized, MRI is recommended. Unfortunately, stopping an antipsychotic medication can be very difficult. If stopping an antipsychotic agent is not an option, it might be possible to switch to aripiprazole, which has both dopamine agonist and antagonist properties, making it the atypical antipsychotic of choice in situations of problematic hyperprolactinemia. But again, for a patient well-controlled from a psychiatric perspective, medication changes come with what may be unacceptable risks. No change should ever be made without careful consultation with the patient's mental health care provider. If a medication change is not possible, the Endocrine Society guidelines recommend MRI. However, in the case of some antipsychotic agents that can result in prolactin elevation in close to 100% of patients, this would result in significant unnecessary testing leading to incidental findings and increased morbidity. In these cases, the degree of prolactin elevation can help guide next steps. It is often thought that medication-induced hyperprolactinemia is limited to prolactin elevations less than 100 ng/mL (<4.3 nmol/L). That said, risperidone and phenothiazines

can result in prolactin elevations well over 200 ng/mL (>8.7 nmol/L). In patients on an antipsychotic agent known to increase prolactin who have a prolactin concentration less than 100 ng/mL (<4.3 nmol/L), many clinicians would not routinely recommend MRI. To rule out hypothyroidism as a contributor and to assess another aspect of pituitary function, measuring TSH and free T_4 would be reasonable. For patients with higher prolactin elevations, especially those on risperidone or paliperidone, it may also be appropriate to defer MRI, especially if a temporal link with the hyperprolactinemia and starting the medication can be established. But for the remainder of patients, MRI is reasonable to rule out underlying pituitary pathology.

Treatment

Treatment of antipsychotic-induced hyperprolactinemia is focused on symptoms rather than on correcting the abnormal lab value. In an asymptomatic patient with regular menses and gonadal function, no treatment is indicated. If the patient is experiencing hypogonadism, replacement therapy with estrogen or testosterone is appropriate for symptoms and for bone protection. If possible, from a psychiatric perspective, switching to a different antipsychotic agent or lowering the dosage of the current medication may also be effective options. While treatment with dopamine agonists such as cabergoline or bromocriptine can normalize prolactin in some patients, use of these agents should be avoided because activating the dopamine receptors that antipsychotic medications are designed to block can lead to severe exacerbations of the underlying psychiatric condition.[4]

While most cases of prolactin elevation with antipsychotic medications are medication related without pituitary pathology, it is also possible to have an underlying prolactinoma. There is no clear evidence to suggest antipsychotic medication use causes prolactinomas; however, it may be that an underlying prolactinoma is exacerbated by these medications. For microadenomas, treatment is the same as it is with purely medication-induced hyperprolactinemia. In addition, at least initially, an annual pituitary MRI should be obtained to assess for tumor growth. If a patient has a macroadenoma or the tumor is showing growth, an attempt should be made to switch to aripiprazole, which has resulted in excellent responses in terms of improved prolactin and lack of tumor growth,[1,4] There are also case reports of treatment with cabergoline or bromocriptine in addition to continued use of an antipsychotic agent, but as mentioned above, this runs the risk of exacerbating the underlying psychiatric disorder and should only be done in very close consultation with the patient's psychiatrist. If the medical therapies are not possible or not successful, surgical resection can be considered for macroadenomas.

Antipsychotic Agents and Metabolic Alterations

At baseline, patients with schizophrenia have an increased risk of obesity, diabetes mellitus, and cardiovascular disease.[5] Second-generation antipsychotic medications have a whole host of metabolic effects that can exacerbate that underlying risk.[1-3,5-7] In 2003, the FDA required a warning label for these adverse events, and in 2004, the American Diabetes Association, American Psychiatric Association, and North American Association for the Study of Obesity teamed up to create a guidance document recommending routine testing of glucose and lipids in patients on these medications.[8]

As with hyperprolactinemia, there is significant variation in the degree of metabolic effects seen with the different antipsychotic agents. While it was initially thought these effects were limited to only a few medications, it is now recognized to a certain extent they all can have unwanted metabolic effects, including weight gain, glucose dysregulation (including diabetes and diabetic ketoacidosis), hypertriglyceridemia, and metabolic syndrome. Evidence suggests olanzapine, clozapine, zotepine, and chlorpromazine result in some of the

largest weight gains,[2,3,5,6] which can be rapid and significant (>7% of baseline weight). While there is clear evidence for a class effect on the other metabolic effects, clear and consistent comparative data between medications for these effects are lacking. As with weight gain, these effects can be rapid, with studies showing a doubling in triglycerides in 2 weeks and acute decompensation with diabetic ketoacidosis.[5] An important observation is the heterogeneity of effects across individuals. It appears that as of yet, not well-understood underlying genetic factors significantly contribute to the degree of metabolic effects seen in a given individual.[3,5,7] For example, weight gain of 30% or more of body weight is not uncommon in some patients, but for other patients on the same medication weight gain may be minimal.

The mechanism for these metabolic changes is likely multifactorial.[5,7] Effects on central neurotransmitters no doubt affect appetite, leading to weight gain which in turn leads to increased insulin resistance, dyslipidemia, and potentially diabetes. While no doubt impacted by weight gain, glucose dysregulation also occurs independent of weight gain with an increased incidence of diabetic ketoacidosis in patients without weight gain. There is evidence for direct effects on insulin signaling and glucose transport, including effects on skeletal muscle glucose transporters impairing glucose effectiveness and direct effects on the pancreatic β cells impairing insulin secretion. The latter is thought to contribute to the increased incidence of diabetic ketoacidosis.[7] Second-generation antipsychotic agents are also thought to stimulate AMP-kinase in the hypothalamus leading to downstream changes such as effects on hepatic gluconeogenesis. It also has been proposed that changes in the gut microbiome and epigenetics may contribute to these changes.[5,7]

Management of Metabolic Changes
In addition to the guideline from the 2004 consensus conference, almost 20 other monitoring guidelines exist with inconsistent recommendations[9] on appropriate monitoring of patients to catch the unintended metabolic

effects early. Unfortunately, data suggest those monitoring guidelines are not consistently followed, perhaps in part due to inconsistencies in recommendations and poor patient follow-up in this population. There remains much that can be done with respect to better screening and evaluation. Providers treating patients who are started on new antipsychotic medications or have a medication change should be on the lookout for any acute metabolic changes. Close monitoring for changes in BMI and new-onset diabetes is important, although recommendations for the timing of these evaluations vary. Given the significant patient variability and what can be very rapid-onset changes, earlier initial evaluation (eg, 4-6 weeks after start of treatment) maybe most appropriate with less frequent follow-up thereafter.

For patients who do experience metabolic derangements from these medications, the initial treatment should be a change in medication, if possible, to an agent with a potentially better adverse effect profile. Ziprasidone and aripiprazole are thought to be the most weight-neutral options with less diabetes-related adverse events than with other antipsychotic agents.[5,6] In addition to lifestyle modification, other therapeutic options that have had success include traditional treatments such as metformin and GLP-1 receptor agonists for diabetes and weight gain, as well as statin therapy for dyslipidemia. Recognizing these metabolic adverse events early is probably the most important intervention, which allows for subsequent treatment and medication adjustments.

Liothyronine as Augmentation Therapy for Depression

Major depressive disorder can be fatal, with suicide currently the 10th leading cause of death in adults in North America. Strategies for treatment-refractory depression include augmentation therapy with nonantidepressant medications such as liothyronine (T_3).[10] Numerous studies have examined liothyronine as augmentation therapy given as an add-on after a trial of a traditional antidepressant such as a tricyclic antidepressant or selective serotonin reuptake inhibitor. Older uncontrolled, nonblinded studies suggest there may be improved response rates with liothyronine in combination with tricyclic antidepressants, although liothyronine toxicity is common. Data for liothyronine in combination with selective serotonin reuptake inhibitors show mixed results. Perhaps the greatest enthusiasm for liothyronine use came after results of the Sequenced Treatment Alternatives to Relieve Depression (STAR*D) trial published in 2006.[11] This 35 million-dollar, multiarmed study assessed the effectiveness of medications or cognitive therapy in treatment of refractory depression. One study arm compared augmentation therapy with lithium vs liothyronine after 2 failed trials of other medications. The authors concluded that, "T_3 has slight advantages over lithium in effectiveness and tolerability. T_3 also offers the advantages of ease of use and lack of need for blood level monitoring." Limitations of the study were that it was nonblinded, was without a placebo control, and had no assessment of thyroid function before or during treatment. An assessment of thyroid function exploring a correlation between TSH suppression and efficacy could have been very informative in guiding subsequent studies and therapy. Despite limitations on the data supporting liothyronine use, psychiatric textbooks and the American Psychiatric Association major depressive disorder guidelines in 2010 recommend the use of liothyronine for refractory depression without recommendations for monitoring thyroid function.[12] The dosing recommendation is typically 25 mcg daily increased to 50 mcg daily after a week, but it is also suggested in the psychiatric literature that dosages above 50 mcg daily may be appropriate, with some publications citing dosages as high as 150 mcg daily.

More recently, it has been recognized that many psychiatrists and endocrinologists feel uncomfortable treating euthyroid patients with liothyronine without adequate monitoring.[11-12] Subsequent guidelines now recommend safety monitoring. The psychiatric recommendation for efficacy is a TSH value at the lower limit of the normal range or lower in the absence of symptoms. It is also recommended to assess bone mineral density by DXA every 2 years while on therapy. These recommendations will hopefully limit the number of cases of unintended severe adverse events due to hyperthyroidism while helping to treat a life-threatening condition—depression. Future studies should focus on a clear safety assessment of liothyronine treatment and explore the hypothesis that there is a correlation between the degree of TSH suppression and efficacy of treatment for depression.

Clinical Case Vignettes

Case 1

A 43-year-old woman with controlled but severe schizophrenia is treated with paliperidone injection every 3 months. Her primary care provider measured prolactin, which was elevated at 125 ng/mL (2-18 ng/mL) (SI: 5.4 nmol/L [0.1-0.8 nmol/L]). She is referred to you for evaluation. Concentrations of creatinine, TSH, and free T_4 are normal. She has no galactorrhea but has not had menses for 2 years. She is not bothered by this and has no complaints. MRI reveals a 2-mm pituitary lesion.

Which of the following is the best next step?

A. Treat with a dopamine agonist (cabergoline or bromocriptine)

B. Ignore the prolactin

C. Start an oral contraceptive pill or other estrogen replacement

D. Ask the psychiatrist to switch her antipsychotic agent to something less likely to elevate her prolactin

Answer: C) Start an oral contraceptive pill or other estrogen replacement

While it is always important to not just treat a number (eg, the high prolactin) for the sake of making ourselves feel better, in this case, the patient is not menstruating and has not for several years. While she may not be symptomatic, there will clearly be adverse effects on her bones, making ignoring the prolactin (Answer B) an inappropriate option. While treating with a dopamine agonist (Answer A) may be potentially appealing, starting one of these medications while being treated with an agent that is acting as a dopamine antagonist is a little like stepping on the gas and the brake at the same time and carries with it the potential for exacerbating her psychiatric condition. Communicating with the psychiatrist (Answer D) is always a good option. However, administration of a depot formulation of an antipsychotic agent suggests more severe disease, and if her psychiatric condition is currently well controlled, switching medications will no doubt carry significant risk. With the MRI findings, it is unclear whether the patient even has a prolactinoma. Other than lack of menses, there is no clear risk of the elevated prolactin. Therefore, providing estrogen for bone health (Answer C) would be the best option for this patient.

Case 2

A 50-year-old man with hypertension, HIV, hypogonadism, major depressive disorder, and obesity is admitted to the hospital with chest pain and a non–ST-elevation myocardial infarction. Telemetry reveals paroxysmal atrial fibrillation. He is discharged on medical therapy and referred to an endocrinologist because of inpatient laboratory testing that documented the following:

TSH = 0.02 mIU/L (0.37-4.42 mIU/L)
Free T_4 = 0.52 ng/dL (0.65-1.80 ng/dL)
(SI: 6.7 pmol/L [8.4-23.2 pmol/L])

Which of the following could be going on?

A. Pituitary tumor with central hypothyroidism

B. Euthyroid sick

C. Laboratory error

D. T_3 thyrotoxicosis

E. Any of the above

Answer: E) Any of the above

This could be any of the proposed options (Answer E). Central hypothyroidism should always be a consideration with an inappropriately low TSH level in the setting of a low free T_4 level. In a sick hospitalized patient, those results could also be consistent with euthyroid sick syndrome. Laboratory error should also be considered with unusual thyroid function test results. For this patient, further testing in the outpatient setting showed he had T_3 thyrotoxicosis with the following lab results:

TSH = <0.01 mIU/L (0.37-4.42 mIU/L)
Free T_4 = 0.57 ng/dL (0.65-1.80 ng/dL)
    (SI: 7.3 pmol/L [8.4-23.2 pmol/L])
Free T_3 = 7.62 pg/mL (2.3-4.2 pg/mL)
    (SI: 11.7 pmol/L [3.5-6.5 pmol/L])

A review of the patient's medical history revealed that he had been started on liothyronine 1.5 years earlier for refractory depression. The dosage had slowly been increased to 75 mcg once daily. The patient endorsed weight loss (which he was happy about) and improved mood on the liothyronine. He was very reluctant to decrease the dosage or stop the medication. In such instances, dialogue between the patient's endocrinologist and psychiatrist is crucial reviewing the relative risks.

Case 3

A 38-year-old obese man (BMI = 31 kg/m²) with type 2 diabetes and schizophrenia is having worsening auditory hallucinations and aggressive behavior for which olanzapine is started. You have been following him for several years for his diabetes, which is currently treated with metformin, glipizide, and a GLP-1 receptor agonist with reasonable control and a hemoglobin A_{1c} level of 7.5% (58 mmol/mol). Given his severe psychiatric condition and risk of hypoglycemia, you have established a goal hemoglobin A_{1c} level less than 8.0% (<64 mmol/mol).

He sees you 5 weeks later and is disheveled and significantly less interactive. He has no glucose meter with him, but he reports polyuria and polydipsia. Point-of-care blood glucose and hemoglobin A_{1c} measurements are 420 mg/dL (23.3 mmol/L) and 9.1% (76 mmol/mol), respectively. He has gained 24.2 lb (11 kg) (10% of his body weight).

Which of the following is the most likely cause of his worsening glycemic control?

A. Weight gain due to poor diet adherence because of worsening schizophrenia

B. Poor adherence to diabetes medications due to worsening schizophrenia

C. Olanzapine

D. New-onset latent autoimmune diabetes of adulthood (LADA) on top of his underlying type 2 diabetes and insulin resistance

Answer: C) Olanzapine

Weight gain is clearly a driving factor in the patient's worsening diabetes control. The rapidity with which he has gained such a significant amount of weight is very suggestive of an olanzapine adverse effect (Answer C) rather than what is seen with typical poor dietary adherence (Answer A). While poor medication adherence (Answer B) can definitely be seen in this setting, that might, if anything, be associated with weight loss given the worsening glycemic control with glucosuria and caloric loss in the urine. Although anything is possible, new-onset latent autoimmune diabetes of adulthood (Answer D) is highly unlikely, but it was needed as a fourth option for this syllabus! Independent of the weight gain seen, olanzapine can also have effects on insulin resistance and pancreatic function contributing to this worsening glycemic control. It is important to identify patients who have these rapid and profound changes early to consider psychiatric medication changes to prevent more severe outcomes such as hospitalization for hyperglycemia and diabetic ketoacidosis in ketosis-prone patients.

References

1. Henderson DC, Doraiswamy PM. Prolactin-related and metabolic adverse effects of atypical antipsychotic agents. *J Clin Psychiatry.* 2008;69(Suppl 1):32-44. PMID: 18484806

2. Young SL, Taylor M, Lawrie SM. "First do no harm." A systematic review of the prevalence and management of antipsychotic adverse effects. *J Psychopharmacol.* 2015;29(4):353-362. PMID: 25516373

3. Smith RC, Leucht S, Davis JM. Maximizing response to first-line antipsychotics in schizophrenia: a review focused on findings from meta-analysis. *Psychopharmacology.* 2019;236(2):545-559. PMID: 30506237

4. Melmed S, Casanueva FF, Hoffman AR, et al; Endocrine Society. Diagnosis and treatment of hyperprolactinemia: an Endocrine Society clinical practice guideline. *J Clin Endocrinol Metab.* 2011;96(2):273-288. PMID: 21296991

5. Abosi O, Lopes S, Schmitaz S, Fiedorowicz JG. Cardiometabolic effects of psychotropic medications. *Horm Mol Biol Clin Investig.* 2018;36(1). PMID: 29320364

6. Huhn M, Nikolakopoulou A, Schneider-Thoma J, et al. Comparative efficacy and tolerability of 32 oral antipsychotics for the acute treatment of adults with multi-episode schizophrenia: a systematic review and network meta-analysis. *Lancet.* 2019;394(10202):939-951. PMID: 31303314

7. Kowalchuk C, Castellani LN, Chintoh A, Remington G, Giacca A, Hahn MK. Antipsychotics and glucose metabolism: how brain and body collide. *Am J Physiol Endocrinol Metab.* 2019;316(1):E1-E15. PMID: 29969315

8. American Diabetes Association; American Psychiatric Association; American Association of Clinical Endocrinologists; North American Association for the Study of Obesity. Consensus development conference on antipsychotic drugs and obesity and diabetes. *Diabetes Care.* 2004;27(2):596-601. PMID: 14747245

9. De Hert M, Vancampfort D, Correll CU, et al. Guidelines for screening and monitoring of cardiometabolic risk in schizophrenia: systematic evaluation. *Br J Psychiatry.* 2011;199(2):99-105. PMID: 21804146

10. Touma KTB, Zoucha AM, Scarff JR. Liothyronine for depression: a review and guidance for safety monitoring. *Innov Clin Neurosci.* 2017;14(3-4):24-29. PMID: 28584694

11. Nierenberg AA, Fava M, Trivedi MH, et al. A comparison of lithium and T(3) augmentation following two failed medication treatments for depression: a STAR*D report. *Am J Psychiatry.* 2006;163(9):1519-1530. PMID: 16946176

12. Rosenthal LJ, Goldner WS, O'Reardon JP. T3 augmentation in major depressive disorder: safety considerations. *Am J Psychiatry.* 2011;168(10):1035-1040. PMID: 21969047

A Little Help From My Friends: The Endocrinology–Dermatology Interface—How Do We Help Each Other?

Joy Y. Wu, MD, PhD. Department of Medicine, Division of Endocrinology, Stanford University School of Medicine, Stanford, CA; E-mail: jywu1@stanford.edu

Matthew A. Lewis, MD, MPH. Department of Dermatology, Stanford University School of Medicine, Redwood City, CA; E-mail: mlewis5@stanford.edu

Learning Objectives

As a result of participating in this session, learners should be able to:

- Learn the mechanisms involved in the development of glucocorticoid-induced osteoporosis.

- Identify patients with inflammatory skin conditions at high risk for bone loss as a result of glucocorticoid therapy.

- Explain the therapeutic options for prevention of glucocorticoid-induced osteoporosis.

Main Conclusions

- Glucocorticoid treatment is an integral component of the management of inflammatory skin conditions, but it can be associated with rapid bone loss and increased fracture risk.

- Patients treated with high-dosage or long-term glucocorticoids should be screened for osteopenia/osteoporosis by DXA scan.

- Patients treated with glucocorticoids should be counseled on adequate calcium and vitamin D intake and exercise.

- For those at high risk of fracture, pharmacologic options include bisphosphonates, denosumab, and teriparatide.

Significance of the Clinical Problem

In treating inflammatory skin diseases, particularly pemphigus, bullous pemphigoid, dermatomyositis, and vasculitis, high-dosage prednisone (1 mg/kg) is often used in the first 3 to 6 months of therapy with a slowly tapering dosage while steroid-sparing agents are taking effect. Due to time constraints and knowledge gaps, dermatologists may not begin appropriate therapy to prevent bone loss at the initiation of glucocorticoid therapy.

Glucocorticoid treatment results in bone loss due to suppression of bone formation by osteoblasts and enhanced bone resorption by osteoclasts.[1] This bone loss occurs rapidly, often within the first 6 months of treatment, and the risk of fractures correlates with the dosage and duration of glucocorticoid therapy.

Barriers to Optimal Practice

- Although awareness of glucocorticoid-induced adverse effects is high, dermatologists already managing the complexities of inflammatory skin diseases lack the time and familiarity with DXA interpretation and medications for glucocorticoid-induced osteoporosis to additionally manage bone loss.

- There is a growing treatment gap in osteoporosis, in part driven by concerns regarding rare adverse effects such as osteonecrosis of the jaw and atypical femur fractures, with the result that treatment rates are declining and fracture rates are rising.[2,3]

- A lack of professional relationships between dermatologists/rheumatologists and endocrinologists may result in referral delays.

Strategies for Diagnosis, Therapy, and/or Management

The 2017 American College of Rheumatology Guideline for the Prevention and Treatment of Glucocorticoid-Induced Osteoporosis recommends that clinical fracture risk assessment should be performed within 6 months of starting glucocorticoid treatment.[4] For adults 40 years and older, and for adults younger than 40 years with history of osteoporotic fracture or significant risk factors for osteoporosis, fracture risk should be estimated with FRAX (https://www.shef.ac.uk/FRAX/tool.jsp) adjusted for glucocorticoid dosage (multiply the risk calculated with FRAX by 1.15 for major osteoporotic fracture and 1.2 for hip fracture if glucocorticoid treatment exceeds 7.5 mg daily) with bone mineral density (BMD) testing if available. Fracture risk assessment should be repeated yearly.

Fracture risk is categorized as follows:

- High fracture risk

  - Adults ≥40 years of age with prior osteoporotic fracture(s), hip or spine BMD T-score ≤ –2.5 in men aged ≥50 years or postmenopausal women, or FRAX (glucocorticoid-adjusted) 10-year risk of major osteoporotic fracture ≥20% or hip fracture ≥3%

  - Adults <40 years of age with prior osteoporotic fracture(s)

- Moderate fracture risk

  - Adults ≥40 years of age with FRAX (glucocorticoid-adjusted) 10-year risk of major osteoporotic fracture 10% to 19% or hip fracture >1% and <3%

  - Adults <40 years of age with hip or spine BMD Z-score < –3 or ≥10% bone loss over 1 year and continuing glucocorticoid treatment ≥7.5 mg daily for ≥6 months

- Low fracture risk

  - Adults ≥40 years of age with FRAX (glucocorticoid-adjusted) 10-year risk of major osteoporotic fracture <10% or hip fracture ≤1%

  - Adults <40 years of age on glucocorticoid treatment only

All adults taking prednisone at a dosage of 2.5 mg daily or higher for 3 or more months should optimize calcium and vitamin D intake and lifestyle modifications (balanced diet, weight maintenance in the recommended range, smoking cessation, weight-bearing or resistance training exercise, limited alcohol intake). For those with moderate fracture risk, there is a conditional recommendation for pharmacologic treatment, with oral bisphosphonates preferred; alternatives include intravenous bisphosphonates, denosumab, or teriparatide (*Table*). For those with high fracture risk, there is a strong recommendation for pharmacologic treatment, with oral bisphosphonates preferred; alternatives include intravenous bisphosphonates, denosumab, or teriparatide.

Table. Medications Approved for the Treatment of Glucocorticoid-Induced Osteoporosis

Medication	Pros	Cons
Oral bisphosphonates: • Alendronate • Risedronate	• Safe and effective	• Gastrointestinal reflux disease • Patient concerns over adverse effects • Contraindicated with estimated glomerular filtration rate <35 mL/min per 1.73 m²
Intravenous bisphosphonate: • Zoledronic acid	• Convenient (once yearly)	• Patient concerns over adverse effects • Contraindicated with estimated glomerular filtration rate <35 mL/min per 1.73 m²
Anti-RANKL monoclonal antibody • Denosumab	• Marked increase in BMD • Can be used in renal insufficiency	• Cannot be stopped abruptly • Caution with immune-compromised patients
Anabolic • Teriparatide	• Builds new bone	• Daily self-injection • No hip fracture risk reduction • Limited to 2 years due to osteosarcoma in rodents

Clinical Case Vignettes

Case 1

A 38-year-old woman with severe pemphigus vulgaris affecting her oral mucosa and 20% of her body surface area has been referred for consultation regarding management of bone loss. Baseline BMD testing revealed a T-score of –1.6 at the femur and –1.4 at the lumbar spine. She has been on prednisone for 2 months, starting at a dosage of 70 mg daily (1 mg/kg) and gradually tapering 10 mg every 2 weeks. Her current dosage is 40 mg daily. Two months ago, she also was started on mycophenolate mofetil, 1000 mg twice daily, and she will receive rituximab infusions next week. She is taking calcium, 1200 mg daily, and vitamin D₃, 800 IU daily. The dermatologist hopes to have her off prednisone after 6 months if the rituximab will put the pemphigus into remission. She is menstruating and has no history of fractures.

Which of the following is the most appropriate treatment for bone loss to recommend now?

A. Continue calcium, 1200 mg daily, and vitamin D₃, 800 IU daily

B. Start alendronate

C. Start calcitonin

D. Start teriparatide

Answer: A) Continue calcium, 1200 mg daily, and vitamin D₃, 800 IU daily

Since this patient is younger than 40 years, has not had any fractures, and does not have a Z-score less than –3, she is at low risk for fracture and therefore should be counseled on adequate calcium and vitamin D intake (Answer A) and appropriate lifestyle modifications. Should a repeat DXA scan in 1 year demonstrate greater than 10% bone loss while she is taking prednisone exceeding 7.5 mg daily, it would be appropriate to consider adding pharmacologic therapy at that time.

Case 2

An 80-year-old man with bullous pemphigoid is referred for management of bone loss. Recent BMD testing reveals a T-score of –2.0 at the femur and a T-score of –1.8 at the lumbar spine. He has been on prednisone for 6 months, starting at 30 mg daily for 1 month, 20 mg for 1 month, 10 mg for 1 month, then 5 mg daily for the past 3 months. He has been unable to reduce the dosage below 5 mg daily without flaring. He is not taking calcium or vitamin D. The dermatologist's plan is to continue prednisone, 5 mg daily, as a long-term treatment. He has no history of fractures.

Which of the following is the most appropriate treatment for bone loss to recommend now?

A. Perform BMD testing again in 2 years

B. Start calcium, 1200 mg daily, and vitamin D₃, 800 IU daily, and estimate fracture risk by FRAX adjusted for glucocorticoid dosage

C. Start teriparatide

D. Start denosumab

Answer: B) Start calcium, 1200 mg daily, and vitamin D₃, 800 IU daily, and estimate fracture risk by FRAX adjusted for glucocorticoid dosage

Although this patient's DXA score is within the osteopenia range, given his advanced age, his risk of fracture should be estimated by FRAX (Answer B). There is no need to increase the FRAX estimated fracture risk since his glucocorticoid dosage is less than 7.5 mg daily. Based on his estimated fracture risk, pharmacologic therapy may be indicated as discussed above.

References

1. Hardy RS, Zhou H, Seibel MJ, Cooper MS. Glucocorticoids and bone: consequences of endogenous and exogenous excess and replacement therapy. *Endocr Rev.* 2018;39(5):519-548. PMID: 29905835

2. Compston J. Reducing the treatment gap in osteoporosis. *Lancet Diabetes Endocrinol.* 2020;8(1):7-9. PMID: 31757770

3. Khosla S, Cauley JA, Compston J, et al. Addressing the crisis in the treatment of osteoporosis: a path forward. *J Bone Miner Res.* 2017;32(3):424-430. PMID: 28099754

4. Buckley L, Guyatt G, Fink HA, et al. 2017 American College of Rheumatology guideline for the prevention and treatment of glucocorticoid-induced osteoporosis. *Arthritis Rheumatol.* 2017;69(8):1521-1537. PMID: 28585373

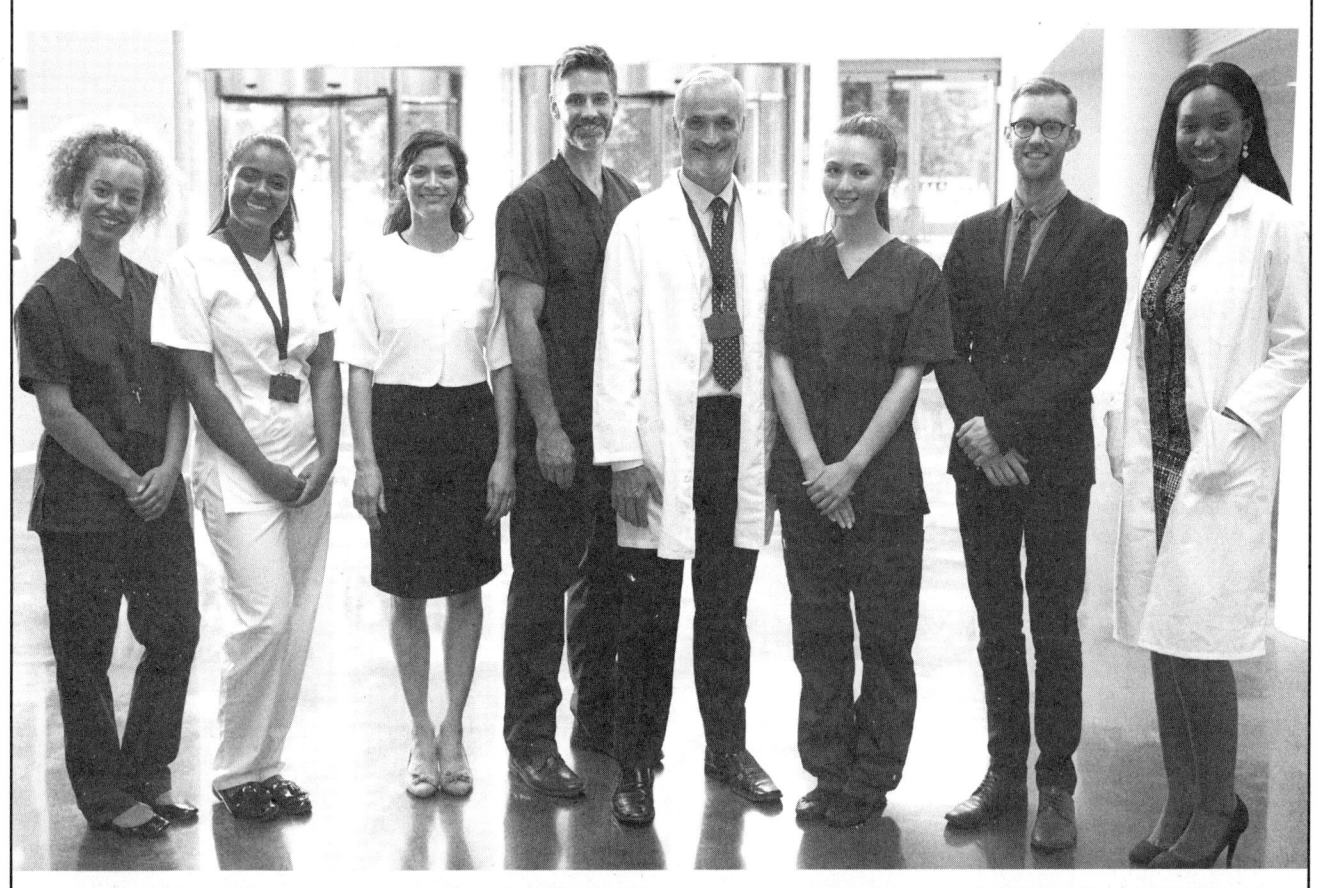

NOTES